A Patient's Workbook for Functional Neurological Disorder

This self-help workbook offers guidance for people coping with functional neurological disorder (FND), as well as their partners, families, friends, and healthcare professionals. It uses a visual metaphor based on the groundbreaking new Pressure Cooker Model to help you understand the condition and to reduce the symptoms. Firmly rooted in neuropsychological principles, this model is practical and relatable, bridging the gap between theoretical and clinical models of FND.

The Pressure Cooker Model focuses on the person with FND, as well as the contribution of the person's environment, interactions, relationships, and surroundings to FND, and looks to improve recovery, reduce stigma and increase FND awareness, providing a radical shift in thinking about FND. Grounded in neuropsychology, this book helps people understand their FND triggers, as well as their emotional and physical symptoms, and offers many strategies for self-care and building healthy relationships.

The book is accompanied by an extensive set of entirely free online resources and templates to help people with FND manage a range of genuine and disabling functional neurological symptoms, from motor symptoms such as tremors, functional weakness, and gait difficulties, to sensory symptoms such as tingles and numbness, and cognitive symptoms such as memory and concentration difficulties or brain fog, and dissociative seizures. It is valuable reading for anyone with FND, their partners, families, and friends, as well as healthcare professionals in any field working with people with FND.

Egberdina-Józefa van der Hulst, PhD, DClinPsy, is a principal clinical psychologist working in the National Health Service in the United Kingdom. She has extensive experience with providing highly specialist clinical neuropsychology input to people with FND, brain injury, and complex trauma, and is passionate about undertaking systemic work, including facilitating family support, group reflections, and complex case discussions.

A Patient's Workbook for Functional Neurological Disorder

Helping to Release the Pressure

Egberdina-Józefa van der Hulst

Routledge
Taylor & Francis Group

LONDON AND NEW YORK

Cover image: Josué Borges Expósito

First published 2025
by Routledge
4 Park Square, Milton Park, Abingdon, Oxon OX14 4RN

and by Routledge
605 Third Avenue, New York, NY 10158

Routledge is an imprint of the Taylor & Francis Group, an informa business

© 2025 Egberdina-Józefa van der Hulst

British Library Cataloguing-in-Publication Data
A catalogue record for this book is available from the British Library

ISBN: 978-1-032-31282-8 (hbk)
ISBN: 978-1-032-31283-5 (pbk)
ISBN: 978-1-003-30897-3 (ebk)

DOI: 10.4324/9781003308973

Typeset in Times New Roman
by Apex CoVantage, LLC

Access the Support Material: www.routledge.com/9781032312828

This book is dedicated to my parents Gerrit and Halina van der Hulst-Wasieczko

Contents

1 Using psychology to understand functional neurological disorder (FND)

Introduction

Welcome to this book about FND! The book intends to support you with navigating through your FND journey by introducing you to a brand-new model of FND, the Pressure Cooker Model, that will help you learn everything you need to know about FND, make sense of this condition, and take away any confusion you may experience. The book will provide you with a wide range of self-help techniques for yourself, your family, your partner, your friends, your healthcare professionals, and everyone who plays an important role in your life. Although the book will explore a biopsychosocial perspective on FND, what you will learn as you start reading the book is that FND is a condition that affects both the person and their environment, and that as a consequence, everyone contributes to FND and has a responsibility for recovery. This book is written for every person with and without FND, whether you have been newly diagnosed and are at the start of your journey, whether you have had FND for a long time and are looking for new ways of approaching the condition, or whether you are a loved one or healthcare professional – you have arrived at the right spot.

In contrast to what people sometimes think, FND has always been around. When we look back in history, we can see that FND even emerged in biblical times, many thousands and thousands of years ago (540 BC):

> Immediately the fingers of a human hand appeared and wrote on the plaster of the wall of the king's palace, opposite the lampstand. And the king saw the hand as it wrote. [6] Then *the king's colour changed*, and *his thoughts alarmed him; his limbs gave way, and his knees knocked together.*
>
> (Book of Daniel 5, verses 5 and 6; Crossway Bibles, 2008)

What is interesting about this verse is that the language has not changed much in the modern day. In current clinical practice, people with FND still frequently report their legs 'giving way', and this can happen in the context of panic episodes that are characterised by 'alarming thoughts'. History provides us with plenty of other examples of FND. In ancient Greek civilisation, a soldier turned blind during a battle after witnessing a traumatic event. Going back even more (1900 BC), when looking at papyrus, we can see the Egyptians spoke about unexplained symptoms in a woman experiencing eye problems and pain (see Raynor & Baslet, 2021, for more information on the history of FND).

Since FND is often viewed as a condition of the mind and the body, it is unsurprising that clinicians and scholars from a wide variety of disciplines have all tried to understand and treat the condition.

Historically, treatment for people with FND has mostly been psychological. The idea was that 'if you are unable to find a neurological cause' then it must mean 'it is between the ears'. For decades, unhelpful terms for FND, including 'hysteria' and 'pseudoseizures', floated around.

DOI: 10.4324/9781003308973-1

Over the years, psychological approaches to FND have certainly been refined, with cognitive-behavioural approaches becoming very popular and showing the largest evidence base for the effectiveness in treating FND.

Parallel to these developments in the clinic, other psychologically informed theoretical approaches looked at thinking processes and the impact of the social environment on these thinking processes in people with FND. These 'cognitive' theories highlighted the important role of increased attention and misinterpretation of physical symptoms to help explain FND.

More recently, biologically informed approaches have started to gain more ground in the world of FND. Research from the 'biological' fields of neurology, physiotherapy, brain imaging, and immunology have increased our knowledge on the mechanisms of FND. All these theoretical and clinical approaches have been vital for understanding some of the reasons FND happens and persists.

More similarities than differences?

Although we are used to looking at FND and neurological conditions in terms of **differences** (functional vs organic, mind vs body, and hardware vs software), there are plenty of similarities! Both types of conditions:

* Are **genuine** and **real**.
* **Are neurological and affect the entire neurological system**, including leg weakness, dissociative seizures, tingles, pins and needles, shaking, speech and swallowing difficulties, memory and other thinking issues. These are symptoms that you can also see in people with 'organic' neurological disorders, such as stroke, epilepsy, multiple sclerosis, head injury, or dementia.
* Cause **major disabilities**, greatly impact on a person's **day-to-day activities**, and may require **equipment** to help you function, like a wheelchair.
* Are treated by a multidisciplinary team and can **benefit from a period of neurorehabilitation**, including psychology, physiotherapy, occupational therapy, speech and language therapy.
* **Cause or worsen other biological issues**: sleep, fatigue, continence issues with your bladder, or opening your bowels.
* Can also require you to take **medications**.
* Lead you to be in touch with a lot of **healthcare professionals** or visit the accidents and emergencies department.
* **Come with physical risks to the person**, including falls, losing your way, or mismanaging medications.
* Can stop you from having a **job**, **driving**, and doing **enjoyable** and **leisure activities** (e.g. sports), 'living your life to the fullest'.
* Can result in **difficult thoughts and feelings**, including depression, anxiety, and anger. Pre-existing psychological difficulties can become amplified (e.g. untreated post-traumatic stress disorder) after developing either of those conditions and **adversely impact on self-esteem**.
* Influence your **personal relationships** and **family functioning**.
* Affect your **social networks** and can result in **social isolation**.

However, there are also some differences!

The nature of neurological symptoms is different for people with FND

A person with dissociative seizures will experience seizure-like episodes that can be captured on a video. In contrast to a person with epilepsy, the dissociative seizures are not accompanied by an abnormal electrical storm of activity in the brain. The symptoms of FND (for example, weakness and numbness in your legs) are not consistent with neurological changes that you can trace back to an injured area in the brain or the spinal cord and that you may see appearing on a brain scan in the hospital, in the same way and quality as for a person with, for example, a stroke, dementia, or multiple sclerosis.

Full recovery is possible

Although this does not always happen, FND is reversible, and people with FND can fully recover from the condition, because the neurological wiring has not been damaged or affected as in a person with organic neurological illness, resulting in a loss of brain cells in a stroke, but not in FND.

A bigger role for psychological and social factors

Psychological, interpersonal, and social factors often tend to play a much larger role in the start and ongoing development of FND ('emergence and maintenance') than in organic neurological conditions and therefore need some more thought.

It is true that in a subset of people with traumatic brain injury, psychosocial factors have likely played a major role in the person acquiring the injury in the first place. Think about someone who may have experienced a lot of childhood adversity, struggled in life, misused drugs and sustained a brain injury as a result of a drug overdose. This person may have come from a complex trauma background and not had the opportunities to learn helpful coping strategies throughout their life. However, the acquired brain injury is caused by a physical trigger, in this case a drug overdose. A stroke is caused by an identifiable biological trigger, such as a blood clot. Epilepsy can be caused by a variety of different biological reasons, for example, a tumour, whereas FND is not.

Even if a clear physical trigger is identified in FND – think, for example, about an accident or spinal surgery that preceded the onset of FND – there is often a considerable overlap with psychological factors that drive the symptoms. For example:

- The way people felt that they were treated in the hospital following an accident.
- Simultaneous family dynamics at the time of the accident.
- The accumulation of stressors over time, with the accident the drop that made the bucket overflow – 'one too many'.

As you will come to learn in this book, FND symptoms are often impacted by the responses and behaviours from individuals in the social world around us which maintain the FND.

Hurtful healthcare experiences

In contrast to what people with organic neurological illness often report, people with FND invariably report hurtful healthcare experiences ('10 out of 10 times'). Later in this book, we will see why this is relevant and look at ways in which these difficult healthcare experiences can prolong and maintain the FND.

A new and practical model of FND: the Pressure Cooker Model!

This book will focus on the description of a new treatment model of FND: the Pressure Cooker Model. It is a biopsychosocial model, which means that it takes into account every biological, psychological, and social factor that plays an important role in FND.

The Pressure Cooker Model differs from previous FND models because it ties together the various strands of research and clinical features into one coherent 'FND story', but with a big emphasis on the 'P' (psychological) and the 'S' (social) factors, because FND is not caused by the same type of brain changes as in a stroke and there are strong links between emotions, the social world, and FND.

Although the Pressure Cooker Model places a bit more emphasis on psychosocial factors, the model ensures that the 'bio' parts of FND are not neglected and fully covered. After all, people with FND show genuine and real *physical* symptoms; therefore, these must take centre stage in the Pressure Cooker Model. Since FND is often viewed as a condition that is on the cusp of body and mind and a person with FND does not exist in a social vacuum but is surrounded by a social world and relationships with other people, any model of FND should equally pay attention to biological, psychological, and social processes.

Before we delve into all that the Pressure Cooker Model has to offer us, let us provide you with some more information about psychology to iron out any misunderstandings that often exist about the profession and provide you with compelling reasons for the important role of psychology in FND. Instead of focusing on medically unexplained neurological symptoms, Chapter 1 hopes to make a case for shifting your thinking towards the idea of **psychologically explained neurological symptoms**.

Psychology: an essential part of the multidisciplinary team for FND

Psychology is only one cog in the giant wheel of FND rehabilitation and often part of a wider treatment team. It is important to understand what position psychology holds within a team that treats people with FND. The nature of FND treatment is 'multidisciplinary'. This means that FND tends to be treated by multiple disciplines that each tap into the biological, psychological, and social factors important in FND. Look at the Figure 1.1 for an overview of the different disciplines that are commonly, and sometimes more occasionally, involved in FND.

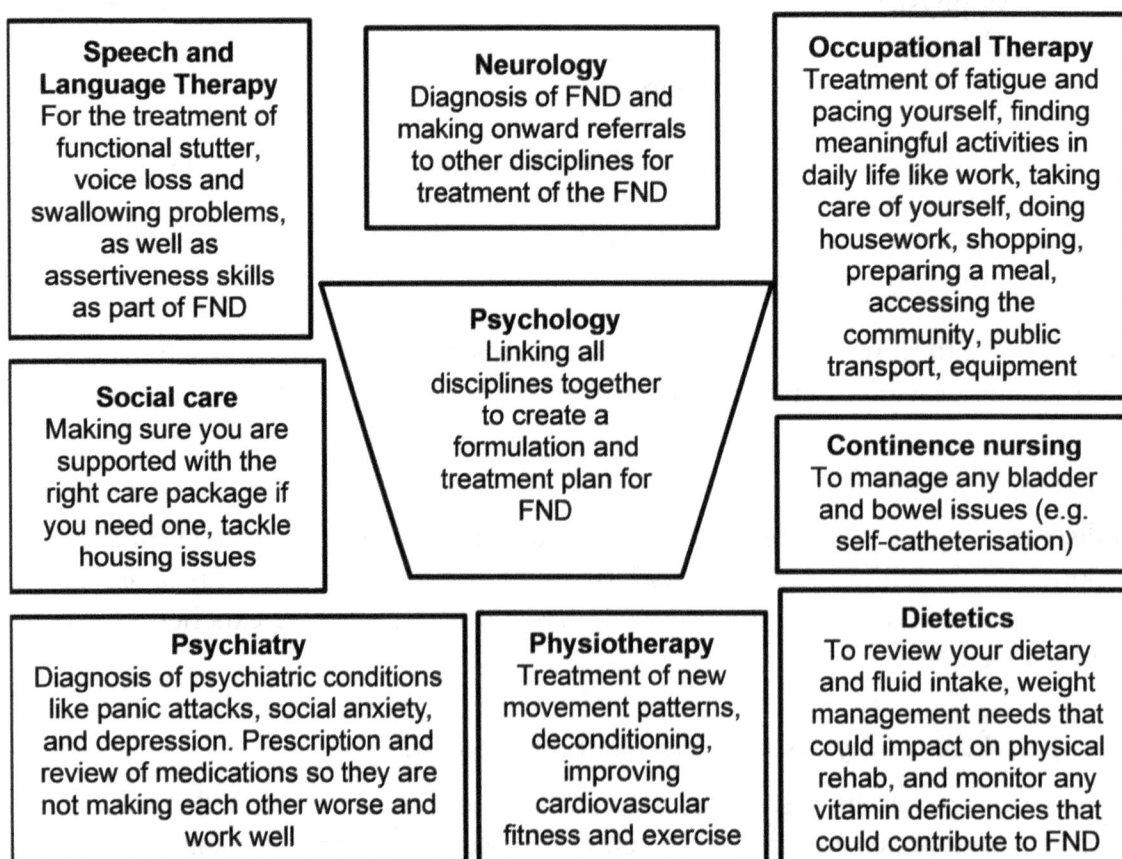

Speech and Language Therapy
For the treatment of functional stutter, voice loss and swallowing problems, as well as assertiveness skills as part of FND

Neurology
Diagnosis of FND and making onward referrals to other disciplines for treatment of the FND

Occupational Therapy
Treatment of fatigue and pacing yourself, finding meaningful activities in daily life like work, taking care of yourself, doing housework, shopping, preparing a meal, accessing the community, public transport, equipment

Psychology
Linking all disciplines together to create a formulation and treatment plan for FND

Social care
Making sure you are supported with the right care package if you need one, tackle housing issues

Continence nursing
To manage any bladder and bowel issues (e.g. self-catheterisation)

Psychiatry
Diagnosis of psychiatric conditions like panic attacks, social anxiety, and depression. Prescription and review of medications so they are not making each other worse and work well

Physiotherapy
Treatment of new movement patterns, deconditioning, improving cardiovascular fitness and exercise

Dietetics
To review your dietary and fluid intake, weight management needs that could impact on physical rehab, and monitor any vitamin deficiencies that could contribute to FND

Figure 1.1 Multidisciplinary treatment of FND.

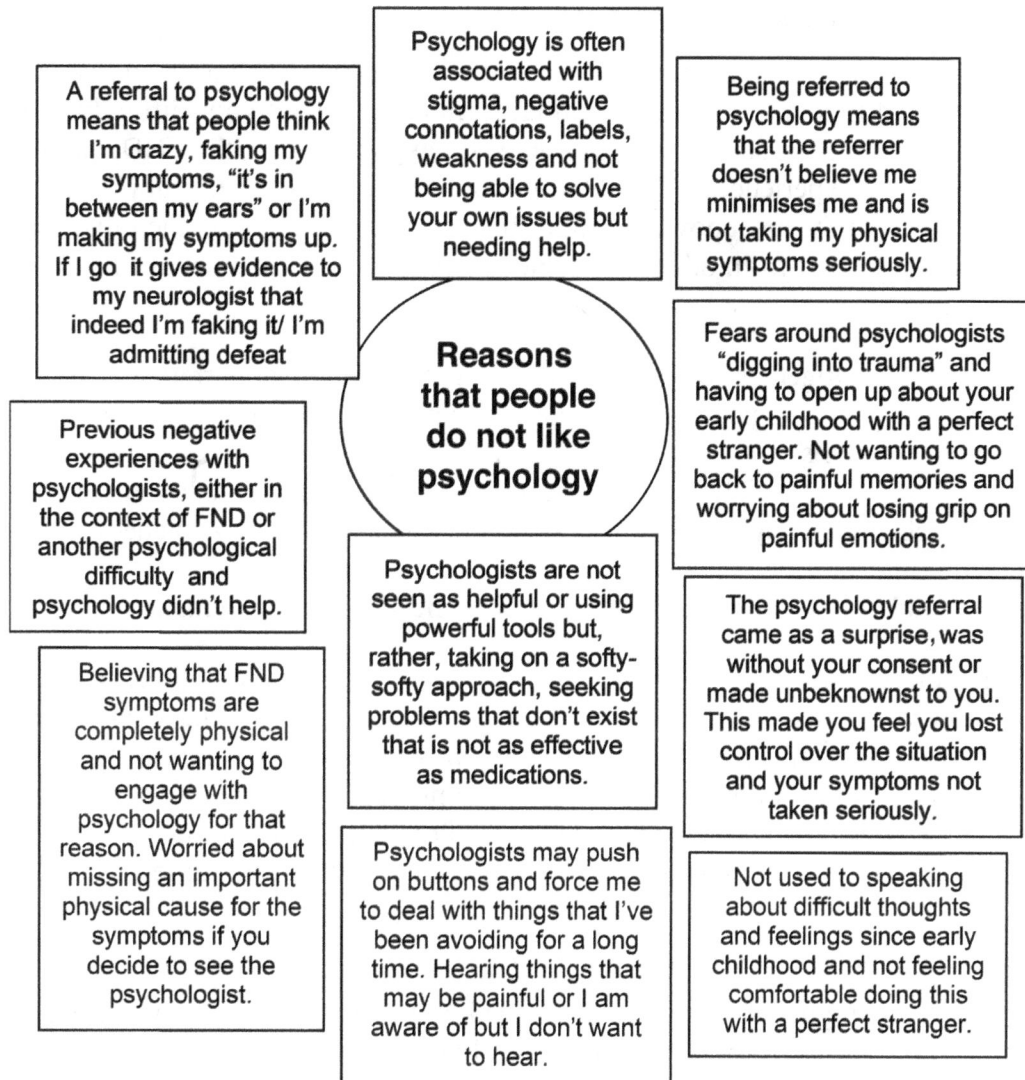

Reasons that people do not like psychology

A referral to psychology means that people think I'm crazy, faking my symptoms, "it's in between my ears" or I'm making my symptoms up. If I go it gives evidence to my neurologist that indeed I'm faking it/ I'm admitting defeat

Psychology is often associated with stigma, negative connotations, labels, weakness and not being able to solve your own issues but needing help.

Being referred to psychology means that the referrer doesn't believe me minimises me and is not taking my physical symptoms seriously.

Previous negative experiences with psychologists, either in the context of FND or another psychological difficulty and psychology didn't help.

Fears around psychologists "digging into trauma" and having to open up about your early childhood with a perfect stranger. Not wanting to go back to painful memories and worrying about losing grip on painful emotions.

Believing that FND symptoms are completely physical and not wanting to engage with psychology for that reason. Worried about missing an important physical cause for the symptoms if you decide to see the psychologist.

Psychologists are not seen as helpful or using powerful tools but, rather, taking on a softy-softy approach, seeking problems that don't exist that is not as effective as medications.

The psychology referral came as a surprise, was without your consent or made unbeknownst to you. This made you feel you lost control over the situation and your symptoms not taken seriously.

Psychologists may push on buttons and force me to deal with things that I've been avoiding for a long time. Hearing things that may be painful or I am aware of but I don't want to hear.

Not used to speaking about difficult thoughts and feelings since early childhood and not feeling comfortable doing this with a perfect stranger.

Figure 1.2 Reasons people with FND may not like psychology.

People who experience problems with seizures, walking, abnormal movements, memory, and concentration often see a neurologist or a physiotherapist first rather than a psychologist. That is not surprising and is definitely the correct thing to do: you need to undergo the appropriate physical investigations to confirm the diagnosis of FND and exclude any other medical conditions. Psychology often comes in later in the process and is often the least liked component of the multidisciplinary treatment of FND. At times, people with FND and their closest family even fiercely reject psychological therapy. This is completely understandable. Let us look at Figure 1.2 next to find out about the reasons commonly reported by people with FND.

1.1 eResource alert!

It is often believed that all psychologists do is talk, listen to your life story and your early childhood, read people's minds, fix mood and adjustment issues provide therapy, and advise people on coping strategies. However, their role, especially in the field of FND, is much bigger than that. If you are curious about the various roles of an 'FND psychologist' and what a psychological assessment in FND exactly entails, then check out the eResource.

What is psychological formulation of FND?

Once a psychologist has gathered information about you and the FND during an assessment, your information is pulled together to create an initial formulation about your difficulties. A psychological formulation can be described as a **personal theory** about you, the FND, and the psychological symptoms you experience. A formulation can be viewed as **'your story'** (see Table 1.1).

Formulation is one of the most powerful tools that psychologists have at their disposal, and it is what sets psychology apart from other disciplines involved in the treatment of FND. A formulation is powerful because it:

- Summarises and ties together complex information into a coherent narrative.
- Gives clarity and psychological containment to what sometimes look like overwhelming and unmanageable problems.
- Is developed together, is collaborative in nature, and makes you feel that you are a team working on your problems. A psychologist will share their ideas with you and check what you, 'the expert on you', thinks.
- Importantly, guides and maps out the steps that you need to follow to make improvements.

Initial formulations are not set in stone and can be subject to change. Sometimes, as the psychologist gets to know you better, new information may come to light during the sessions that changes the formulation. At other times, the initial formulation is confirmed as more information is gathered about your difficulties. Formulation is a dynamic process between you and the psychologist.

In the rest of the book, you will be introduced to the Pressure Cooker Model of FND, which will help you and your family make your own formulations about your difficulties.

What happens in psychological therapy?

Once an initial psychological formulation about the FND is shared and in place, you and the psychologist agree on a series of therapy sessions. Did you know that the act of tying together the different strands of information that have been gathered during the assessment and sharing the

Table 1.1 Important elements of a formulation

Formulation element	Example(s) in FND
The "problem"	Not being able to walk
What made you vulnerable towards developing FND in the first place	The type of upbringing you experienced and traumatic events that may have happened
What may have happened right before the FND developed and why the FND developed now	An accident, physical injury, psychological event, or a string of stressful events that built up over years
Reasons why the FND is still going	Not expressing your emotions
	Lack of enjoyable activities in your life
Things that help and support you in managing the FND	Accepting the FND diagnosis
	A positive view of psychology
	A supportive family

formulation can be an intervention in itself? The formulation may give someone so much clarity about their FND that the steps that follow in therapy become a lot easier to complete.

Consider Miriam's story:

Miriam presented to the FND psychology clinic with a hand tremor that was diagnosed a few weeks before. The first time that Miriam noticed the tremor was several months ago. During the initial assessment, the psychologist asked Miriam about any stressful experiences that were happening in her life. Miriam mentioned that her husband was diagnosed with a serious, life-threatening illness some time ago. The psychologist asked when her husband was diagnosed and was particularly interested to find out whether the FND symptoms started after her husband's diagnosis. Miriam explained that soon after the couple had received the news, her hand tremor started. The psychologist drew a timeline on a big piece of paper, with dates of her husband's diagnosis and the start of her symptoms. Miriam looked at the timeline, and suddenly, it dawned on Miriam that there was a relationship between her husband's news and the emergence of her hand tremor. This experience was a very powerful 'eye opener' for Miriam. She realised that since her husband's diagnosis, she had been continuously 'on the go' to care for him and had not had a space to express her own anxiety about the situation and their future.

So what makes (psychological) therapy effective in FND?

1.2 eResource alert!

Read here for more background details on all the factors in Figure 1.3 that make psychology a helpful experience.

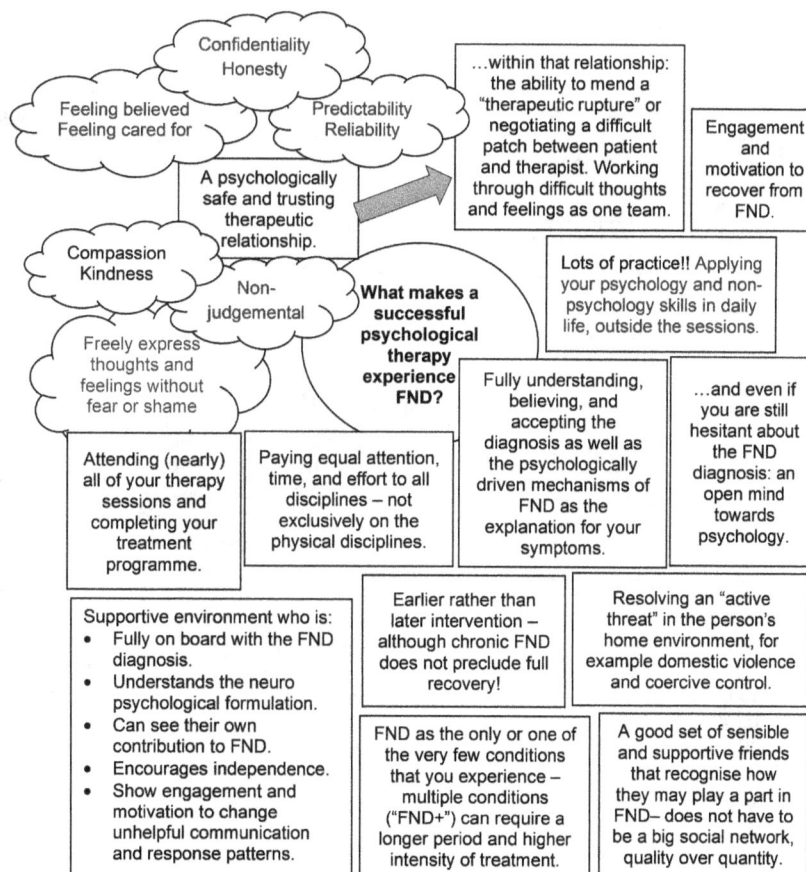

Figure 1.3 Positive factors in psychological therapy for FND.

Common myths and misunderstandings about psychology

In the following section, we will revisit a range of myths, misunderstandings, worries, and fears about psychological treatment that people with FND and their families have reported and encountered.

Psychology means it is in between your ears

Technically speaking, yes. Everything we think, feel, and do on a daily basis is in between our ears because of our brain! Speaking, walking, eating, sleeping, waking up, but also thinking, feeling, planning, predicting, connecting, recognising emotions – it all comes from the same brain. Figure 1.4 shows you a range of important physical and psychological functions that are supported by the brain.

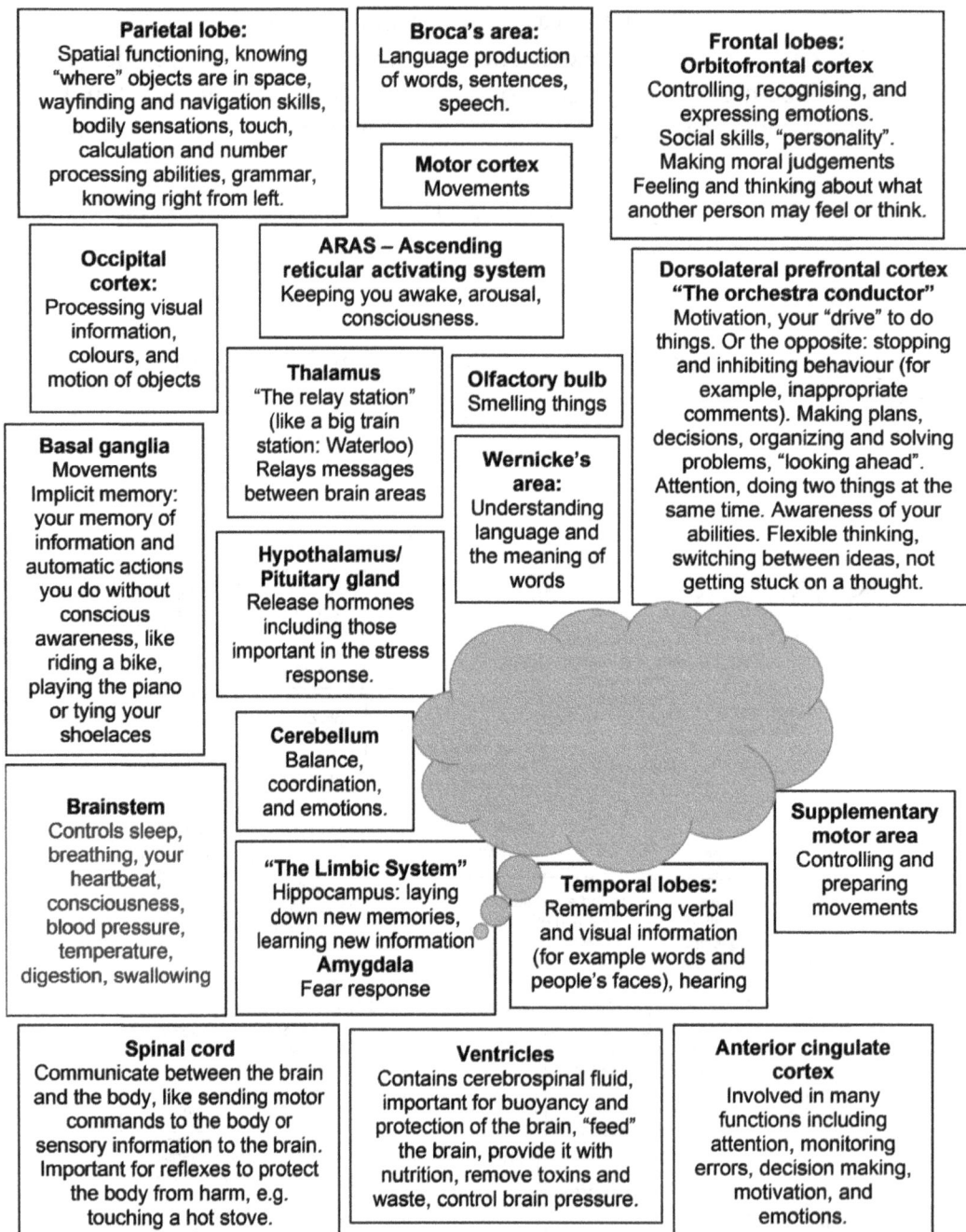

Parietal lobe:
Spatial functioning, knowing "where" objects are in space, wayfinding and navigation skills, bodily sensations, touch, calculation and number processing abilities, grammar, knowing right from left.

Broca's area:
Language production of words, sentences, speech.

Motor cortex
Movements

Frontal lobes:
Orbitofrontal cortex
Controlling, recognising, and expressing emotions.
Social skills, "personality".
Making moral judgements
Feeling and thinking about what another person may feel or think.

Occipital cortex:
Processing visual information, colours, and motion of objects

ARAS – Ascending reticular activating system
Keeping you awake, arousal, consciousness.

Thalamus
"The relay station" (like a big train station: Waterloo) Relays messages between brain areas

Olfactory bulb
Smelling things

Dorsolateral prefrontal cortex
"The orchestra conductor"
Motivation, your "drive" to do things. Or the opposite: stopping and inhibiting behaviour (for example, inappropriate comments). Making plans, decisions, organizing and solving problems, "looking ahead". Attention, doing two things at the same time. Awareness of your abilities. Flexible thinking, switching between ideas, not getting stuck on a thought.

Basal ganglia
Movements
Implicit memory: your memory of information and automatic actions you do without conscious awareness, like riding a bike, playing the piano or tying your shoelaces

Wernicke's area:
Understanding language and the meaning of words

Hypothalamus/ Pituitary gland
Release hormones including those important in the stress response.

Cerebellum
Balance, coordination, and emotions.

Brainstem
Controls sleep, breathing, your heartbeat, consciousness, blood pressure, temperature, digestion, swallowing

"The Limbic System"
Hippocampus: laying down new memories, learning new information
Amygdala
Fear response

Temporal lobes:
Remembering verbal and visual information (for example words and people's faces), hearing

Supplementary motor area
Controlling and preparing movements

Spinal cord
Communicate between the brain and the body, like sending motor commands to the body or sensory information to the brain. Important for reflexes to protect the body from harm, e.g. touching a hot stove.

Ventricles
Contains cerebrospinal fluid, important for buoyancy and protection of the brain, "feed" the brain, provide it with nutrition, remove toxins and waste, control brain pressure.

Anterior cingulate cortex
Involved in many functions including attention, monitoring errors, decision making, motivation, and emotions.

Figure 1.4 Important functions and skills supported by the brain.

A referral for psychological treatment for FND means that

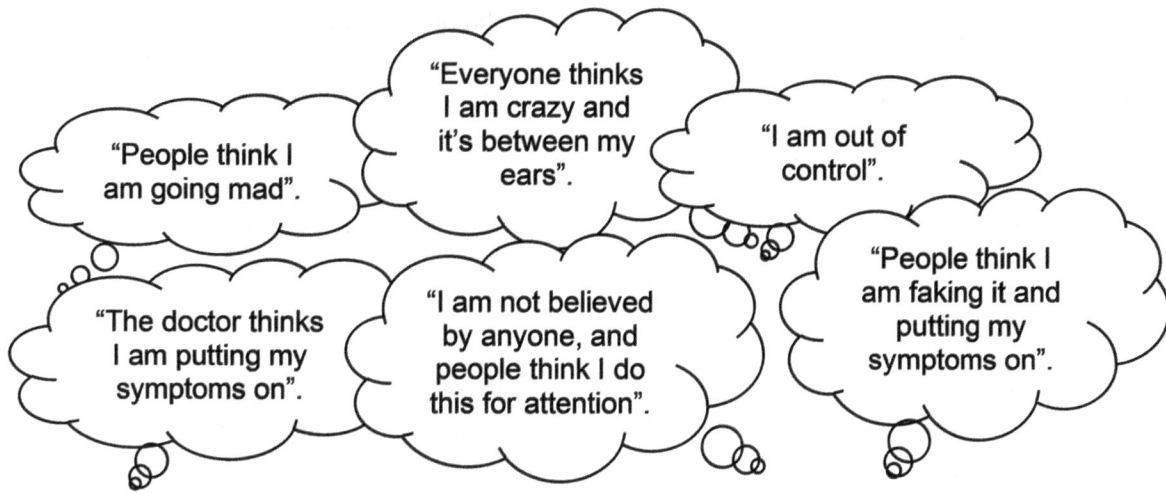

Figure 1.5 Common beliefs in FND.

Probably the most often reported beliefs by virtually every person with FND! Very sorry to hear that you may have been thinking these thoughts yourself; that must have been a difficult and lonely experience for you. In true psychology fashion, shall we try to challenge these thoughts?

Challenge #1: an unhelpful way of thinking – the mind–body distinction

People generally tend to think in terms of 'either/or' and artificially separate the two concepts: if the problem is not caused by physical or neurological factors, then surely it must be . . . psychological . . . and that's a bad thing.

Here are some examples to show you that the mind and body are far more integrated and tied together than we normally think:

- Stress causes physical changes in the human body (see Chapter 8).
- Early trauma can impact on brain development.
- People with organic neurological illnesses (think about Parkinson's disease, multiple sclerosis, or Alzheimer's dementia) likewise can experience stress and psychological difficulties, either because an area in the brain that supports emotions is affected or in the context of psychological adjustment to a serious illness.

FND completely challenges the notion of a sharp mind–body distinction and does not fit neatly into existing categories. It is much more useful to think of FND as maintained by a combination of physical, psychological, and social factors, each equally as important. The Pressure Cooker Model will help you think more from this 'biopsychosocial' perspective.

Challenge #2: another unhelpful belief – FND is not real

Your symptoms are clearly real. Whether you experience an organic tremor due to Parkinson's disease or a functional tremor because of FND, both affect your body, and you can clearly perceive the shaking with your own eyes happening in front of you.

Reframe this belief as 'not my problem' but a problem created by the system around you:

- Although FND awareness has come a long way, people in personal and healthcare contexts still do not always shy away from making crude remarks about FND.

- Do not underestimate the power of non-verbal communication. Eye rolling, angry and disapproving looks, lack of compassion, and 'careless care' are, sadly, still a reality.
- Fears of not being believed by people around you can have roots in traumatic childhood experiences. Some people have endured similar disbelief by important people in their life (parental figures) and almost 're-experience' these worries. Read more about 'systemic re-traumatisation' in Chapter 9.

*Challenge #3: psychological difficulties are undeservedly associated with stigma
and shame, however . . .*

Let us normalise psychological healthcare!

- Psychological difficulties are extremely common in the general population.
- Psychology is hardly a thing anymore: general society seeks more access to psychological treatment nowadays.
- People in the spotlight are a lot more open about psychological difficulties, including members of the royal family, celebrities, and people on social media.
- Opening up about difficult thoughts and feelings is an essential emotion regulation skill.
- Psychological healthcare is a necessary and vital part of our everyday routine, in the same way that we need to eat and drink as part of our daily physical healthcare to sustain ourselves.

I have had psychological treatment for FND in the past, and it didn't help – this is not for me

If psychological therapy has not given the results that you had initially hoped for, it is understandable that you lost faith in the power of psychology for FND. Let us explore a few reasons for unsuccessful psychological therapy experiences in FND.

Reason #1: therapeutic relationship

You did not 'click' with, did not trust, or were suspicious of the psychologist. The therapeutic relationship did not really develop into a safe psychological space. It is important to note that people with FND can struggle to establish a therapeutic relationship because of previous life experiences and that 'relationships' are exactly the area to tackle to help overcome the FND.

Reason #2: insufficient practice and application of strategies

Let us suppose you did finish the therapy but you found the application of your strategies in day-to-day life too difficult. Maybe you did not finish the course of therapy because you struggled to tolerate emotions that had been buried for a long time. As expected, psychology tends to make you initially feel worse, not better, and some people decide to leave midway, at the height of their emotions.

Reason #3: lack of FND specialist therapy

Some people are referred to community or secondary mental health teams rather than FND specialist services without access to a full multidisciplinary team, particularly the physical disciplines. The therapy was delivered by a psychologist without specialist training in FND, limited clinical FND experience, and perhaps not sufficiently sensitive to the intricacies of FND. It is also possible that the psychologist felt lacking in skill set to treat FND, and this showed during therapy.

Reason #4: circumstances around the psychology referral

Unfortunately, and to the detriment of the therapeutic relationship, people are sometimes unaware of any psychology referral or feel heavily coaxed into attending sessions by referrers against their preferences. That will set the stage and start you off on the wrong foot. Understandably, it will be harder to fully engage in something that you felt pressured into. Some services may also be wary of people with FND and use language such as 'complex', 'refractory', and 'chronic' in referral letters that you are copied into. This could create the impression of hopelessness and a lack of belief that any treatment, including psychology, will be effective.

Reason #5: lack of readiness for therapy

Maybe you were not ready yet to fully engage with psychological therapy as you experienced major doubts, for example, about the FND diagnosis and pending telemetry or other crucial investigations. Maybe your psychologist tried to shoehorn you into a therapy model but you were not feeling it or needed some 'preparatory work' on dissociation.

Reason #6: inappropriate length, intensity, or breadth of psychological therapy

The course of therapy that was offered to you may have been too brief, low-intensity, and too individually focused to bring about change. People with FND and their families can develop long-standing patterns of unhelpful coping and responding. Undoing entrenched patterns is going to take time, and there is no 'quick fix' or 'shortcut' to this process. Health services cannot always offer long treatment episodes or provide couple and family-based therapies, especially important if the FND is associated with relationship and family difficulties. Even short-term FND or group programmes do not guarantee lasting recovery, and it is not unusual for a person to experience setbacks or lose the gains following discharge.

Reason #7: not feeling believed

Maybe you did not feel believed by anyone so far. A psychology referral through your mailbox totally cements your 'beliefs about not being believed'. Other unhelpful non-verbal or verbal communications that you have been exposed to along your journey and that suggest disbelief may have further eroded your views on the value of psychology for FND.

Reason #8: other therapies were a better match

If you have had challenging psychological therapy experiences before, then more physical disciplines like occupational therapy or physiotherapy that focus less on emotions or do not require emotion language to the same extent as psychology does can feel a lot more comfortable, easier to engage with, and less threatening, perhaps creating the unhelpful impression that psychology is not that necessary for FND.

Reason #9: team factors

Incomplete multidisciplinary teams in the context of staff funding, recruitment, and retention issues are normal in the world of FND. However, FND recovery can stall when you make progress in psychological therapy but there is no physiotherapist available to work on long-term deconditioning, muscle wasting, and develop a normal walking pattern. Vice versa, a lack of psychologist can equally hamper FND recovery in physiotherapy programmes when previously buried emotions, trauma, and interpersonal issues suddenly come up during exercises. For optimal FND recovery, all disciplines need each other!

Reason #10: systemic factors outside the person and therapist's influence

There is a scarcity and geographically poor distribution of FND specialist services in the United Kingdom. Furthermore, long waiting lists, often spanning multiple years rather than months, are a common occurrence. By the time that a person is finally able to access psychology, the FND symptoms could have worsened and become harder to recover from.

FND means that I have physical symptoms – I need physical, not psychological, treatment

This is a very understandable way of thinking. After all, FND presents with physical symptoms that impact on a person's day-to-day functioning, including your ability to walk, take care of yourself, run your household, sustain yourself, do sports, go to your job, maintain relationships, and enjoy a social life. Everything about FND feels very physical, not psychological. However, FND experts generally agree on a multidisciplinary treatment approach to FND (Demartini et al., 2014; Russell et al., 2022), and there are at least two good reasons to think about the psychological side of things in FND.

Reason #1

People may feel that physical treatment is sufficient because they may not identify with the emotions and psychological features of FND, a phenomenon called dissociation or 'cutting off emotions'. You may identify the physical and behavioural symptoms of anxiety but not connect with the underlying emotion because of dissociation. If this applies to you, it makes sense that you prefer physical over psychological treatment (see Chapter 7 to learn more about dissociation).

Reason #2

Researchers and clinicians have identified an increased focus of attention on physical symptoms as one of the factors that 'feed into the FND' (Edwards et al., 2012; Nielsen et al., 2015). Therefore, focusing on only the physical side of treatment may actually keep the FND going rather than help improve the condition, since the psychological reasons that contribute to FND are not being addressed (see Chapter 8 to learn more about self-focused attention).

Psychologists only want to talk about your early childhood experiences, open up your traumas, and create problems that do not exist

Psychologists in movies

Although many people with FND, researchers, and clinicians agree that there is an association between trauma, upbringing, any other childhood adversity, and FND, it is true that not everyone will identify with these links. Trauma experiences may set the stage for the development of FND; however, not every person with FND will have experienced a traumatic or abusive background, challenging upbringing, or view their life experiences in this way.

Popular culture and movies have also focused on the image of the psychologist as a person who primarily works with traumatised patients, 'cracks the patient', and 'digs' into childhood experiences. This romanticised idea of what a psychologist does in day-to-day practice does not reflect reality well. It may potentially be dangerous to do what movie psychologists do.

Trauma therapy starts with learning new coping strategies or 'stabilisation'. Sometimes, people want to disclose or talk about the trauma, and sometimes people choose not to. Once coping strategies are in place and well-practiced, then if the person wishes, the clinician is in agreement, and there is a clear clinical need, traumas can be further explored in therapy.

Psychologists work with a wide range of therapies, and only a few of these will focus heavily on childhood experiences during your treatment (see Chapter 3 and the eResource for more information on the different types of psychological therapy in FND).

There are good reasons to shine a light on some of your early experiences

Only a few psychological therapies focus heavily on early childhood experiences. That is not to say that all the other therapies will never ask you about your childhood. On the contrary, it is reasonable to expect some questions about your early experiences. It is entirely up to you to decide whether you would want to talk about your upbringing during your sessions. However, it probably is a good idea to explore childhood experiences, particularly for the following reasons.

IF YOU EXPERIENCE INTERPERSONAL TRIGGERS FOR FND

People with significant day-to-day interpersonal difficulties and complex trauma often report adverse childhood experiences. Interpersonal triggers for FND can, in some people, be related back to early and later adverse interpersonal experiences; therefore, speaking about 'the past' can be of great benefit for your FND recovery (see Chapter 7).

IF YOU CARRY AN UNSPEAKABLE DILEMMA

It is not uncommon for people with FND to carry unspeakable dilemmas (Griffith et al., 1998). In a nutshell, this refers to a 'secret' or a piece of information that weighs heavily on you and that you have not yet expressed to people close to you, maybe for years or even decades. It is called a dilemma because bottling it up causes you a lot of pain, hurt, or difficult feelings, but releasing it would likely do the same for your environment, with potentially irreversible psychological and social consequences for you, including rejection, ostracisation, and a big aftermath. Why is this important?

Releasing an unspeakable dilemma can greatly improve FND symptoms.

Sometimes, unspeakable dilemmas are a 'public secret', meaning, that everyone is fully aware but no one is openly talking about it. At other times, people may have buried the dilemma so deeply into their minds that they are not or are minimally aware of the contents.

Thoughts, feelings, and memories associated with the unspeakable dilemma may suddenly become 're-activated' by a recent 'critical' trigger event. Some unspeakable dilemmas stem directly from childhood experiences, and for that reason, opening up about childhood experiences can be therapeutic and help recovery (see Chapters 5 and 6).

Find out where current unhelpful thoughts and coping strategies come from

Early experiences shape the beliefs we hold about ourselves, other people, the world around us, and the way we see our future. Some people do not remember much of their childhood or consistently note that their childhood was happy and carefree and do not agree with other people exposed to similar events (like a sibling sharing a completely different, more negative side). That said, people with FND quite often have developed a belief and coping system that, although protective whilst growing up, loses its functions in later life. People with (and without!) FND frequently report early childhood coping mechanisms repeating into adulthood, particularly:

- Keep self to self ('bottling things up').
- Pushing on ('just do').
- Cutting off emotions ('dissociation').

Psychological treatment means that there is something wrong with my personality and that I have done the FND to myself

On the contrary, nothing could be farther from the truth:

- It is always the person who carries and experiences the FND symptoms who is referred for psychology and, unfortunately, never the environment.
- In the clinical field, there is little awareness about the strong influence of systemic factors maintaining the FND.
- Service infrastructures for FND are not really set up for family work. It is often an 'add-on' rather than the main focus of treatment for example, a carer/couple's session at the end of therapy, or one family education session in a group programme). Couples and family therapy resources are limited and hard to access.
- Because of time, resource, and funding constraints, most services will focus their care and attention solely on individual treatment of the person with FND.
- All this creates the **false impression that FND is a 'person problem'** and that the causes of FND should be ascribed to the person only.

Luckily, the Pressure Cooker Model has a radical new view: the model is big on thinking about social factors and firmly believes that FND is the joint product of both the person and the environment. If you want to treat FND effectively, achieve maximum potential for recovery, and obtain long-term gains, you need to focus on the person as well as important individuals close to the person. How about replacing this question with the following statement?

Everybody needs psychology – FND or no FND!

I have not experienced trauma or stress in my life; surely, I won't need psychological treatment for FND?

It can be frustrating, and anger-provoking, being asked repeatedly whether you are stressed or anything stressful happened when you developed FND, especially if you do not identify with

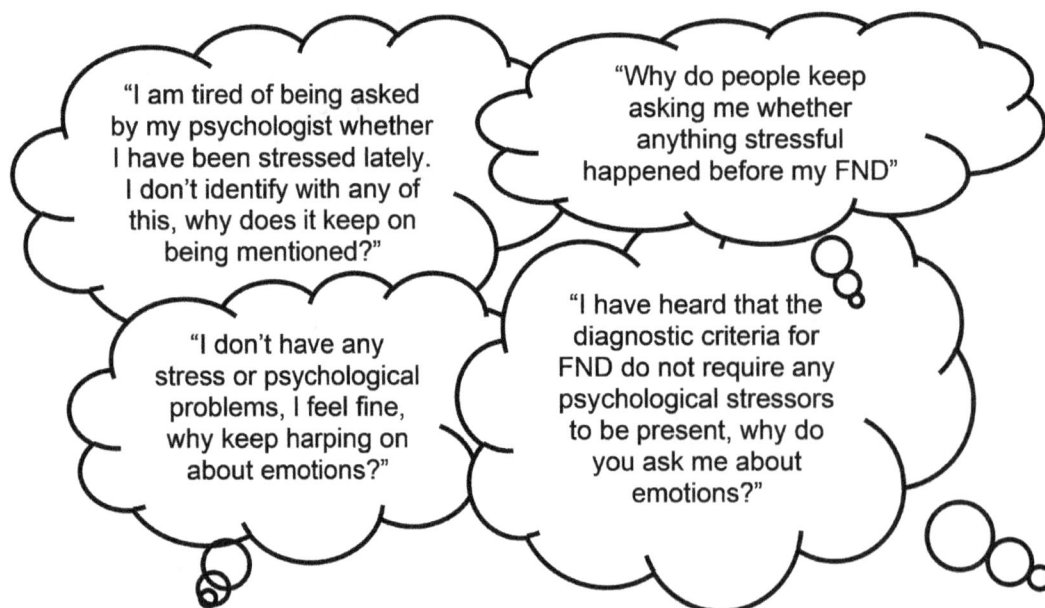

Figure 1.6 Questions about stress that can feel frustrating for people with FND.

stress. However, the reality is that day-to-day life is full of stresses. Ask a random person on the street whether any of these could cause them stress, anxiety, or other negative emotions, like anger and low mood, and you will receive a resounding yes to quite a few of these examples:

- An argument with a partner or family member.
- Childcare arrangements breaking down whilst you need to be at an urgent appointment.
- Being late for work because of a traffic jam.
- Increasing bills.
- Your boiler breaking down.
- Shop not having an item that you need.
- A health problem that does not go away.
- An annoyingly loud neighbour who will not stop.
- Barking dogs.
- Constant rain and becoming soaking wet when you are out and about.
- Some person parked in your designated space.

Some people experience more frequent or severe stress in their lives than others:

- Serious health problems that warrant direct medical attention and may pose a threat to life.
- An unwell family member who needs continuous care.
- An unexpected house move or eviction.
- Job loss.
- Divorce or an ex-partner who does not cooperate with childcare.
- Domestic violence and abuse in the home environment.
- Car accident.

This list could be endless and is certainly not exhaustive. The point of making the list is: *a stress-free life does not exist.* (And if you do think you have cracked the code to a 100% stress-free life, share the news as widely as possible!).

I have heard that not everyone with FND needs psychology – is that true, and could I be one of the people that does not need it?

Psychological stress is not always viewed as essential for a diagnosis of FND. In light of scientific and practice-based evidence, this is quite a bold statement to make. Let us first start with a brief discussion of why erring on the side of caution ('psychology is needed for every person with FND') is better than incurring the risk of some people who truly need it but lose out because of this viewpoint.

People with FND often do not report stress for one or more of the following reasons:

- Dissociation, an inability to identify, or lack of awareness of stress or anxiety.
- Confusion about emotions (anger vs anxiety is common).
- Unsure of what you feel inside (chest pain vs anxiety, tiredness vs low mood).
- Not having the words to describe emotions ('alexithymia'; Demartini et al., 2014).
- Shame and embarrassment about unmet emotional needs around not feeling cared for, heard, or noticed by other people.
- Mental health stigma.
- Not wanting to come across as 'weak'.
- Not wanting to burden loved ones.
- Worries about not being believed.

- Healthcare professionals not always able to recognise subtle signs of dissociation or psychological distress.
- Not trusting healthcare professionals at the beginning of therapy or during a one-off review visit.

Not offering psychology to everyone with FND is denying a person the possibility of gaining insight and awareness into important maintaining factors of FND and, ultimately, living life to the fullest. Even people who are currently FND-free may benefit from learning more about psychology to help curb potential later setbacks.

I am the one with FND, so why does my social environment need to be involved? I would rather not have them involved

Some people prefer not to involve family or partners in FND treatment:

- Treatment is viewed as a private matter.
- People feel self-conscious or embarrassed about the psychological aspects of FND, with some family members believing symptoms were part of a stroke or brain injury.
- Strong negative family views around emotional expression.
- Deteriorated or estranged family relationships.
- Family does not believe in FND and may not engage or be helpful in treatment.
- Not wanting to burden family.
- Person may be in danger due to coercive control or other forms of domestic violence.

A partner, family, friends, and a supportive social network can be helpful in psychological therapy – especially if they 'buy' into the FND diagnosis and management – for several reasons:

- The Pressure Cooker Model is **made for everyone involved in FND**; it is important that your family, loved ones, or anyone that you interact with regularly practice and apply their own skills, all in the pursuit of recovery from FND.
- It may help to **find interpersonal triggers and break family relationship and response patterns** that contribute to FND, for example, arguments, communication difficulties, a relationship that has deteriorated, or some unspeakable dilemma that has not yet been released.
- It can **help foster your independence**, particularly when a lot of chores and tasks have been taken out of your hands or your family is overinvolved and hypervigilant about the FND.
- Psychological therapy can also help **relieve 'carer burden' and social isolation** in people that care for you and have not had much time to pursue their own personal activities.
- To **educate on FND and address any misinformation**, particularly if your environment does not buy into the diagnosis or believes that you have had a stroke that resulted in permanent brain injury.
- To **act as your 'FND ally'**. A psychologist can be particularly helpful in exploring and reducing the impact of negative comments from family members on the person, for example, family not believing the person or thinking that the symptoms are 'for attention' and 'put on'.

The Pressure Cooker Model firmly believes that in FND, 'everybody has a problem and everybody needs treatment'.

I have no social support network/my family is not very supportive: if social factors impact on FND, will psychological therapy be helpful at all, and will I ever recover from FND?

Definitely helpful and definitely a chance for recovery! Psychologists are used to looking beyond the individual and often have a 'holistic' view of the person with FND and their relationships with

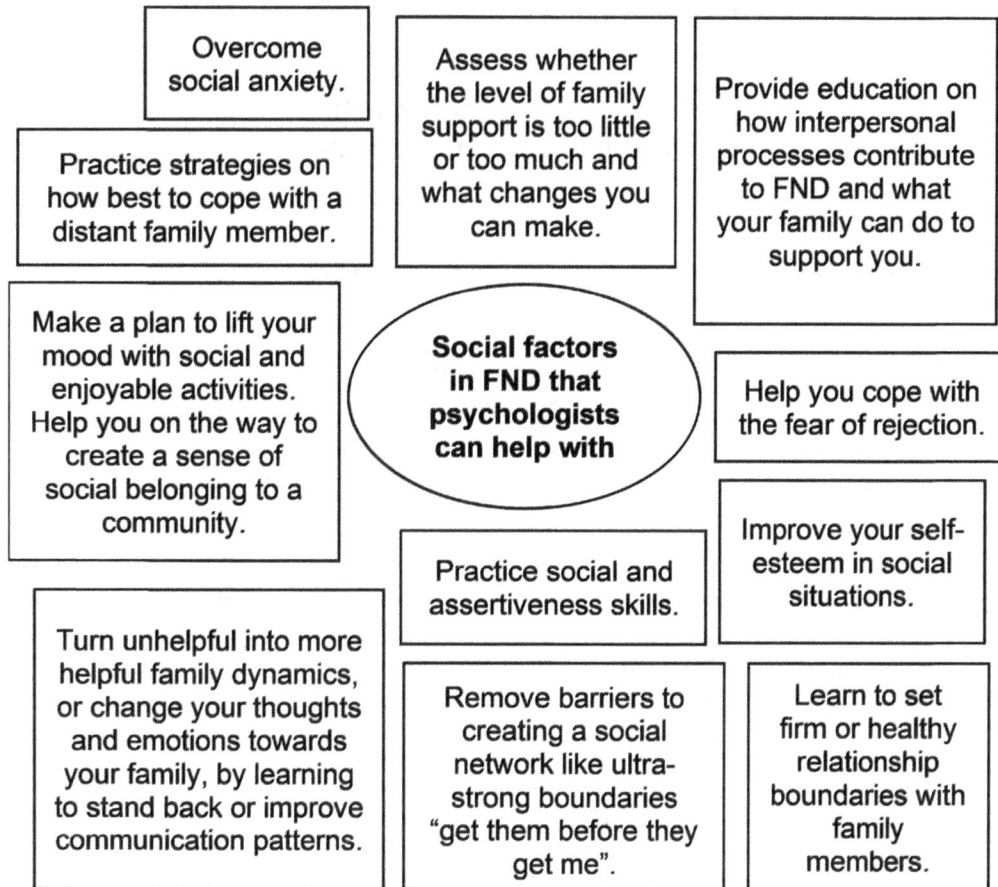

Figure 1.7 Treatment examples of social maintaining factors in psychological therapy.

the social environment. Psychologists are very well capable of helping you explore barriers that stop you from growing a social network or cope with an unsupportive family (see Figure 1.7).

I have had FND for decades ... will I ever get better?

FND is reversible even if you have had it for 10 or 20 years! There are many reasons you may still struggle with FND:

- You never had access to FND specialist psychological therapy.
- FND specialist treatment was too short to undo long-standing movement, relationship, and behaviour patterns.
- Lack of FND services in your local area.
- Late diagnosis due to a lack of awareness on FND preventing early intervention.
- Self-fulfilling prophecy: if healthcare professionals view you as 'chronic', and 'unlikely to recover', and focus on adjusting to illness rather than on a cure, why would you even believe in recovery?
- Necessity is the mother of invention: years of trying to seek help with services withdrawing and discharging you forced you to develop your own routines and coping strategies to keep FND at bay. Despite FND still being a problem, you are relatively happy and stopped searching for treatment.
- Lack of trust in the healthcare system after many harrowing experiences stopped you from seeking help, prolonging your symptoms.

I have been diagnosed with FND+: a personality disorder/brain injury/autism – am I not too complex, severe, or beyond help?

No one with FND is beyond help! Experiencing these additional conditions does not preclude recovery but may highlight to your psychologist to make some changes to the type, quality, and length of the treatment (see Figure 1.8).

I don't think my FND can be minimised by a Pressure Cooker Model

Valid point. You are right: no psychological or theoretical model could ever fully capture the complexities and intricacies of FND (or any condition, for that matter!). Everybody is unique, and FND has many layers to it – no doubt about that. The Pressure Cooker Model does not aim to minimise people's problems. Rather, it has been created to help and not to hurt.

However, you have to start your journey of recovery somewhere:

- A clear metaphor will help you visualise complex processes in FND more easily.
- Using a shared language will support you and your family with understanding FND and communicate some of the maintaining factors of FND during treatment.
- The Pressure Cooker Model helps join up the work of every discipline involved in your treatment and develop one coherent narrative of a person's FND journey and symptoms.

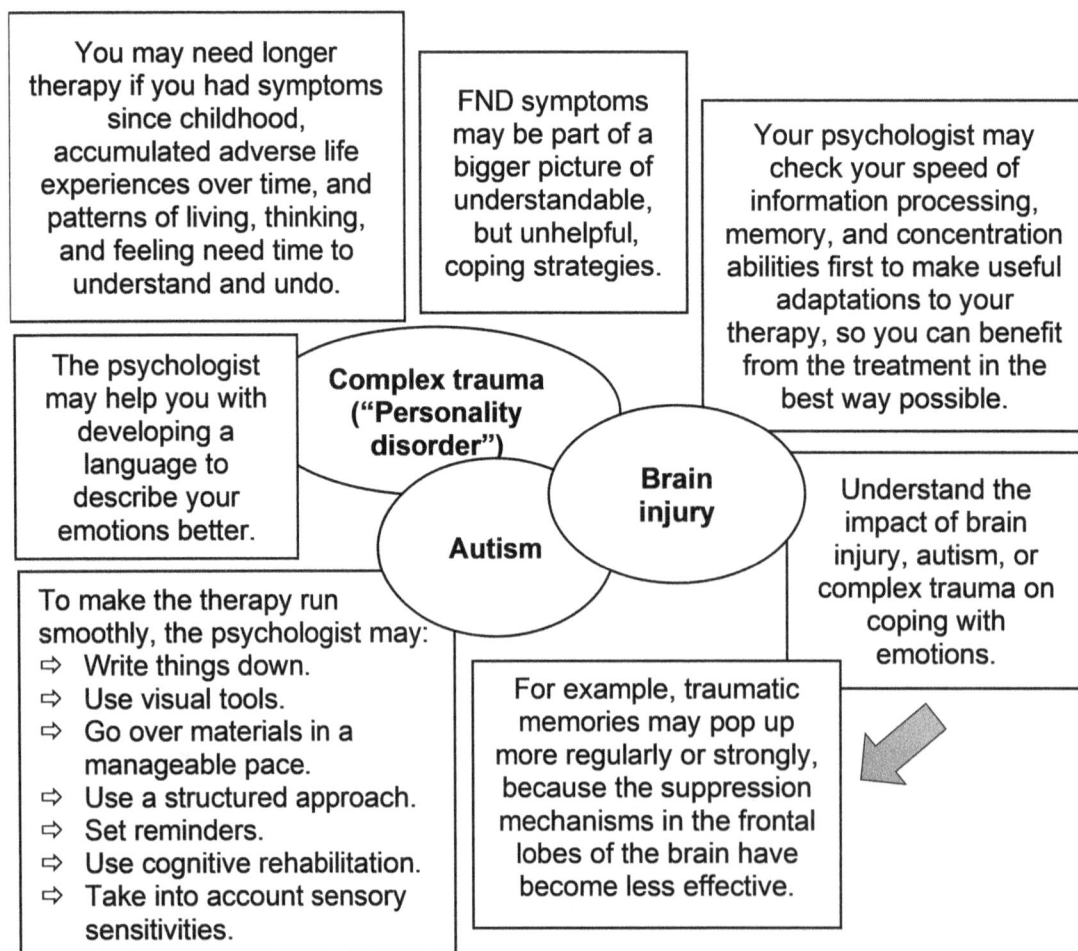

You may need longer therapy if you had symptoms since childhood, accumulated adverse life experiences over time, and patterns of living, thinking, and feeling need time to understand and undo.

FND symptoms may be part of a bigger picture of understandable, but unhelpful, coping strategies.

Your psychologist may check your speed of information processing, memory, and concentration abilities first to make useful adaptations to your therapy, so you can benefit from the treatment in the best way possible.

The psychologist may help you with developing a language to describe your emotions better.

Complex trauma ("Personality disorder")

Brain injury

Autism

Understand the impact of brain injury, autism, or complex trauma on coping with emotions.

To make the therapy run smoothly, the psychologist may:
⇨ Write things down.
⇨ Use visual tools.
⇨ Go over materials in a manageable pace.
⇨ Use a structured approach.
⇨ Set reminders.
⇨ Use cognitive rehabilitation.
⇨ Take into account sensory sensitivities.

For example, traumatic memories may pop up more regularly or strongly, because the suppression mechanisms in the frontal lobes of the brain have become less effective.

Figure 1.8 Things to think about in psychological therapy for people with 'FND+'.

I think I am doing all the right stuff, including faithfully attending all my sessions, completing, and following my treatment plan, with an FND specialist team: why am I not getting better?

Definitely, do not give up, and please do not think you are not trying hard enough! Let us look at some reasons that, despite your good efforts, and all the stars aligned, the treatment is not working out:

- **You have not had the number of sufficient sessions yet to see change.** Although physical improvement can happen fast in FND, the psychological bits tend to 'lag' and take more time. Early childhood coping strategies, repeated over years, need time and patience to undo.
- Sometimes, the **process of therapy is far more revealing than the contents.** Completing homework can be quite a logical endeavour: it is structured, you fill out forms, and it keeps you busy and active. This logical approach ('intellectualisation') can become a way to avoid or cut off emotions rather than actively engage and 'feel' difficult thoughts and feelings on an emotional level – without us realising it!
- **Not everyone practices and applies their strategies in day-to-day life.** Unfortunately, the real work takes place in the 167 hours that you are not with your therapist and starts at home, where the FND triggers and barriers often appear.
- **Fear of the unknown** (see Chapter 7). If after years of FND you learn to walk again . . . where are you going to walk to? What are you going to do with your new life, independence, time?
- You have yet to **uncover hidden triggers** that continue to drive the FND symptoms, particularly the not-so-obvious interpersonal and family-related triggers (see Chapter 7 for a trigger list).

The rocky road in the middle

'I started psychological therapy, and you are making me feel worse!' and variations to this statement. Strange as it sounds, no reason to be alarmed!

- You are confronting long-time avoided life issues head-on.
- Letting through buried emotions may result in a worsening of distress.
- You are actively reconnecting with your emotions.
- It may feel sudden and come as an emotional shock.

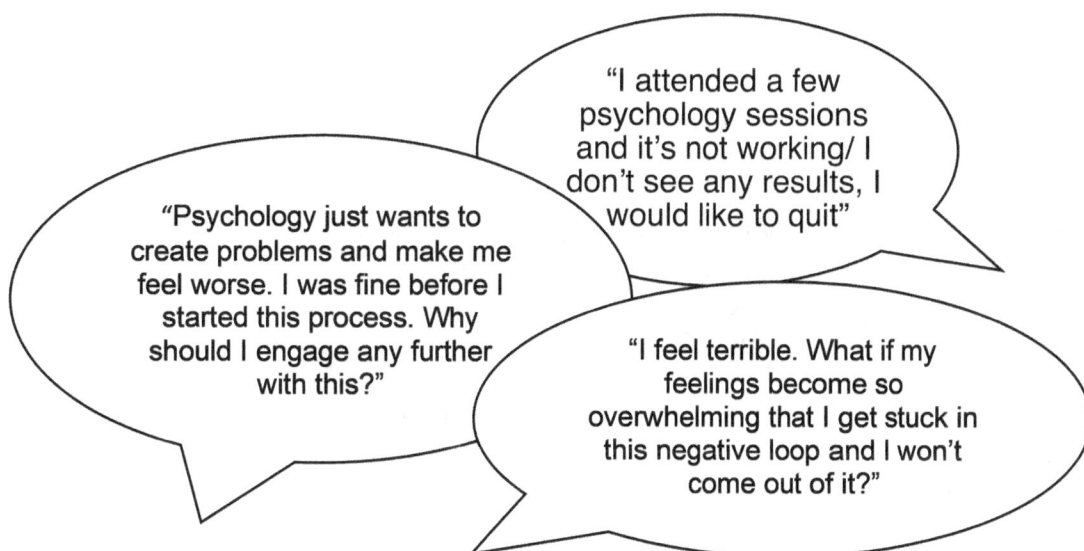

Figure 1.9 Statements people make when psychology does not seem to work.

Progress in Occupational Therapy and Physiotherapy:

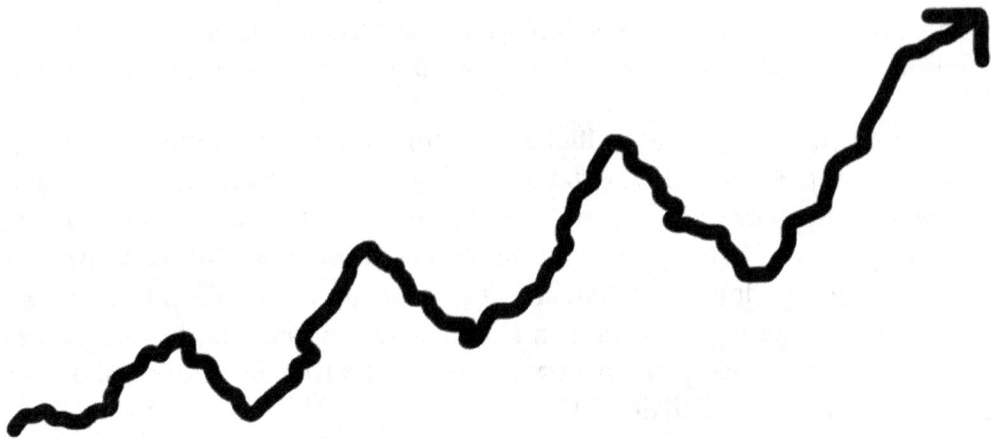

Figure 1.10 Typical recovery pathway for non-psychology disciplines in FND.

The Psychology graph:

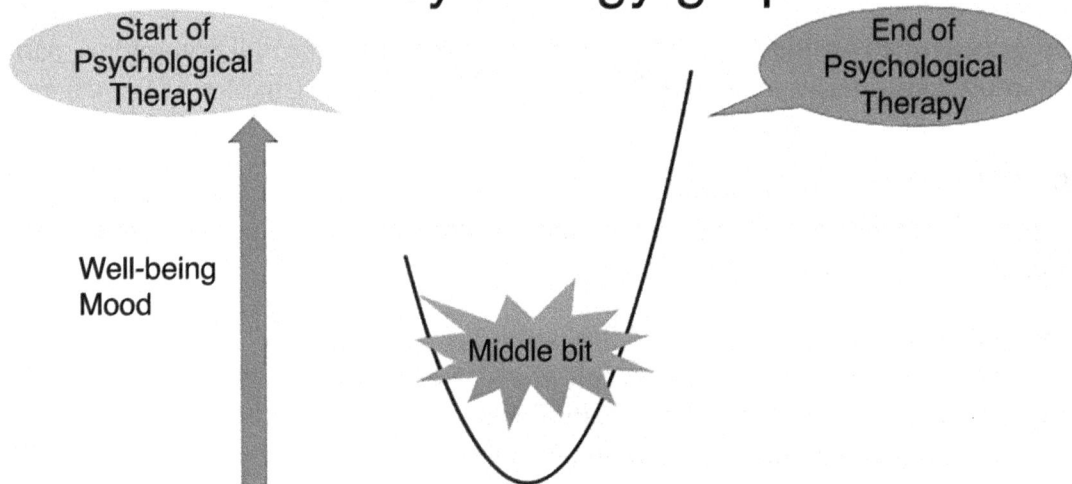

Figure 1.11 Typical recovery pathway for psychology in FND.

- It is a temporary and expected phase that will pass.
- Although unpleasant, your therapy is working.

In clinical practice, people with FND often show very different trajectories of progress ('recovery pathways') across disciplines (see Figures 1.10 and 1.11).

If you are 'at the height of the emotion', do not stop therapy earlier than recommended! The psychologist will guide you through the 'wild storms'. Otherwise, you risk:

- Not experiencing that negative emotions reduce over time.
- Not consolidating what may be the beginnings of helpful strategies for FND.
- Being left with a poor impression of psychology.
- Not building the confidence to test out that you can cope independently with strong emotions.
- Missing out on other potentially helpful strategies.
- Worsening the FND without refuge to a support system as provided by your psychologist.
- Not learning the core skills in FND: express your emotions and tolerate a storm of discomfort, thoughts, and emotions before the storm turns into FND.

Using this book

1.3 eResource alert!

Read here about some potential misgivings about this book and an outline of what this book tries to achieve instead.

The football coach analogy

A good approach is to think of this book as your football coach that is coaching you from the side lines of the field.

The coach teaches you strategies, exercises, and what pitfalls to watch out for when you are on the field busy trying to aim to ball in the goal. From the sidelines, your coach actively encourages you, gives you an occasional much-needed pep talk, and shouts motivational and positive one-liners to keep you going and not give up in the face of tiredness, pain, and perhaps feelings of defeat and helplessness against a strong opponent – which in your situation is the FND. Coaches can only do so much: they cannot run on the field and kick the ball into the goal for you. In the end, it is you who will keep running after the ball for hours, sometimes in extended time; change tactics; keep an oversight on the game; communicate with your football allies on the field; and eventually, after much practice, bypass the keeper and kick the ball straight into the goal. This means that you are doing all the hard work, and any credit is due to your efforts.

In the next chapters, you will learn more about a tool called the Pressure Cooker Model of FND that may help you in your journey to kick the 'FND ball' into the goal. The book has an educational slant and is written to provide you with lots of information on FND 'straight from the clinic' and based on 10+ years of clinical experience from the author. Some of it may ring familiar, while other pieces of information you may not have learned yet. This book is intended as an FND resource to help you on your way to recovery.

The book will offer you and your environment a lot of strategies that you can practice to help manage FND. Yes, that is right: the book is aimed at people with and without FND. The grand theme underlying the Pressure Cooker Model is that:

Everyone contributes to FND.
Therefore, everyone contributes to recovery from FND.

Online e-materials

The ultimate goal of the Pressure Cooker Model is to raise much-needed awareness on a lesser-known side to FND that holds one of the most important keys to recovery: social, relationship, and interpersonal factors. To support you with the process of reading and working through this book, you will be offered a large online eResource. These materials are freely available without any cost to you. All you need to do is to register on the following websites and start downloading. There are no restrictions to the number of times you can download the materials: you can have as many copies as you want!

- www.routledge.com/9781032312828
- www.drvanderhulst.com

The eResource contains supplementary materials that support and provide more elaboration to the contents of the book. In addition, questions will help you, your partner, your family, your friends, and healthcare professionals to better engage with the book. The questions are definitely not meant as a knowledge test, a full-blown exam, or in some way trying to catch you out! There is no grade at the end, and you are not required to complete all questions, although it will be helpful. The questions are intended to help you reflect on thoughts, feelings, memories, and ideas that pop up whilst reading the book. Engaging more deeply with the book in this way will also aid your memory for FND management strategies. You can make as many notes as you wish.

FNDictionary

Quite a lot of new and unfamiliar terms are explored in this book. Luckily, you can always consult the 'FNDictionary' for short descriptions of terms (listed in alphabetical order) in the eResource.

Pressure Cooker Values

Chapter 10 contains a set of 'Pressure Cooker Values', a useful group of statements that summarise important concepts and principles of the Pressure Cooker Model and FND 'in a nutshell'.

Memory and other cognitive strategies

Before you carry on, it may be a good idea to look at this 1.4 eResource straight away to read more about some useful cognitive rehabilitation strategies to support your reading and help you work effectively through this book, so you get the most out of it.

What to do with very difficult thoughts and feelings

Please read the 1.5 eResource on what to do when you experience difficult thoughts and feelings around hurting yourself. Sometimes a 'taboo' topic, but definitely not a subject that this book shies away from. As you work through the book, people can experience a temporary resurgence of intense emotions, particularly after having avoided or cut off feelings for quite a while. It is important that you know what you and your family can do to support you and what strategies are available.

References

Crossway Bibles. (2008). *The ESV study Bible: English standard version*. Wheaton, Ill: Crossway Bibles.

Demartini, B., Batla, A., Petrochilos, P., Fisher, L., Edwards, M. J., & Joyce, E. (2014). Multidisciplinary treatment for functional neurological symptoms: a prospective study. *Journal of Neurology, 261*, 2370–2377.

Demartini, B., Petrochilos, P., Ricciardi, L., Price, G., Edwards, M. J., & Joyce, E. (2014). The role of alexithymia in the development of functional motor symptoms (conversion disorder). *Journal of Neurology, Neurosurgery & Psychiatry, 85*(10), 1132–1137.

Edwards, M. J., Adams, R. A., Brown, H., Pareés, I., & Friston, K. J. (2012). A Bayesian account of 'hysteria'. *Brain, 135*(11), 3495–3512.

Griffith, J. L., Polles, A., & Griffith, M. E. (1998). Pseudoseizures, families, and unspeakable dilemmas. *Psychosomatics, 39*(2), 144–153.

Nielsen, G., Stone, J., Matthews, A., Brown, M., Sparkes, C., Farmer, R., ... & Edwards, M. (2015). Physiotherapy for functional motor disorders: a consensus recommendation. *Journal of Neurology, Neurosurgery & Psychiatry, 86*(10), 1113–1119.

Raynor, G., & Baslet, G. (2021). A historical review of functional neurological disorder and comparison to contemporary models. *Epilepsy & Behavior Reports, 16*, 100489.

Russell, L., Butler, L., Lovegrove, C., Owens, C., Roberts, L., Yates, P., ... & Price, C. (2022). *Developing a multidisciplinary pathway for functional neurological disorders in a UK National Health Service: The Exeter model. ACNR, Advances in Clinical Neuroscience and Rehabilitation*.

2 The history of the Pressure Cooker Model

Welcome to making it this far already to Chapter 2! Let us provide you with an in-depth description of the exciting journey of the Pressure Cooker Model of FND. In Chapter 2, you will have a chance to read about a group of amazing people with FND, various historical events, and pivotal clinical observations that led up to the development of the Pressure Cooker Model. Since its inception, the model has undergone several major transformations, as it has moved through four different clinical FND services. The unique characteristics of each of these clinical environments helped shape and refine the Pressure Cooker Model to a fully fledged clinical tool that can help people overcome FND. Are you curious to learn more? Let us delve into the world of metaphors and show you that the Pressure Cooker Model is much more than just a metaphor.

Metaphors in FND

Psychological processes can sometimes be abstract, intangible, and hard to grasp. For example, what is dissociation, attachment, a core belief, and even just the concepts of emotions and thoughts? One way to understand psychological processes better is to make them more concrete, relatable, and visual by using metaphors. Metaphors are often used in clinical practice for people with FND. The following three metaphors have been popular in the field of FND:

- The perception of FND as **'a software, not a hardware, problem'.** The software represents the functioning of the nervous system, whilst the hardware refers to the structure of the nervous system. According to this definition, people with FND tend not to show injuries or changes to the basic wiring of the nervous system (although recent brain imaging studies have perhaps somewhat challenged this view, bear in mind that this research comes with provisos – read about this in Chapter 3). What is important to know is that scans and EEG recordings of your brain come back as normal, and the tests that neurologists perform do not yield any results that would indicate organic neurological abnormalities. This definition suggests that something has gone awry with the *functioning* rather than the *structure* of the nervous system in people with FND.
- The idea that in FND **the messages from the brain are somehow not passed on appropriately or effectively to the rest of the body.** The faulty messaging subsequently results in your legs or your arms not working.
- The concept of **FND as a disconnect between the mind and body**, with therapies for FND attempting to 'reconnect' the mind with the body.

Metaphors are a well-intended means to help people with FND and their healthcare professionals understand the intricacies of FND. Clinicians often use metaphors to explain and communicate the diagnosis for the first time. This helps lift the veil on something that may be quite confusing and overwhelming. It provides a common initial language to describe what is happening to the person. In addition, it makes people feel believed, validated, and taken seriously. There is something not

DOI: 10.4324/9781003308973-2

working well in your body, and finally you feel that this is recognised by a healthcare professional. This is often a welcome experience after a long period of disbelief and uncertainty.

Despite these benefits, there are also several drawbacks to the metaphors:

- Metaphors can give **mixed messages**. For example, a person with FND and their family may be left wondering whether they have neurological injury or irreversible changes in their nervous system. This leads to unhelpful ideas, such as 'I will experience FND for the rest of my life', and 'There is nothing I can do about neurological problems in my brain'.
- Metaphors provide tangible and relatable descriptions of FND. However, they can be quite **vague** and **do not offer any explanation** for the mechanism or maintaining factors of FND. What and where exactly the mechanism is not functioning properly or breaking down is unclear, for example, what exactly are the contents and features of the messages that are not being passed on from the brain to the rest of the body? This situation leaves people often wondering and confused. They know what FND is not (a neurological condition caused by organic factors, like a stroke or a blood vessel that is blocked or ruptured), but simultaneously, the metaphor does not offer a clear explanation of what FND is.
- Metaphors **do not provide any ideas and solutions to treatment** or lay out a plan of steps to help you remediate FND symptoms.
- Metaphors are **always about the person with FND** and unhelpfully locate the problem within the individual, despite research clearly showing that FND has major social components that warrant a closer look at the contribution of the person's environment to FND.

Okay, so metaphors may have helped to some extent in FND but clearly have drawbacks. We therefore need to look at other ways to help understand FND. In the history of psychology, mechanical models that represent psychological processes have always been popular with clinicians. Could mechanical models be of use in FND?

From stress buckets . . .

Let us make a little sidestep from FND to psychosis to explain how a mechanical model can help with understanding phenomena that may initially be difficult to grasp.

People with psychosis often report experiences of people or things that they can see, hear, or think but other people may not. In the field of psychosis, the stress bucket model (Brabban & Turkington, 2002) has become one useful way to explain these phenomena to people with psychosis and their families. The stress bucket is filled with water. The bottom of the bucket has a series of holes. The water in the bucket represents all sorts of stressors important in psychosis, including *psychological* stresses (issues with relationships and family), *social* stressors (problems with employment or your financial situation), as well as *biological* stressors (issues with health and sleep). The holes at the bottom represent positive coping strategies to help manage the stressors, such as engaging with enjoyable activities, relaxation, as well as expressing difficult thoughts and feelings with people you are close to and trust.

Stress buckets differ between people. For some people, stress buckets may be filled up halfway: there is some water (i.e. some life stressors), but the bucket will not overflow because there are sufficient holes to let the water out (i.e. enough positive coping strategies to deal with and 'offset' the stressors). Other people's stress buckets are completely filled with only a few tiny holes that are able to let out the water: their buckets are at a tipping point of nearly overflowing. These people may experience a lot of stress in their life with very few coping resources to manage. When too much stress has built up in a vulnerable person's bucket, the bucket may overflow: the person may be at an increased risk of developing psychosis.

Do you see how a 'mechanical' metaphor that represents psychological, social, and biological processes can be used to explain a condition like psychosis to other people? Not only can the stress bucket help with understanding the mechanisms of psychosis, but the model also clearly tells us where to intervene to manage or prevent psychosis. For example, we could make more holes in the bucket to release the water (i.e. develop a number of extra coping strategies) or make the existing holes bigger (i.e. use our existing coping strategies more regularly). We could also try to find the tap and stop the water from streaming into the bucket (i.e. address relationship problems and sleeping difficulties).

... To pressure cookers

Pressure Cooker Models are another type of mechanical model that have always been around. Schreiber and Seitzinger (1985) used a pressure cooker to visualise stress and trauma processes in police forces. Their pressure cooker consisted of a heat, water, and a valve element. Each of the elements represented a concept that was important for understanding and managing stress – for example, 'constructive release' via the valve reflected things like exercise or meeting up with a friend. The 'heat' or amount of stressors could be 'adjusted'. Other pressure cookers have been used to describe the psychological processes involved in anger (French, 2001) using very similar elements, for example, a lid, steam release, flames, and matches.

In comparison to stress buckets, pressure cookers are objects with more features on them. For that reason, pressure cookers are probably better suited to describe conditions with multiple biological, psychological, and social layers, such as FND. In the next section, we will look at the origins and subsequent development of the Pressure Cooker Model into a fully fledged treatment model for people with and without FND.

The ten-year development of the Pressure Cooker Model of FND

The following section will describe the history and the process of development of the Pressure Cooker Model. The model's journey was heavily shaped by a vast number of clinical experiences in FND services and the many valuable conversations between people with FND, people without FND, healthcare professionals, and the clinician.

Phase 1: pre–Pressure Cooker Model

Laying down the foundations of the Pressure Cooker Model: the top 3 coping habits in FND

People with FND often report a **top three** of characteristic coping habits. Check out Figure 2.1 to see how coping habits make a person feel emotionally settled and psychologically safe.

2.1 eResource alert!

Read here about three stories of people with FND that illustrate these coping habits in more detail.

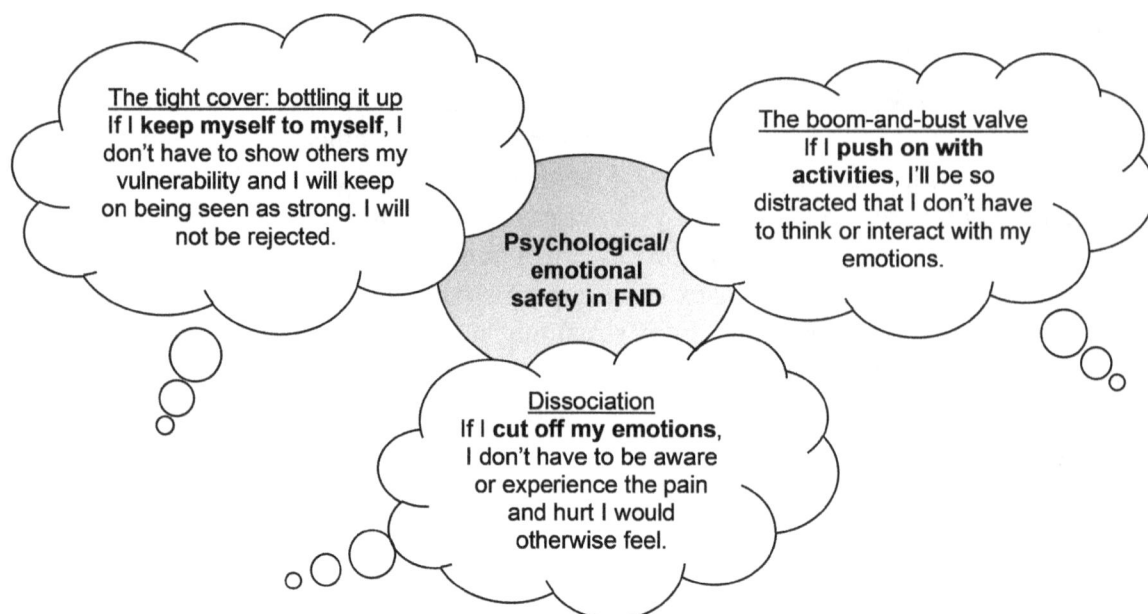

Figure 2.1 Coping habits and psychological safety in FND.

The FND coping triangle and the power of repetition

Coping habits do not just spontaneously fall down from the sky on people. When people with FND looked back on their childhoods and were asked the question **'How did you cope with emotions when you were a child?'** the answer was often (at least one out of three):

- I bottled things up. I **kept myself to myself**.
- I just **blotted it out** of my mind. I can't remember much of my childhood.
- I don't know . . . I just did. I **pushed on** . . . got on with things.

There is nothing wrong or faulty about any of these coping strategies. Growing up, sometimes under very difficult circumstances, people often developed these **'survival' strategies**, out of necessity, **to protect a person's emotional and physical well-being**.

That said, people **repeated and rehearsed** coping strategies over the years, and ultimately, these strategies became long-term, ingrained habits (see Figure 2.2).

Everything seemed to go well for years, until something more substantial happened in the person's life, and their existing coping habits, previously useful, were now suddenly insufficient in dealing with overwhelming or copious amounts of distress. What worked so well in the past did not work so well any longer. This is when the FND tended to set in as an 'emergency' coping strategy that quickly and effectively managed a person's discomfort.

Although this top three of coping strategies is **similarly reported by people without FND**, keep in mind that many other maintaining factors – other than early, repeated childhood coping habits – will impact on whether someone develops FND or not. Keep reading the book to find out about all the maintaining factors you need to know about!

Relationships and FND: could there be a possible link?

People in therapy often spontaneously and consistently brought up one topic during sessions: **relationships**! A psychological space to explore **challenging relationship dynamics** often led to

Sticky foods

Lack of verbal and/or emotional
expression in childhood

| "I kept myself to myself" | "I cut off my feelings"
(dissociation) | "I just pushed on and
didn't think about it" |

Tight cover

Lack of verbal and/or
emotional expression in
adulthood

e.g. "I keep myself to
myself"

Overpressure plug

Dissociation in
adulthood

e.g. "black-outs"

"dissociative
episodes"

**Blocked or Dysregulated
Valve**

Reduced stress release or

boom-and-bust cycle

e.g. "I push on"

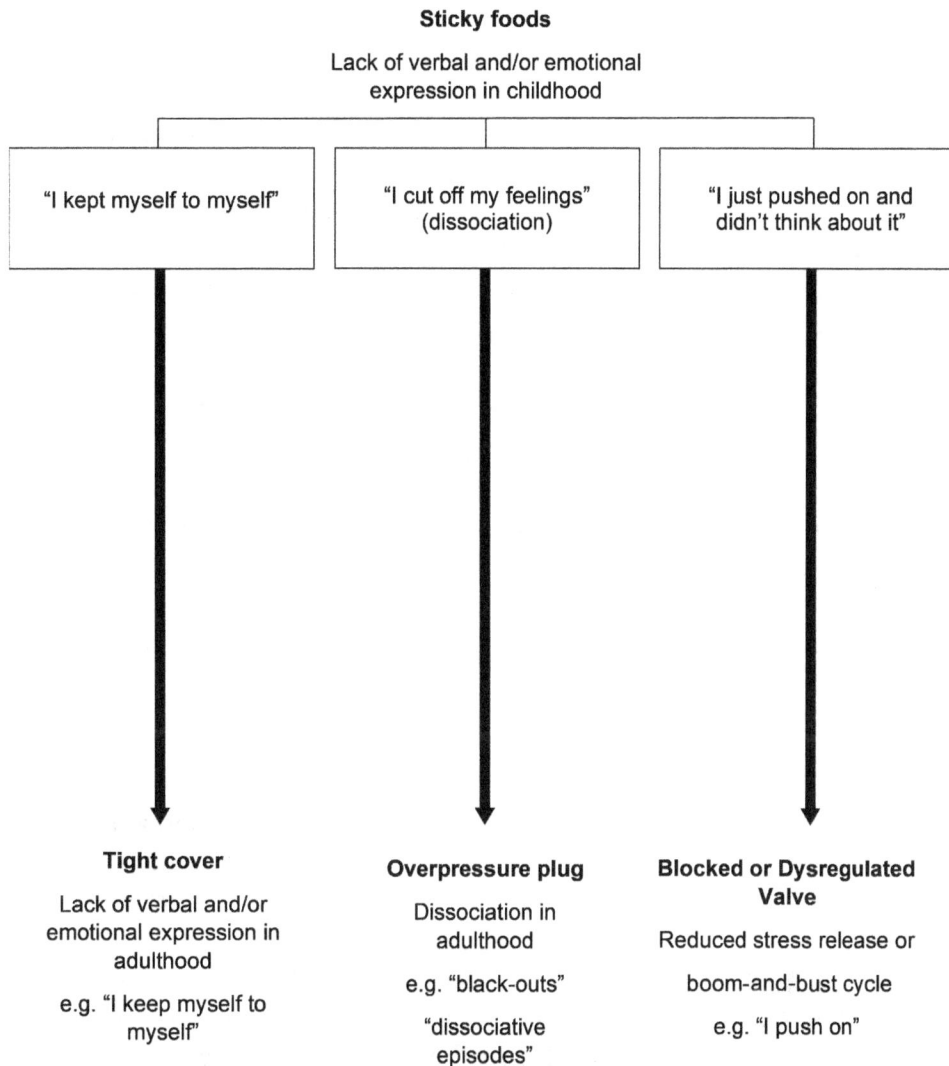

Figure 2.2 How early childhood coping strategies repeat into adulthood.

Source: Graphic design by Josué Borges Expósito.

'breakthroughs' and insight into what exactly maintained FND. Relationships were clearly meaningful, and some people started making **links between relationships and FND**.

What type of relationship issues emerged?

- Relationships on the verge of breakdown with a complicated web of interactions and a negative impact on the existing family unit.
- A perceived or real lack of emotional support from family members or bosses.
- Poor communication skills between family members or partners, particularly bottling up difficult thoughts and feelings and conflict-ridden exchanges.
- Inequality or mismatch of emotional needs being met within a relationship, with one emotionally more sensitive partner expressing a need for more connection from the emotionally distant or unavailable partner, who is unable to provide it.
- An inability to meet the high expectations around household and job chores within the relationship that was set by a demanding partner not meeting the emotional needs of the person with FND.
- A new person introduced into an existing family unit, causing turmoil and wreaking havoc to existing relationships, conflicts, and arguments with colleagues at work.

In quite a few of these situations, a clear link could be made between the relationship troubles that someone was going through and the start or intensity of the FND symptoms. For example:

- Developing functional weakness for the first time soon after a new unwanted person arrived in their family environment that they felt unhappy about (but did not verbally express).
- Whenever a person's partner or family member was not communicating nicely to them, with FND symptoms immediately worsening during these difficult interactions.
- Someone with relationship problems whose FND immediately increased whenever their partner approached them physically.

It was also striking that people with FND, and with significant relationship problems, would most often attend the clinic on their own. There were various reasons for partners or family not being involved. For example:

- Exploration of sensitive and personal issues were often associated with these same partner or family relationships.
- Partners had no interest in coming to the sessions.
- Family members did not believe and distanced themselves from the person with FND.
- Practical issues around work, transport, or childcare.

The need for connection?

Therapy sessions were often supported with book materials on FND. Interestingly, these materials were often not even mentioned or quite quickly pushed aside, in favour of a face-to-face conversation with the therapist. People visiting the service clearly expressed a preference to 'talk' rather than to 'read' and discuss book materials in the sessions. Therefore, therapy sessions focused on exploring the relationship issues that people brought, with the book materials as a helpful guide. Once more, this seemed to highlight the importance of relationships in FND on multiple levels. The question arose whether the FND could be described in a cohesive framework that somehow would tie all these clinical observations together and would support people with brain fog and concentration problems to remember the different bits and pieces of FND. Read the next section to find out how these early observations lay the foundations for the birth of the Pressure Cooker Model.

Phase 2: simple Pressure Cooker Model

The first 'launch': initial conceptualisation of the Pressure Cooker Model

A basic version of the Pressure Cooker Model for FND was officially trialled in 2016 during a psychological therapy session in an FND clinic. Let us look at Sarah's life situation to explain how this process came about.

THE BEGINNING

WHERE DID IT ALL GO?

Sarah's life consisted of constant 'pushing on' and unreasonable demands placed on her by people in her environment without a way to relieve any of these pressures:

- She made long hours at work.
- After work, she spent time on any needs and crises that arose in her family.
- Sarah had dropped all her hobbies and interests.

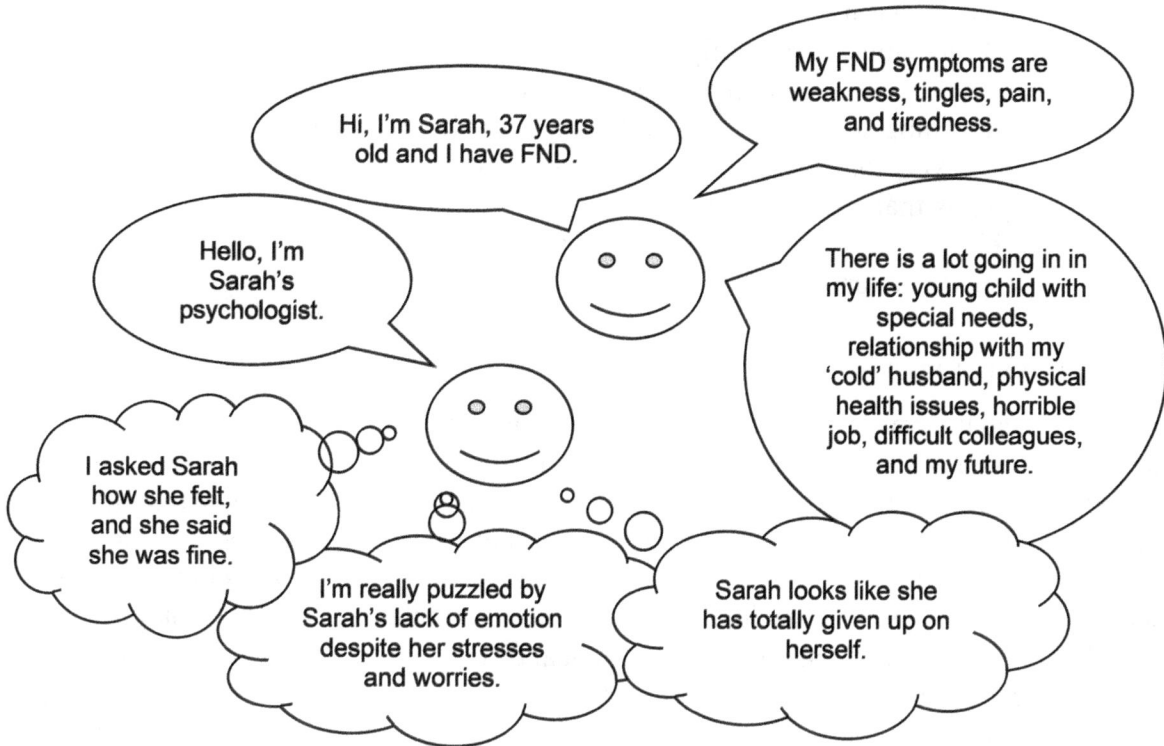

Figure 2.3 Introducing Sarah and her psychologist.

- Her social network was limited to only one vague friend whom she had not seen in months and was not regularly in touch with.
- Her only contacts involved day-to-day interactions with her family and colleagues at work. Definitely not the happiest of exchanges, which often made Sarah feel on edge.
- Her marriage was in hot water, and her husband had distanced himself from her. Sarah was unable to talk to her husband about any life challenges.

Although Sarah was surrounded by family and colleagues, she was isolated and cut off, with no one to turn to. The question arose: Where did all of Sarah's worries go?

A ROADBLOCK: STUCK IN THERAPY

Despite weeks of therapy, Sarah did not progress. She continued to report the same symptoms and problems, week after week. Therapy had stalled, and this 'stuckness' was defined by the following observations:

- Despite many explanations and psychoeducation on FND symptoms by the psychologist, Sarah remained puzzled and confused about FND.
- Sarah was unaware that she had a problem with identifying and connecting with her emotions that she struggled to access. As a result, the psychologist was unable to fit her psychological difficulties into existing cognitive-behavioural therapy (CBT) treatment models, as these models required Sarah to identify with her emotions.
- New symptoms emerged for Sarah on a weekly basis. Each time the psychologist felt they were onto something, 'clinician hopes' were dashed, and the psychologist needed to recalibrate again and seek a new avenue of treatment.

- The psychologist felt a sense of discomfort right before seeing Sarah and was regularly switching off during the sessions, particularly when Sarah reported a string of physical symptoms and felt an increasing urge to give up. It was as if Sarah's dissociative symptoms and hopelessness mirrored the psychologist's own thoughts, feelings, and behaviours.
- In addition, the psychologist did not have any recourse to resources to quickly check out the physical symptoms that Sarah reported: Were they part of the FND or totally unrelated? The psychologist felt isolated – again, in a similar way as Sarah was likely feeling in the context of her lack of support network.

SARAH WAS CONNECTING WITH 'SOMETHING'

Despite Sarah and the psychologist not progressing together on their therapy journey, Sarah was a conscientious patient who attended her weekly sessions and diligently engaged with her homework. She never cancelled and was always on time, even when she was clearly sick and sniffling. There was no sign of Sarah being disinterested in the contents of what was discussed, nor did she appear to be 'forced' by her environment to attend. Although her medical doctor had referred her to the service, she was in full agreement with the FND diagnosis and the need for psychological intervention. Furthermore, Sarah lived at quite a geographical distance from the service; attending her sessions took a great chunk out of her day and represented somewhat of a sacrifice. The psychologist felt that, although Sarah was not making any big or observable strides in therapy, she clearly was connecting with 'something' in the process that was meaningful to her – even if she was unable to verbalise what that 'something' was that pulled her towards setting time aside to attend the sessions.

THE BIRTH OF THE PRESSURE COOKER MODEL

After carefully considering Sarah's motivation to attend the sessions and several moments of deep self-reflection on the direction that the therapy was taking, the psychologist went back to the drawing board. Several characteristics in Sarah's presentation stood out to the therapist:

- **Sarah's sessions always revolved around FND symptoms.** There was something unusual about Sarah's reports on the symptoms. Large parts of the session were often devoted to the exploration of Sarah's symptoms. Furthermore, new symptoms frequently appeared, and symptoms could come and go and were highly variable. Instead of focusing on the contents of the symptoms (what symptoms Sarah experienced), the psychologist realised that the process was probably more meaningful (the big role that the symptoms played in Sarah's life, the constant upheaval of discovering a new symptom, the general unpredictability of the symptoms). 'Big impact', 'constant upheaval', and 'unpredictability' – perhaps this was what Sarah was experiencing on a deeper, emotional level? Could the symptoms symbolise Sarah's only language of expressing emotions?
- **Sarah's lack of understanding on the mechanics of FND.** A question that often came up in sessions was, 'Why [did I develop FND]?' Sarah explained the FND and its underlying mechanisms by using confusing metaphors that focused on physical processes, leaving out any psychological or social aspects of FND, and that failed to provide a treatment plan. Although the psychologist had formed a narrative around the 'why' and 'how' of Sarah's FND symptoms, translating these ideas into a simple language that would support Sarah's understanding of FND (or help Sarah make an informed decision to 'refute' the narrative that the clinician had in mind) made this a complex question that was not easy to respond to.
- **Sarah had no one to turn to.** Sarah demonstrated reduced verbal emotional expression and lacked close, psychologically safe relationships with other people in her life that would allow verbal emotional expression.

- **Sarah's activity levels were all over the place.** Sarah's daily activities were not a steady, reasonable, and manageable stream, with some slight variation depending on life's demands. A slightly varying but constant level of activity can be psychologically very containing and provide a sense of control, as well as a stress buffer. In contrast, Sarah's activity levels varied widely and were characterised by a boom-and-bust pattern (this, and other common activity patterns in FND, will be discussed in Chapter 6). Sarah demonstrated a tendency to work extreme hours for prolonged periods of time ('boom', high activity), intermixed with long recovery periods of inactivity that required her to take sick leave from work ('bust', low or minimal activity). Sarah's daily life seem to be devoid of any regular rest breaks.
- **What ticked Sarah and what made her life enjoyable?** Sarah did not report regularly engaging with enjoyable activities; she had dropped hobbies and sports and could not identify any passions or interests. There was no 'me' time available to work on her individual and personal life goals. Sarah had lost complete touch with her identity: What ticked Sarah? What could contain her psychologically during stressful times in her life?
- **Sarah had no sense of social belonging.** Another striking element in Sarah's story was the absence of social belonging. Although Sarah was part of the family unit, she was slowly succumbing to family stress. Her husband distanced himself from Sarah's symptoms, and her marriage was defined by the antithesis of social belonging. Outside her family and work, Sarah was not connected to friendship circles, communities, or clubs consisting of people with similar interests that elicited positive emotions.
- **Did Sarah display an FND coping triangle?** Sarah's habits of pushing on, not speaking, as well as cutting off her emotions were developed early in her life. It was as if these coping strategies had repeated over time and were still fully present in Sarah's life. Her childhood was characterised by a harsh and strict upbringing, with two parents that met her physical needs but were not sufficiently attuned to her emotional needs. Since a young age, Sarah was required to work hard and contribute to the family, with big responsibilities ascribed to her that were probably beyond what would be expected for a child her age. There was no room for emotional expression; Sarah had no one to turn to if she experienced difficult thoughts and feelings.

These observations were not unique to Sarah. In fact, this specific combination of features was observed across the vast majority of people with FND who visited the clinic. It was more surprising to encounter a person with FND who did not demonstrate these features. The psychologist came to the realisation that, although cognitive-behavioural therapy models were useful to some degree, none of the existing models were able to fully accommodate these FND-specific features. Something about these models needed to change if we wanted to improve our understanding and treatment of people with FND.

THE FIRST LAUNCH OF THE PRESSURE COOKER MODEL

The psychologist had noticed some similarities between FND and mechanical models that were commonly used to understand and treat psychological problems other than FND:

- The stress bucket for psychosis (Brabban & Turkington, 2002)
- Stress in the police force (Schreiber & Seitzinger, 1985)
- Anger in adolescents (French, 2001).

Although at first glance these areas seem widely apart, each of these mechanical models had several things in common:

- The core of the models focused on an emotion, 'stress', or a psychological symptom.
- The idea of contents (water, food) held in some form of container (a bucket or a pan).

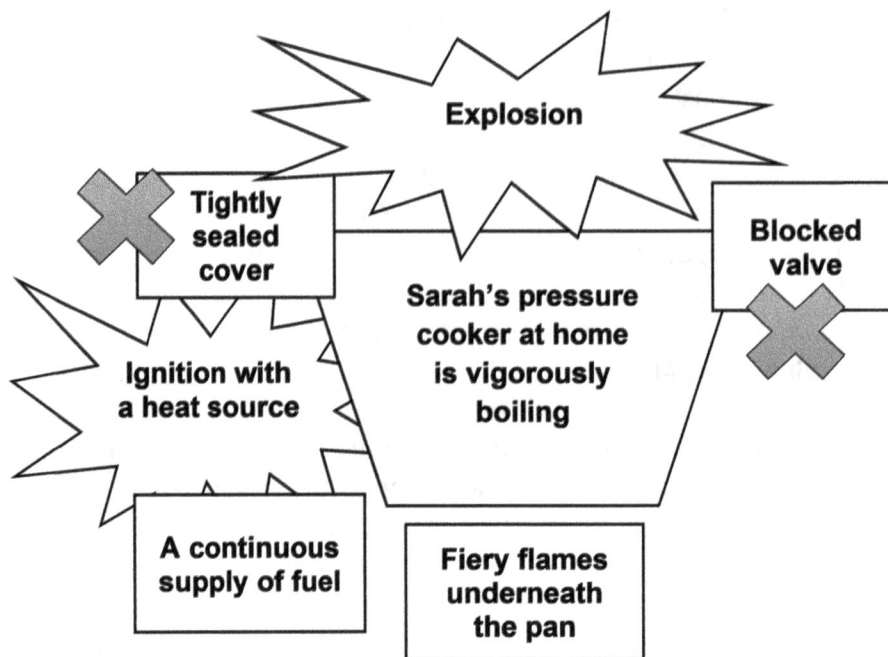

Figure 2.4 A basic Pressure Cooker Model.

- A sense of 'mechanical malfunction', build-up, blockage, or overflow of contents.
- A need to release the contents using a channel, such as a valve, a hole in the bucket, or opening a cover.
- The use of a visual metaphor to explain complex psychological concepts.
- Simple language.

During a therapy session quite late in the treatment course, Sarah and the psychologist continued to 'revolve' around each other in opposing directions: Sarah kept focusing on and bringing up new symptoms, whereas the psychologist kept trying to shoehorn Sarah into a treatment model, even though the psychologist knew that this attempt at treating Sarah's problems would soon bite the dust. In the middle of the session, the psychologist made the radical decision to push aside all models and start anew by drawing a pressure cooker container on a piece of paper that was specifically adapted for some of the FND-specific features that Sarah presented with and that could support the formulation of Sarah's difficulties. Sarah was asked to think about what would happen to the scenario depicted in Figure 2.4.

- **Question 1:** What would happen to a boiling pan if your fuel source supply was continuously feeding the flames under the pan but you found yourself in a situation with a tightly sealed cover and a blocked valve? (Sarah rightly responded that the pan would explode.)
- **Question 2:** How is the pan preventing itself from exploding at the moment? The clinician spontaneously added a third channel on the pressure cooker pan (the overpressure plug) to illustrate how the boiling contents were released so that the pan did not break down. This plug represented the FND.
- **Question 3:** In what other ways could we prevent an explosion of the pan? By opening the cover and unblocking the valve so that we do not need to engage the overpressure plug (the focus initially was on the top parts of the pressure cooker).

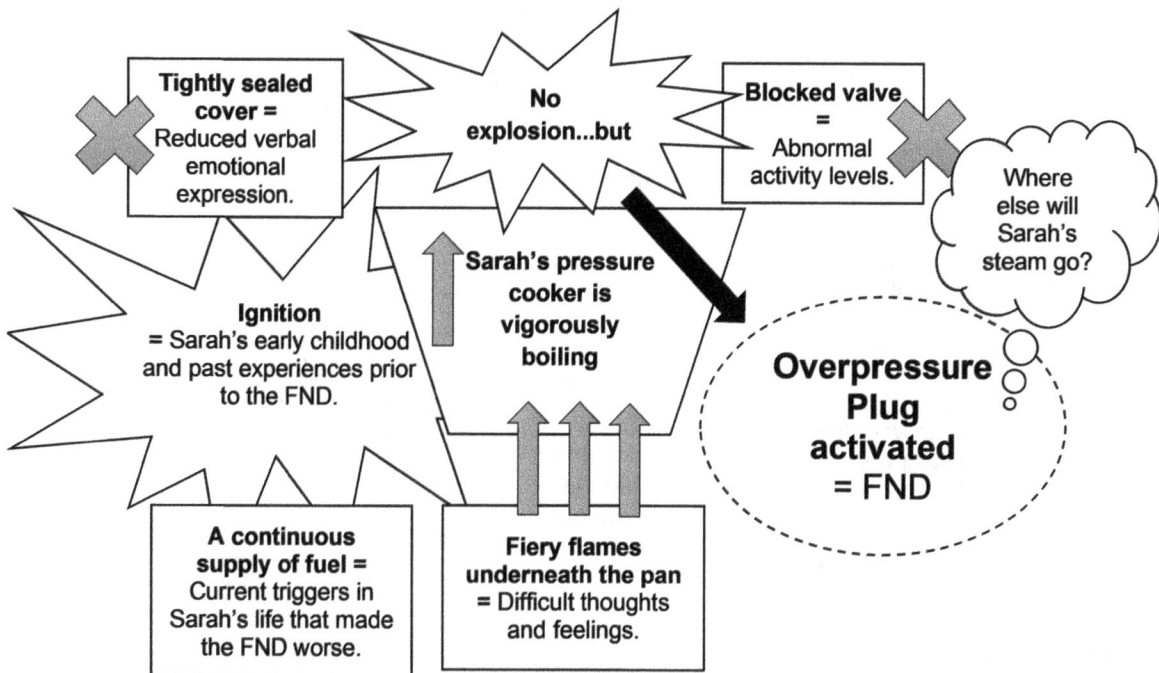

Figure 2.5 Sarah's Pressure Cooker Model.

The mechanical elements of Sarah's pressure cooker pan were subsequently associated with psychological processes important in FND to help Sarah's understanding of her condition. See Figures 2.5 and 2.6 for this basic version of the Pressure Cooker Model.

After sharing the formulation depicted in Figure 2.6, Sarah acknowledged that she had gained a much better understanding of the mechanisms of FND. With the help of the pressure cooker pan, Sarah learned that the FND supported her with coping and reducing ('internally regulate') her unpleasant internal state that she was unable to label.

Whenever Sarah experienced or spoke about her physical symptoms at length, what she was really saying was: 'I'm hurting, I'm anxious, help me.' In her early years, Sarah had not learned to connect with her emotions. How was she able to learn if she did not have the 'emotional role models' to glean these skills from? Cutting off and keeping her emotions to herself whilst pushing on were three coping habits that helped Sarah survive her challenging family circumstances.

Although these survival skills were the best thing she could have done, the downside was that after years of disconnecting from her emotions, she completely lost touch with emotions which felt foreign to her. Her physical symptoms appeared to be the only 'currency' that she had at her disposal and that allowed her to relate to her feelings and somehow communicate these unpleasant feelings to her environment.

The explanation of FND using the basic Pressure Cooker Model turned out to be a powerful moment in therapy for both Sarah and the clinician. By the end, Sarah's FND and mood symptoms had slightly improved. Even though Sarah had not fully recovered in the eyes of the psychologist, this was not consistent with Sarah's own view of her progress. Importantly, she expressed feeling very happy about how the psychological therapy had 'panned out' for her. This felt as a genuine reflection, as Sarah was smiling and appeared more energetic. She had made the first steps towards starting her journey of discovering her interests and connecting socially with a friend she had not seen in a long time. Sarah left the service with a better understanding of the mechanics of FND.

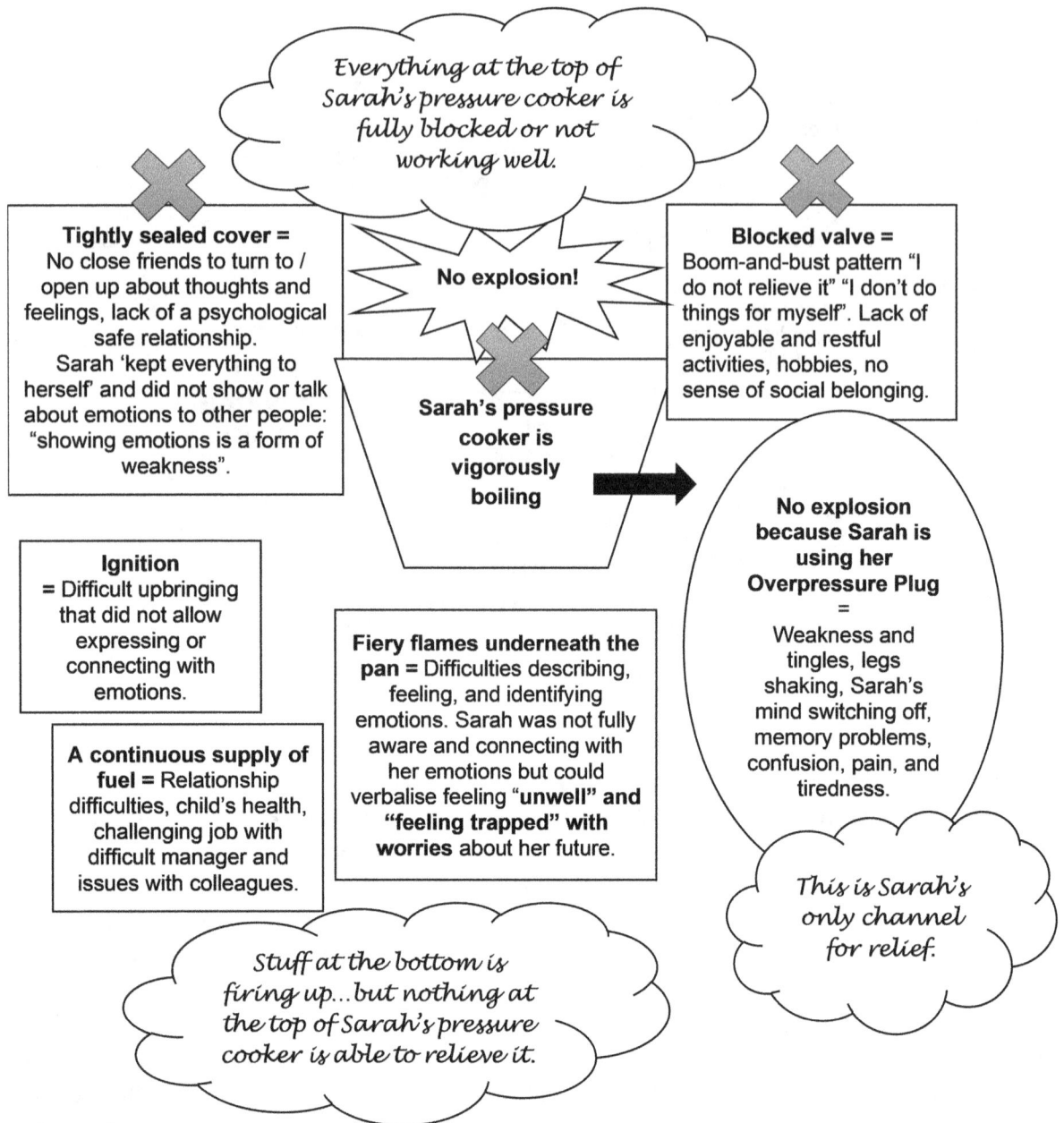

Figure 2.6 Sarah's Pressure Cooker Model, but now completed with details from her own life.

Subsequent development of the Pressure Cooker Model

Following this initial positive experience with the Pressure Cooker Model, the psychologist started to apply and share the formulation more frequently with other people with FND. Along the way, more FND-specific features were added onto the pan:

- The **warning light** represents the increased self-focused attention on physical symptoms, an important maintaining factor of FND and extensively written about in the scientific literature of FND.
- The **heat** represents the 'temperature' of emotions, ranging from cold (not feeling and dissociating from them) to hot (feeling completely caught up in your emotions, or strong, intense emotions that quickly change between hot and cold).

The model seemed to be particularly effective for people whose symptoms and beliefs did not fit into traditional cognitive-behavioural therapy (CBT) models and who experienced poor emotion awareness, an inability to describe emotions in words, as well as high levels of dissociation. One person commented that 'talking' (about emotions, that is, 'opening the cover') was the single most important thing that they could identify that had helped them to recover from FND symptoms. This was certainly an accurate observation, although they had also started to reconnect with friends that they had lost contact with over the years ('unblocking the valve'). The following equation seemed to apply:

learning to talk and connect with emotions (**'opening the cover'**)
+ creating a sense of social belonging (**'unblocking the valve'**)
= reducing the risk of FND (**'no need to engage with the overpressure plug'**)

PRESSURE COOKER MODEL: GROUP THERAPY

The Pressure Cooker Model was not only useful during individual therapy sessions; the model also proved to be a great tool to adapt and trial for use in a group therapy format for people with FND. The first ever 'Pressure Cooker Model' group consisted of a small number of people with FND (mostly with dissociative seizures) and their loved ones, who occasionally attended the group too. Although one person with a highly technical skill set commented on the inherent design flaws of the pressure cooker pan, this person took the model fully on board and gained a better understanding of the mechanics of FND!

2.2 eResource alert!

Are you curious to read about the Pressure Cooker Model group therapy and how this was received by people with FND and their loved ones? Check out the eResource to read more about the many positive comments that people have made about the group therapy.

UNFOLDING SOCIAL PROCESSES IN THE PRESSURE COOKER MODEL GROUP

As can be seen from Figures 2.7 and 2.8, the group therapy experience revealed a range of interesting 'interpersonal' beliefs about other people, especially around not being believed and feeling alone in your journey with FND.

The group therapy was socially very inclusive and encouraged partners, family members, and friends to join in. Although there were no specific questions asked about what participants thought of their significant other's contributions to the group process, Figure 2.8 shows their spontaneous comments.

BEHAVIOURAL ACTIVATION: REDISCOVERING AND RECLAIMING A SENSE OF SOCIAL BELONGING

The valve is a very important element in the Pressure Cooker Model, and it would be too simplistic to view the valve as just representing a person's activity levels and not look any further. As we will discover in Chapter 6, **the valve is strongly connected to social functioning**. This is relevant to FND: one of the most striking features of people visiting the clinic was **social isolation, a reduction in social activities, limited social networks, and no sense of social belonging**

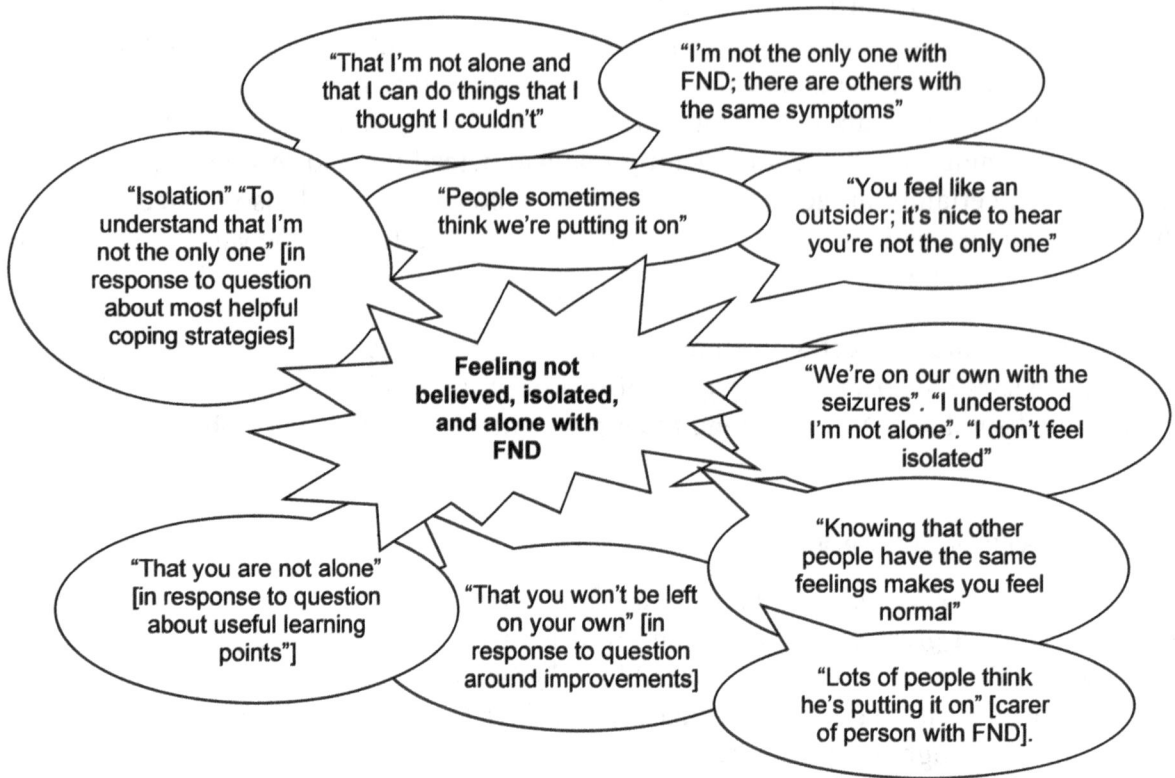

Figure 2.7 Isolation, loneliness, and not feeling believed in FND.

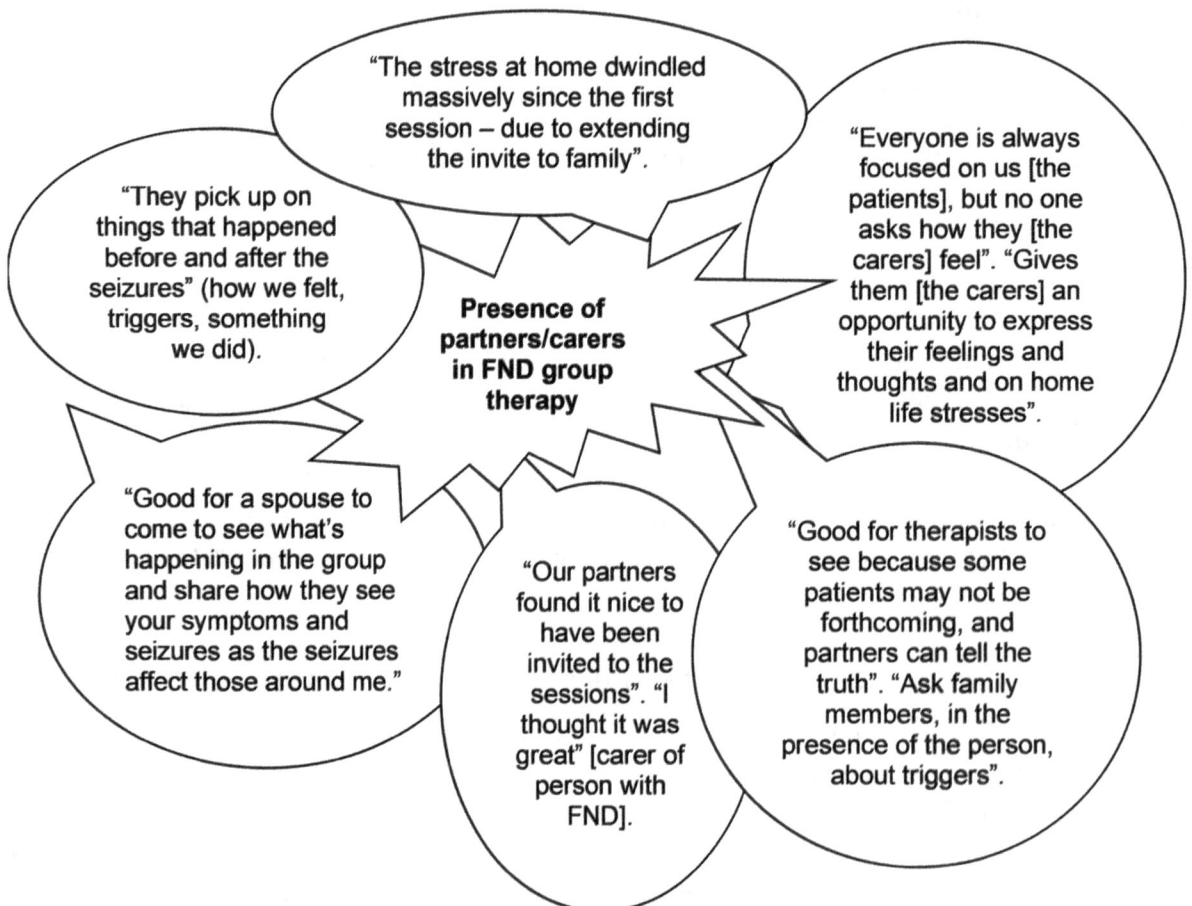

Figure 2.8 Positive qualities about involving carers in the Pressure Cooker Model group therapy.

to a community, including occasionally 'the family'. This was often due to a myriad of factors, including:

- **Physical disabilities** and **physical symptoms** restricting access to the community – not limited to FND but also including fatigue and pain.
- **Depression** and a very understandable **lack of motivation,** as well as **low levels of energy** to seek out the company of others.
- **Social anxiety** and anxiety associated with not having been out and about for a long time and having to get used to people, crowds, and sensory overload.
- **Interpersonal difficulties** due to **complex trauma** or **autism,** making it harder for someone to communicate and establish social connections with other people.
- **A sudden event** that stopped the person from having friends, for example, a separation from a partner or an argument with an entire group or a community turning against the person.
- **Embarrassment** and a **fear of rejection** around reconnecting with friends after a long period of absence or silence on messages.
- **Family members not knowing how to respond** or **connect** to the person with FND, who may now be in a wheelchair and needing support with personal care. Occasionally, partners and family members felt embarrassed about the person with FND and were less inclined to take the person out.
- A small subset of people with FND may be the victim of **coercive control** and **domestic violence**.

'Behavioural activation' is a treatment focused on helping the individual reintroduce enjoyable and meaningful activities in their life (doing things that 'activate' a feeling of happiness). Enjoyable activities include creative endeavours, sports, finding a new hobby, or pursuing an interest.

The quest for enjoyable activities can generate a positive 'side effect' of meeting and connecting with new people and become a powerful tool at remediating social isolation as well as alleviate FND symptoms. People seemed to make the **strongest improvements** if they were **not only actively engaged with psychological therapy** and able to **build a firm therapeutic relationship** with the clinician but were also **able to 'generalise' these relationship skills** through **building or rekindling relationships outside the therapy space** and develop more openness towards participating in a social life or becoming part of a community. Chapter 6 will explore the concept of social belonging in great detail.

Another important lesson learned from behavioural activation was that even if people were not aware of emotions and continued to struggle connecting, which is arguably a longer process, **at least unblocking the valve by increasing their level of enjoyable activities** could already bring about some **significant changes** in their **well-being and FND symptoms**.

DOUBLE REINFORCEMENT: A HARD-TO-SPOT PHENOMENON IN THE CLINIC

Clinical observations of people with FND who were accompanied by their family on their appointments, lifted an interesting veil on the direct impact of the social environment on FND.

- **Reinforcement.** The responses from a partner or a family member to a dissociative episode were often well-intended and came from a good heart but were unfortunately reinforcing the symptoms and increasing the risk of their reoccurrence in the future.

    Lola was diagnosed with dissociative seizures and always attended the psychology sessions with her partner. At all times, Lola preferred her partner to be present, and when one-to-one sessions were proposed, to which her partner happily agreed, Lola was reluctant and expressed anxiety. It was not uncommon for Lola to experience a seizure in the session, especially when difficult life events, thoughts, and feelings were explored. The moment Lola would feel the first upcoming signs of a seizure, her partner would jump out of their chair, immediately approach and hug Lola tightly, pat her on the back, and speak reassuring words to her. After about 10–15 minutes, the seizure would gradually stop, and Lola was ready to re-engage with the session again. In this example, the seizure supported Lola with coping with her distress by finding psychological safety with her partner. But her partner, feeling sorry and empathy for Lola, felt equally distressed and wanted nothing more for the seizures to stop as quickly as possible.

- **Intermittent reinforcement.** The role of intermittent reinforcement from the environment in the maintenance of FND symptoms. Intermittent reinforcement in FND means that a person often receives a mixture of positive responses to the FND (e.g. family comforting and reassuring the person during a dissociative episode) as well as negative responses (e.g. person not feeling believed, getting dismissed, or being treated in a rude manner by healthcare professionals). Learn about the dangers of intermittent reinforcement in Chapter 9.
- **Invalidation.** Unusual or unhelpful responses from the environment to a person displaying hurt or a difficult emotion in the therapy session, for example, telling the person to stop crying, not comforting the person, exhibiting frustrations at witnessing emotions in the person with FND.
- **Disbelief at FND.** Family members did not always understand the diagnosis of FND or fully believed that their loved one had FND rather than an organic neurological condition. Some people helped to vigorously advocate for an organic instead of a psychological explanation causing the FND symptoms. 'Are you sure that they do not have epilepsy? Is this absolutely clear? I noticed a new symptom and looked this up on the internet. I wonder whether this medical diagnosis can explain their symptoms?'
- **Overzealousness.** Family members 'exposing' or 'selling' the person with FND out in front of the clinician, particularly around keeping certain aspects of the FND or emotions hidden. Occasionally, the person was heavily encouraged by their loved ones to attend the sessions without the person wanting to be there themselves and not saying much during the sessions.
- **Abnormal relationships** playing out 'live' in the therapy room: conflicts, disagreements, and arguments between partners; palpable coldness and distance; enmeshed relationships and ensuring the proximity of family members; signs of coercive control or abuse by a partner.
- **Other social effects on dissociative seizures.** FND symptoms would not unusually flare up in more public situations, for example, in a clinical area, on busy hospital grounds, or during group therapy. On one occasion, a group of people diagnosed with dissociative seizures all simultaneously experienced a seizure in a waiting room.

Although awareness of the social aspects of FND was starting to gradually increase, at this stage of its development, the Pressure Cooker Model did not yet have a specific element dedicated to the impact of the social environment and relationships on the FND. The next section will describe the process by which this 'inkling' developed into a fully fledged idea to become one of the core principles of the model.

Phase 3: refinement of the Pressure Cooker Model

The Pressure Cooker Model was subsequently taken into the realm of treating people with symptoms at the more complex end of the FND spectrum. How was this complexity manifested? And was the Pressure Cooker Model not too basic for people experiencing complex FND?

- **Chronic and enduring FND symptoms** experienced over many years, occasionally over multiple decades, sometimes starting in childhood, without the person having had access to a proper diagnosis or specialist support and often with heaps of equipment and home adaptations, or a comprehensive care package.

- **Severe FND** characterised by both arms and legs paralysed ('functional tetraplegia'), with patients understandably very dependent on other people for their personal care needs, as well as patients with high-frequency or severe dissociative seizures that caused people to seriously injure themselves and others around them.
- **Unusual and rare symptoms**, including severe dystonia; speech problems, including an inability to speak at all; tics; foreign accent syndrome; severe bladder dysfunction; and functional amnesia, where the person forgot their entire life.
- **Multiple conditions affecting the body, brain, and the mind.** For example, experiencing FND but also fibromyalgia, chronic fatigue syndrome, Ehlers–Danlos or POTS (postural orthostatic tachycardia syndrome), as well as people with FND who are on the autism spectrum or have learning difficulties.
- **FND+.** People with **functional overlay** who also experienced a brain or spinal injury on top of the FND that required a careful and complex disentangling of the contributions of each condition to the symptoms.
- A **complex trauma background** with people struggling interpersonally, which often played out in therapy sessions.
- **Strong emotions** caused by symptoms and behaviours that often provoked high levels of anxiety and anger in the staff around the person with FND, for example, a lack of engagement, falls, deliberate self-harm, anger outbursts, or difficult family interactions.
- **Quickly morphing, changeable, and fluctuating symptoms** in a person that required a lot of support from staff, for example, a period of experiencing a lot of falls, followed by fewer falls but a period of increased pain symptoms, followed by self-harm, followed by more dissociative seizures, and so on.

The Pressure Cooker Model as a tool for engagement with psychology

Engagement with psychology sessions and adopting a psychological way of thinking on FND was not always easy for people! Read this **2.3 eResource alert!** for a list of totally understandable fears and reservations about psychological therapy reported by people with FND.

Engagement with psychology proved difficult for another important reason: the use of standard CBT models did not always agree with the psychological difficulties and symptoms that people with FND experienced, especially people with more severe forms of FND.

DANIEL'S STORY

In the following section, you will learn more about Daniel, his family, and his treating team. The Pressure Cooker Model viewed the FND in Daniel's situation as a problem that affected **the person** as well as **the entire system around the person** and **the interpersonal dynamics between everyone who was part of that system**.

Looking at FND in this way, we can say that **'everyone has FND'** – not just the person that experiences the actual physical symptoms, like Daniel. The person with FND is simply the 'carrier' of the symptoms, reflecting underlying problems in relationships with the multi-layered systems that include as well as surround the person. On multiple occasions throughout the book, this broader definition of FND will be explored. Let us take a look at Daniel first and get to know his story.

Daniel's background   Daniel was a young gentleman in his early 30s who attended a multidisciplinary rehabilitation programme to help him tackle the FND.

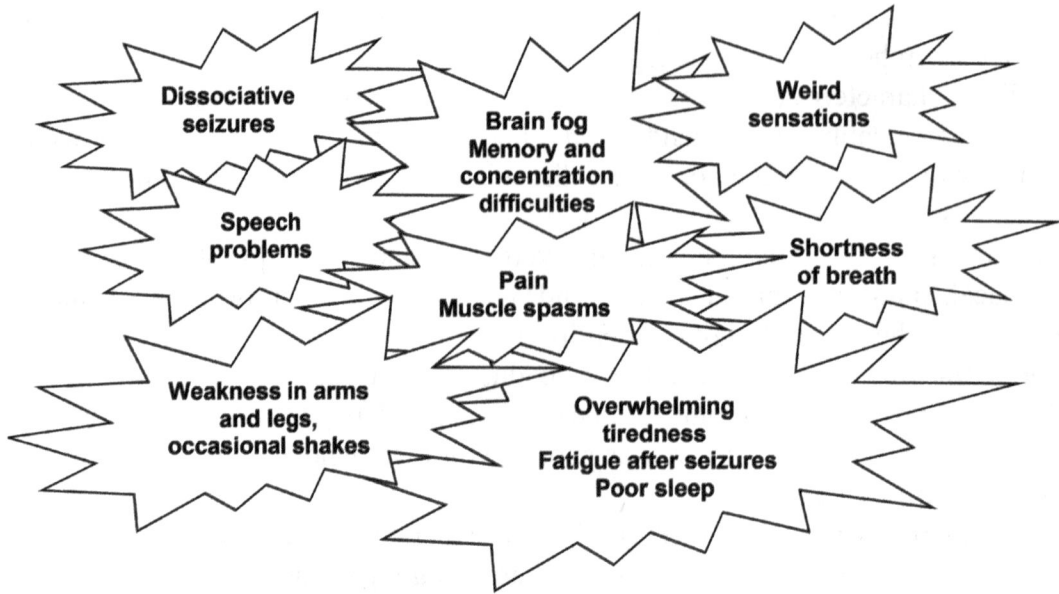

Figure 2.9 Daniel's most bothersome symptoms.

His symptoms (see Figure 2.9) developed around five years prior following a small collision with a motorbike on the sidewalk in front of his house. Just in case, an ambulance was called, and Daniel was brought to the emergency department. Fortunately, Daniel had not sustained any serious injuries, apart from a few bruises that healed up quickly. After a brief check-up in the hospital, Daniel was discharged home with an FND diagnosis and some equipment, but no referrals or follow-up care.

After the accident

Kayleigh's views   With all the focus on Daniel's health and his difficulties with expressing himself, it was really important to gauge Kayleigh's views too. Although everybody had adapted to this new way of living, Kayleigh bore the brunt of caring and experienced all kinds of conflicting thoughts and feelings, all normal and understandable (see Figure 2.11).

What did the FND look like?   In the hospital, Daniel would often spend days on end in his bed sleeping and unrousable. When woken up by staff, he occasionally experienced a dissociative seizure on the spot. Dissociative seizures could happen anywhere and anytime:

- In the gym.
- Outdoors.
- Sometimes with people present.
- Sometimes without people around when alone in his bedroom.
- At night-time.
- During the daytime.
- Following a meal.
- In the middle of a conversation.
- After a phone call.
- When watching television.
- And in many more situations, different times of day, locations, and circumstances.

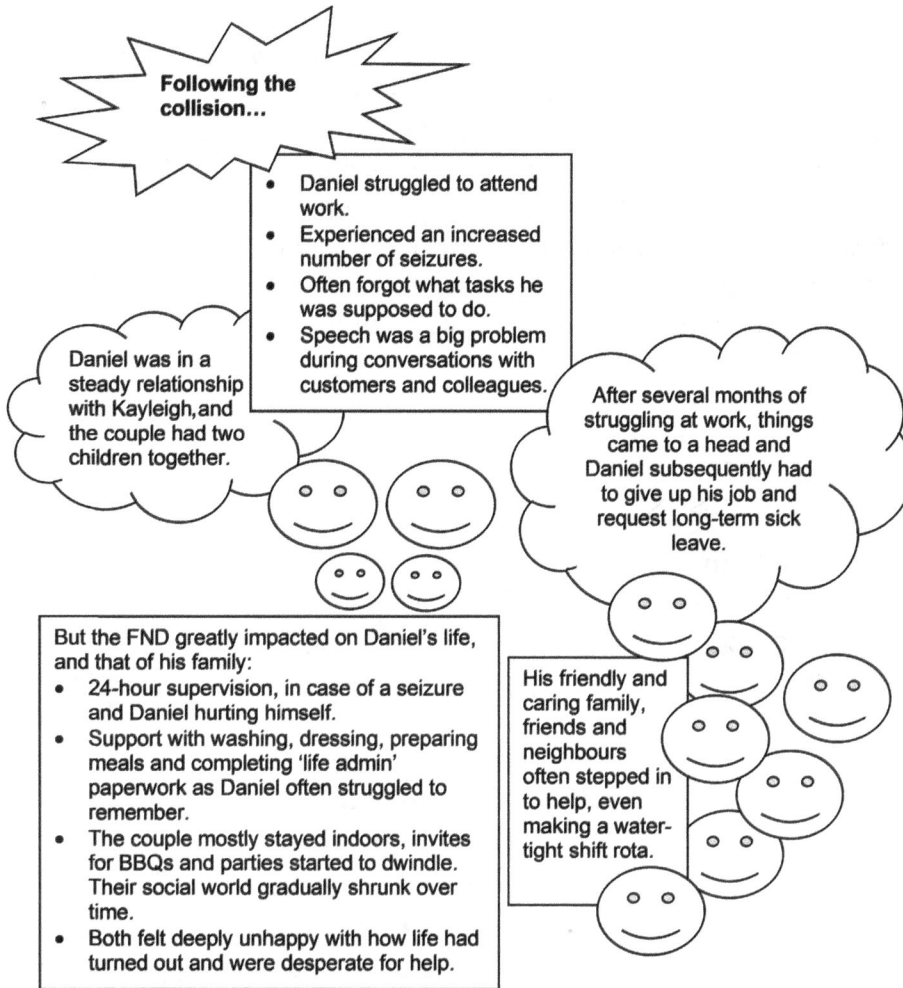

Figure 2.10 The impact of the accident on Daniel's and Kayleigh's lives.

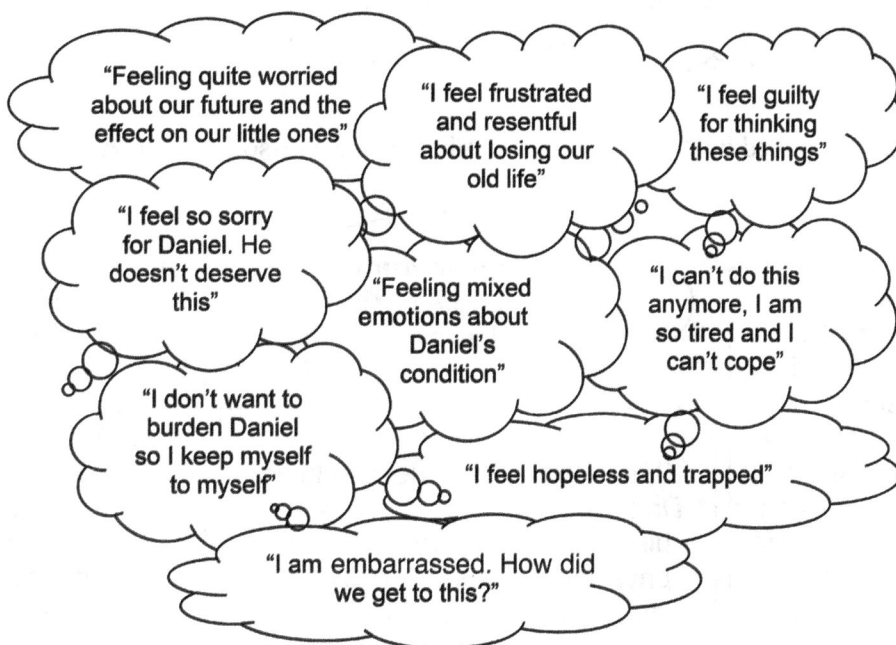

Figure 2.11 Kayleigh's thoughts and feelings about Daniel's symptoms.

Daniel and his family had 'no clue' where the seizures came from and were unable to identify any triggers. Each time, the episodes would start off in the same way (see Figure 2.12).

A typical dissociative seizure could last for seconds to minutes or go on for hours. After those 'heavy-duty' seizures, Daniel would feel wiped out and would spend days, sometimes weeks, mostly in bed 'in recovery mode' until he felt a bit better again – but never the same as his previous baseline, long before he developed the symptoms of FND. During particularly tough episodes, Daniel would end up hurting himself by accident, and he would often forget what had happened. He sustained bruises and cuts on occasion. As you can see in Figure 2.13, different people reacted in different ways to the dissociative seizures.

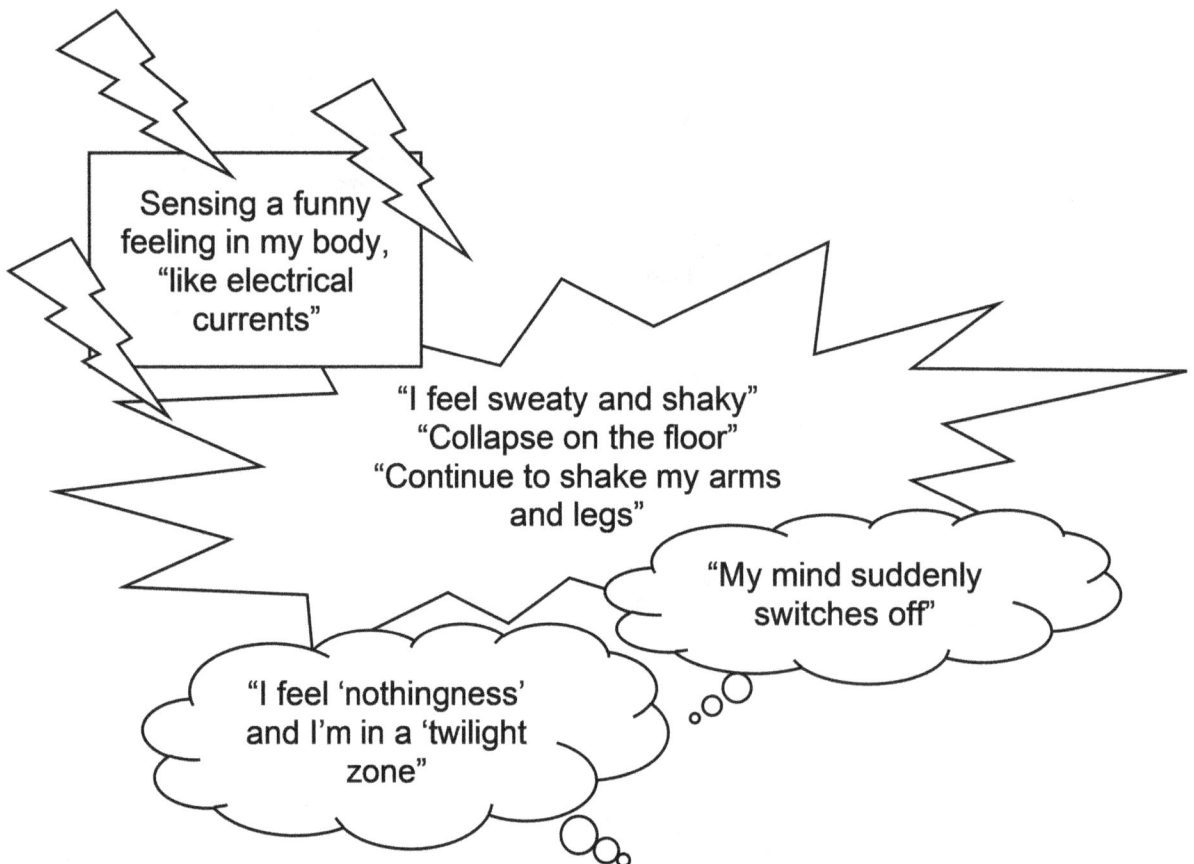

Figure 2.12 What happened in Daniel's body and mind during a dissociative seizure.

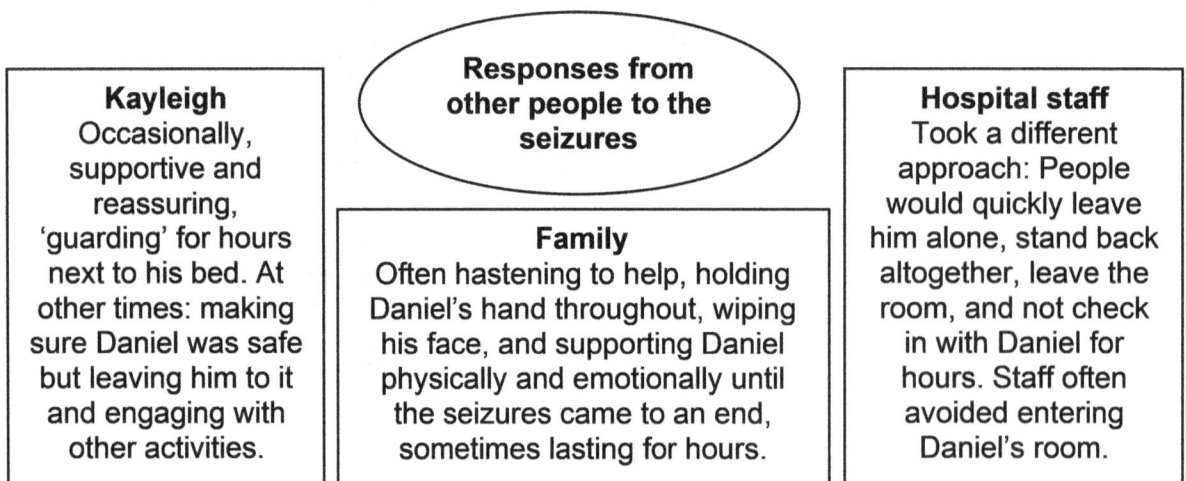

Figure 2.13 The variety of responses from people to Daniel's dissociative seizures.

As you can see, people's responses to the seizures vastly differed! This was problematic for various reasons:

- Some responses can help manage seizures in the short term but almost always prolong seizures in the long run.
- Contradictory responses (e.g. simultaneous reassurance but avoidance by different people) can make it difficult to reduce the seizures in the future.
- There was no 'captain steering the ship'. The variety of responses was confusing for Daniel and anyone close to him: everybody was doing something different, and nothing had been working so far.
- Adverse effects on Daniel: missing out on chunks of his rehabilitation, risks to his safety and psychological well-being, as well as reduced quality time with his family, as this was often spent on managing seizures.
- Adverse effects on his family and friends: some people started to avoid Daniel, became tired, were unable to do their own activities, and felt hopeless or frustrated about the situation.

None of the responses were fully 100% helpful in Daniel's situation, but each had useful elements in them. In the end, a seizure management plan is *always* based on a firm neuropsychological formulation that is not 'one-size-fits-all' but individually tailored to the person's and the environment's unique characteristics and FND symptoms. It is handy to have a 'template' ready that can guide you, and this is something that you will learn to do with the Pressure Cooker Model (as the template) throughout this book.

The responses from Daniel's environment tended to be on the extreme ends of care: either 'enmeshed and too much' or 'distant and too little'. Again, there is no blanket rule on seizure guidelines, as this should always be based on a neuropsychological formulation, but for Daniel's situation, you will learn that the middle response was probably the more helpful one.

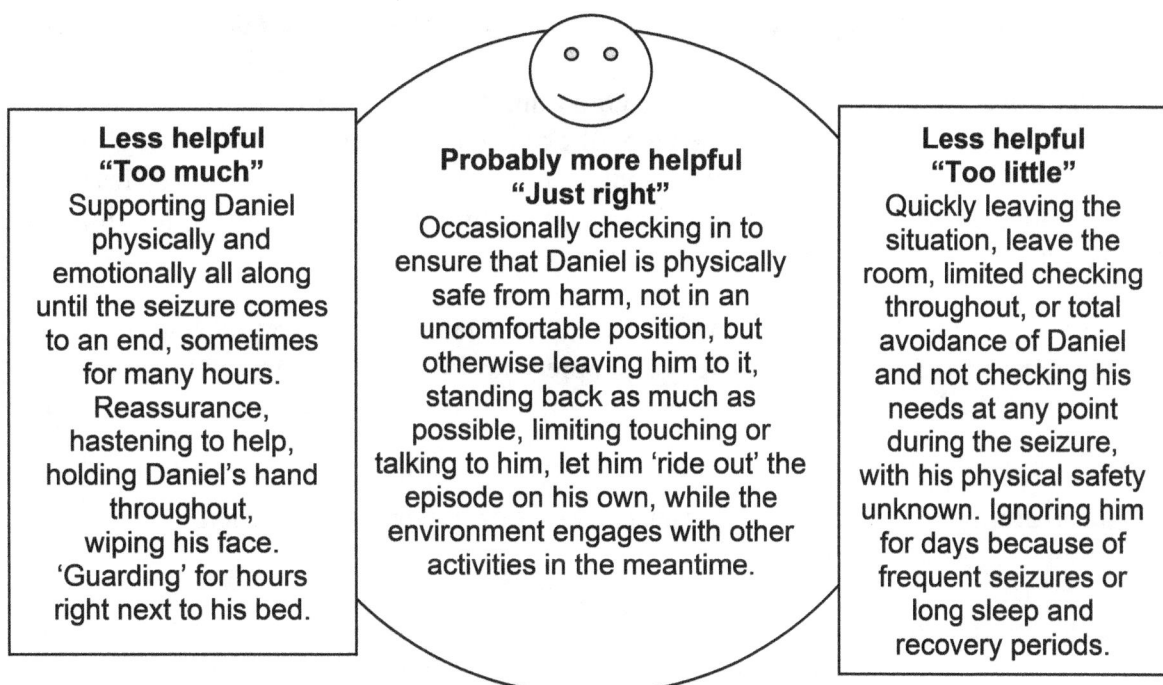

Less helpful "Too much"
Supporting Daniel physically and emotionally all along until the seizure comes to an end, sometimes for many hours. Reassurance, hastening to help, holding Daniel's hand throughout, wiping his face. 'Guarding' for hours right next to his bed.

Probably more helpful "Just right"
Occasionally checking in to ensure that Daniel is physically safe from harm, not in an uncomfortable position, but otherwise leaving him to it, standing back as much as possible, limiting touching or talking to him, let him 'ride out' the episode on his own, while the environment engages with other activities in the meantime.

Less helpful "Too little"
Quickly leaving the situation, leave the room, limited checking throughout, or total avoidance of Daniel and not checking his needs at any point during the seizure, with his physical safety unknown. Ignoring him for days because of frequent seizures or long sleep and recovery periods.

Figure 2.14 Three types of responding to dissociative seizures.

A mixture of emotions was felt by the people around Daniel

- **Anxiety, fear, fright, and shock** – about witnessing the seizure unfolding and not being able to control or manage the seizure.
- **Empathy, compassion, and feeling sorry** – about Daniel feeling unwell and suffering.
- **Embarrassment** – for how the seizure looks, what other people may think, and wanting to put a stop to it as quickly as possible (think about seizures that may happen in public places, where crowds can quickly form).
- **Anger and frustration** – about the seizure management taking up time, resources and effort that cannot be spend on other people or activities.
- **Sadness** – in relation to Daniel feeling unwell/missing opportunities and wanting him to be better as quickly as possible.

Daniel tried everything to stop the seizures, but the strategies proved ineffective

- **Distraction** and **reality grounding techniques**. For example, listening to his favourite songs, counting all the colours that he could spot in a picture, working a puzzle, smelling a scent.
- Listening to **relaxation** and **breathing exercises** via his earphones.
- Trying **relaxation exercises** with another person.
- Doing a **light physical exercise** to try to stop a seizure in its tracks before it developed into something bigger.
- Holding a **squeeze ball** or using **elastic bands**.

Daniel and his family felt at a loss. Things felt totally out of their control, and they expressed concerns about Daniel's future. Was he going to be like this forever? There were many reasons these psychological strategies did not work well for Daniel:

- Daniel was feeling too unwell and overwhelmed to have a good go at actively practicing the strategies. Just like building physical muscles in the gym, growing 'mental muscles' needs time, effort, and a clear mind to learn and practice the principles.
- The strategies were too superficial to meet Daniel's deeper needs and address the roots of his psychological issues.
- None 'hit the core' of Daniel's problems. One thing that stood out from the list of strategies was the individual focus: the strategies are all exclusively geared towards 'fixing' something internally in Daniel's mind and body – applied by Daniel himself. As you will learn later in Daniel's story, most of the reasons for 'treatment failure' had something to do with Daniel's social environment.

Before exploring these 'social' factors in more detail later, let us first take a closer look at one of the most common characteristics of people with FND in therapy (often, this applies to their families too, since coping strategies tend to be shared or passed on from generation to generation):

- A reduced ability to experience and describe emotions in words (also called 'dissociation' and 'alexithymia', respectively).

How did the psychological sessions go for Daniel?   Attempts at meeting with Daniel for psychology sessions were sometimes unsuccessful. He was either asleep or could only tolerate very brief sessions, around a maximum of 15 minutes, before expressing that he wanted to leave or experiencing FND symptoms that stopped any further meaningful therapy. Speech problems were a barrier that prevented Daniel from speaking about any difficult thoughts and feelings, which he did not feel were applicable to him – he could not remember a time that he felt low in mood or fearful. Writing was a problem due to his arm weakness. Even if he managed to hold a pen, the writing process was uncoordinated and characterised by Daniel writing letters that were hardly readable. Sometimes, Daniel experienced a dissociative seizure in the session.

Cognitive-behavioural therapy did not go smoothly   A traditional CBT model was initially used as part of Daniel's psychological therapy. Even during moments of relative calm and manageable FND symptoms, the CBT model was difficult to apply to Daniel's problems, and he did not engage well with the model. Earlier CBT, from years ago, had not worked, and this was not surprising: CBT models require a person to have 'emotion language'.

However, Daniel experienced quite the opposite: he demonstrated great difficulty putting his emotional experiences into words. Daniel did not have the emotional language available to express his emotions and would often refer to emotions using physical symptoms ('My chest hurts' whilst appearing visibly anxious). Although his symptoms fit in the 'hot cross bun' (see Figure 2.15, which follows) that is often used in psychological therapy, it was hard to see how all of Daniel's thoughts, feelings, behaviours, and physical symptoms connected and formed a 'story'; they did not seem to link up in one coherent narrative for Daniel and the psychologist to make sense of. How could all this end up in Daniel's experience of FND?

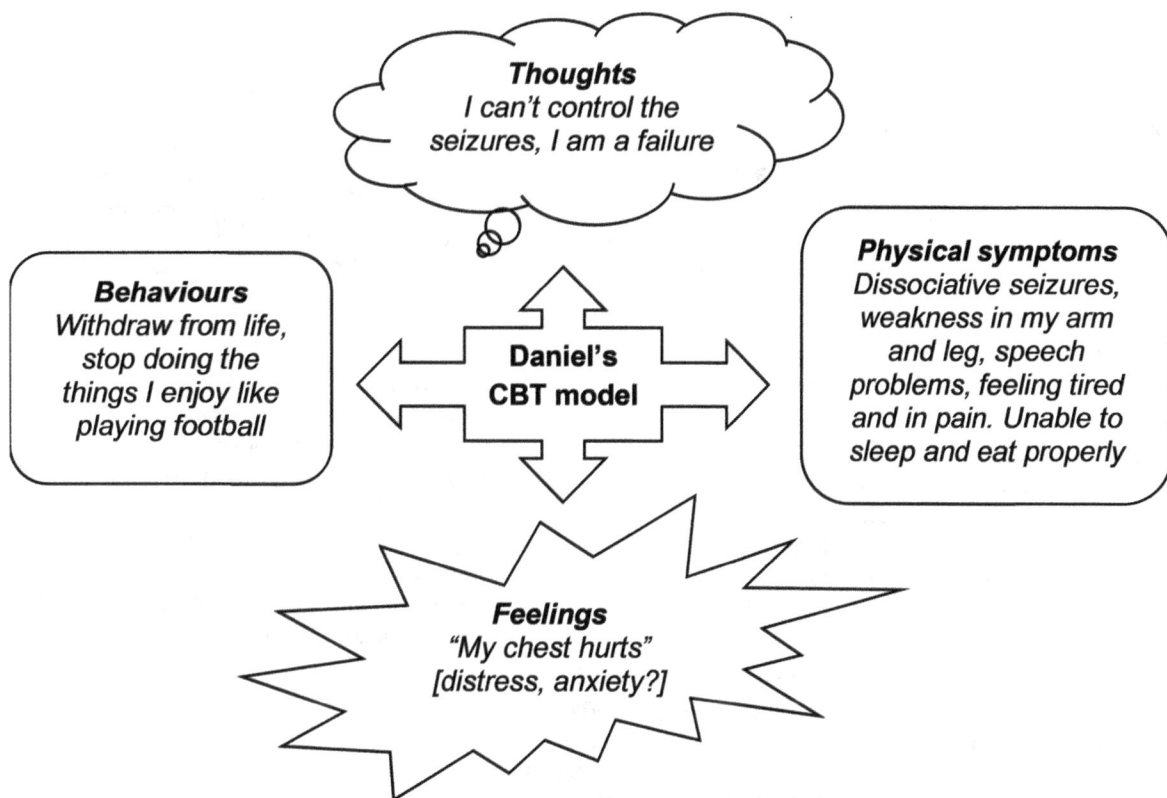

Figure 2.15 The hot cross bun model of CBT ('Daniel's story of FND').

Daniel's prior healthcare experiences were terrible

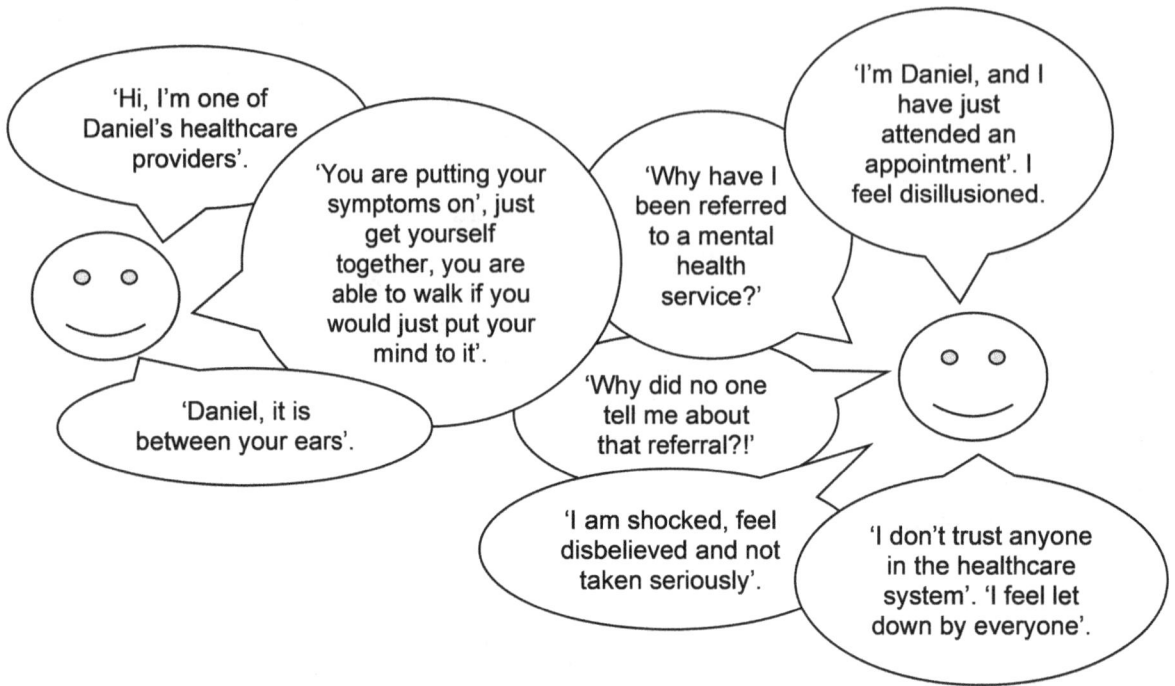

Figure 2.16 Daniel's unpleasant healthcare experiences.

Daniel is making minimal progress across other disciplines

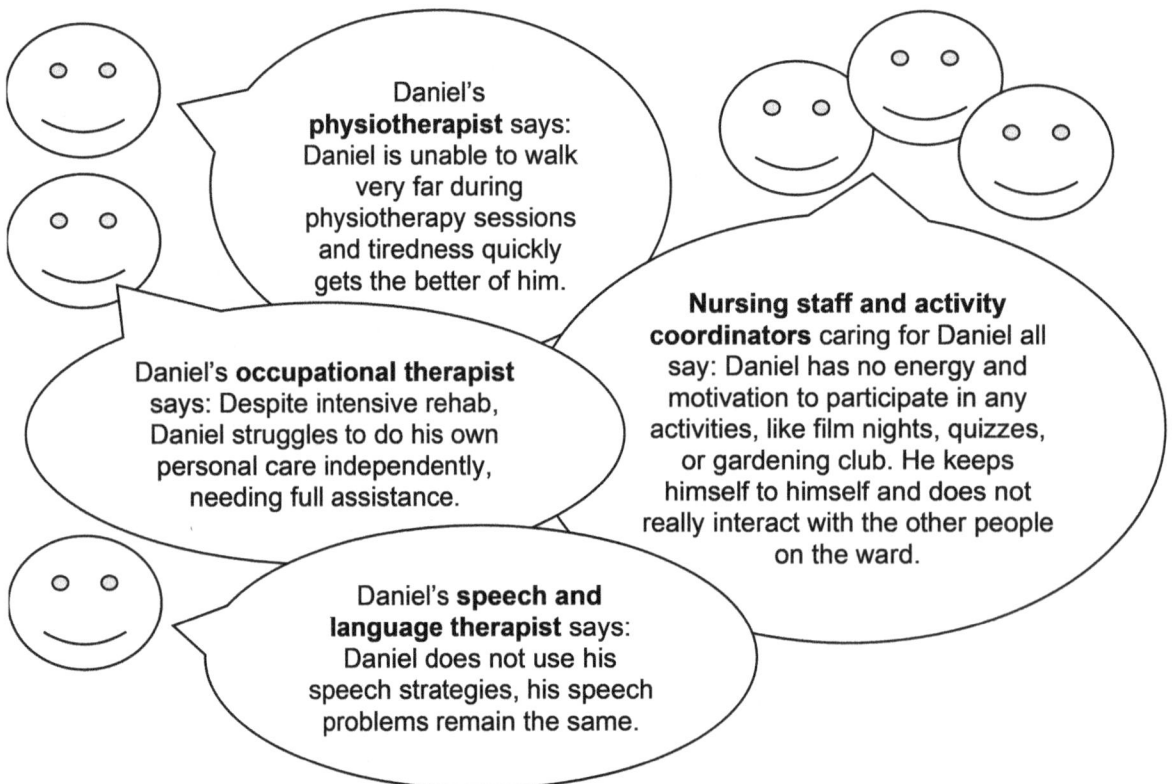

Figure 2.17 Daniel's multidisciplinary team: comments about Daniel's progress.

The team feels at a loss

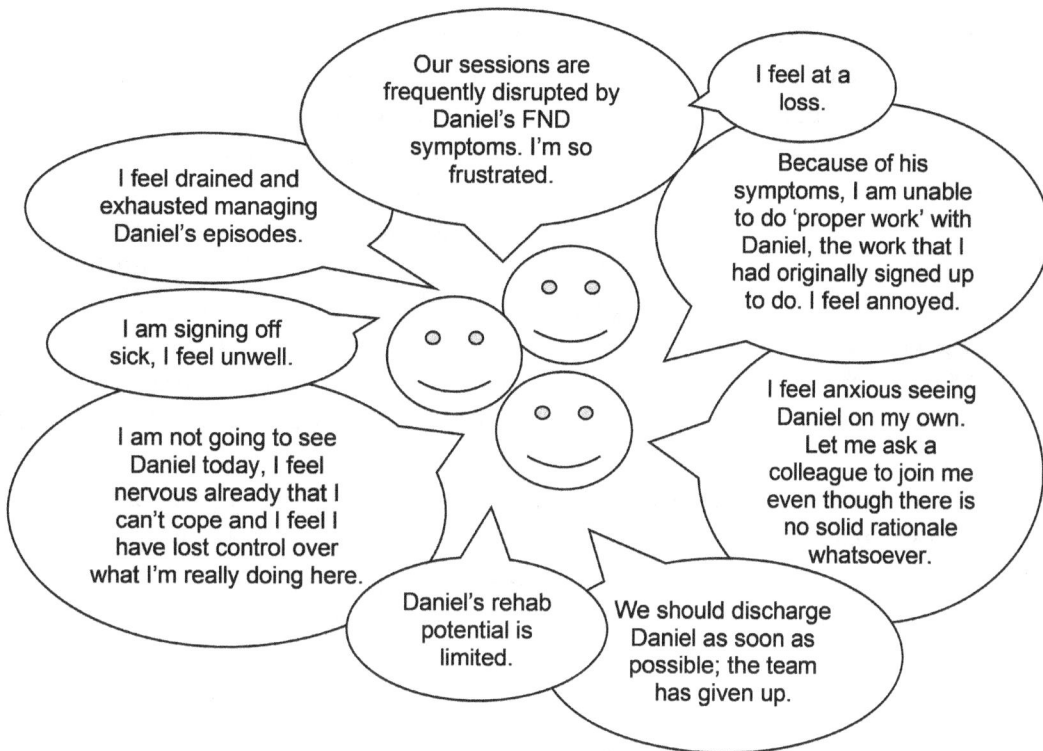

Figure 2.18 Daniel's multidisciplinary team: beliefs, emotions, and responses.

A RADICAL CHANGE IN WORKING: INTRODUCING THE PRESSURE COOKER MODEL

Where to go next in Daniel's treatment? Daniel's team gathered to think more deeply about the team's beliefs, emotions, and responses (see Figure 2.18). A big question that popped up was: 'Where was the collaboration in Daniel's treatment?'

'Something' (the treatment) was being done to Daniel in a '**one-way street**' manner as opposed to developing a 'two-way street' collaboration. Admittedly, Daniel found it hard to communicate his needs, wishes, and preferences to the team, due to the FND symptoms standing in the way, but the team struggled to actively take into account Daniel's 'voice' and put measures in place to make the working relationship more reciprocal. In addition, Daniel was often 'babied': any tasks, demands, chores, and responsibilities were taken out of his hands. Although everyone agreed that reducing the seizures as quickly as possible was a top priority, no one had bothered to check with Daniel's views on the seizures and his personal wishes for treatment.

A radical change in thinking   Maybe it was time for a radical change in approach towards Daniel's difficulties? A temporary Pause button was pressed on the CBT model. Instead, the Pressure Cooker Model was introduced as a means to facilitate Daniel's initial engagement with a different way of thinking about the FND.

Daniel's first step: exploring the Pressure Cooker Model together   Daniel and his family expressed a great deal of confusion about FND and struggled to get to grips with the mechanisms of FND. Therefore, the first goal was to increase Daniel's insight into FND without specifically referring to his own situation.

'**What are the mechanics of FND?**' The Pressure Cooker Model, with its elements, was shared with Daniel – without any pressure to add details from his own personal experience on the sheet. Initial sessions simply focused on exploring the various elements and talking about the mechanics of FND without focusing on Daniel's own situation. The model showed Daniel the connection between emotions and FND, particularly in the presence of other, blocked channels for emotional expression (keeping the cover closed and a blocked valve). Daniel was asked: What happens when there is a lot of fuel, flames, and heat under the cooker but the cover is tightly sealed and the valve is blocked? He correctly responded that the cooker was going to explode if it did not quickly find a different channel to release the boiling steam (the tiny overpressure plug representing the FND).

'Shall we take a look at how the Pressure Cooker Model might look like in other people with FND?' The next stage involved 'externalising the problem', which meant that Daniel applied the Pressure Cooker Model on another person with FND for him to see how the mechanisms work and how FND can emerge in other people. He was given a story of a person with FND with similar symptoms and asked to complete the model with support of the psychologist. After completion of the Pressure Cooker Model, Daniel was asked about his views on the 'pressure points' for this person. This helped Daniel familiarise himself with the model.

'What did your Pressure Cooker Model look like when you felt at your happiest?' Daniel was asked to think back about a time when he felt happy. He subsequently practiced completing a Pressure Cooker Model for himself during a time of happiness in his life and no FND symptoms, more than five years ago. This helped Daniel check out the things he did that he was not doing now.

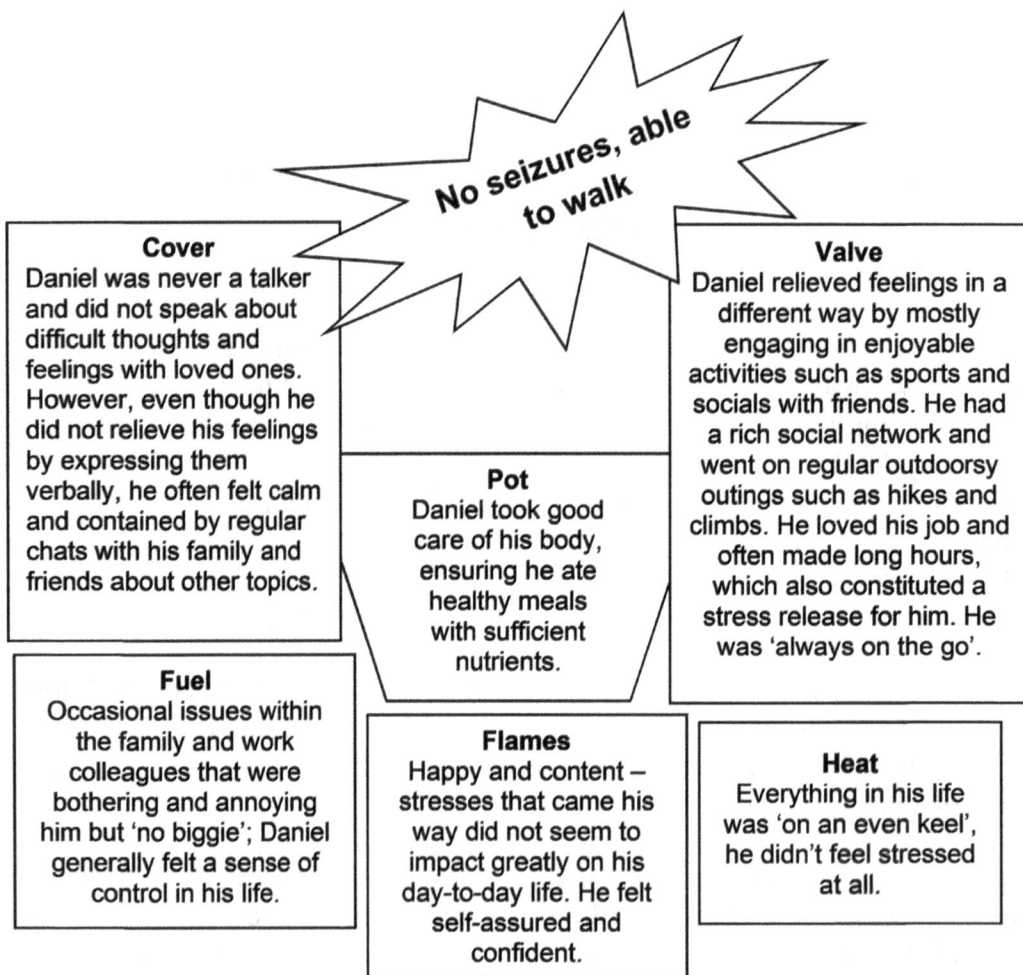

No seizures, able to walk

Cover
Daniel was never a talker and did not speak about difficult thoughts and feelings with loved ones. However, even though he did not relieve his feelings by expressing them verbally, he often felt calm and contained by regular chats with his family and friends about other topics.

Valve
Daniel relieved feelings in a different way by mostly engaging in enjoyable activities such as sports and socials with friends. He had a rich social network and went on regular outdoorsy outings such as hikes and climbs. He loved his job and often made long hours, which also constituted a stress release for him. He was 'always on the go'.

Pot
Daniel took good care of his body, ensuring he ate healthy meals with sufficient nutrients.

Fuel
Occasional issues within the family and work colleagues that were bothering and annoying him but 'no biggie'; Daniel generally felt a sense of control in his life.

Flames
Happy and content – stresses that came his way did not seem to impact greatly on his day-to-day life. He felt self-assured and confident.

Heat
Everything in his life was 'on an even keel', he didn't feel stressed at all.

Figure 2.19 Daniel's Pressure Cooker Model of happiness.

'What needs to be changed to feel better from FND?' Daniel analysed what bits may need to be changed for the FND to go away – not necessarily referring to Daniel's own situation in the first place, but just generally: look at the Pressure Cooker Model and consider what bits may need changing in order to feel better from FND. What parts on the pot need opening and unblocking? Daniel pointed to the top parts of the pressure cooker: although this was exactly the thing that he was the most uncomfortable with, he acknowledged his pressing need to learn to speak about difficult thoughts and feelings (open the cover) and socially connect again (unblock the valve). *Without doing these things in the moment, he was only naming and acknowledging the problems without delving into specifics.*

In the beginning phases of this new slant towards therapy, Daniel was still struggling to speak and write. Initially, his sessions were kept very brief but regular to help Daniel learn to tolerate the presence of the psychologist without feeling the pressure of opening up. Despite his disabilities, he was able to make his needs sufficiently known and to communicate with the psychologist who helped complete the relevant sections in the model with him. One day, Daniel took a pen in his own hand and drew a cover element: it was not just tight – it was locked shut with dozens of padlocks. Both Daniel and the psychologist knew that this was the start of a new bumpy journey.

2.4 eResource alert!

Check out the eResource to read about Daniel's journey of learning more about dissociation with the psychologist. You can also jump ahead to Chapter 7.

Team Daniel: elements of the therapeutic relationship   Relationship and interpersonal triggers are very common in FND. Although it was not entirely clear at this point what was bothering Daniel exactly and driving the FND symptoms, his arrival on the ward showed that it was difficult to establish a relationship with him initially and that he struggled to engage and connect with anyone. That was a clue towards suspecting that perhaps something relational or traumatic was going on for Daniel that deserved attention. Furthermore, as you will learn later, Daniel had a history of long-standing rejection since early childhood. If Daniel would not be aware of the difference between therapeutic and personal relationships, then the psychologist placing strong boundaries might be taken as rejection by Daniel, and that would impact negatively on the therapeutic relationship.

2.5 eResource alert!

It is not always easy to distinguish a therapeutic from a personal relationship, like a family bond or a friendship. Read and learn about the important differences between a therapeutic and a personal relationship.

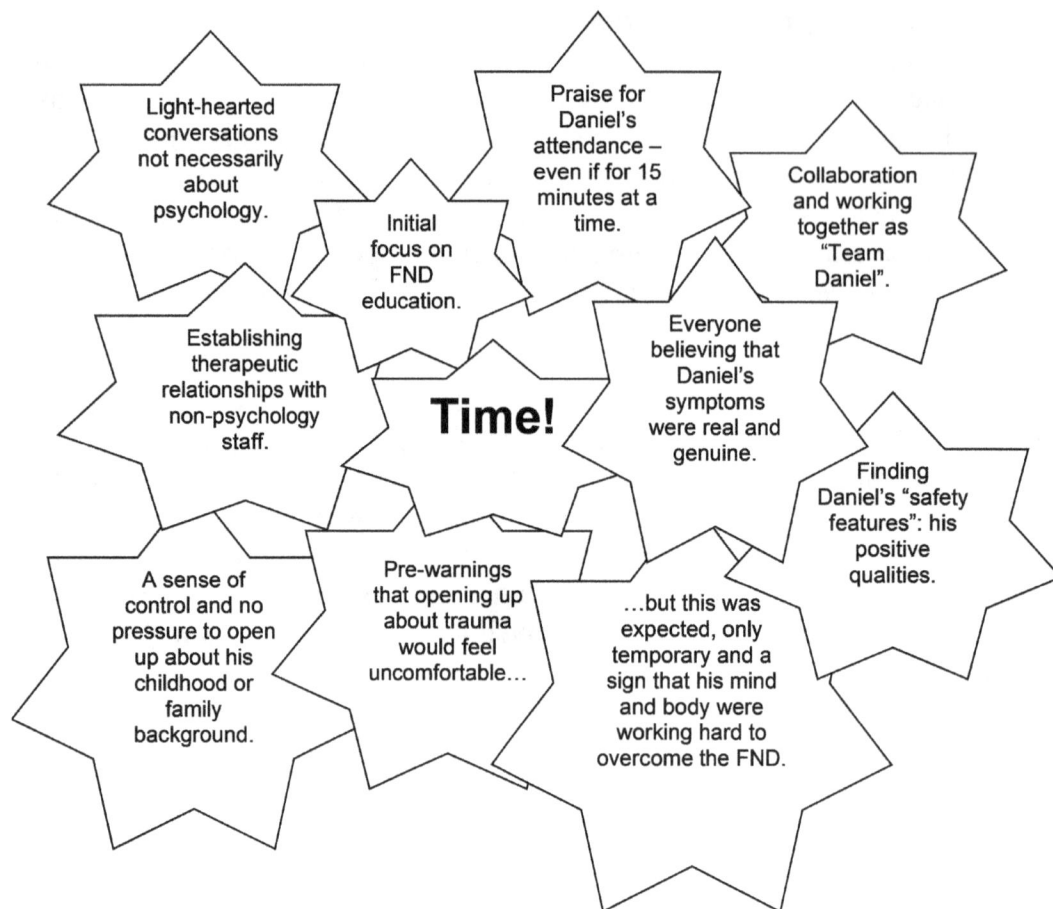

Figure 2.20 'Star ingredients' for building a strong therapeutic relationship between Daniel and his psychologist.

DANIEL'S PRESSURE COOKER STORY: OPENING THE PADLOCKS

Daniel was carrying around a heavy load of personal and traumatic experiences and memories that weighed deeply on him but that he was not expressing ('padlocks').

Even though everybody close to him knew Daniel was struggling with these secrets and Daniel knew that his loved ones and some staff knew, this did not relieve his distress and symptoms in any way. It was as if he carried the padlocks with him without having access to the code to open each one of them. Not knowing the code ('not knowing how to express emotions in relation to the difficult memories safely') was the difficulty, rather than the mere existence of these padlocks ('memories'). Daniel needed to release these secrets on his own, but he worried about losing control, because he already felt so 'out of control'. Building the therapeutic relationship, with Daniel feeling sufficiently psychologically safe and in control, was going to be the key to opening the padlocks on the cover and overcoming the FND.

Daniel's Pressure Cooker Model formula was as follows:

keep opening up about how I feel (open my cover) + plan in sufficient enjoyable activities, keep my normal routine, as well as not overdo it (unblock/regulate my valve) = I will be able to reduce the risk of FND (my mind and body not needing to use the overpressure plug)

Now, sceptics may say, 'Maybe Daniel was starting to get used to the staff and naturally getting better'. But Daniel made it clear during a team meeting that, in his view, it was psychology that contributed the most to his breakthrough. Read more about Daniel and Kayleigh's journey of FND in Chapter 10.

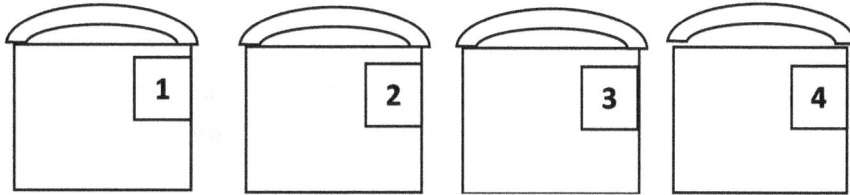

Figure 2.21 Daniel's tightly shut padlocks.

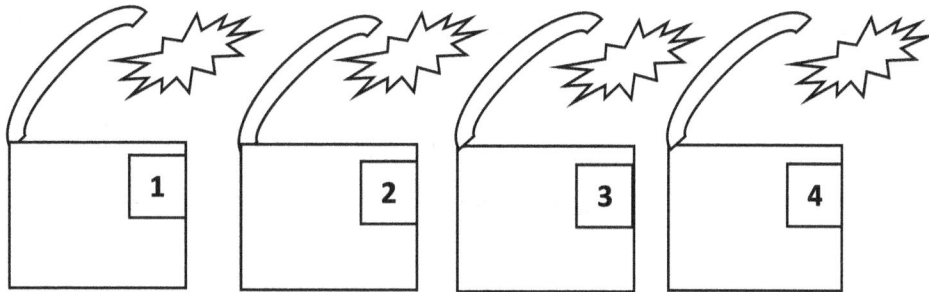

Figure 2.22 Daniel's opened-up padlocks.

THE PRESSURE COOKER MODEL AS A GROUP THERAPY: KATE'S EUREKA MOMENT

Daniel's treatment results were very promising. Not only was the refined version of the Pressure Cooker Model suitable for 'one-to-one' work (just the person with FND with the psychologist), but the model also turned out to be great in group therapy settings too! With a few tweaks and adaptations, a new group therapy programme was developed. Although the group was focused on FND education and coping strategies, a group is never just about its 'contents'. Let us read about one of the group participants, Kate, next to highlight this point further.

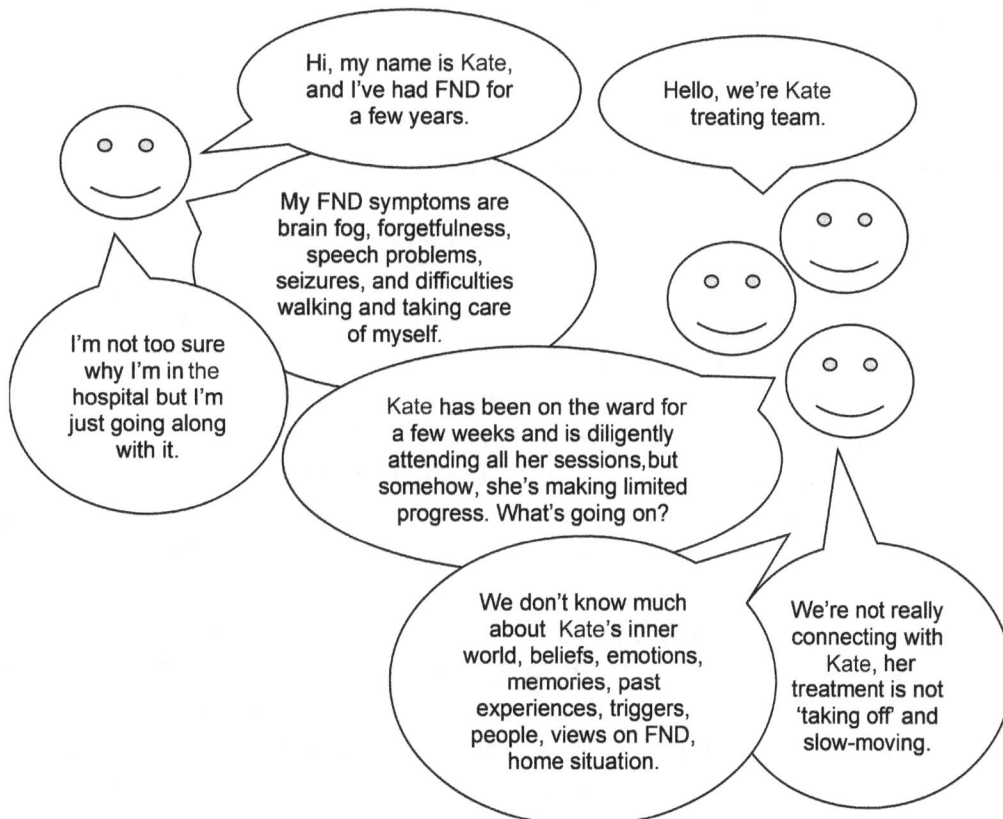

Figure 2.23 Introducing Kate's background story and her treating team.

Kate was subsequently invited to the Pressure Cooker Model group. Much to everyone's surprise, staff and patients alike, Kate became one of the most avid contributors to group discussions! The group process was pivotal in transforming Kate's mindset and helping her come out of her shell. Group therapy also had a 'knock-on' effect on Kate's individual therapy sessions. She felt psychologically safe to share memories and experiences that had long been bothering her. Kate flourished because she built new relationships with people around her who impacted positively on her self-esteem; she felt accepted and validated. In addition, she was particularly full of praise about the Pressure Cooker Model. Kate felt that the model was a powerful tool that helped her understand FND for the very first time as a coherent, meaningful story and that she had a new language to explain FND to other people.

THE PRESSURE COOKER MODEL AS A MULTIDISCIPLINARY APPROACH TO FND

But that was not all. Kate was in an inpatient setting that was characterised by a strong tradition of multidisciplinary team working – unlike other areas of the health service, where FND teams are often 'incomplete', with disciplines missing.

This was very different from the current situation Kate was in, where she had access to the full multidisciplinary team. Kate felt that all disciplines involved in her treatment came together in the Pressure Cooker Model, and this greatly helped her understand the rationale underlying her multidisciplinary treatment. Although each of the elements of the Pressure Cooker Model was associated with a psychological process, every element was also uniquely tied to a 'non-psychology' discipline. The Pressure Cooker Model is a 'biopsychosocial' model and consists of elements that represent the body, mind, and social processes – and not just emotions (see Figure 2.24).

Kate's new-found understanding of FND and her positive attitude towards the Pressure Cooker Model helped her make sense of her treatment in hospital and demonstrated its value for use in multidisciplinary settings. There are plenty of reasons that a multidisciplinary approach is important for the treatment of FND:

- As the Pressure Cooker Model shows, **FND is a biopsychosocial condition**. This means biological, psychological, and social aspects all play an important role in the maintenance of symptoms. The treatment should therefore also be biopsychosocial, or else, we would not address all aspects of FND!
- **FND is different for everyone.** There is a huge range of symptoms that people can present with. Some people may have more problems with walking, while others will have difficulties with losing awareness during a dissociative seizure but less so with moving around. It is therefore important that a team caters for all kinds of symptoms.
- There may sometimes be **roadblocks and bumps on the road** during the treatment journey. For example, a person having physiotherapy may struggle to progress their exercises due to anxiety. The psychologist can then jump in and support with strategies. Vice versa, a person may do well in psychological therapy but has not walked in a long while and perhaps developed deconditioning. The expert knowledge from a physiotherapist will be helpful in taking the first steps.
- As people make progress in one discipline, **'new problems' may appear** in another discipline that need solving. A common one is establishing a new routine. Getting better from FND also means changing your routine and 'starting a new life' with new meaningful activities and life pursuits. The occupational therapist will be incredibly helpful to support you with building a normal routine without booming and busting. Medications may also need changing and tweaking as people start to feel better.

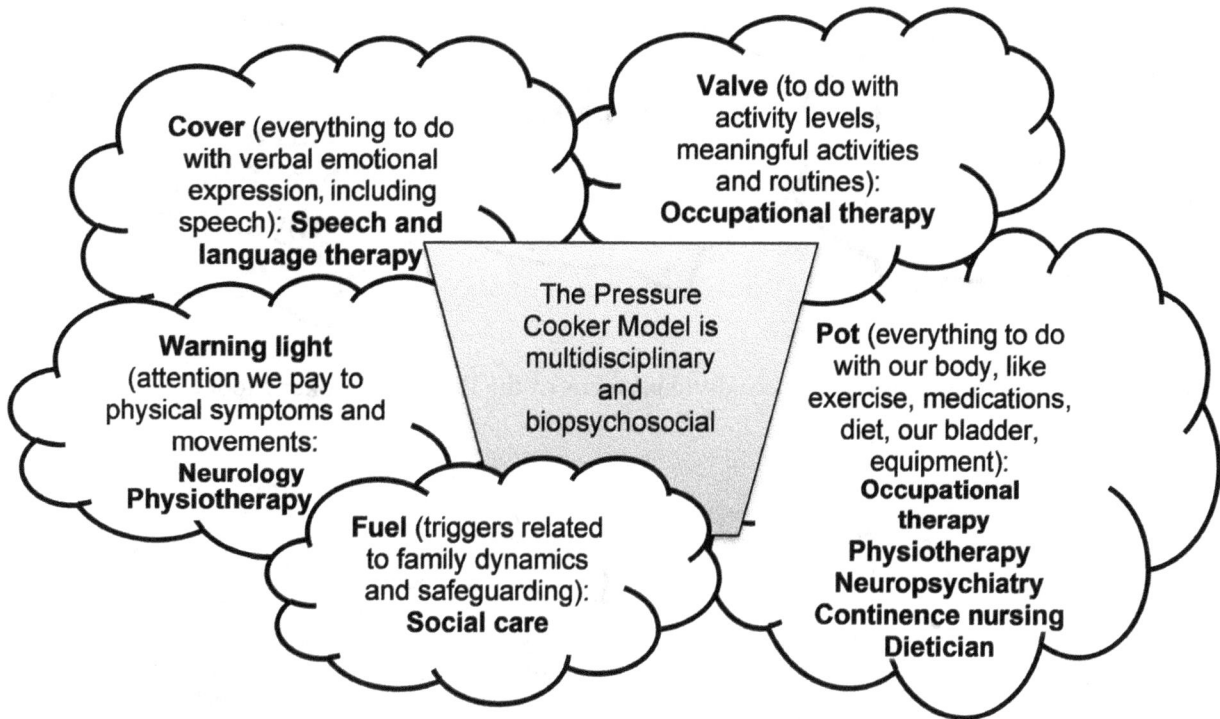

Figure 2.24 The Pressure Cooker Model: a biopsychosocial model of FND.

A WATERSHED MOMENT: THE POWERFUL EFFECTS OF SYSTEMIC RE-TRAUMATISATION

During a group therapy session, Steve, one of the participants with FND, appeared low in mood and disappointed. Steve was grappling with several tough questions (see Figure 2.25).

An awkward silence followed. Indeed, the way the group therapy had been structured strongly suggested that people with FND were viewed as the sole cause of their own problems and assumed to somehow have the power to sort this out by themselves, if they wanted to recover.

Steve's comments ignited a spontaneous discussion that was not planned and 'on the menu' for that session. Something about the emotional temperature in the room was telling everyone, 'This is extremely important, do not let go of this opportunity for a deep discussion'.

The group protocol was subsequently abandoned, and a therapeutic space was provided for people to share their healthcare experiences in a safe environment. Most experiences revolved around the time in the run-up to the FND diagnosis – 'The first time I was told I had FND' – and the immediate aftermath in the wake of the diagnosis. Invariably, people reported a whole range of negative experiences, beliefs, and emotions about past challenging interactions with healthcare professionals. Anger, frustration, sadness, and fear were most often described in relation to these interactions, in addition to high levels of confusion, which, technically speaking, is not an emotion but nevertheless important to mention here.

The common denominator themes that connect all these comments include themes around:

• Feeling rejected
• Feeling abandoned or being left to your own devices
• Not feeling cared for, feeling insignificant
• Not being believed or taken seriously
• Differential treatment, being singled out

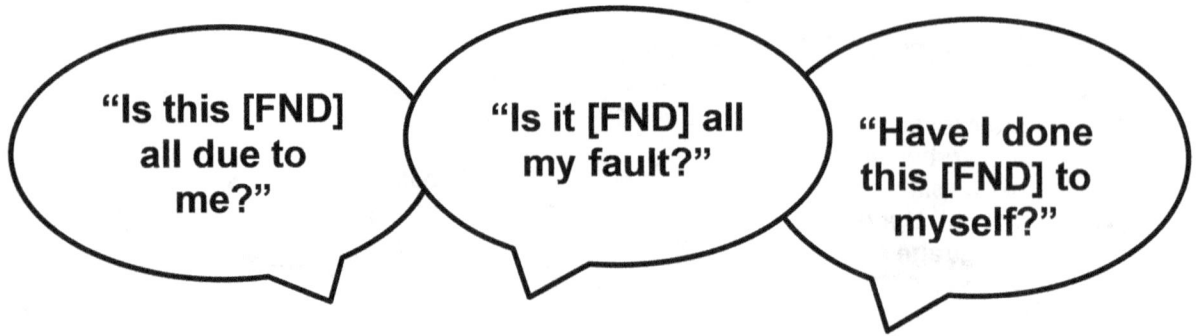

Figure 2.25 Steve's questions about the individual focus of the Pressure Cooker Model.

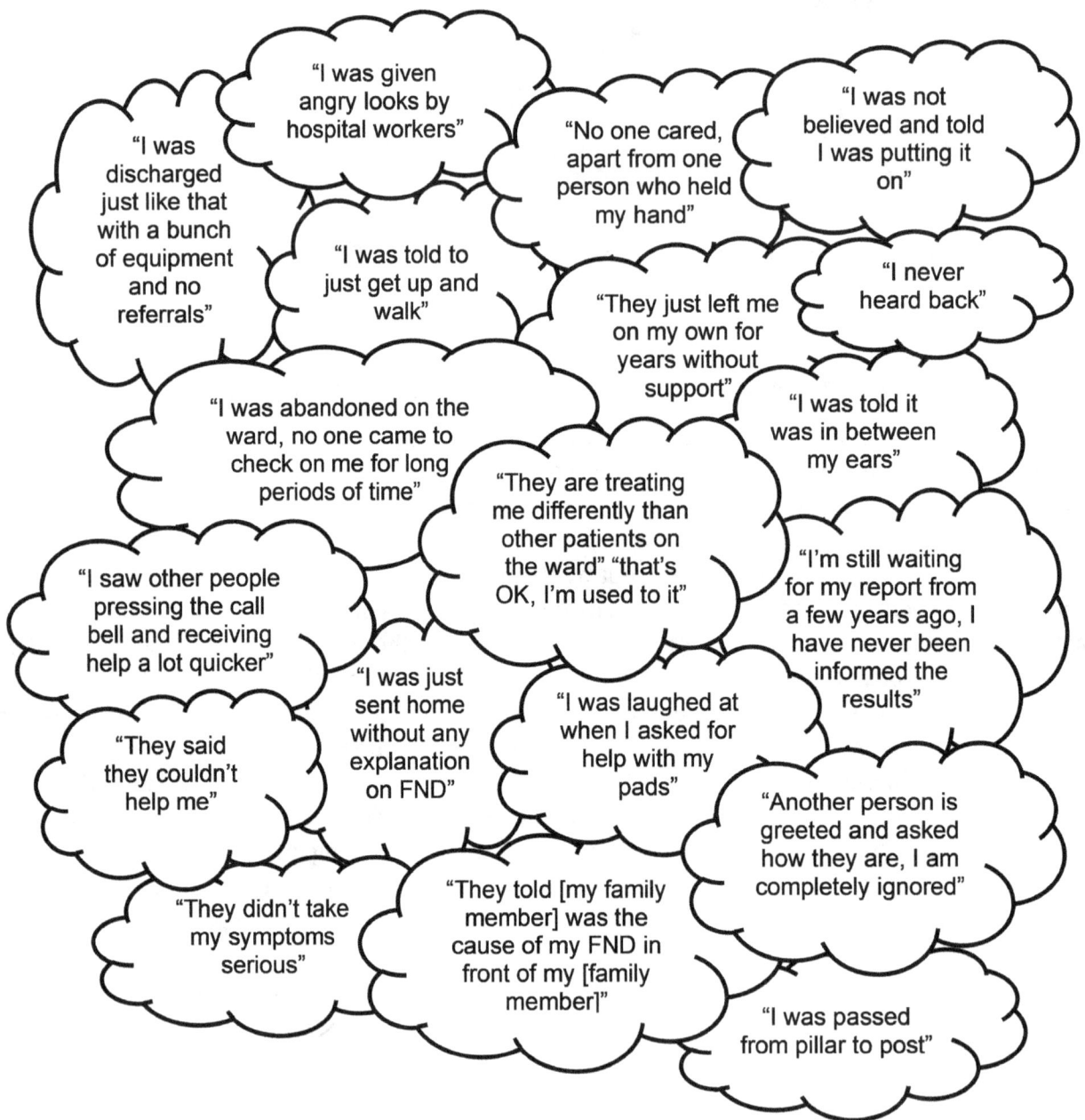

Figure 2.26 Adverse healthcare experiences reported by people with FND.

After this pivotal group session, it became clear that it was important for any clinician working in FND to be increasingly more attuned, sensitive, and aware of people's healthcare experiences – not just their experience of the FND itself.

- The **psychological hurt** that these healthcare experiences cause is already a sufficient reason for exploration.
- Knowing that FND is strongly connected to emotions, the **additional burden** that these negative healthcare experiences bring can make FND worse.
- These healthcare experiences can **affirm some of the negative beliefs and emotions** that people with FND already experience. If you have depression and hold depression-related beliefs about yourself ('I am less than others', 'I am different', 'People hurt you'), then these healthcare experiences dangerously provide 'the evidence' for those beliefs to be strengthened in a person who is trying to battle those beliefs.

However, there was more to the story.

- In a few people with FND, not feeling believed by a healthcare professional **mimicked their early rejection experiences in childhood**, particularly around parents not believing the child's pain, sickness, or fatigue, as well as parents not believing the child's report of abuse. On a less-conscious level, people's childhood emotions were re-triggered.
- Another subset of people had experienced an accident with relatively minor or no injuries. The accident was often linked to the FND that emerged soon after. However, some people reported negative or even a hostile treatment from healthcare professionals during their admission. It was not so much the accident itself **but rather the responses that made people feel upset, angry, sad, and rejected and contributed to the FND**. The responses from healthcare professionals resembled and retriggered earlier adverse life experiences.

The other side of the coin

But what about staff treating people with FND? What were they thinking and feeling? Could it be that people with FND were simply *perceiving* these healthcare interactions as negative rather than reflecting *reality*? After all, healthcare professionals are supposed to care, be compassionate, and not reject; that is why they often enter healthcare professions: to help people. Observations of staff working with people with FND lifted an interesting veil on this matter. Take a look at Figure 2.27.

As you can imagine, these behavioural responses from staff members can cause the following thoughts and feelings in people with FND:

- Feeling rejected
- Feeling abandoned or being left to your own devices
- Not feeling cared for, feeling insignificant
- Not being believed or taken seriously
- Differential treatment, being singled out

It is a scary idea to think that the previously discussed healthcare experiences from people with FND actually match up quite neatly with a few of the staff behaviours listed in Figure 2.27. It appears that difficult healthcare experiences are a full-blown reality for many people with FND.

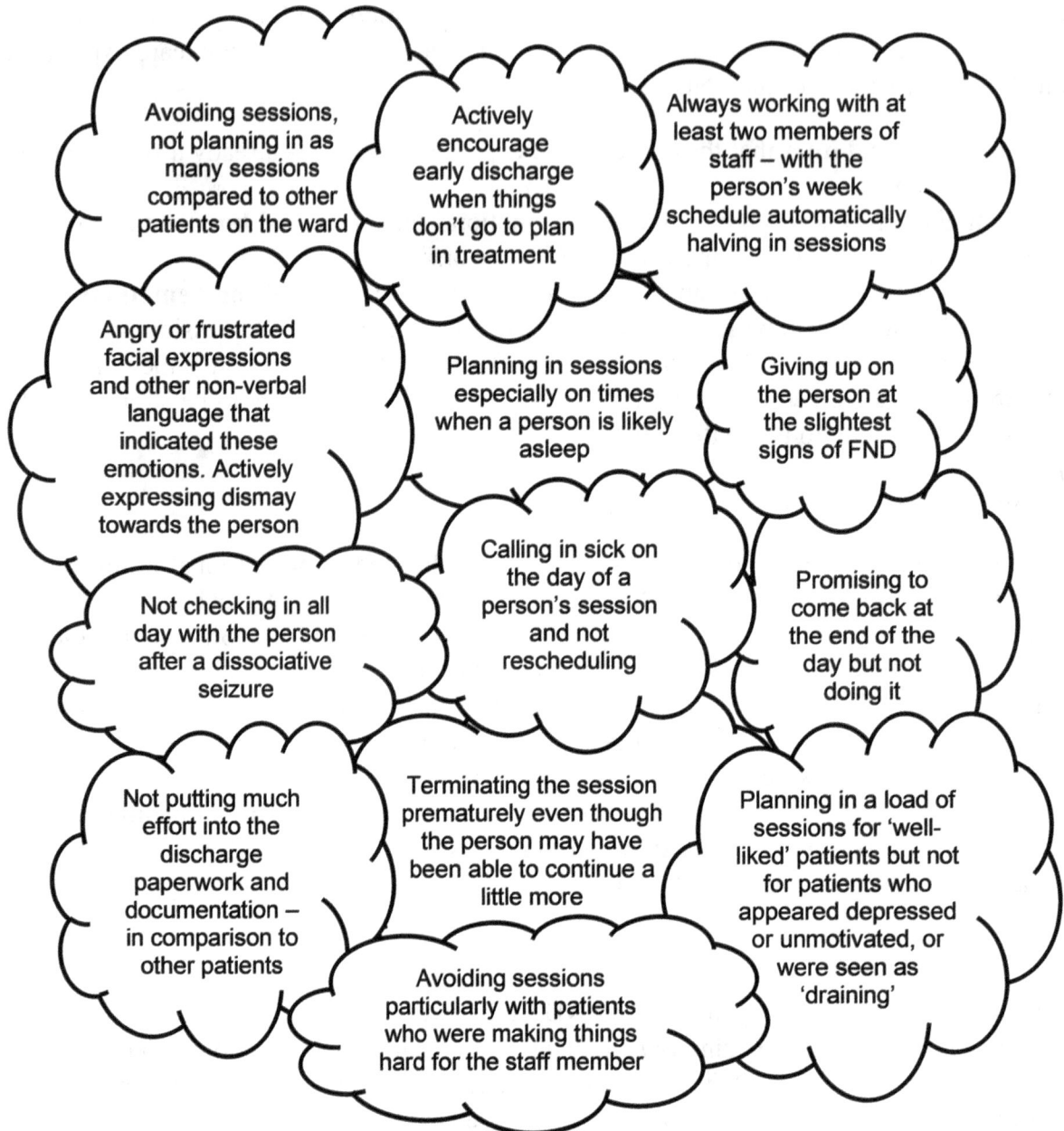

Figure 2.27 Observations of behavioural responses of staff to people with FND.

If you start thinking about what emotions may underlie these patient and staff experiences, we can conclude that these are pretty similar. Yes, that's right: both people with FND and healthcare workers who treat people with FND experience the same emotions during their interactions: anger, frustration, sadness, and fear. Emotions are intricately linked to thoughts (see Figure 2.28).

It seems that everybody who was part of these healthcare interactions was becoming 'triggered'– not just people with FND. **It was clearly a two-way street**. In Chapter 9, we will explore more of these 'mirror' themes and delve deeply into the concepts of 'reciprocal reinforcement' and 'systemic re-traumatisation'.

This increased awareness on interpersonal dynamics between the person with FND and staff members changed the format of psychological therapy on the ward. Therapy did not only focus on the FND, but in addition, these healthcare interactions were also explored in more detail and represented a good starting point in therapy. People with FND did not always feel convinced that bringing up staff interactions was relevant to their FND recovery (see Figure 2.29).

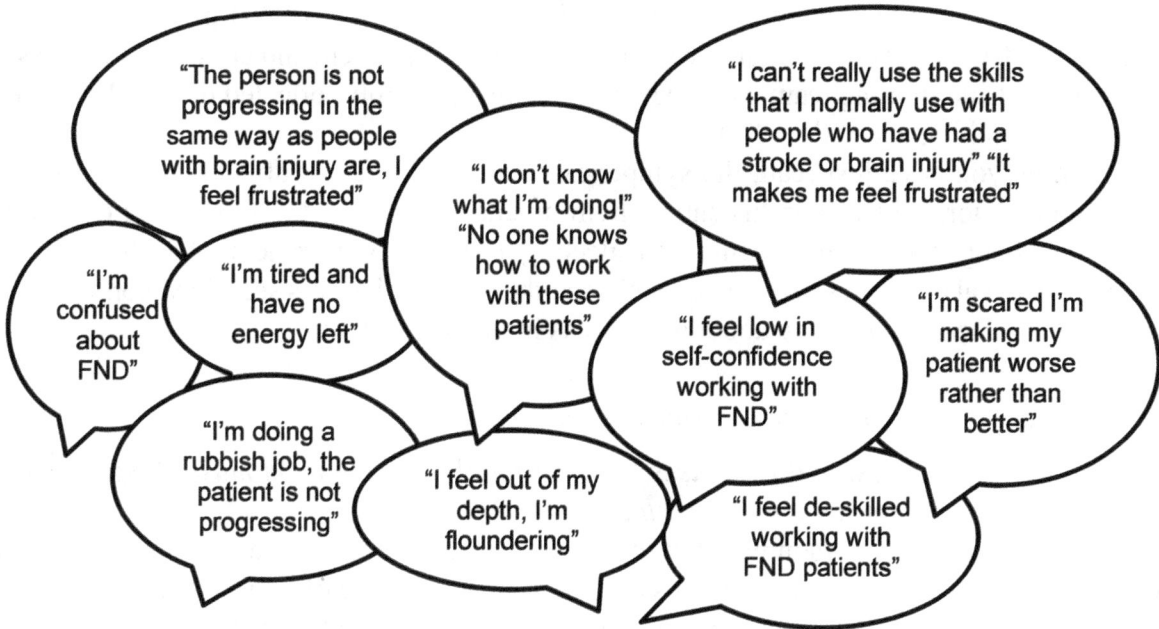

Figure 2.28 Thoughts reported by healthcare employees working with people with FND.

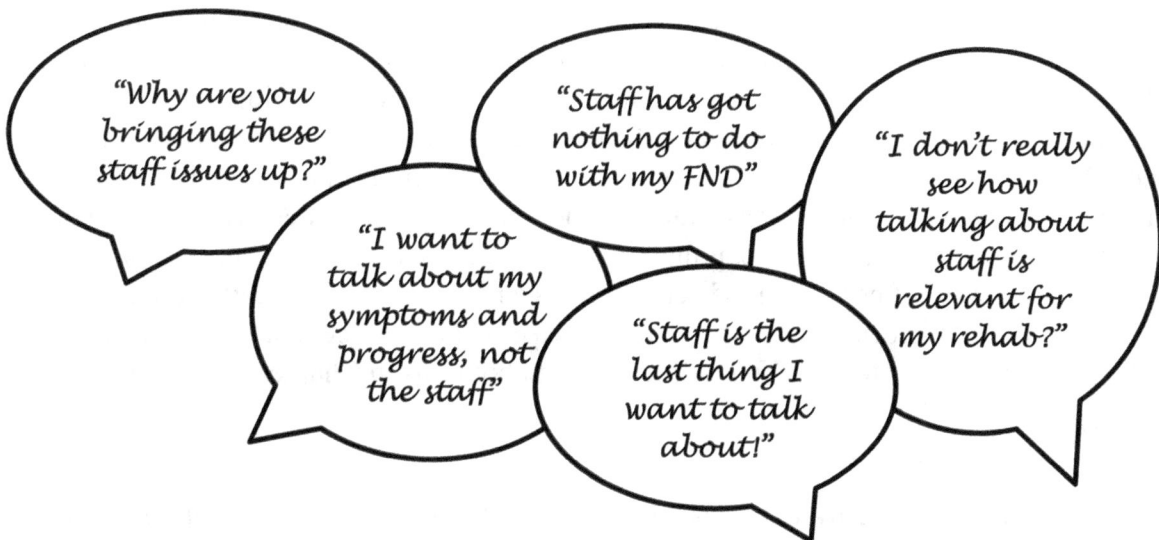

Figure 2.29 Questions and comments from people with FND when encouraging the discussion of current healthcare interactions.

However, after exploring these interactions in more detail, people often realised and acknowledged that interpersonal dynamics played an important role in the persistence of the FND symptoms. The development of increased insight into these interpersonal processes helped people uncover other areas of their lives that posed similar difficulties.

Phase 4: full version of the Pressure Cooker Model

Do you remember Daniel? Given what you have just read, a big question about Daniel's treatment is: 'Did the individual focus on Daniel's treatment do him any favours?'

The treatment seemed to be completely focused on **'Daniel and his FND problem'**. This was completely understandable. After all, the symptoms were quite severe and causing a lot of disruption. His family and treating team were exhausted, which probably reflected the level of severity and psychological impact of the FND.

However, as you have just read, the symptoms clearly did not just affect Daniel himself but equally had a major influence on his entire environment. Were we not missing a big opportunity for potential change and improvement by 'neglecting' Daniel's environment? Was there anything in the interpersonal dynamics between Daniel and other people that was somehow contributing to the FND? Let us learn a bit more about these ideas in the next section.

Pressure cooker principle #1: reciprocal reinforcement

*Could the **beliefs**, **feelings**, and **responses** from his family and the team make things worse for Daniel? Were these responses somehow related to the FND?*

Daniel was not the only person who felt that the symptoms were outside his control. One thing that became very apparent during Daniel's treatment was the sense of hopelessness and the high level of distress that the FND symptoms, without exception, generated in the people in his environment. It was as if Daniel's inner turmoil and high arousal levels were reflected in 'mirrors' around him: his environment was experiencing similar levels of internal discomfort.

Understandably, and well-intentioned, some people were trying to help and support Daniel emotionally and physically with a lot of reassurance, hoping that this would stop the seizure and his discomfort sooner rather than later, and help Daniel feel supported throughout a difficult time. Not only was the reassurance focused on helping Daniel, but reassuring him also simultaneously (and probably less consciously) helped people in his environment cope with their own discomfort and reduce their anxiety about witnessing the seizure and seeing Daniel in an unwell state. The sooner Daniel would 'get over' the seizure, the sooner his environment would 'get over' their own anxiety. However, people's reassurance responses also directly negatively impacted on the seizures by 'reinforcing' this as a coping strategy. Daniel missed out on many opportunities to learn alternative ways of coping with discomfort: his environment was already doing that for him. This interpersonal 'mirroring' process is called **'reciprocal reinforcement'** and is central to FND and the Pressure Cooker Model. You will learn a lot about this in Chapters 9 and 10.

Pressure cooker principle #2: systemic re-traumatisation

*Did Daniel's **prior healthcare experiences** impact, in any way, on progress in rehab? Were his current healthcare experiences doing any damage?*

Without a shadow of a doubt, Daniel's prior experiences with healthcare professionals left a mark on him and did not create much trust in the system. What was worse, members of his current team started to distance themselves from his care. This knocked Daniel's confidence, and he rightfully perceived this as a rejection. This is important for various reasons. If we think about the strong association between FND and emotions, then having more negative emotions added into the mix could make FND symptoms potentially worse. Furthermore, as you will come to learn later in Daniel's story, his childhood had been difficult and was characterised by rejection and invalidation from his parents. The responses from his current healthcare team had the potential to re-trigger Daniel's old hurts, adding more negative emotion, and therefore more FND. Hence, the answer to the preceding question is a resounding 'yes'. Learn more about this phenomenon called 'systemic re-traumatisation' in Chapter 9.

Pressure cooker principle #3: intermittent reinforcement

*What can we say about the **mixed responses** to the seizures that Daniel experienced?*

Kayleigh, Daniel's family, and his treating team provided a range of different responses to the seizures. Occasionally, the seizures were met with people's reassurance, while at other times, people avoided Daniel as much as possible. We could think of this situation as innocuous and not bearing much impact on the seizures. After all, it made sense that his environment was trying to figure out the best way to approach Daniel and manage the seizures. This would understandably come with 'trial and error'. However, this mixture of reassurance and avoidance of the seizures risked what is called an 'intermittent reinforcement' schedule (Wagner, 1961; Kendall, 1974). Providing occasional reassurance ('every once in a while' – by a subset of people in Daniel's environment) increased the chances that the seizures would happen more often and made it harder to overcome the seizures in the future. You will learn about intermittent reinforcement in more detail in Chapter 10.

THE LAUNCH OF A HYBRID MODEL OF FND

As you have just seen, (1) if the person with FND and the environment have strong and/or negative beliefs, emotions, behavioural patterns, and responses towards each other and (2) we know that FND and emotions are interconnected, (3) then it is reasonable to assume that the environment influences the person with FND, their emotions, and may play a vital role in keeping the FND going:

> What if FND is the result of an emotion-regulation problem between the person with FND and their environment, either partially or fully?

Emotion regulation in this context means the way that people cope with their own emotions by influencing each other's emotions, beliefs, and responses. This concept of emotion regulation will be revisited many times throughout this book. The important thing to remember is that, in relationships, a person with FND and their environment are influencing each other, and it is a two-way, not a one-way, street. If we assume that this is, indeed, the case in FND, shouldn't we also be thinking about treating the environment? Are we not missing a trick if we just leave the environment for what it is and completely focus on the person? These thoughts and questions led to a radical new way of thinking about FND:

- Unless the environment is also treated, a person with FND who is in treatment may not be able to fully achieve their potential in treatment and recover from the symptoms, or fully achieve their potential but may be at risk of keeping their gains only *temporarily, for a shorter period of time*, and perhaps lose some of these gains following discharge or later down the line, particularly when returning to the same environment that has not changed alongside the person.

Adopting this way of thinking had several far-reaching consequences for the Pressure Cooker Model, which was ready for the next exciting stage in its development. The central question asked was:

> Could the Pressure Cooker Model be tweaked in such a way that it would also be possible to use the model in people without FND, with a particular focus on partners, family members, and healthcare professionals?

This new-found awareness on the crucial influence of the environment on FND necessitated further changes to the Pressure Cooker Model; hence, two brand-new features were added to ensure that the model was equally applicable to the environment:

- **'The kitchen'**, representing the environment around the person with FND and consisting of all the pressure cookers of the individuals in the person's environment that are assumed to directly interact with each other.
- A new view on what the **overpressure plug** entails during the treatment of FND, representing a broader set of coping strategies that included FND, amongst other forms of coping.

TWEAKING THE OVERPRESSURE PLUG AND THE INABILITY TO TOLERATE DISTRESS: FINDING PSYCHOLOGICAL SAFETY

Psychological safety is an extremely important concept in the Pressure Cooker Model, both for people with and without FND:

- People with FND occasionally report a range of past strategies that quickly brought down distress, intense emotions, turmoil, discomfort, arousal, or any other unnamed unpleasant internal state.
- It is important to not only look at these strategies individually. Instead, explore the 'process' and 'go beyond contents'. Ask yourself the questions: **What ties these strategies together,** and what is the **underlying theme** that connects each one of them?

Figure 2.30 shows that each strategy helps the individual change from a state of 'psychological unsafety' to feeling 'psychological safety' and relief. For these reasons, coping strategies that restore psychological safety quickly and effectively are sometimes hard to let go off. Why would you if it helps you feel better in a short space of time?

Throughout the years, it became apparent that people with FND were not the only group using these coping strategies in day-to-day life to manage feelings! People without FND (family, partners, friends, and healthcare professionals) were equally at risk of using the strategies just mentioned, as well as a whole host of additional strategies (see Figure 2.31).

Of course, many of these responses are very well-intended and not always about the environment feeling anxious, stressed, or worried. The point is that people with and without FND

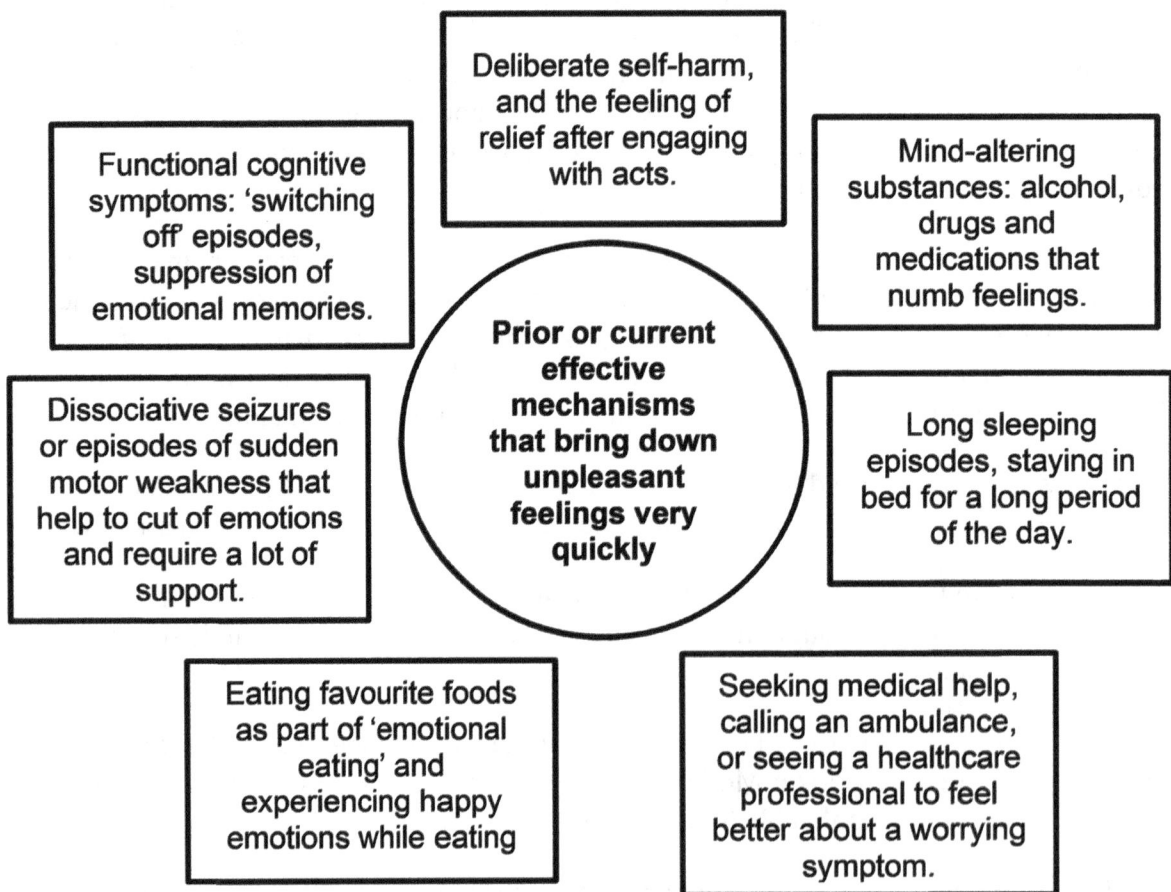

Figure 2.30 Understandable but unhelpful emotion coping strategies in some people with FND.

Verbal and physical reassurance during dissociative seizures, e.g. holding hands, staying close, calming the person, orienting the person to time and place.

Excessive caring, 'mollycoddling', walking the extra mile, dropping everything to accommodate the person as quickly as possible.

Or the opposite: **distancing** from the person, **avoidance** at all costs, passing the person on to another professional, stopping contact.

Taking activities out of the person's hands, 'baby-ing' Doing everything for the person, taking chores out of their hands, just in case they may get tired – but you feel reassured nothing bad will happen.

Effective mechanisms that bring down unpleasant feelings in the environment very quickly

Hypervigilance, lots of **supervision**, always making sure you're monitoring the person, overprotective behaviours, in case of a seizure or fall, and preventing them to hurt themselves.

Hours of searching on the internet, logging symptoms, ensuring that all avenues for help have been exhausted, making lots of appointments with healthcare professionals.

Strongly advocating for the person, accompanying the person to every health appointment, to feel more in control of a condition that can be quite unpredictable.

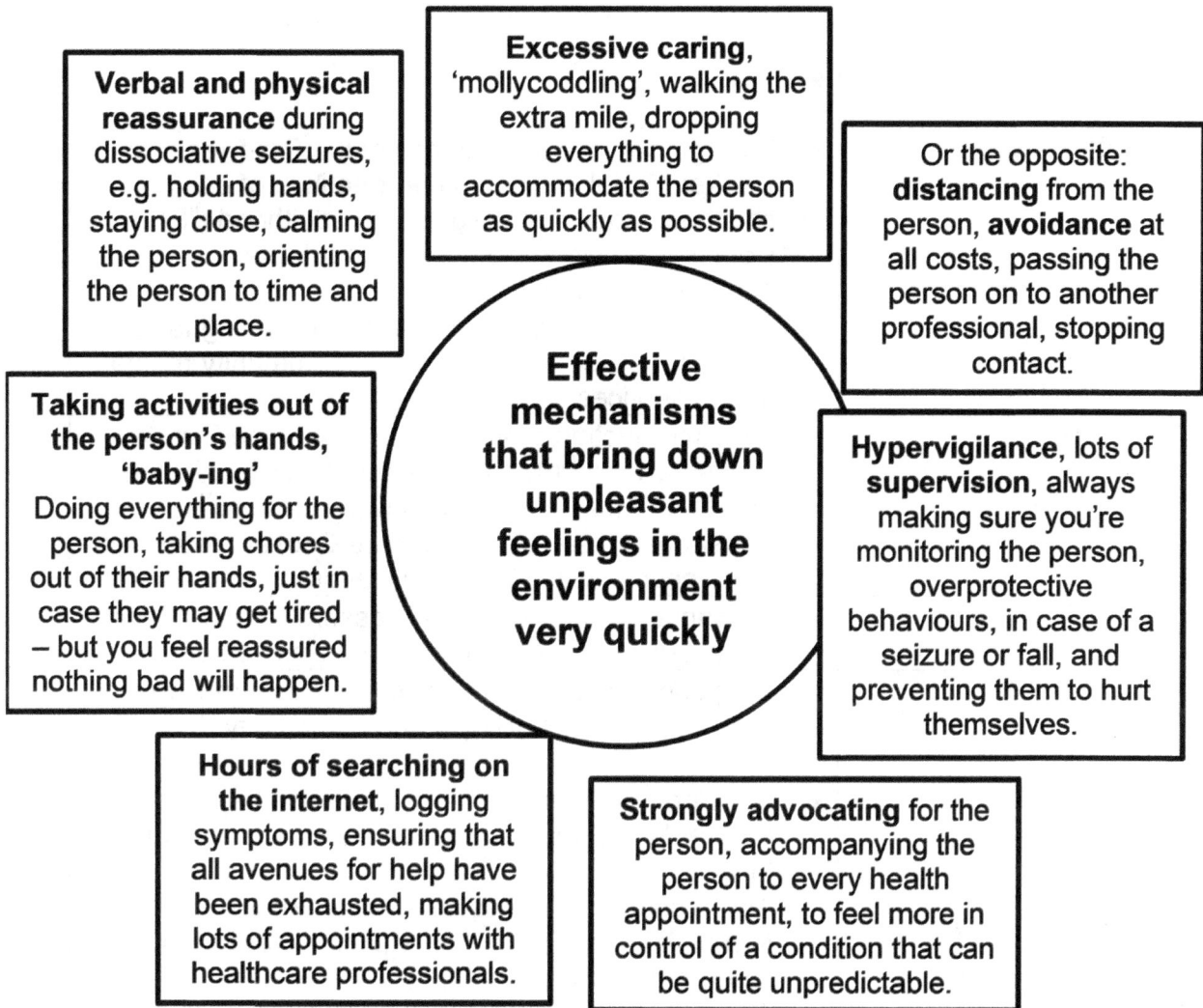

Figure 2.31 Understandable but unhelpful emotion coping strategies in people without FND.

frequently experience the same feelings of 'psychological unsafety' and attempt to reduce this discomfort by making use of effective and fast-acting mechanisms **to reach a state of 'interpersonal' safety.**

Key points on the Pressure Cooker Model timeline

Development of the Pressure Cooker Model: is it all done?

Today, the Pressure Cooker Model is a fully fledged model that is able to formulate the difficulties of the person with FND, people in their environment, as well as the interpersonal dynamics that emerge between all participants who are part of the FND story. As it stands, the Pressure Cooker Model, in its current form, is believed to be comprehensive, detailed, widely applicable to people with and without FND, and assumed to involve most of the factors important in the emergence and maintenance of FND symptoms.

Despite these advantages, the model's development is far from over. Theories take time to stew and brew. The Pressure Cooker Model, which has been developed for over a decade, is no exception. A newly launched model does not remain static and will certainly not be the finished product. The field of FND is exponentially growing, and new discoveries are made on a regular basis.

Table 2.1 Stages and key events throughout years of development of the Pressure Cooker Model

Time	Key events
2012– 2016	• Laying down the foundations of the Pre-Pressure Cooker Model, including the repetition of early childhood coping strategies into adulthood ("FND Coping Triangle") and the important role of relationships in FND. • Two presentations on FND and maintaining factors to clinical colleagues in different community mental health services.
2016	• First introduction of a basic version of the Simple Pressure Cooker Model to a person with FND in a one-to-one psychological therapy session. • Subsequent use of the Pressure Cooker Model with more people with FND in clinical practice.
2017	• Presentation of the Simple Pressure Cooker Model to trainee clinical psychology university students.
2017-2018	• Adapting the basic version of the Pressure Cooker Model for group therapy in the community (two cycles).
2018-2021	• Development of the refined version of the Pressure Cooker Model for use in people with and without FND. • Active sharing of Pressure Cooker Model formulations during multidisciplinary ward rounds in a neurorehabilitation setting. • Adapting the refined Pressure Cooker Model for a revised group therapy programme for delivery of three cycles (ward-based).
2019	• Presentation of the Pressure Cooker Model to clinical psychologists specialising in neuropsychology.
2019, 2020	• Further two presentations on the Pressure Cooker Model to multidisciplinary and nursing teams – psychology and non-psychology - of all levels, ranging from student, junior to senior.
2023	• Finalised and fully-fledged Pressure Cooker Model.

With time, more clinical observations, as well as an increasing amount of scientific research, the Pressure Cooker Model will undoubtedly become more refined and accurately convey the intricacies that are part and parcel of FND.

References

Brabban, A., & Turkington, D. (2002). The search for meaning: Detecting congruence between life events, underlying schema and psychotic symptoms. *A Casebook of Cognitive Therapy for Psychosis, 59*, 76.

French, R. (2001). *Getting along and keeping cool: A group program for aggression control*. Perth: Rioby Publishing.

Kendall, S. B. (1974). Preference for intermittent reinforcement. *Journal of the Experimental Analysis of Behavior, 21*(3), 463–473.

Schreiber, F. B., & Seitzinger, J. (1985). The stress pressure cooker: A comprehensive model of stress management. National Emergency Training Center. *Police Chief, 52*(2), 40, 45–49.

Wagner, A. R. (1961). Effects of amount and percentage of reinforcement and number of acquisition trials on conditioning and extinction. *Journal of experimental Psychology, 62*(3), 234.

3 Rationale for developing the Pressure Cooker Model

Throughout centuries, FND has been regarded as a 'complex' condition affecting the mind and the body, simultaneously fascinating and baffling both clinicians and researchers. As a result, the field has generated a multitude of different theories, models, and ideas about FND.

In this chapter, you will learn more about important theoretical advances and observations from clinical practice that contributed to the field of FND and ultimately formed the basis for the development of the Pressure Cooker Model. Although it is beyond the scope of this book to discuss each FND theory in detail, Chapter 3 will provide you with a brief overview on historical ideas of FND, followed by an in-depth discussion of the three major streams of thinking about the mechanisms and maintaining factors of FND: theoretical (cognitive/attentional), biological, and clinical (including CBT). All these ideas have been invaluable for advancing the field and the development of treatments for FND. The Pressure Cooker Model has borrowed several influential ideas and aims to integrate some of these features into the model.

3.1 eResource alert!

Before delving more deeply into Chapter 3, you may find the eResource on 'theory and research basics' helpful to support your understanding of what theories are, why they are developed, and how they are tested. Consider this a crash course!

The history of FND

The Pressure Cooker Model uses concepts, ideas, and techniques from a wide range of models in FND – including historical ideas that have proven to be beyond valuable. To understand the rationale and the need for this new model, it is important to learn about the remarkable history that preceded its development. Many scholars and medical professionals have made a lasting impact on FND history.

Jean-Marie Charcot, a French neurologist (1825–1893), was a famous neurologist and widely regarded as the 'godfather' of neurology, who made many discoveries in the field of neurology, for example, multiple sclerosis and motor neurone disease, which are both due to brain injury. Charcot also treated people with 'hysteria' (FND at that time was known under the now-pejorative and outdated term 'hysteria'). He believed that FND was due to hereditary causes and a disorder that affected the nervous system that was both progressive and irreversible. Throughout his career, however, Charcot somewhat changed his ideas about FND and considered a more prominent role of psychological influences and traumatic events on the development of FND.

Josef Breuer, a physician from Vienna, Austria (1842–1925), treated a famous patient with FND called Anna O. She experienced a range of symptoms, including paralysis, loss of sensation,

DOI: 10.4324/9781003308973-3

pain, problems with her vision and speech. Breuer's treatment focused on 'talking' to Anna O, including about her symptoms, and recalling trauma memories connected with her symptoms under hypnosis, which positively impacted on the FND. Talking had such a positive influence on her symptoms that Anna O described this as the 'talking cure'. Breuer coined the term the 'cathartic method'. *Catharsis* is the process by which a hidden trauma that is unconscious to the person is expressed and released out in the open.

As you will learn in Chapter 6, the cover of the Pressure Cooker Model represents a person's level of verbal and emotional expression. The cover is one of the most important elements that is often found to be shut and tight in people with FND. For various reasons, people may struggle to express emotions and bottle up their emotions and difficult events that happened to them – one such reason is the unspeakable dilemma. In the clinic, it is not unusual to see a person with FND recover from their condition and improve their psychological well-being after they have developed a strong therapeutic relationship with their therapist, which has increased their insight and 'consciousness' into their unspeakable dilemma or a past traumatic event, and are subsequently able to release it to their therapist in a psychologically safe space. There is a strong association between bottled-up emotions and FND.

One of Breuer's famous protégés was **Sigmund Freud**, another neurologist from Austria (1856–1939), who also happened to have been one of Charcot's students. We know Freud from his major contributions to the field of psychoanalysis. He believed that FND was the result of unconscious conflicts and repression of memories. He placed a large emphasis on sexual trauma, sexuality, and the impact of early childhood experiences on the development of FND and many other psychological conditions. To improve people's symptoms, Freud used various therapeutic methods, including 'free association', or the act of talking openly and freely in a 'no-holds-barred way' about anything that came up in a person's mind, as well as dream analysis. Another important concept in the context of psychoanalysis was 'transference', which refers to the process of projecting, redirecting, or 'transferring' your feelings, wishes, or expectations about another person, for example, from an earlier relationship, onto the therapist. 'Countertransference' is the opposite phenomenon, when a therapist 'transfers' their feelings onto the person with FND. This has been regarded as a very important process in the therapeutic relationship.

Several of Breuer's and Freud's discoveries (Breuer & Freud, 1893) have played an important role during the development of the Pressure Cooker Model. For example:

- The contribution of **early childhood experiences** to FND, represented by the ignition element – including trauma for some (but not all) people with FND. For more information on this topic, jump ahead to Chapter 5.
- The **act of talking openly and freely** about things that bother a person with FND in a psychologically safe relationship (see, for example, Macmillan, 1977). This will come back again when we explore the cover element in Chapter 6.
- The idea that people can be **less or not at all conscious** of their emotions and memories and the notion that memories can be 'suppressed' or dissociated from to help the person not think about them or feel the emotion associated with these events. You will learn more about dissociation and functional cognitive symptoms in Chapter 7.
- The concept of **transference** and **countertransference** between a person with FND and other people in their environment, including partners, family members, and healthcare professionals. You will learn about the role of 'reciprocal reinforcement' and 'systemic re-traumatisation' in FND and the kitchen environment in Chapters 9 and 10.

Pierre Janet (1859–1947) was another highly influential figure in the field of FND and a French psychiatrist, philosopher, and psychologist who studied and worked under Charcot at a famous hospital in Paris in the 1880s. He is best known for his comprehensive work on dissociation and hypnosis treatment for FND, as well as investigating the association between a person's history of traumatic experiences and current symptoms, like FND (Janet, 1907; Janet, 1920). Janet also looked into the role that physical illness, fatigue, and attention mechanisms played in FND (e.g. Janet, 1889; van der Hart & Horst, 1989), three important elements that many contemporary theorists and clinicians have described and encountered in FND.

You can consider Janet as one of the 'founding fathers' of dissociation. Janet was not the only scholar interested in this phenomenon, though; Freud also looked into similar unconscious processes. Janet provided meaningful descriptions of this important psychological 'defence' mechanism that essentially helps people protect themselves from feeling difficult and overwhelming emotions, as well as memories, in the context of traumatic experiences, by putting that information outside conscious awareness. The effects of trauma may manifest through, for example, a person's behaviours, movements, perceptual abilities, and altered sensations without the person being aware or having any memory of it. This is the definition of *dissociation*, a core concept in the world of FND. Janet's work comes quite close to the idea of the loss of awareness and memory that many people with dissociative seizures often report.

Finally, a mention on '**behaviourism**'. This is the branch of psychology that places great emphasis on how a person's behaviour is shaped and heavily influenced by the environment, spearheaded by the 'fathers of behaviourism': **Ivan Pavlov** (1849–1936) and **B. F. Skinner** (1904–1990). Behaviourism developed in response to psychoanalytic theories you just briefly read about, for example, as developed by **Sigmund Freud**. Although behaviourism in its purest form is certainly not an approach that is advocated by the Pressure Cooker Model, the model does use helpful and evidence-based psychological principles from this line of thinking (see, for example, Pavlov, 1927; Skinner, 1963).

Operant conditioning

Skinner developed a theory about how behaviours increase or decrease in frequency depending on the consequence that follows the behaviour. This is called operant conditioning (Skinner, 1963). What might that mean, particularly for FND? Let us look at two examples of **negative reinforcement**, a concept that is very important in FND, particularly for people who experience dissociative seizures.

Imagine that you experience a headache. Pain is a trigger that causes discomfort. You take a painkiller ('the behaviour'). Soon, your headache disappears after a few minutes ('the consequence'). You may have learned that whenever you experience a headache, taking a painkiller will provide quick and effective relief. The tablet takes something unpleasant away (the pain); therefore, next time you experience a headache, chances are that you will reach for a tablet again to make it go away.

Now imagine that you experience dissociative seizures. A trigger (trauma reminder of an accident you were involved in) causes you discomfort or distress. This results in a seizure ('the behaviour', a coping strategy). Soon, you experience relief from the discomfort that the trauma reminder caused you ('the consequence'). In the same way as taking a tablet for a headache, a dissociative seizure can take away something unpleasant for a lot of people experiencing these episodes, for example, discomfort, emotions, arousal, stress, upset, and so on. The seizure helps the person feel relief from uncomfortable feelings and achieve a state of psychological safety.

In their theory of dissociative seizures, Brown and Reuber (2016) very clearly describe this characteristic reduction in arousal following a dissociative seizure. This process resembles the psychological process of **negative reinforcement** by Skinner (1963) that we have just discussed. In behaviourist terms, the relief from arousal, anxiety, or another unpleasant state is classified as a 'reward' or 'reinforcement', a positive consequence. Next time you encounter the trauma trigger and feel discomfort, the chances of experiencing another seizure will have increased, as your body and mind have now learned that the seizure helps to feel quick relief and safety.

3.2 eResource alert!

Interested in learning more about behaviourism? Read the eResource about another influential behaviourist scholar, Dr Ivan Pavlov. The resource also contains more examples and information about the principles of reinforcement learning in people with and without FND.

The next section is a whistle-stop tour of influential and contemporary models in FND. Any theory of FND has perks and drawbacks – none is perfect. Describing drawbacks is not intended to 'bash' theories of FND and all the hard work of researchers, scholars, and clinicians. It is important to provide you with a balanced view and help you think about how these theories spurred on the development of the Pressure Cooker Model.

Theoretical models of FND

One group of influential models has focused on **cognitive ('thinking')** and **attentional factors** as important agents in FND. Theoretical frameworks have meant a lot for the advancement of the field and have been invaluable for many different reasons. Let us discuss the three most famous theoretical models and read about why they have made a big mark.

The Integrative Cognitive Model (ICM; Brown, 2004; Brown, 2006)

The ICM is a model that was originally developed for medically unexplained symptoms (also called 'MUS', an umbrella term that includes FND as one of the conditions). According to this theory, MUSs are caused by memory representations that are 'activated' and bias an attentional system to select faulty information. What does that mean?

Let us take a look at 'rogue representations', a central concept in the ICM. Rogue representations emerge when a person 'misinterprets' sensory information and experiences this misinterpretation as real symptoms, leading to the experience of FND.

An easy way to understand this idea is to explore visual illusions that have been extensively researched in the field of psychology. Have you heard of the Hermann grid (1870) before? Look at Figure 3.1. What do you notice about the grid?

Figure 3.1 Hermann grid illusion.

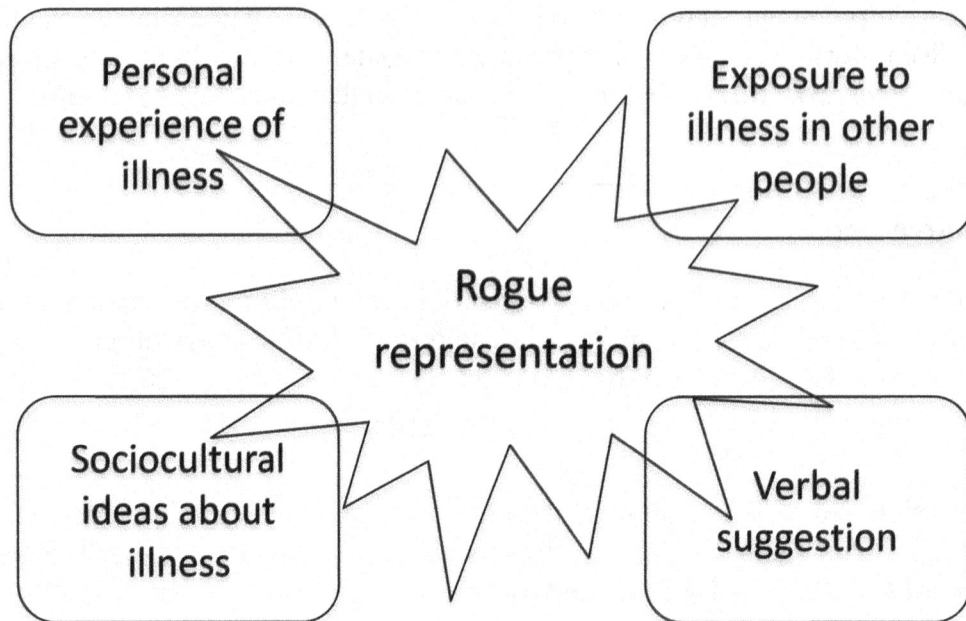

Figure 3.2 Origins of rogue representations.

Most people will see a 4 × 4 grid of black opaque squares, as well as small flickering grey circles located on the intersections. Can you see the grey blobs too? They suddenly disappear when you look straight at an intersection. The reality is, there are no grey blobs printed, only black squares, and that is it! Yet we 'misinterpret' this information through our senses as 'real' grey blobs. And they definitely feel as a real experience. You can think of rogue representations and FND symptoms in similar ways. It is as if the brain plays tricks. Figure 3.2 shows you what sources rogue representations are believed to originate from.

It turns out that rogue representations will activate more strongly through **increased self-focused attention** on symptoms which maintain MUS or FND. The ICM is an elegant theory that does an excellent job at explaining the **involuntary nature** and **real and genuine experience** of FND or MUS in the absence of pathology or an identifiable organic cause in the body. The description of a tangible mechanism has done a lot for the field and helped professionals take people with FND seriously (although admittedly there is still a long way to go).

Brown and Reuber (2016): the Integrative Cognitive Model applied to dissociative seizures

The ICM-DS is another theory that provides a beautiful explanation of how dissociative seizures appear and unfold. Figure 3.3 shows how (1) the perception of cues with a threatening meaning and (2) the prospect of a seizure together activate a **'seizure scaffold'**.

A 'seizure scaffold' is a mental representation of the dissociative seizure: how your mind views, interprets, and understands the dissociative episode. It is believed that this mental representation can be influenced by many things, for example, your previous experience of illness, traumatic experiences, and 'seizure models' (a close family member or someone you have seen in the media with epilepsy).

A dissociative seizure effectively reduces the unpleasant arousal that so often builds up and precedes a seizure and subsequently feeds this information back into the seizure scaffold, until the next dissociative seizure appears and the same process repeats.

In their integrative model for dissociative seizures, Brown and Reuber (2016) very clearly describe how a high level of arousal can lead to a dissociative seizure via a complex interplay

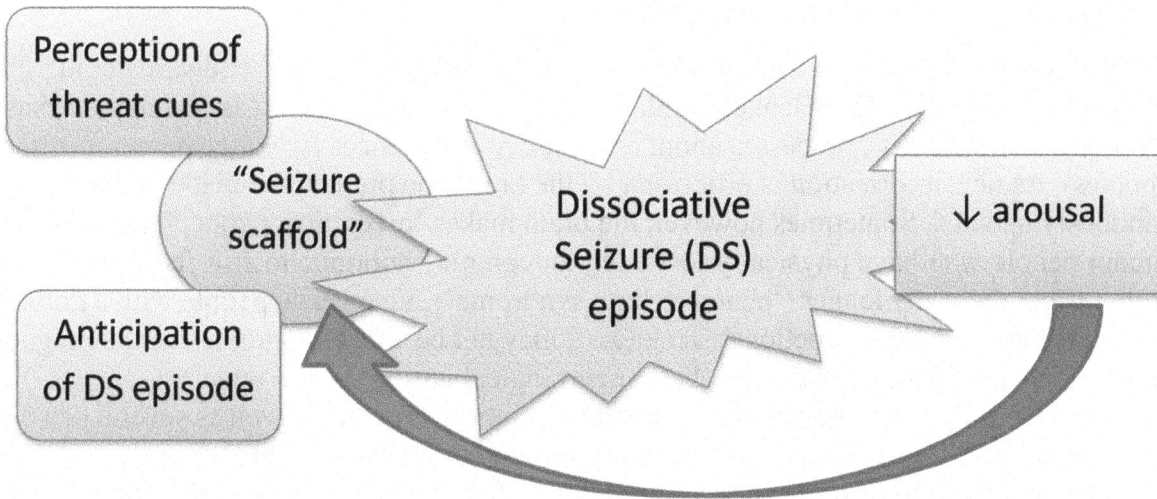

Figure 3.3 A very simplistic schematic depiction of the ICM applied to dissociative seizures.

of cognitive, emotional, and behavioural events. In a sophisticated manner, the model also mentions that elevated arousal is not always necessary for a dissociative episode to emerge in some situations, a phenomenon that people with dissociative seizures sometimes report ('I didn't feel anything, suddenly my brain switched off', 'I was happy before I experienced the seizure').

The model is appealing because it is able to integrate a range of processes that are specific to dissociative seizures. For example:

- The idea of **prediction** and **anticipation** of a seizure that a lot of people with dissociative seizures experience ('I feel funny and queasy, things feel unreal around me, this means I'm going to have a seizure').
- **Perception of threat cues** and **trauma reminders** around you, in the context of previous trauma experiences. For example, a person may have developed dissociative seizures following an accident on the road. Every time the person sees a roundabout (threat cue or trauma reminder), they may start to feel uncomfortable and develop a seizure.
- The impact of prior exposure to **'seizure models'**. Let us explain what that means. We know that a subset of people with FND have previously been in a healthcare profession; were required to care for an ill family member in their personal life, perhaps whilst growing up; or have had an illness experience themselves prior to developing dissociative seizures, for example, 'organic' seizures caused by an abnormal electrical storm in the brain. The theory is good at accounting for how these 'modelling' experiences can increase the chances that you develop seizures later in life.
- The **subjective, personal experience of something that feels like a loss of consciousness** that is so often reported by people with dissociative seizures. The idea that it is possible to experience **'panic without panic'** in FND (please also see Goldstein & Mellers, 2006). A person may experience the physical symptoms of a panic attack but may not be able to fully connect with underlying panic feelings due to **dissociation**, a central concept in FND. This acknowledgement can truly resonate with people who may not have always been believed.
- Not only does the model focus on psychology-only factors, but it also highlights a variety of **biological**, **psychological**, and **social factors** that can 'shape' and impact on the dissociative seizures, including prior physical injury (biological), unhelpful thinking processes such as misinterpretation (psychological), and seizure models around you (social). This takes away the psychological pressure from people that it is not all psychological and 'in the head'.

Bayesian model of FND (Edwards et al., 2012)

Have you ever heard of "predictive processing" or "predictive coding"? (Edwards et al., 2012; Keller & Mrsic-Flogel, 2018; Bennett et al., 2021; Drane et al., 2022). It is understood that the brain engages in predictive processes about our sensory experiences (what we perceive or feel in our bodies). As new information is processed by the brain, the predictions made by the brain are continuously updated. Sometimes however, the brain makes 'prediction errors'. Think for example about people who have physically lost a leg though may continue to still feel their leg even though it is not there any longer ('phantom limb syndrome'). Vice versa, people with a numb and paralysed leg due to FND ('functional weakness') may not be able to feel or move their leg, even though it is physically present and the 'basic neurological wiring' is still intact.

An influential theory that describes the 'predictive coding' process, as well as several key thinking processes in FND proposed a 'Bayesian formulation' of brain function (Edwards et al., 2012) that emphasises the role of prior knowledge in FND. According to the Bayesian model, **abnormal prior beliefs** about **illness** contribute to the generation of FND symptoms.

Like the Integrative Cognitive Model, the Bayesian model ascribes an important role to **attention** in FND. Known as one of the biggest maintaining factors of FND and a well-documented phenomenon in research, **heightened self-focused attention allocated to physical symptoms** is a common finding in people with FND (Brown, 2006; Van Poppelen et al., 2011; Edwards et al., 2012; Stins et al., 2015).

The **abnormal beliefs about illness** are subjected to **heightened self-focused attention** and lead to **misattribution of agency**: voluntary experiences are perceived as involuntary by people with FND.

The Bayesian model has also been influential in highlighting how the social environment can influence our thinking processes and create **abnormal expectations**, **beliefs**, or **misattributions** about illnesses. Let us look at some examples of how social experiences can impact on our thinking:

• A healthy person with a family member recently diagnosed with dementia goes into another room of the house . . . and forgets what item they were after. The person may misattribute an innocuous, everyday memory difficulty to a more serious, irreversible memory condition because of their prior exposure to dementia in the family.

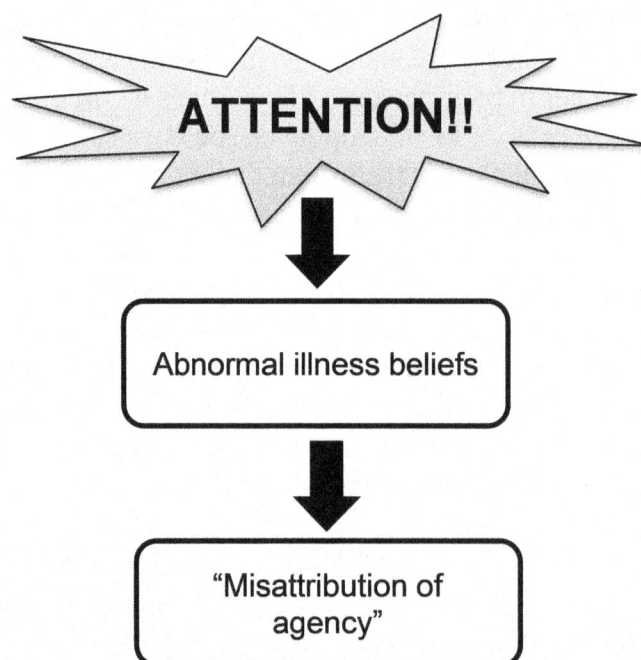

Figure 3.4 A very simplistic schematic depiction of the Bayesian model of FND.

- A person who works with people with progressive neurological conditions on a daily basis may immediately believe that a twitch in their foot is due to a serious neurological illness, because they have been exposed to this illness so often.
- Having witnessed an epileptic seizure, stroke, or heart attack in a family member before may make a person anxious about being afflicted with a similar type of acute illness when they suddenly feel weird body sensations, lose their train of thought, and notice things feel unreal in the world around them.

Abnormal expectations about illness may come from a variety of social sources and predispose an individual to develop abnormal illness beliefs

- **Health scares, diseases, and other medical problems** reported in the **media**, newspapers, movies, the internet, podcasts, social media, blogs, documentaries, and medical programmes on TV about illnesses, a radio interview with an ill person, the news coverage on the Covid-19 pandemic, and so forth. Exposure to illness is everywhere and influences, consciously and unconsciously, our thoughts, feelings, and behaviours, occasionally resulting in FND symptoms that resemble the conditions that people have been exposed to.

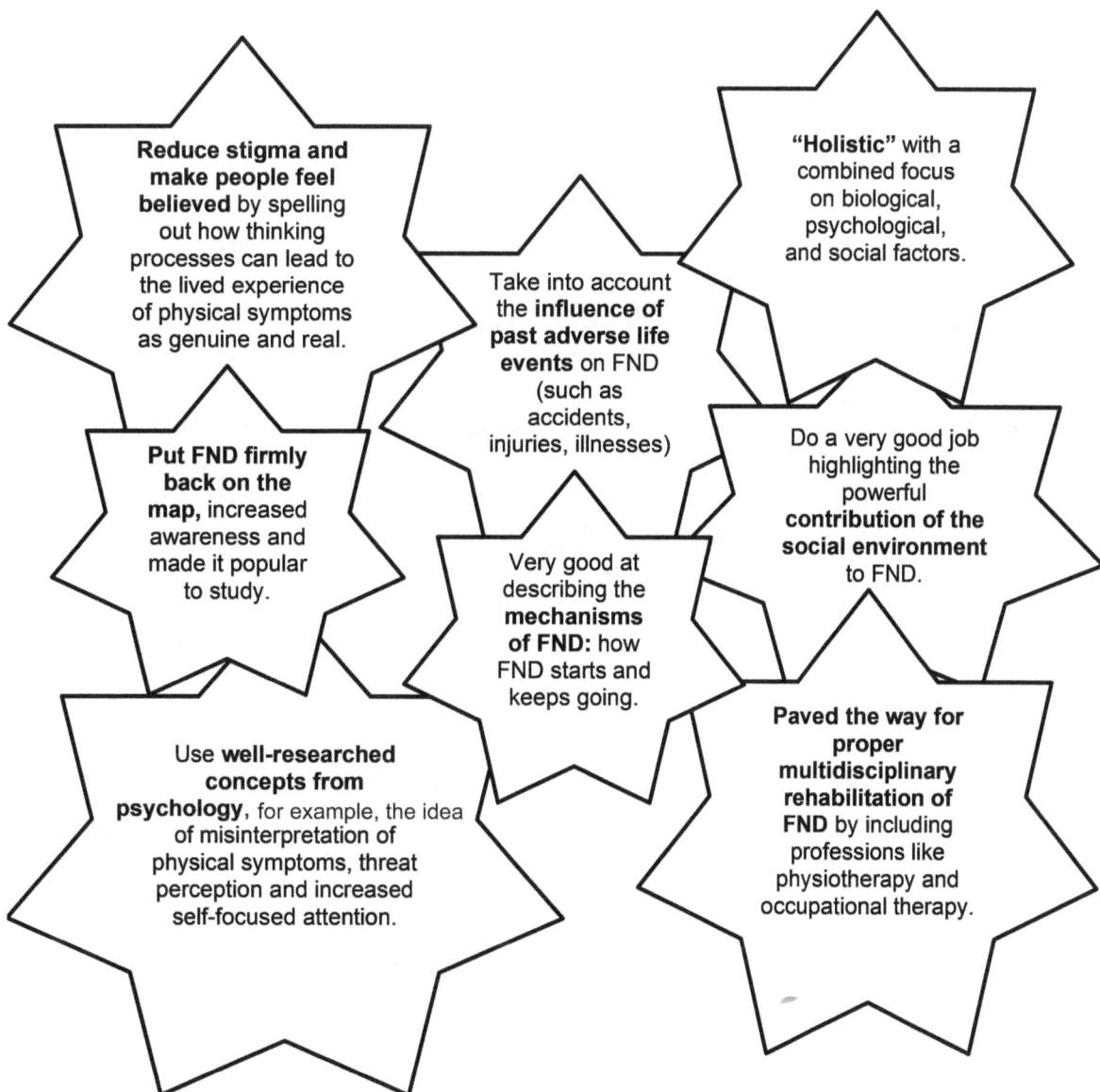

Figure 3.5 Star qualities of theoretical models in FND.

- **Exposure to physical illnesses** or **health scares** in **personal relationships**, for example, a sick family member, friend, neighbours, colleagues, other people in your vicinity or local community.
- Some people with FND **cared for an ill person** or a **family member** for longer periods and witnessed neurological symptoms 'up close and personal', such as epilepsy, dystonia, and stroke.
- Your **own personal experience** of physical illness. Sometimes, people who have had epileptic seizures in childhood may develop non-epileptic episodes in adulthood, long after the childhood seizures disappeared. Other people experience both epileptic and non-epileptic seizures.
- Holding down a **job in the hospital** or in a **healthcare profession**; for example, as a nurse, paramedic, medical or allied health student, or carer, you will be in contact with ill people.
- **Cultural expectations** and views on illness, for example, on what a seizure looks like (lots of shaking, movement, and eyes closed).

What are some of the issues with theoretical models in FND?

- Explain FND very well but are less helpful in treating the FND in the clinic.
- Theory–practice links are not as strong as for Cognitive Behavioural Therapy (CBT). Some practical strategies are available to treat FND but not for all maintaining factors.
- Psychological processes and emotions are highlighted, but CBT/clinical models probably do a better job at explaining them.
- Tend to focus on anxiety (threat, stress, trauma) and view 'anxiety' in 'general' terms, but there are a lot of different types of anxiety: panic, social anxiety, as well as fears of rejection, recovery, 'the unknown', and of FND setbacks (see Chapter 7).
- Do not focus on other important emotions, like low mood, anger, guilt, and embarrassment, often associated with family/personal relationship dynamics and which explain why some FND symptoms keep going.
- Although the impact of the social environment is highlighted, not much attention is paid to family/personal relationship dynamics, as well as childhood and adulthood coping strategies, all factors that contribute to FND.
- Language can at times be complex, abstract, technical, and not always patient-friendly, causing confusion, particularly for people with brain fog and memory problems.
- Theoretical models are often focused on only one specific FND subtype – dissociative episodes or motor FND – but are less good at explaining a mixture of FND symptoms, which is probably the most common presentation in clinics.

Clinical models for FND: cognitive-behavioural therapy (CBT)

CBT is probably the most famous clinical model used in FND treatment and will therefore be our focus of attention. CBT is based on cognitive and behavioural learning theory. Therapy aims to change your thinking processes and any unhelpful behaviours in order to relieve your distress (Beck, 1967, 1976).

The hot cross bun of CBT

Most CBT models will look at **four areas** to understand and treat psychological difficulties, with some CBT models considering a fifth area: the social environment. Clinicians call this the 'hot cross bun'. All areas of the hot cross bun are connected to one another (see Figure 3.6).

Physical
What you feel in
your body
"hot and sweaty"
"dissociative
seizure"

Emotional
What you feel
"anxiety, fear, or an
unpleasant feeling
building up inside"

Cognitive
What you think,
what goes through
your mind
"I'm going to have a
seizure"

Behavioural
What you do or
don't do
"Staying indoors to
avoid seizures in
public"

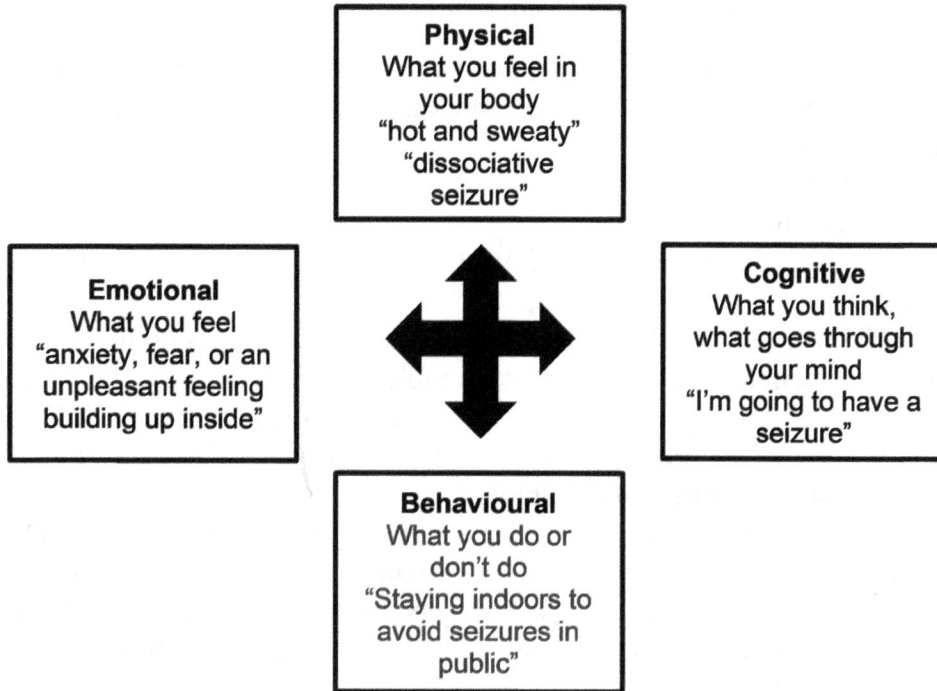

Figure 3.6 A hot cross bun formulation of dissociative seizures.

Have a look at the positive aspects of CBT models in Figure 3.7

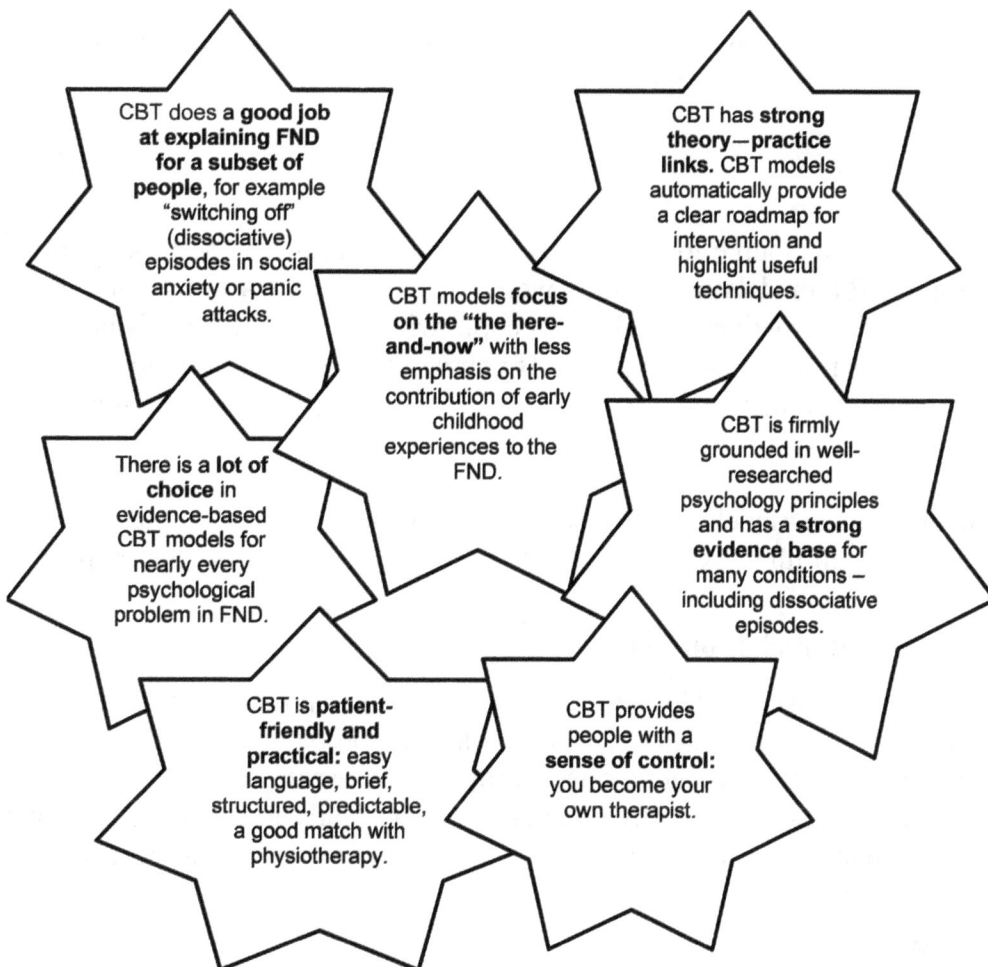

CBT does a **good job
at explaining FND
for a subset of
people**, for example
"switching off"
(dissociative)
episodes in social
anxiety or panic
attacks.

CBT has **strong
theory—practice
links.** CBT models
automatically provide
a clear roadmap for
intervention and
highlight useful
techniques.

CBT models **focus
on the "the here-
and-now"** with less
emphasis on the
contribution of early
childhood
experiences to the
FND.

There is a **lot of
choice** in
evidence-based
CBT models for
nearly every
psychological
problem in FND.

CBT is firmly
grounded in well-
researched
psychology principles
and has a **strong
evidence base** for
many conditions –
including dissociative
episodes.

CBT is **patient-
friendly and
practical:** easy
language, brief,
structured, predictable,
a good match with
physiotherapy.

CBT provides
people with a
sense of control:
you become your
own therapist.

Figure 3.7 Star qualities of CBT models in FND.

What are some of the issues with CBT models in FND?

- Requires you to have a good understanding and awareness of emotions and thoughts.
- You need to be open towards psychological thinking and feeling comfortable speaking about/connecting with emotions.
- Although there are a lot of CBT models, most people's FND symptoms will simply not fit into CBT models that easily.
- FND mechanism of action is sometimes a mystery: How do psychological difficulties exactly lead to FND?
- There is no unifying CBT model for FND, and existing models miss quite a few of the important psychological maintaining factors (for example, dissociation, reduced verbal emotional expression, boom-and-bust cycle, social isolation, and the social functions of FND).
- **Focus strongly on the person** and not so much on the social aspects of FND, including responses from your environment to symptoms.
- **Highly focused on psychology** and not so much on the physical aspects of FND.
- Focusing on the 'here-and-now' may be **too superficial** in FND because past relationships, early coping strategies (dissociation), and adverse childhood experiences play an important role in FND.
- CBT models are probably **too logical** and risk encouraging dissociation and disconnection from emotions – the opposite of what is needed for people with FND.
- Often **too focused on content rather than process**. What does this mean? Learning concrete strategies to stop panic attacks or social anxiety is one part of therapy for FND, but the other essential part has to do with therapeutic processes: learning to form an attachment and a relationship, opening up about emotions regardless of what these are, feeling accepted by a non-judgemental person who 'hears' you.
- The effectiveness for CBT is **mostly proven** for people with **dissociative seizures**. However, a lot of people experience a mixture of FND symptoms.

3.3 eResource alert!

Please consult this eResource for more background reading on the perks and drawbacks of theoretical and CBT models in FND, as well as two approaches in psychology that have proven to be good alternatives to CBT for people with FND: dialectical behaviour therapy and the psychodynamic school of thought. If you would like to learn more about other psychological approaches (there are so many!), keep reading this eResource for a summary.

If theoretical and clinical models are not the complete answer, could biologically informed models perhaps be more helpful in explaining and treating FND? Let us find out in the next section!

Biologically informed models of FND

A few theories of FND have lifted biological processes up as important factors in the development of FND. These approaches, although not 100% biological, probably have adopted a stronger biological slant towards FND than other theories and are therefore categorised under 'biological models of FND'. In the end, no theory or treatment of FND will fully focus on just biological factors. Let us explore some recent scientific papers and interesting biologically informed views on FND.

A diathesis–stress model of FND

Keynejad et al. (2019) adopted a **'diathesis–stress'** approach towards FND. **'Diathesis'** refers to a genetic or biological vulnerability or predisposition that people may be born with. **'Stress'** refers to difficult or traumatic life events that have happened to the person. According to this theory, some people may have a higher, while others have a lower, biological vulnerability towards developing FND. This diathesis–stress model views FND as the result of a combination of biological vulnerability and stressful or traumatic life events. In particular, the authors highlight that the threshold for a person to develop FND symptoms in life can be reached as a result of different combinations between (1) biological risk or vulnerability, (2) childhood 'maltreatment', and (3) a 'precipitating' stressor (this is a stressful event in a person's life that tends to happen immediately before and sets off the FND).

Stress and biology in FND

The biological impact of stress responses may relate to FND. Although these studies are exciting, work on this area has only just begun, and the results of these studies should be interpreted cautiously.

Hypothalamic-pituitary-adrenal ('HPA') axis dysregulation

The HPA axis is a complex sequence of events that unfolds in the brain and the body, and involves stress hormones that can impact on our physical health and immune system, mood, thinking skills, sleep and fatigue levels. Like the fight-or-flight response (see Chapter 8), the HPA axis forms a crucial part of the body's response to stress. It involves several important brain areas, including the hypothalamus and pituitary gland, as well as the adrenal glands (on top of your kidneys). Studies on FND found increased cortisol ('stress hormone') levels that was associated with trauma and stressful life events in people with dissociative seizures and the motor type of FND (Bakvis et al., 2010; Apazoglou et al., 2017), although others did report an effect (Maurer et al., 2015).

Allostatic load

The idea of **allostatic load** refers to the cumulative effects and burden ('build-up') of exposure to prolonged, repetitive, and frequent stress and life events on the body, for example, on the heart, inflammation, and the nervous system. Although the jury is still out on whether increased allostatic load plays a role in FND, it is nevertheless an interesting idea, since people with FND report stressful and traumatic events, sometimes life-long and from childhood onwards (see Keynejad et al., 2019; Popkirov et al., 2019; and Silverberg & Rush, 2024, to read more on allostatic load and FND).

The amygdala and the freezing response

People with FND can occasionally present with a total lack of movement and become 'floppy' during a dissociative seizure or experience a period of sudden 'whole body' functional weakness in the legs and arms as part of functional motor disorder, resembling a **freezing response** to threat. Interestingly, one brain imaging study (Aybek et al., 2015) showed increased activation in an area called the periaqueductal grey in people with FND. This area is important for the freezing response of anxiety. The periaqueductal grey is also connected to the amygdala, a key brain area involved in anxiety. This study also found increased activation in the **amygdala** in response to negative emotions in people with FND (Aybek et al., 2015), whilst another study found a similar effect during movement (Voon et al., 2011).

Brain imaging studies in FND

In more recent years, researchers have turned their attention towards uncovering changes in the structure and function of the brains of people with FND. **Brain imaging investigations** ('taking a photograph of your brain') have made major strides in the field of FND. Another closely related and upcoming area of interest in FND is **neuropsychology**, which studies the relationships between the brain and thinking skills (like memory, attention and planning), mood as well as behaviour.

3.4 eResource alert!

Want to know more about brain imaging and neuropsychology research in FND? Why not check out this eResource to learn about important findings in these fields.

Positive aspects of biological approaches to FND

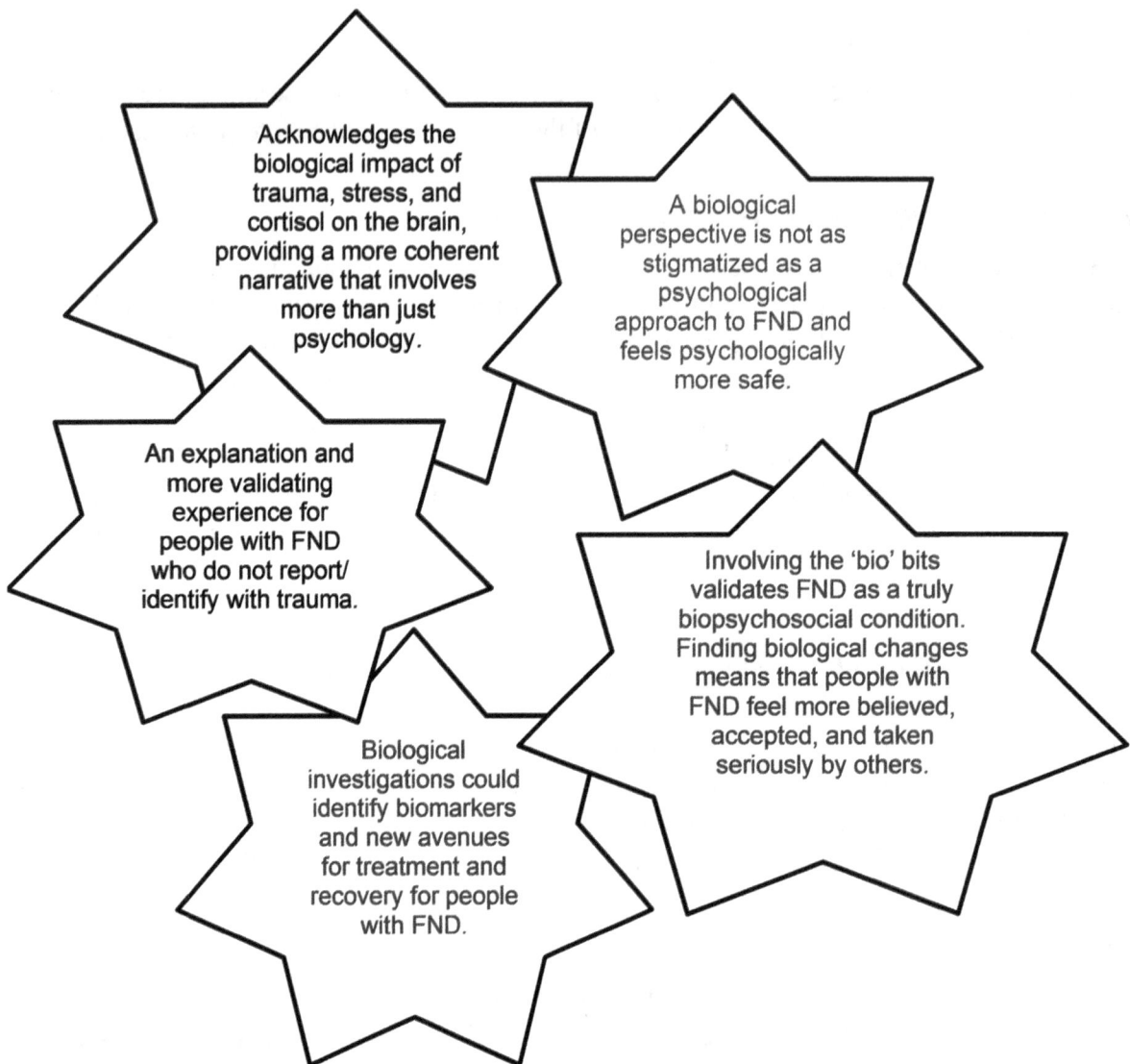

Acknowledges the biological impact of trauma, stress, and cortisol on the brain, providing a more coherent narrative that involves more than just psychology.

A biological perspective is not as stigmatized as a psychological approach to FND and feels psychologically more safe.

An explanation and more validating experience for people with FND who do not report/ identify with trauma.

Involving the 'bio' bits validates FND as a truly biopsychosocial condition. Finding biological changes means that people with FND feel more believed, accepted, and taken seriously by others.

Biological investigations could identify biomarkers and new avenues for treatment and recovery for people with FND.

Figure 3.8 Star qualities of biologically informed models in FND.

Drawbacks of biological approaches to FND

- Brain imaging studies in people with FND suffer from a **wide range of methodological problems** which **limit our confidence in the conclusions**, including:
  - Correlation does not mean causation.
  - Other causes, like age and epilepsy, may better explain the brain changes found in FND (Asadi-Pooya & Homayoun, 2020; Sharma et al., 2022).
  - Brain changes may not be permanent but reversible over time (see Vuilleumier et al., 2001). Most studies use cross-sectional designs (like 'a snapshot' in time) rather than longitudinal (multiple observations over a longer period).
  - Not everyone finds the same, or any, brain changes.

- Statistical errors with investigations 'finding' an abnormality in the brain, but in reality, there is no abnormality ('a false alarm').
- Low sample sizes.
- Risk of overinterpretation and confusion about FND, with people believing that they may have brain injury, in a similar way as someone with a stroke. See **eResource** 3.5 to learn how the course of FND recovery is often very different from stroke recovery.

- Biological approaches locate the problem in the individual and may increase, rather than decrease, stigma and blame.
- Despite its important role in FND, the impact of the social environment, interpersonal processes, and relationships on symptoms may be entirely missed. You could therefore miss out on helpful opportunities to learn psychological and family communication strategies.
- By heavily focusing on biology, self-focused attention on physical symptoms, one of the major maintaining factors of FND (Edwards et al., 2012), becomes even further increased than it already is.
- Biological approaches provide a less-hopeful message for FND recovery and reinforce the idea that 'FND is for life', without a clear-cut treatment plan.
- Adds another layer of problems, worries, and distress and may lead to catastrophic thoughts around 'something is seriously wrong with my brain', contributing to more FND.

3.6 eResource alert!

This eResource will provide more background reading on the positive qualities as well as the drawbacks of biologically informed perspectives on FND.

A new model of FND: the Pressure Cooker Model

The Pressure Cooker Model is a newly developed model that takes into account the positive features and drawbacks from all previously described models and tries to combine the 'best of all worlds'! Shall we look at what makes the model so special and useful? Get ready for the top 20 reasons that it is worth giving this model a go.

Top 20 reasons that you should try out the Pressure Cooker Model:

1. **Relatable visual metaphor** that explains complex ideas about FND in an easier way. Great for FND education to your family, friends, and healthcare professionals.
2. **Easier-to-understand language** and concepts that help explain how the FND appears and keeps going, particularly how FND links in with emotions and other psychological processes, and everything else that is important in FND.
3. Although each element is psychosocial in nature, other disciplines involved in your care, like occupational therapy, physiotherapy, as well as speech and language therapy, are fully represented by their own element in the Pressure Cooker Model.
4. **Ties together multiple disciplines involved in FND treatment** into one story using the same language. One coherent narrative helps organise your and your team's thoughts around the FND, how it started and what keeps it going. **Focuses on collaboration, joining up your care, and reducing confusion.**
5. Your personalised 'Pressure Cooker Model' story can be directly applied in a practical way to manage FND. **It guides and maps out your treatment** with strategies that are best suited for you and your family to help tackle the FND.
6. The Pressure Cooker Model believes that **'everybody has FND'**: it does not make much distinction between people with vs without FND. Therefore, the model is **made for everyone,**

including **your family, friends, healthcare professionals**, and anyone else you are close to and interact with on a regular basis. The social environment and relationships play a central role in the Pressure Cooker Model of FND and encourages both the person with and without FND to look at their own contribution to FND.

7. **Biopsychosocial model** that looks at psychological, social, and biological processes all in one model and that does not separate the mind from the body but instead looks at how all these factors together contribute to FND.

8. Uses important **evidence-based principles and techniques** from well-researched clinical models, like CBT, that have proven to be effective in treating FND (e.g. behavioural experiments, 'reinforcement learning'). The Pressure Cooker Model also keeps some of the **features from important FND theories**, for example, how self-focused attention on physical symptoms can keep the FND going.

9. Looks at relationships and other psychosocial aspects of FND. Learning 'life-long' **strategies to repair relationships and relate better to one another** may give hope for a different future with skills that you can always carry with you and don't 'run out' of.

10. Even though the person with FND experiences/carries the symptoms, the Pressure Cooker Model believes that **both the person and the environment equally contribute to FND** and, therefore, together hold the 'key' to resolving FND. Family and healthcare professionals are advised to apply a pressure cooker on themselves.

11. Key processes in FND that have been neglected in other approaches play a central role in the Pressure Cooker Model, for example, **dissociation**, **bottling up emotions**, and **boom-and-bust cycles**.

12. The Pressure Cooker Model **can work with different types of emotions**, like anxiety, depression, as well as internal states that are not clearly defined. Even if you do not identify with emotions, you can still work with the model. Focuses both on 'contents' (*what* emotions does someone feel) and 'process' (*how* do the emotions come out?).

13. We know that **FND comes in all forms and shapes**. Some people experience dissociative episodes, other people have problems with movement or their memory, while most have a mixture of symptoms. For the Pressure Cooker Model, it does not matter what type or symptoms of FND you experience, how often you have the symptoms, how long you have had the FND, how severe or 'complex' the FND is – **it covers the full range of FND symptoms.**

14. FND unfortunately affects everyone: no matter what age you are or whether you experience other conditions like autism, epilepsy, or complex trauma. Luckily, the Pressure Cooker Model is quite flexible and caters to a lot of people.

15. **Can be adapted in many formats:** individual work, in a group, online, in early intervention for just-diagnosed people.

16. **Uses friendly, no-stigma language.** Instead of saying that people with FND 'seek attention', the Pressure Cooker Model says FND has 'social functions' for everyone involved, whether you experience FND or not.

17. Looks at the **detrimental impact** of **difficult healthcare experiences** on FND symptoms and recovery by showing that people with FND and their healthcare professionals think the same things about each other.

18. Has been found **acceptable**, **feasible**, and **positive** by quite a few people with FND, their families, and healthcare professionals alike!

19. Not only focuses on 'what does not go well' and 'what is going wrong'; it also looks at 'what is going well', 'what is right', **people's positive qualities and protective factors** in their quest to overcome FND.

20. Aims to **radically transform FND recovery** by using more positive language and shifting the responsibility for recovery from the individual to the individual-in-the-environment.

3.7 eResource alert!

If you would like to know more about some of the evidence for the individual elements, as well as the mechanism for FND detailed in the Pressure Cooker Model, then this eResource will explain a bit more about the research background.

References

Apazoglou, K., Mazzola, V., Wegrzyk, J., Polara, G. F., & Aybek, S. (2017). Biological and perceived stress in motor functional neurological disorders. *Psychoneuroendocrinology, 85*, 142–150.

Asadi-Pooya, A. A., & Homayoun, M. (2020). Structural brain abnormalities in patients with psychogenic nonepileptic seizures. *Neurological Sciences, 41*, 555–559.

Aybek, S., Nicholson, T. R., O'Daly, O., Zelaya, F., Kanaan, R. A., & David, A. S. (2015). Emotion-motion interactions in conversion disorder: An FMRI study. *PLoS One, 10*(4), e0123273.

Bakvis, P., Spinhoven, P., Giltay, E. J., Kuyk, J., Edelbroek, P. M., Zitman, F. G., & Roelofs, K. (2010). Basal hypercortisolism and trauma in patients with psychogenic nonepileptic seizures. *Epilepsia, 51*(5), 752–759.

Beck, A. T. (1967). *Depression: Clinical, experimental and theoretical aspects*. New York: Harper and Row.

Beck, A. T. (1976). *Cognitive therapy and the emotional disorders*. New York, NY: International Universities Press.

Bennett, K., Diamond, C., Hoeritzauer, I., Gardiner, P., McWhirter, L., Carson, A., & Stone, J. (2021). A practical review of functional neurological disorder (FND) for the general physician. *Clinical Medicine, 21*(1), 28.

Breuer, J., & Freud, S. (1893). On the psychical mechanism of hysterical phenomena. *The Standard Edition of the Complete Psychological Works of Sigmund Freud, 2*(1893–1895), 1–17.

Brown, R. J. (2004). Psychological mechanisms of medically unexplained symptoms: an integrative conceptual model. *Psychological Bulletin, 130*(5), 793.

Brown, R. J. (2006). Medically unexplained symptoms: A new model. *Psychiatry, 5*(2), 43–47.

Brown, R. J., & Reuber, M. (2016). Towards an integrative theory of psychogenic non-epileptic seizures (PNES). *Clinical Psychology Review, 47*, 55–70.

Drane, D. L., Fani, N., Hallett, M., Khalsa, S. S., Perez, D. L., & Roberts, N. A. (2021). A framework for understanding the pathophysiology of functional neurological disorder. *CNS spectrums, 26*(6), 555–561.

Edwards, M. J., Adams, R. A., Brown, H., Parees, I., & Friston, K. J. (2012). A Bayesian account of 'hysteria'. *Brain, 135*(11), 3495–3512.

Goldstein, L. H., & Mellers, J. D. C. (2006). Ictal symptoms of anxiety, avoidance behaviour, and dissociation in patients with dissociative seizures. *Journal of Neurology, Neurosurgery & Psychiatry, 77*(5), 616–621.

Hermann, L. (1870). Eine erscheinung simultanen contrastes. *Archiv für die gesamte Physiologie des Menschen und der Tiere, 3*(1), 13–15.

Janet, P. (1889). *L'automatisme psychologique: Essai de psychologie expérimentale sur les formes inférieures de l'activité humaine*. Paris: Félix Alcan.

Janet, P. (Ed.). (1907). Lecture I: The problem of hysteria. In *The major symptoms of hysteria* (pp. 1–21). Macmillan Publishing.

Janet, P. (1920). General definitions. In P. Janet (Ed.), *The major symptoms of hysteria: Fifteen lectures given in the medical school of Harvard University* (2nd edition with new matter, pp. 317–337). MacMillan Co.

Keller, G. B., & Mrsic-Flogel, T. D. (2018). Predictive processing: a canonical cortical computation. *Neuron, 100*(2), 424–435.

Keynejad, R. C., Frodl, T., Kanaan, R., Pariante, C., Reuber, M., & Nicholson, T. R. (2019). Stress and functional neurological disorders: Mechanistic insights. *Journal of Neurology, Neurosurgery & Psychiatry, 90*(7), 813–821.

Macmillan, M. B. (1977). The cathartic method and the expectancies of Breuer and Anna O. *International Journal of Clinical and Experimental Hypnosis, 25*(2), 106–118.

Maurer, C. W., LaFaver, K., Ameli, R., Toledo, R., & Hallett, M. (2015). A biological measure of stress levels in patients with functional movement disorders. *Parkinsonism & Related Disorders, 21*(9), 1072–1075.

Pavlov, I. P. (1927). *Conditioned reflexes: An investigation of the physiological activity of the cerebral cortex.* Oxford: Oxford University Press.

Popkirov, S., Asadi-Pooya, A. A., Duncan, R., Gigineishvili, D., Hingray, C., Miguel Kanner, A., Curt LaFrance, W., Pretorius, C., Reuber, M. & ILAE PNES Task Force. (2019). The aetiology of psychogenic non-epileptic seizures: risk factors and comorbidities. *Epileptic disorders, 21*(6), 529–547.

Sharma, A. A., Goodman, A. M., Allendorfer, J. B., Philip, N. S., Correia, S., LaFrance Jr, W. C., & Szaflarski, J. P. (2022). Regional brain atrophy and aberrant cortical folding relate to anxiety and depression in patients with traumatic brain injury and psychogenic nonepileptic seizures. *Epilepsia, 63*(1), 222–236.

Silverberg, N. D., & Rush, B. K. (2024). Neuropsychological evaluation of functional cognitive disorder: a narrative review. *The Clinical Neuropsychologist, 38*(2), 302–325.

Skinner, B. F. (1963). Operant behavior. *American Psychologist, 18*(8), 503.

Stins, J. F., Kempe, C. L. A., Hagenaars, M. A., Beek, P. J., & Roelofs, K. (2015). Attention and postural control in patients with conversion paresis. *Journal of Psychosomatic Research, 78*(3), 249–254.

Van der Hart, O., & Horst, R. (1989). The dissociation theory of Pierre Janet. *Journal of Traumatic Stress, 2*(4), 397–412.

Van Poppelen, D., Saifee, T. A., Schwingenschuh, P., Katschnig, P., Bhatia, K. P., Tijssen, M. A., & Edwards, M. J. (2011). Attention to self in psychogenic tremor. *Movement Disorders, 26*(14), 2575–2576.

Voon, V., Brezing, C., Gallea, C., & Hallett, M. (2011). Aberrant supplementary motor complex and limbic activity during motor preparation in motor conversion disorder. *Movement Disorders, 26*(13), 2396–2403.

Vuilleumier, P., Chicherio, C., Assal, F., Schwartz, S., Slosman, D., & Landis, T. (2001). Functional neuroanatomical correlates of hysterical sensorimotor loss. *Brain, 124*(6), 1077–1090.

4 The structure of the Pressure Cooker Model

Pressure Cooker Model: an overview

Have you ever used a pressure cooker at home? Figure 4.1 shows you a simplified version of a pressure cooker that we may find in our kitchens.

As you can see in Figure 4.1, the pressure cooker pot has flames under it, some bubbling contents inside, a cover to make sure the heat does not escape, and a valve to let off steam. The flames underneath are kept alive by some sort of fuel. For the pressure cooker to start boiling its contents, the flames need to be ignited by an ignition source, such as a gas lighter.

If someone ignited the flames under the pressure cooker, added lots of fuel, produced big and hot flames under the pot, turned up the temperature regulator to 'very high', but sealed off the cover very tightly and did not take good care of the blocked valve, the pressure cooker would very likely explode, as is illustrated in Figure 4.2.

Looking back at Figure 4.1 again, there are many ways to intervene to prevent an explosion. For example, you may reduce the fuel, dial down the temperature regulator, loosen the cover, or unblock the valve. All these strategies may help. Later in Chapter 4, you will look at this in more detail. For now, let us consider a slightly more sophisticated pressure cooker.

A detailed pressure cooker

Figure 4.3 shows you a more comprehensive and detailed pressure cooker, with some more elements added in:

- **Safety features** to make sure that the pressure cooker will not explode or perhaps delay that moment as much as possible if the cooker is in peril.
- **Sticky leftover food** from all the previous times that you cooked with the pressure cooker. You tried really hard to get rid of glued food that got stuck to the bottom of the pot, but regular dish soap did not work.
- A **warning light** that flickers when the pressure inside the pot rises.
- The **overpressure plug**, which helps reduce the pressure inside the pot if it builds up to dangerous and uncontainable levels.
- Finally, you will find pressure cooker pots most likely in **kitchen** environments or cupboards.

Pressure cooker of FND: a whistle-stop tour

Now imagine that all of us have our own pressure cooker. Let us suppose that each of the 12 elements of the pressure cooker represents a process in our mind or our body that is important in FND. An element may either be important in starting the FND ('emergence') or play a role in continuing the FND symptoms ('maintenance'). These elements have been identified in research studies

DOI: 10.4324/9781003308973-4

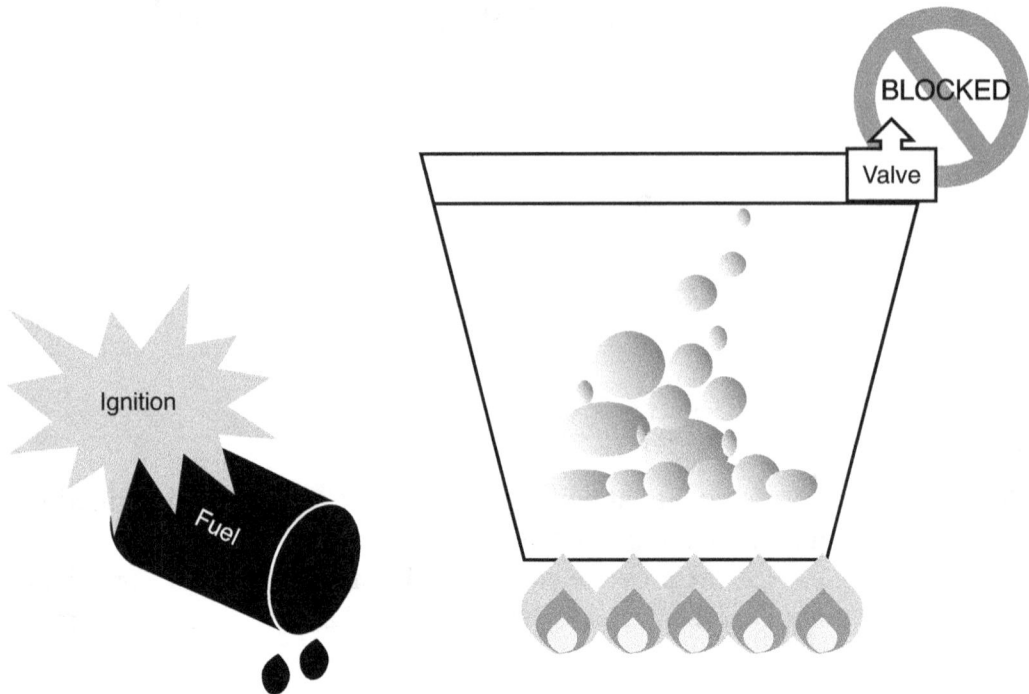

Figure 4.1 Simple version of a pressure cooker at home.

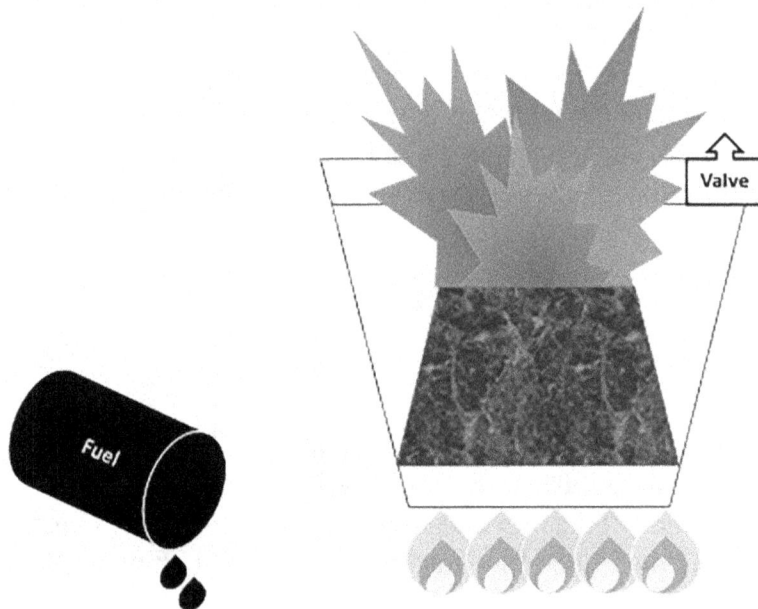

Figure 4.2 Pressure cooker explosion.

with people who experience FND and have also been observed by clinicians working in FND services. In the following section, let us take you on a whistle-stop tour of the Pressure Cooker Model (PCM). You will be shown the first element on its own ('the ignition'). Gradually, as more elements are added, you will see the Pressure Cooker Model built up using a series of graphics.

Element #1: ignition

The PCM starts with the **ignition**. This element represents past life events, early experiences, upbringing, interactions, and relationships that happened **prior to the onset of your first FND symptoms** and that make a person vulnerable towards developing FND at a later point in life.

Safety features
Parts of the pressure cooker that act like "buffers" to prevent or lower the risk of the pressure cooker exploding

Overpressure Plug
Is activated when the pressure in the pot gets too high and the cooker is at risk of exploding

Kitchen environment
The environment where we commonly find a pressure cooker

Cover
To ensure the boiling food does not spill over / keep the heat in the pot

Valve
To release steam from the pressure cooker that is generated during the cooking process

Warning light
The small light that starts flashing when the pressure in the pot becomes too high

Pot
The pot that holds the food contents during the cooking activity

Sticky left-over food
The food contents that got stuck to the bottom of the pot and take some time to scrub off and get unstuck

Ignition
Something that starts or sparks off a flame such as a lighter or hob igniter

Heat
The temperature of the flames, regulated by the temperature control on the hob

Fuel
A burning agent that keeps the flames going, after it has been sparked off, such as gas

Flames
The flames that warm the pressure cooker pot at the bottom

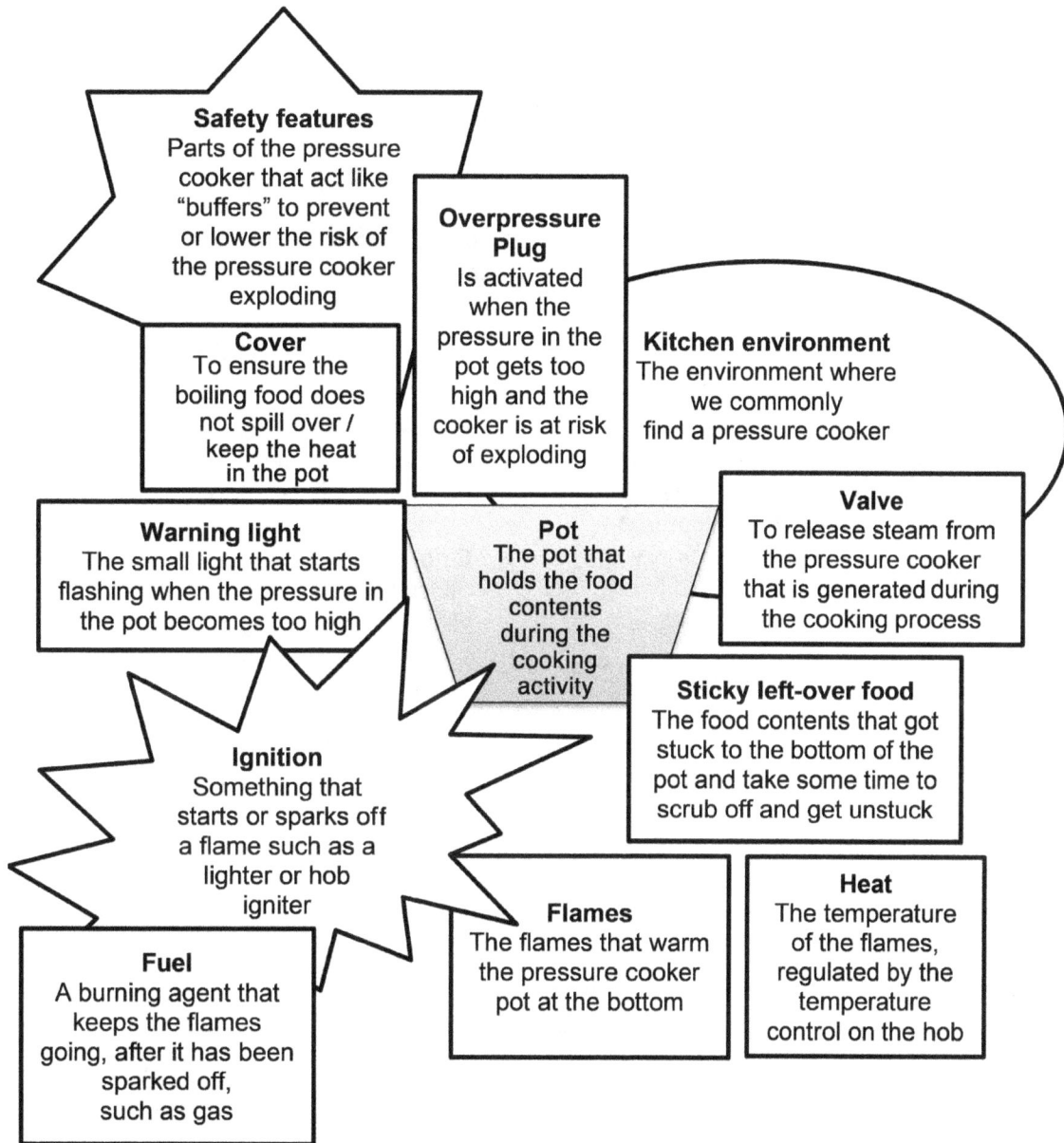

Figure 4.3 Twelve elements you would expect in a normal pressure cooker at home.

Think about challenging or traumatic events in early childhood, bullying during your teenage and school years, a problematic relationship in adulthood, a divorce, work stress, sickness bug, or a car accident requiring a hospital admission. Time-wise, the FND can emerge immediately after these events (after what is called the 'critical incident') or play a significant role in the more longer-term process of 'stewing and brewing' towards developing FND.

All these circumstances can cause a person to experience distress, panic, discomfort, or a state of feeling psychologically unsafe, which the person may not always be aware of. To cope, the person may resort to a process called **dissociation**, and FND may develop.

Not all people with FND report these adverse early life experiences. And people who report early adverse childhood experiences do not all go on to develop FND (but may develop other coping strategies that may be, or may be less, helpful). Although the relationship between adverse early experiences and FND is not a 100% association, it is significant enough for clinicians to often pick this up when working with people with FND. Figure 4.4 shows the location of the ignition element in the model.

Table 4.1 Different types of life events that make up the ignition element

"The past"		
Remote past Very far back in time, in childhood and adulthood		**Recent past** Still before the onset of your first FND symptoms, often right before the FND started
Adverse in nature Obvious traumatic life events	Adverse in nature May be "less obvious" / not always recognised as "clear-cut traumatic" but difficult, somehow different, unhelpful, or out of the ordinary relationships and living circumstances.	**"Critical incidents"** • A **gradual build-up** of challenging life circumstances. The FND shows up after "it all gets too much". • **One-off traumatic** or otherwise difficult event (e.g., accident, virus) which greatly challenges a person's existing coping survival strategies. • **Out-of-the-blue** experience of physical symptoms without any warning or clear trigger.
Childhood abuse experiences Domestic violence	Strict, harsh upbringing Emotional neglect Separation from parent(s) Conflicts and arguments	

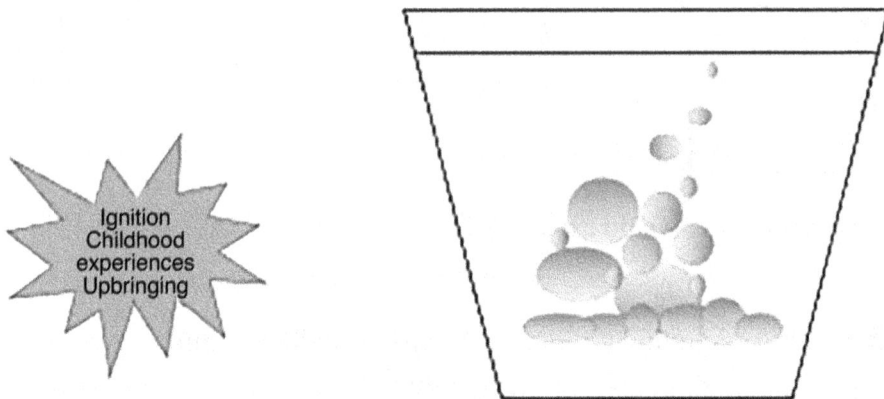

Figure 4.4 The ignition element in the Pressure Cooker Model.

Element #2: fuel

In contrast to the ignition, which highlights often more remote and 'pre-FND' life events and experiences, the fuel element refers to our **current triggers of FND**, which are the things, events, or feelings that spark off FND on a daily basis (see Figure 4.5). People with FND report many different types of triggers. Triggers that commonly set off FND symptoms include **physical** triggers

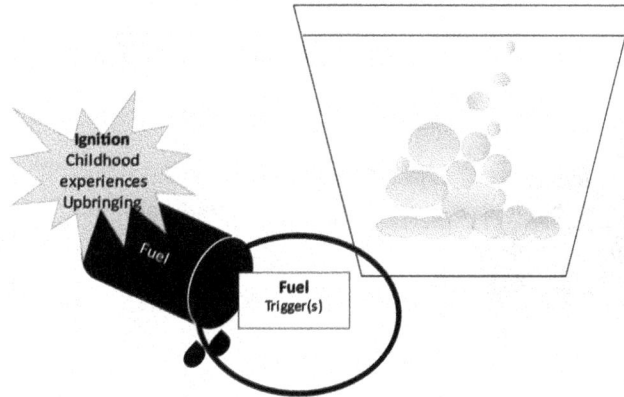

Figure 4.5 The fuel element in the Pressure Cooker Model.

(heat, noise, temperature changes), **environmental triggers** (trauma reminders in people with co-existing post-traumatic stress disorder), **psychological triggers** (worries and anxiety), **bodily triggers** (a funny feeling in your stomach, pain, or dizziness), **interpersonal triggers** associated with other people (family arguments, feeling uncared for), **re-triggers** by conversations with healthcare professionals that make a person feel disbelieved or uncared for and remind the person consciously or unconsciously about their own similar childhood experiences of not being believed or cared for, and many more! Chapter 7 will discuss each type of trigger in more detail and provide strategies to help you overcome them.

Element #3: flames

The flames underneath the pressure cooker represent the **contents of our thoughts and feelings**. Figure 4.6 shows you where you can find the flames in the Pressure Cooker Model.

People with FND experience many different types of thoughts, including **illness beliefs** ('I will always have FND for the rest of my life', 'FND is caused by the flu', 'FND is a condition that you need to learn to live with'); worries about **negative judgements from other people**, particularly about symptoms not being believed by other people, like healthcare professionals or family; unhelpful **thoughts around recovery** and the scary prospect of what the future holds without FND; **worries about setbacks** and what to do when this occurs, on top of **'regular worries'** about day-to-day life – think for example about relationships, housing, work, and financial affairs.

The flames element also reflects our **emotions**. Both people with and without FND experience a range of emotions, such as happiness, sadness, fear, anger, shame, embarrassment, and guilt. However, the features of emotions in people with FND can be different compared to those of people without FND. For example, people with FND may not always be able to describe their mental state or put it in the right words; confuse certain emotions such as anger and anxiety which physically may feel quite similar but are associated with different triggers, beliefs, and behaviours; or only feel the physical but not connect with the 'emotional' or 'experiential' aspects of emotions.

Element #4: heat

Flames can be very hot, flicker and look more yellow, or stop flickering and create a soft amber glow. You can have a lot of flames in a row or a tiny faint flame. A pressure cooker will have a temperature regulator that you can dial up or down. The **heat** element refers to the **strength** and **intensity level of an emotion** or, if it is hard to label the emotion, an unpleasant internal state of

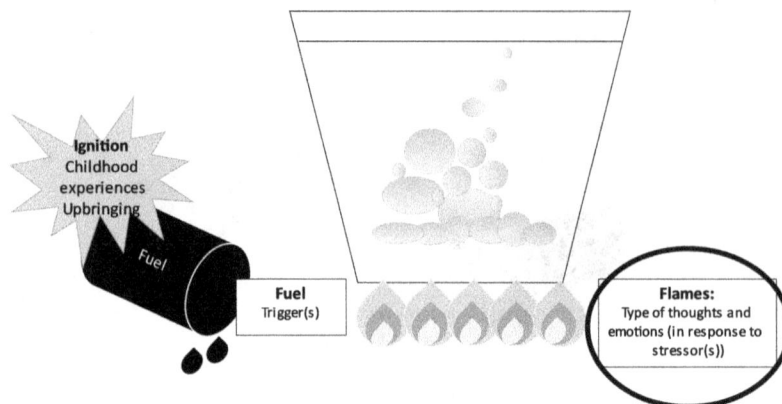

Figure 4.6 The flames element in the Pressure Cooker Model.

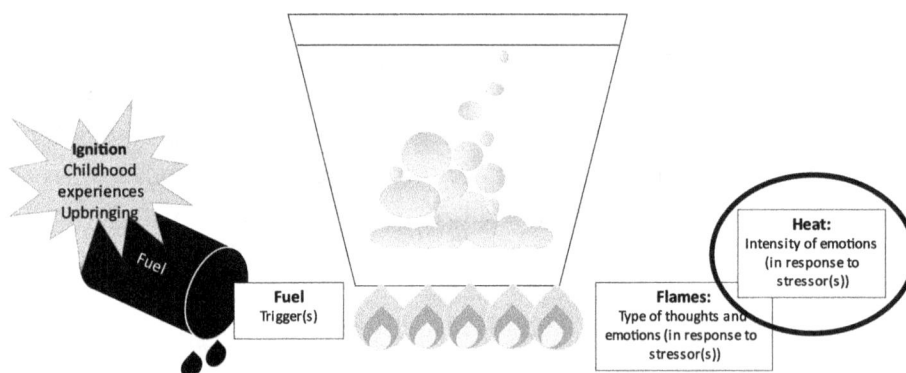

Figure 4.7 The heat element in the Pressure Cooker Model.

being (see Figure 4.7). Three main patterns of heat regulation have been observed in people with FND:

- **Low setting (or the freezing iceberg or ice block)**, representing **dissociation**. Some people with FND report a complete absence of emotion or stress. It is like the temperature setting of the flames is continuously dialled down without any increase in temperature in response to triggers that people without FND will normally find stressful, such as an argument.
- **High-low-high-low setting (flickering flame)**, representing **emotional dysregulation**. People with this setting experience frequent, rapid, and sometimes, extreme changes in the level of intensity and strength of their emotions. It is like the flame temperature regulator is out of control and changes from high to low to high to low in a short space of time.
- **High-to-low setting ('rise-and-fall' or combustion)** represents what happens to people with dissociative episodes. An emotion or internal state may gradually or instantly become very strong and subsequently sharply reduce. It is like the temperature is quickly dialled up to high heat and subsequently reduced for a period of time.

Element #5: sticky leftover food

Sticky leftover food is that stuff in the depths of the pressure cooker pot that has been sitting there glued for a long time and is hard to get unstuck. The **sticky leftover food** element (see Figure 4.8)

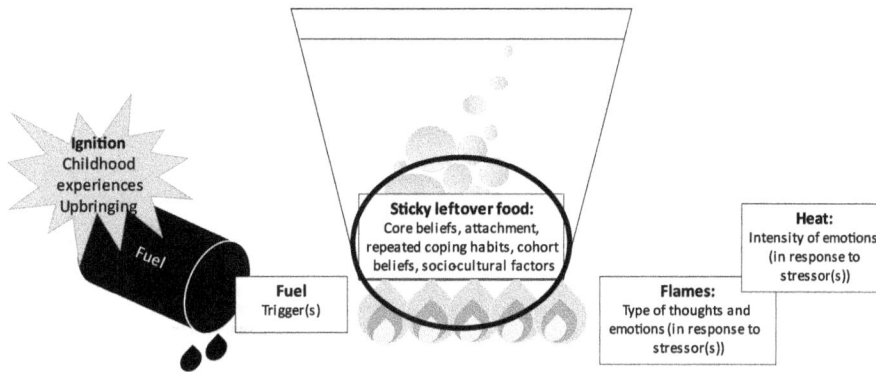

Figure 4.8 The sticky leftover food element in the Pressure Cooker Model.

is rooted in faraway childhood and adulthood life events which, amongst other things, are experiences that heavily shape our **belief system** and how we look at ourselves, other people, the world, and the future that awaits us; **attachment styles** in relationships and how much we trust or not trust other people; **self-esteem** and how we set **boundaries** in relationships with other people; and **childhood coping strategies**.

People with FND often report **three classic types of early coping strategies**:

- **'Bottling up'** or keeping yourself to yourself and not discussing your feelings with anyone else in a psychologically safe relationship.
- **'Just do'** or pushing on with activities.
- **'Cutting off'** or dissociating and disconnecting from your emotions.

All these coping strategies originate in childhood and, in the same way as 'real' sticky food glued for a long time at the bottom of a pressure cooker pot, have often been **repeated over many years into adulthood** and tend to be **quite rigid (but not impossible to change!)**.

As you can see in Figure 4.8, the bottom parts of the Pressure Cooker Model have now all been described. You can consider 'everything below the pot' as the things and events that you encounter daily. Some of us would call this collection of elements 'daily stresses' or simply 'daily life'. The bottom parts of the model are part of the human experience; we all deal with stresses, even if you do not feel it emotionally or in your body.

Later on, you will learn that, even though life throws us stresses and constant pressures, with some people unfortunately experiencing more of this than others, **it is what we do at the top of the Pressure Cooker Model** that, in the end, **will determine how we feel, think, act, behave, relate, and fare in life** in the context of these life events. But before we look at the top parts, let us first move on to the middle group of elements in the Pressure Cooker Model. These elements are strongly associated with the physical and body-related aspects of FND.

Element #6: pot

The **pot** is the physical outer shell of a pressure cooker. Its metal body is the first thing we see and acts as a reservoir holding the boiling food contents together. Some pots have strong, sturdy walls and are able to easily withstand increases in heat and pressure. Other pots have been exposed to conditions that may not be good for the pressure cooker in the long term. For example, the pot may not have been taken care of properly over time; the walls are chipped or scratched, show little hairline fractures, or have been broken, cracked, and patched up again, held together by materials that may not be able to protect it completely from breaking down.

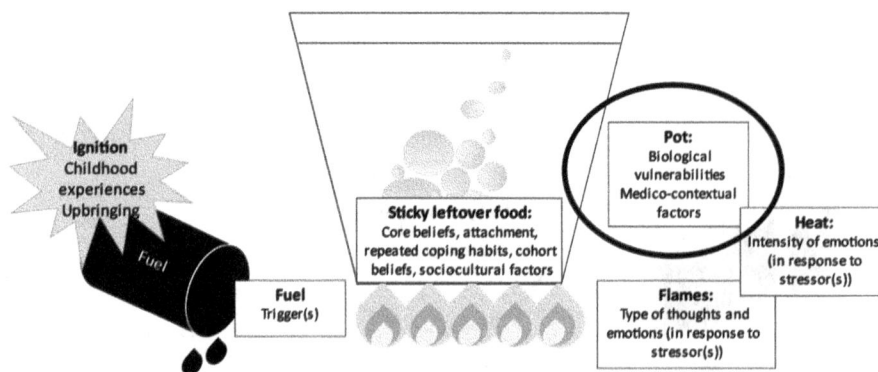

Figure 4.9 The pot element in the Pressure Cooker Model.

In the Pressure Cooker Model, the pot represents all the features that are associated with our own outer shell: the physical body (see Figure 4.9). A model of FND without elements that represent the body is not a proper model! FND is a mind–body condition: both psychological and physical factors need to be incorporated into a model for an accurate description of the condition.

The **FND SELF-CARE acronym** is a useful mnemonic that covers **biological and medical vulnerabilities** that have been consistently identified in the clinic and in research studies as important in the maintenance of FND. Think, for example, about issues with sleep, bladder and bowel functioning, overmedication, and deconditioning, to name a few common problems for people with FND.

Looking at the acronym can also help you and your family gauge the **level of severity and disability of the FND in your day-to-day functioning**, for example, what you can still do and not do for yourself (e.g. walking, personal care, preparing meals, taking care of your house), the type and amount of equipment and home adaptations you rely on, and assess any risks to you and your environment due to the FND, as well as provide an idea of the number of healthcare contacts and professionals involved in your care.

The FND SELF-CARE acronym does not claim to be the 'be-all and end-all' of 'everything physical' in FND, but it does a pretty good job at covering a diverse set of biological vulnerabilities and physical factors that have the potential to keep FND symptoms going if not addressed.

Element #7: warning light

The important role of **increased self-focused attention on physical symptoms in FND** has been highlighted in several major contemporary theories of FND (Brown, 2006; Brown & Reuber, 2016; Edwards et al., 2012) and is an integral part of physiotherapy treatment for FND (Nielsen et al., 2017). This concept is deemed so important because **having too much attention allocated to symptoms can feed the FND and keep it going**. It therefore makes sense 'to pay attention to attention' in the Pressure Cooker Model of FND. The idea of heightened self-focused attention is represented by the warning light element (see Figure 4.10).

We have just looked at the **bottom** and the **middle parts** of the Pressure Cooker Model. Let us now review the **top parts**. Remember what was spoken about earlier? The bottom parts are pretty much 'what happens in daily life', but the top parts are where you can make a big impact on the FND and difference for your quality of life.

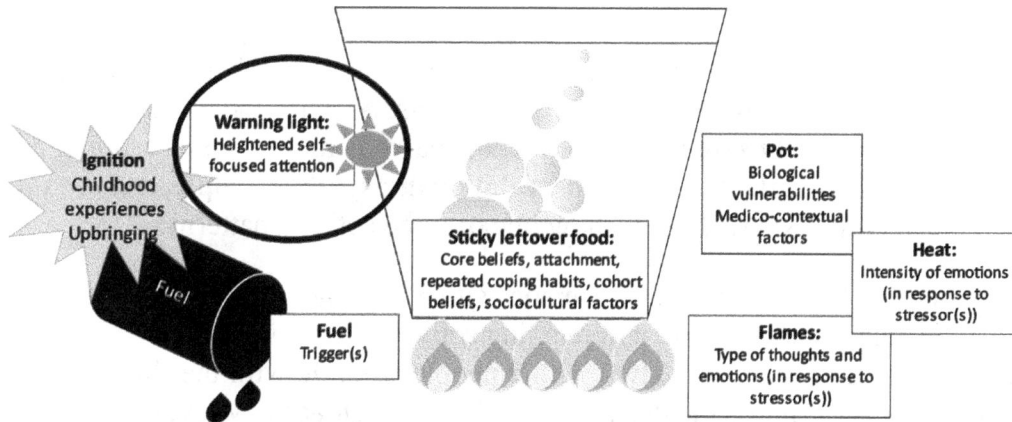

Figure 4.10 The warning light element in the Pressure Cooker Model.

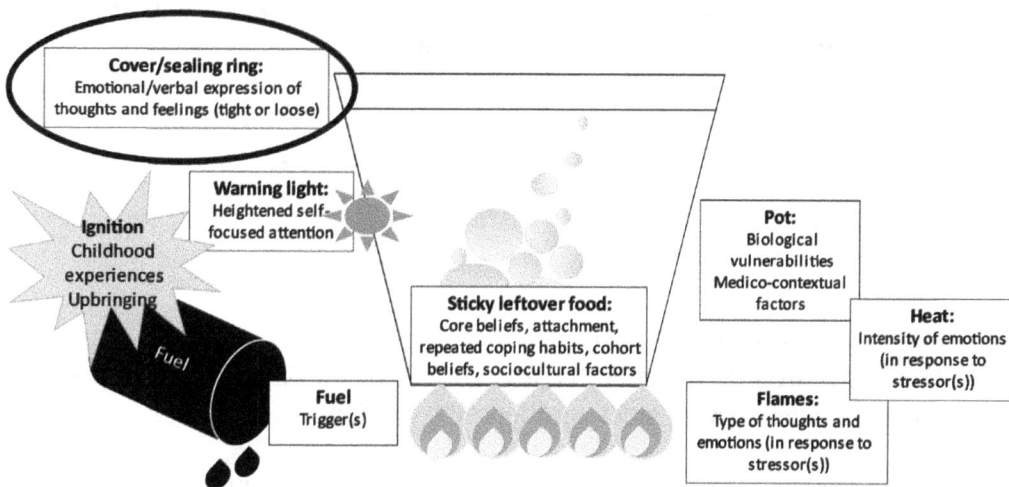

Figure 4.11 The cover element in the Pressure Cooker Model.

Element #8: cover

The **cover** on top of the pressure cooker represents our level of **verbal emotional expression in relationships** and is one of the most important elements in the treatment of FND (see Figure 4.11). Expressing emotions by speaking about them does not mean 'just talking' randomly about emotions. In contrast, it involves **talking about emotions with another person in a psychologically safe relationship** that creates the circumstances for you to feel comfortable expressing them on a regular basis to people that reciprocate and reflect those feelings back to you in healthy ways with appropriate boundaries. That is, in a nutshell, what an 'open cover' represents.

Researchers have documented a relationship between emotional expression and FND symptoms. In particular, **expressing emotions is associated with less FND** (Bowman & Markand, 1999; Alsaadi & Marquez, 2005) (REFs). The opposite situation is often encountered in the clinic: people with FND tend to keep themselves to themselves and exhibit a 'tight cover'. This coping strategy has often been repeated over many years and sometimes passed down from generation to generation.

Element #9: valve

Another crucial element you will find at the top of the Pressure Cooker Model is the valve (see Figure 4.12). This element represents our activity levels. As with the cover and 'talking about emotions' **in psychologically safe relationships**, the valve is more than just 'doing or not doing activities' and **intricately linked to emotions, relationships, other people,** and **the social world around us**. People with FND will often show one of three activity patterns:

- **Bust-after-boom** ('blocked' valve). A person with FND may not have any or have reduced access to enjoyable, social, leisure, and relaxing activities in their life.
- **Boom-and-bust** ('dysregulated' valve). Other people struggle with the 'highs' and the 'lows' of activity and never achieve the desired 'even keel'. High activity levels are alternated with times of no, or minimal, activity, and then the boom-and-bust cycle starts all over again. Over time, the recovery periods may become longer.
- **Boom** ('overused' valve). A subset of people is constantly 'on the go' and experience sky-high activity levels without stopping or regular rest breaks. However, there comes a time when a person becomes less able to manage long periods of relentless activity and the 'bubble bursts'. Boom is often the precursor stage for bust-after-boom.

Abnormal activity levels make it a lot harder for people to feel socially connected to other people in real life, experience a sense of social belonging to a community, and are a major risk of social isolation in FND.

Element #10: overpressure plug

We have arrived at the heart of the Pressure Cooker Model! **The overpressure plug represents a person's FND** (see Figure 4.13). Generally, a good way of thinking about FND symptoms is to divide them up into four categories (most people will experience a mixture):

- **Dissociative seizures:** switching off, absences, loss of awareness and responsiveness
- **Functional cognitive symptoms**: memory and concentration problems, brain fog

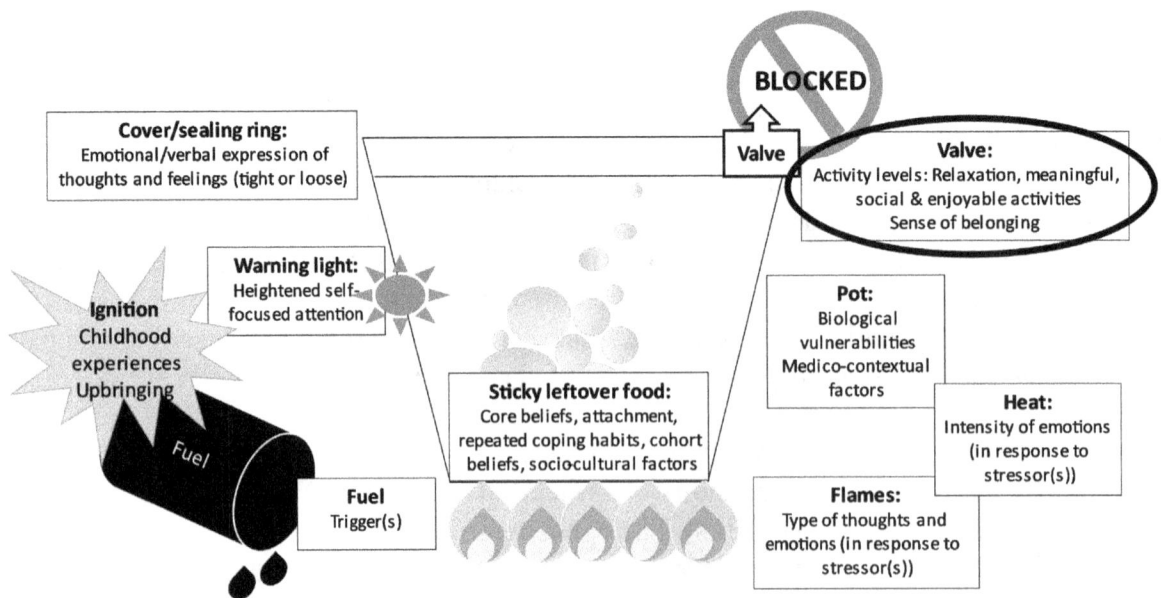

Figure 4.12 The valve element in the Pressure Cooker Model.

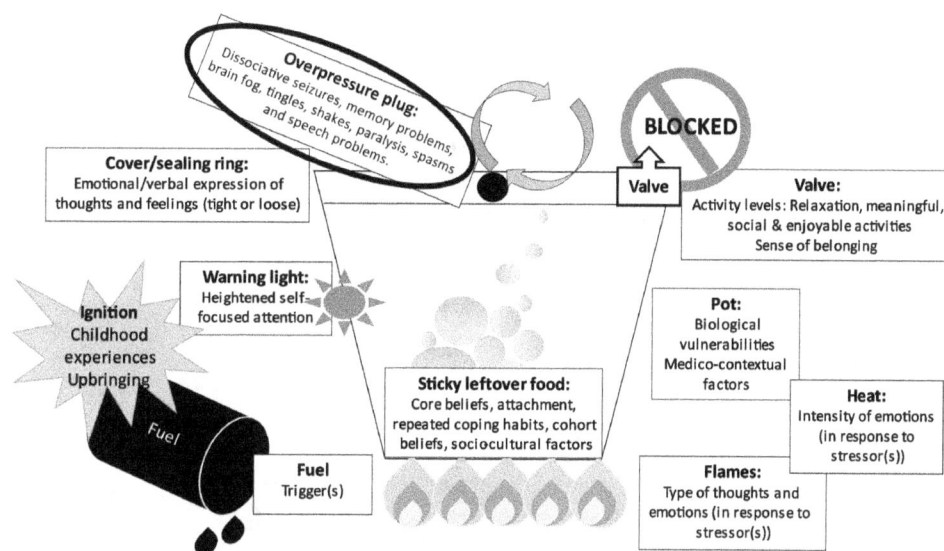

Figure 4.13 The overpressure plug element in the Pressure Cooker Model.

- **Sensory FND features**: altered, reduced, or loss of sensation
- **Motor-type FND**: shakes, weakness, spasms
- Although technically speaking subsumed under 'Motor-type FND', a fifth category concerns **speech problems**, a very common occurrence in FND: stuttering, halting speech, and even muteness.

It is also very common for people with FND to experience a specific combination of a tight cover and simultaneously a blocked, dysregulated, or overused valve. What is more important is that working on **opening a tight cover and regulating the valve decreases the risk of FND**!

Another valid point: the Pressure Cooker Model does not make much distinction between people with and without FND. Did you know that **people without FND have an overpressure plug too?** That includes partners, parents, children, carers, friends, and healthcare professionals. As you may recall, Chapter 2 explored coping mechanisms that **bring down unpleasant feelings very quickly and effectively**.

A dissociative seizure is one example; **providing care and reassurance, either 'too much' or 'too little',** is another example. Although the manifestations may seem entirely different, **the underlying process is exactly the same**: in the end, it all boils down to reducing, regulating, and managing emotions, distress, unpleasant internal states, and arousal.

Element #11: kitchen

As much as mind–body connections are central to FND (the 'psychological' and 'bio' bits), a person with FND does not exist in a social vacuum but is surrounded by a complex social world (see Figure 4.14).

This intricate social web of people represents the kitchen element in the Pressure Cooker Model (see Figure 4.15).

Why is it important to look at the environment in FND? Why bother? Is not the person with FND whom you need to focus the treatment on?

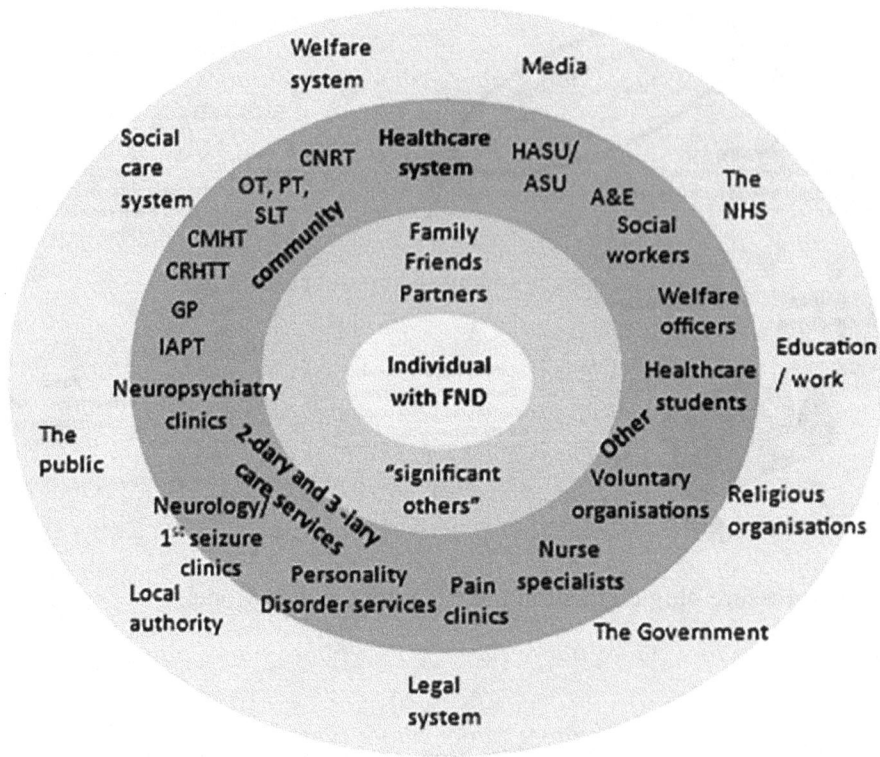

Figure 4.14 Complex web of relationships with people and systems in FND.

Note: CNRT = community neuro rehabilitation team; OT = occupational therapist; PT = physiotherapist; SLT = speech and language therapist; CMHT = community mental health team; CRHTT = crisis resolution and home treatment team; GP = general practitioner; IAPT = improving access to psychological therapies; A&E = accidents and emergencies; (H)ASU = (hyper-)acute stroke unit; NHS = National Health Service.

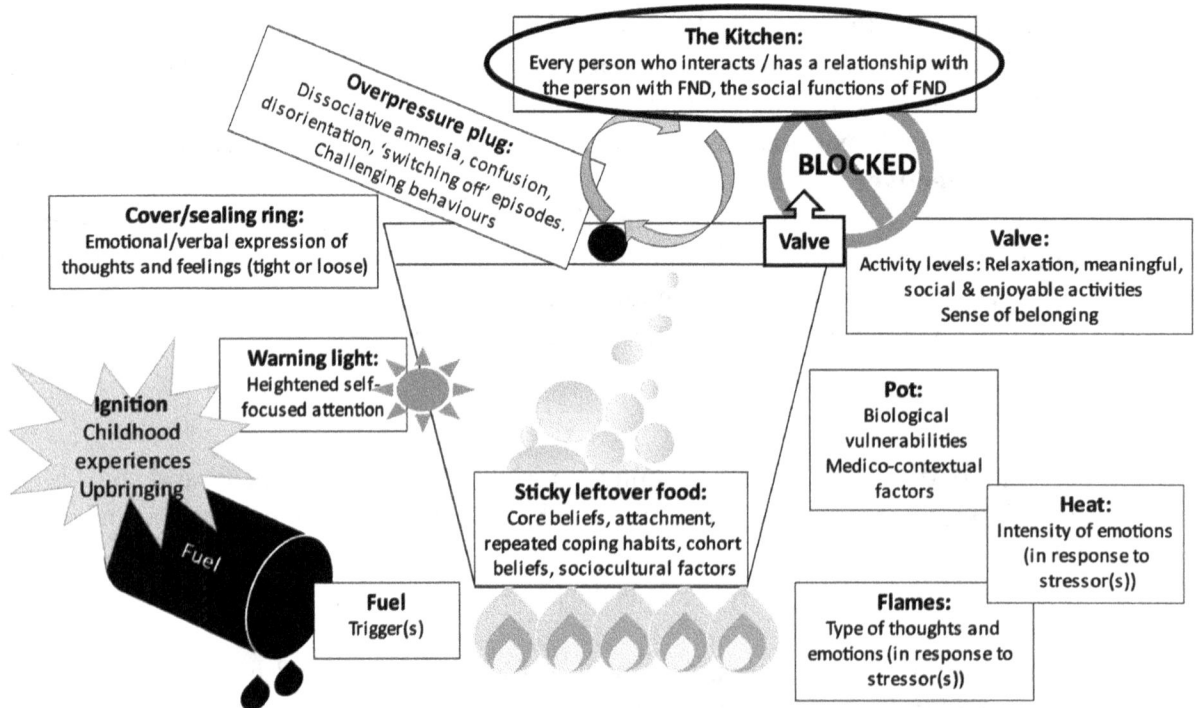

Figure 4.15 The kitchen element in the Pressure Cooker Model.

There are plenty of reasons, but for now, just remember two important points:

1. FND has social functions: it is not a one-way, but a two-way, street.

People with FND are sometimes told truly inappropriate things by other people. The number of times that people report being accused of 'faking symptoms', 'doing it for attention', 'putting it on' (in front of other people), and so on is quite baffling and suggests that the person with FND is somehow doing something bad to themselves and to the environment. But it is not a one-way street at all!

The Pressure Cooker Model believes that FND is maintained by the interactions, interpersonal dynamics, responses, and communication patterns between people with and without FND. This idea is central to understanding:

- Where the FND comes from ('emergence')
- Why it keeps on going ('maintenance')
- How to recover from the condition ('restoration')

In the Pressure Cooker Model, 'everyone has FND' – the person with FND 'carries' the symptoms, but everyone contributes to maintaining the FND and has a unique responsibility for FND recovery. The model is built in such a way that everyone can use it, whether you have FND or not. In fact, it is highly recommended that everyone involved in the person's life uses the Pressure Cooker Model, most definitely partners, family, friends, and healthcare professionals.

2. Healthcare experiences . . .

. . . are a really important topic in FND. As you can see from Figure 4.14, the healthcare world comprises a big chunk of interactions for people with FND. Most professionals in the field agree that healthcare experiences have been nothing short of terrible for quite a few people with FND. The Pressure Cooker Model goes a step further than just acknowledging this difficult reality and believes that these interactions are detrimental for maintaining FND and calls for treatment of both the person with FND and people close to the person – **including healthcare professionals**.

The 12th element: pressure cooker 'safety features'

It makes sense that theories of FND focus on the stuff that is not going well. After all, if you feel unwell with symptoms that greatly impact on your relationships and day-to-day life, it is important to figure out what underlying mechanisms cause these problems in order to be able to help you overcome FND.

However, with so much focus on pathology, illness, symptoms, and 'what is wrong', you would almost forget about a person's protective factors and 'what is going well' in FND recovery! As humans, we are not defined by difficulty only; we equally have positive qualities going for us that we need to connect with. This is an often-forgotten area in FND rehab.

Luckily, the Pressure Cooker Model does something more than just thinking about difficulties. The **safety features** highlight your strengths, your positive qualities, and the protective factors that you can draw on during rehab. It is not only important to shift from an individual to an environmental perspective in FND; it is equally important to describe a more balanced view of strengths and difficulties of a person (see Chapter 1, 'So what makes (psychological) therapy effective in FND?' for a range of important safety features – the list is not exhaustive!).

Tying it all together

Now that you have learned about each element, let us put them all in the Pressure Cooker Model to see what that looks like (see Figure 4.16). Do you remember the 'domestic' pressure cooker

Safety features
Your protective factors in treatment.
What makes you feel psychologically safe already? What positive qualities can help you in your recovery from FND?

Cover
Verbal expression of emotions to another person on a regular basis in a psychologically safe relationship.

Overpressure Plug
Your FND symptoms
FND "aftereffects" like muscle pain and fatigue
Safety behaviours

Kitchen environment
Your relationships with other people including partner, family and healthcare professionals. The social functions of the FND

Warning light
The amount of attention someone pays to the FND symptoms which feeds the FND and keeps it going.

Pot
Everything to do with your body and physical functioning

Valve
Activity levels and sense of social belonging to a community or a group of people.

Ignition
Remote and more recent adverse or traumatic life events in childhood and adulthood – prior to the onset of FND.

Flames
Your thoughts and emotions including worries and believing that other people don't believe your symptoms. A psychological state that you cannot exactly describe but that feels very unpleasant, uncomfortable or distressing.

Sticky leftover food
Coping strategies that you used in childhood, for example, pushing on, keeping yourself to yourself, or dissociation. Strong ingrained beliefs about yourself, others, the world and your future.

Fuel
Current triggers of FND that happen on a regular basis.

Heat
The strength and intensity level of an emotion or an unpleasant state of being.

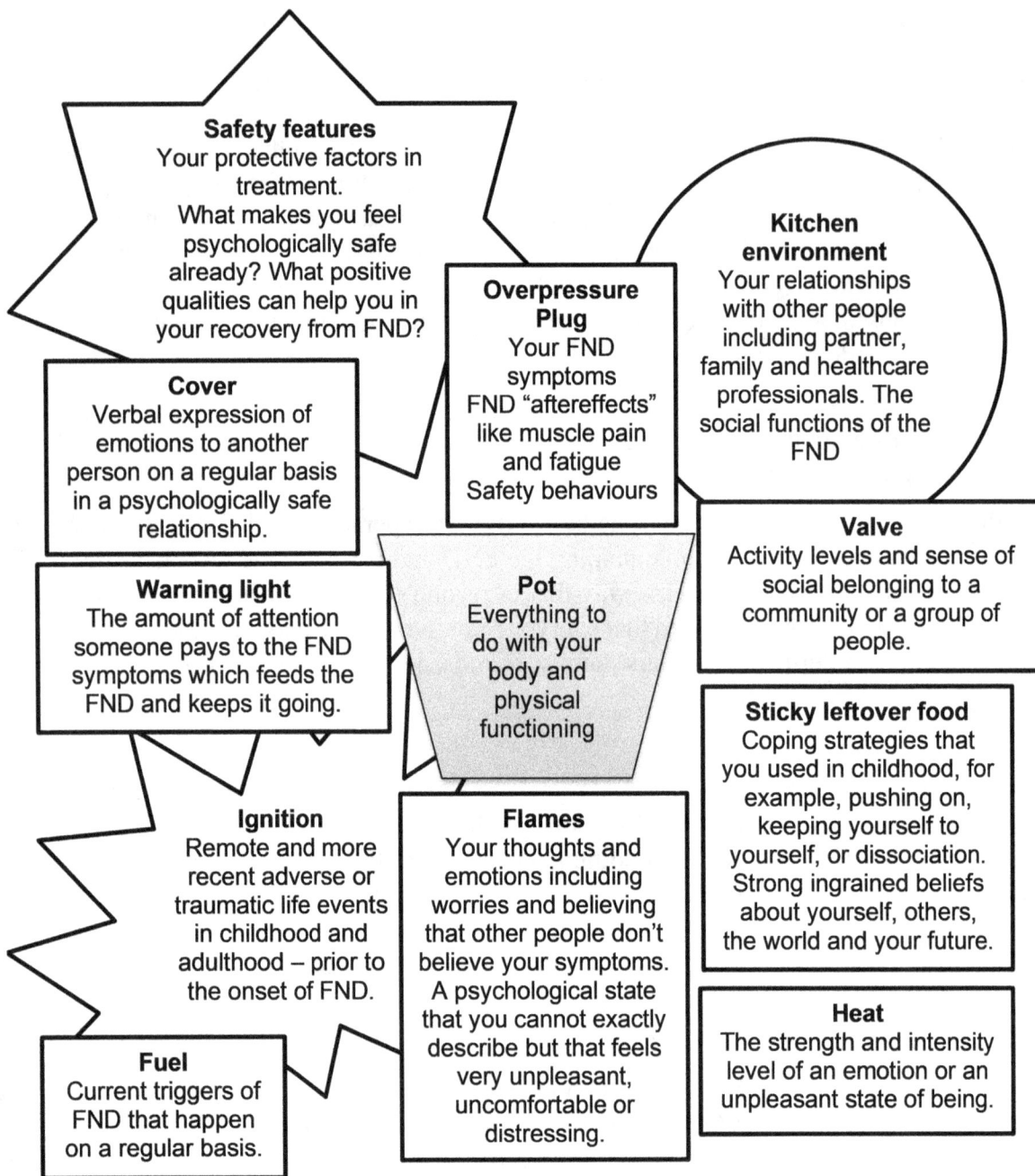

Figure 4.16 The 12 elements of the Pressure Cooker Model of FND.

that you can find in people's homes? Briefly think back of Figure 4.3. Now imagine that each element of the regular pressure cooker is replaced with elements that represent an important part of FND.

A biopsychosocial definition of FND: tying it all together with the Pressure Cooker Model formulation

Now that you have learned about the biological, psychological, and social elements of the Pressure Cooker Model, the question arises: How do all these elements work together to become FND? What are the pressure cooker processes that explain FND? Figure 4.17 shows a brief story that can help with understanding the mechanics of FND.

Have you seen or used a pressure cooker before? Imagine a pressure cooker. It has a pot, a cover, a valve to release steam, a warning light for when the pressure builds up. There are flames under it that need fuel. It might look like this:

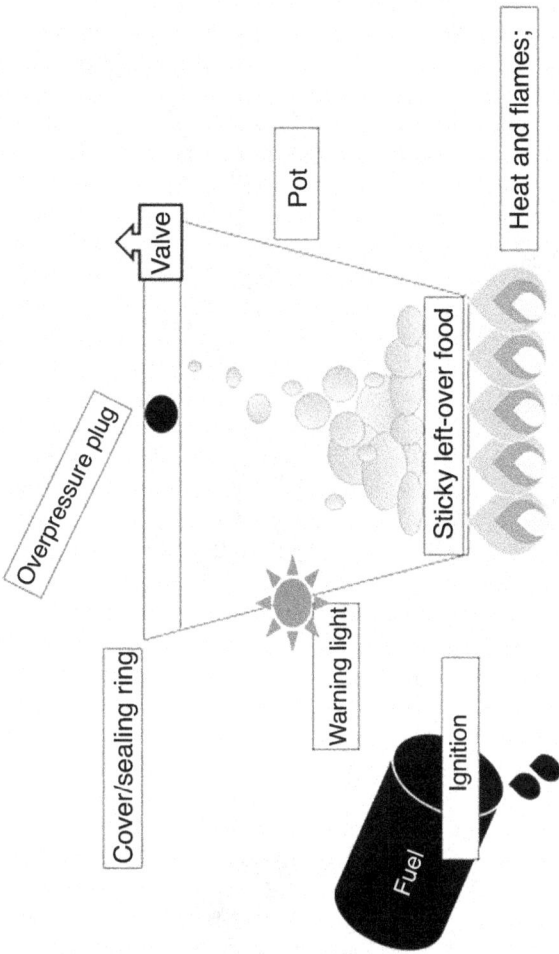

Imagine a pressure cooker, now with a tight cover and a blocked valve. What happens? (The pressure cooker will explode!)

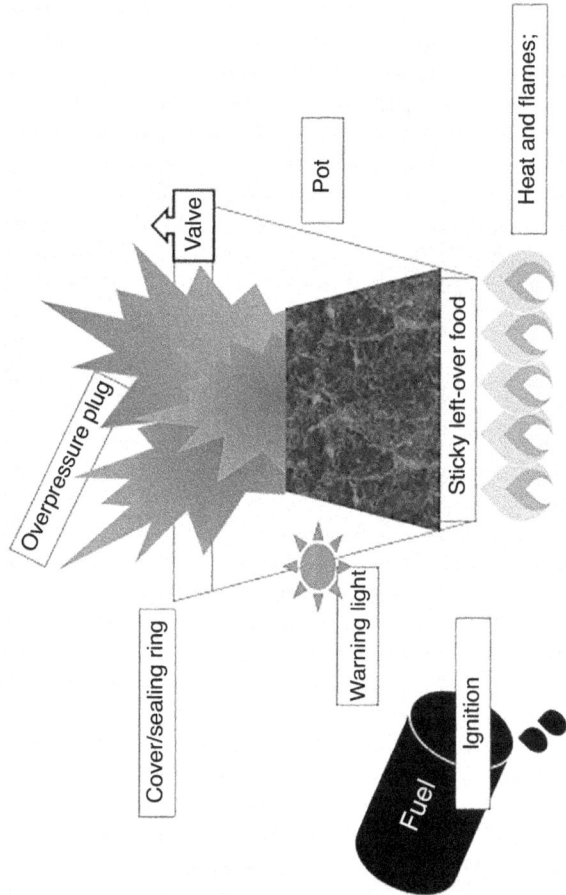

Figure 4.17 The mechanics of FND in the Pressure Cooker Model.

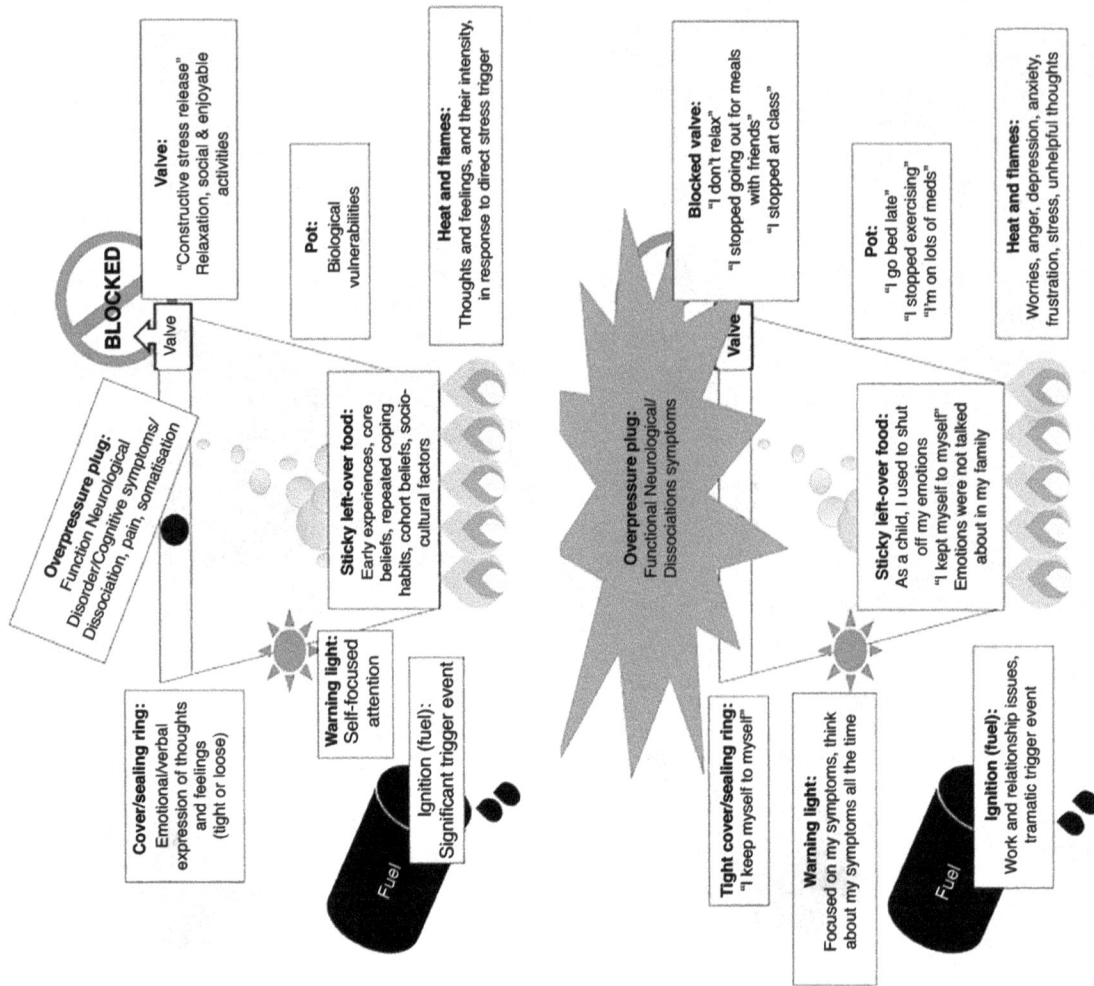

Biological, psychological, and social factors all play an important role in FND. Imagine that every part of the pressure cooker stands for something important in FND, like this:

Valve: "Constructive stress release" Relaxation, social & enjoyable activities

BLOCKED

Pot: Biological vulnerabilities

Heat and flames: Thoughts and feelings, and their intensity, in response to direct stress trigger

Overpressure plug: Function Neurological Disorder/Cognitive symptoms/ Dissociation, pain, somatisation

Sticky left-over food: Early experiences, core beliefs, repeated coping habits, cohort beliefs, socio-cultural factors

Cover/sealing ring: Emotional/verbal expression of thoughts and feelings (tight or loose)

Warning light: Self-focused attention

Ignition (fuel): Significant trigger event

Fuel

You have just been diagnosed with FND. Maybe you have had quite a lot going on in your life, including FND, and now you feel unwell.

From an early age on, you may have had a tight cover and do not really talk about or release your feelings in other helpful ways. You also have a blocked valve. You dropped many hobbies and do not see your friends that often anymore. With a tight cover and blocked valve, where does all your pressure go? Your pressure cooker may look like this:

Blocked valve: "I don't relax" "I stopped going out for meals with friends" "I stopped art class"

Pot: "I go bed late" "I stopped exercising" "I'm on lots of meds"

Heat and flames: Worries, anger, depression, anxiety, frustration, stress, unhelpful thoughts

Overpressure plug: Functional Neurological/ Dissociations symptoms

Sticky left-over food: As a child, I used to shut off my emotions "I kept myself to myself" Emotions were not talked about in my family

Tight cover/sealing ring: "I keep myself to myself"

Warning light: Focused on my symptoms, think about my symptoms all the time

Ignition (fuel): Work and relationship issues, tramatic trigger event

Fuel

Figure 4.17 Continued

References

Alsaadi, T. M., & Marquez, A. V. (2005). Psychogenic nonepileptic seizures. *American Family Physician*, *72*(5), 849–856.

Bowman, E. S., & Markand, O. N. (1999). The contribution of life events to pseudoseizure occurrence in adults. *Bulletin of the Menninger Clinic*, *63*(1), 70.

Brown, R. J. (2006). Medically unexplained symptoms: A new model. *Psychiatry*, *5*(2), 43–47.

Brown, R. J., & Reuber, M. (2016). Towards an integrative theory of psychogenic non-epileptic seizures (PNES). *Clinical Psychology Review*, *47*, 55–70.

Edwards, M. J., Adams, R. A., Brown, H., Parees, I., & Friston, K. J. (2012). A Bayesian account of 'hysteria'. *Brain*, *135*(11), 3495–3512.

Nielsen, G., Buszewicz, M., Stevenson, F., Hunter, R., Holt, K., Dudziec, M., Ricciardi, L., Marsden, J., Joyce, E., & Edwards, M. J. (2017). Randomised feasibility study of physiotherapy for patients with functional motor symptoms. *Journal of Neurology, Neurosurgery and Psychiatry*, *88*(6), 484–490.

5 How adverse life experiences can create a vulnerability towards developing FND

Ignition (layer 1)

Trigger warning

In this chapter, we will explore the relationship between adverse events in a person's life **before the FND** and how these experiences may relate to **the development of FND later in life**.

From an emotional point of view, the contents of this chapter may be difficult for you to read and re-trigger unpleasant thoughts and feelings that you may have buried or avoided for a long time. You may not want to read this chapter at all, read only parts of it, read it with someone you trust and who cares about you, or maybe return to reading it later.

All these options are completely understandable, acceptable, and appropriate.

Not reading Chapter 5 will not stop you from learning about FND. Take as much time as you need for whatever you decide to do. If you do decide to go ahead and read this chapter and it brings up all kinds of difficult thoughts and feelings and it all becomes unbearable to the point that you feel you cannot cope or you are thinking of hurting yourself, *please tell someone you trust, like a partner, family member, friend, or healthcare professional, so you can get the right support*.

The goal of Chapter 5 is not to cause you psychological harm or make you feel bad. It aims to help you understand and make sense of the relationship between difficult life events and FND (see Figure 5.1).

Ignition

The ignition element describes adverse life events that created a vulnerability towards developing FND. Generally, there are two types of ignition events: **remote** and **critical incidents**. Remote events can be viewed as 'setting events', the events that set the stage for FND to develop. Setting events do not always result in FND, but they can be powerful determinants of how we fare later in life, particularly how we cope with our emotions and the types of life experiences we encounter or seek out.

Remote events: adverse early experiences in childhood

You may have noticed that the ignition is 'social' in nature. The events are interpersonal and associated with other people affecting relationships in negative ways. The examples from Figure 5.1 fall into the following broad categories:

- **Conflict**, arguments, and strife in early relationships and family environments – perhaps in combination with an intermittently loving and caring environment, causing confusion about relationships.
- **Separation or losses** of important people, such as parents or other caregivers, including 'psychological losses' and grief in the context of caring for an ill parent (psychologically 'losing' a parent), even if temporary.
- **Overinvolvement** and 'enmeshed' relationship patterns within the family home.
- **Underinvolvement** of parents who were distant and did not tend to emotional needs.

DOI: 10.4324/9781003308973-5

Ignition

Addiction problems in a parent

Military or combat trauma "Shell shock"

Lots of house moves: upheaval and loss of friendships

Having experienced (unexplained) physical symptoms, pain or psychological difficulties / self-harm as a child

Physical, neurological, or mental illness: personal, parent or in a close relative

Learning / neurodevelopmental difficulties in childhood and the social consequences, e.g. parental expectations, bullying

Abuse
Physical
Emotional
Sexual
Assault
Domestic violence
Harassment
Stalking

Sibling rivalry, differential treatment between siblings

Work, study or school pressures – including parental pressures or expectations and overly involved or overprotected caregivers.

School bullying

Conflict-ridden upbringing with arguments / discord, strife, custody battles

Being taken into foster care, separation from the family home

Hospitalisation, surgery, medical interventions, invasive procedures, or hospital care in adulthood or childhood with attachment break

Oppressive, strict, harsh households with physical discipline and emotional neglect

Emotional neglect, unavailable parents, punishment and invalidation of emotions

Loss, bereavement separation, divorce, no contact from a parent in childhood

Due to circumstances, having done a lot of caring for adults or siblings as a child

Tight cover: Keep self to self

Overpressure Plug: FND / dissociation

Valve: Pushing on

Adverse early experiences in childhood that made me vulnerable towards developing FND **Insecure attachment**

Timeline

Things that keep the FND going

Critical incident or gradual build-up of stresses that triggered FND

Sticky leftover food:

Negative core beliefs (Belief system)
Low self-esteem
"I'm worthless"
"I'm not good enough"
"I'm different"
"People will let me down"
"People will abandon / reject me"

Early childhood Survival coping strategies
Learned adaptive coping strategies in response to difficult circumstances
"Keep myself to myself"
"Just push on"
"Dissociation"

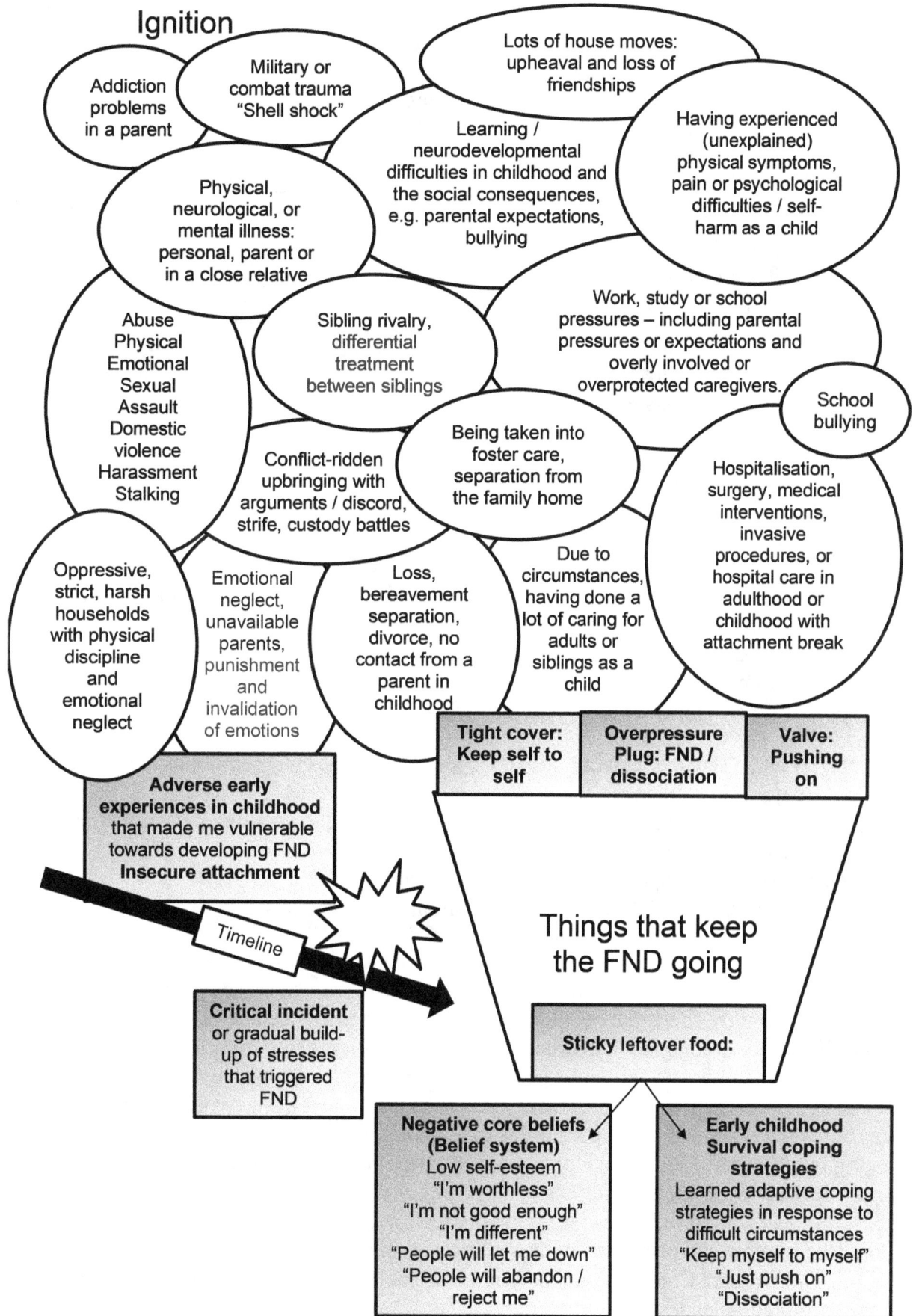

Figure 5.1 Life events reported by people with FND in the clinic or as part of research studies, and their relationship to FND.

- Various forms of **abuse**, including physical, sexual, emotional, and bullying.
- An **invalidating** parent denying your emotions or experiencing their own problems with emotion regulation.
- A **strict, harsh upbringing** without much attention for emotion. Not feeling seen or heard by your parents – emotional neglect.

Awareness of these historic interpersonal experiences should strongly compel us to pay attention to the current social and relationship aspects of FND.

Remote events: adverse experiences later in adulthood

Not only do people with FND often report adverse events in childhood, but similar events are also frequently described in adulthood. Some people have experienced a lot of traumatic events in their life, from childhood onwards and continuing into adulthood. When people have experienced a lifetime of traumatic events or pervasive difficulties in relationships over a long period of time, we call this 'complex trauma'.

A note on complex trauma

Complex trauma is sometimes interchangeably used with the term **'personality disorder'**. Research studies have reported that a subset of people with FND is diagnosed with personality disorder, for example, borderline or dependent personality disorder (Binzer et al., 1997). People with borderline features may present with emotions that quickly go up and down, have difficulties in relationships, and do things that can hurt them. People with dependent features may rely heavily on other people and elicit a lot of care from their environment.

A diagnosis of personality disorder may sometimes help:

- Get **clarity** and a **sense of closure** on why a person struggles with emotions and relationships in day-to-day life.
- People receive **appropriate and timely access** to specialist services that offer longer-term therapy to help them overcome their difficulties.
- Provide an avenue for support with **helpful medications**.
- Communication as it is a **'shared language'** among professionals.

However, the label itself can be **stigmatising** and may suggest that there is something wrong with a person's personality. Society tends to view personality as **fixed**, permanent, and perhaps hard to change.

If you think about the fact that people with FND often experience **low self-worth** (Petrochilos et al., 2020), you can imagine that a diagnosis of personality disorder on top of that can further confirm that low self-worth and make people feel worse about themselves. Furthermore, people who have been diagnosed with personality disorder have often been through very difficult life events and not always had the opportunities to learn helpful coping strategies. These people end up **being labelled for having developed coping strategies** that helped them survive in the past but may now have lost their usefulness. If anything, these people are survivors that simply used the best possible coping strategies for highly distressing life experiences.

Therefore, another and better way of describing personality disorder is using the term **'complex trauma'**. The Pressure Cooker Model does not use labels but instead incorporates many features that are part of complex trauma.

Critical incident

Remote events can set the stage for FND to develop. Let us look at what **critical incidents** are, and their relevance to FND. Table 5.1 shows you what distinguishes the two types of events.

Table 5.1 Crucial differences between remote events and critical incidents in the Pressure Cooker Model

Remote events	Critical incident
Early childhood	Later in life
Often far removed in time from the FND	More recent event and closer to the onset of FND
"Longstanding": often a series of events and associated with relationships	"Acute" or "One-off": often a specific event
Give rise to core beliefs we hold about ourselves, other people, the world, and our future.	Does not give rise to core beliefs but can re-trigger them and start a "maintenance cycle"

People with FND often report a critical incident immediately before the onset of FND symptoms and that somehow appears to have 'sparked off' the FND. For example:

Critical incidents that are biological or physical

- Accident or fall
- Surgery or an invasive medical procedure
- Physical illness, like a nasty viral infection, flu, or cold
- Pain
- Physical injuries – both minor and major
- Health scare in yourself or people close to you
- Vaccination experience that caused anxiety-provoking or unexpected physical symptoms
- Adverse event associated with medication

Critical incidents that are psychosocial

- **Trauma**: assault, domestic violence, exploitation by partners, witnessing trauma, a scary and life-changing event that threatens your livelihood and well-being
- New job or **job difficulties** (e.g. bullying, loss or rejection, overloaded with work in the presence of reduced assertiveness, ongoing work stress), school exams with no access to stress releasing strategies
- Lot of **caring** commitments in the family home or a job in healthcare
- People that have hurt you in the past are **suddenly back in your life**, seek contact, or live close to you
- A **new loss**: relationship break-up, social circle falling apart, losing friendships, bereavement, miscarriage, childbirth (a loss of your old life without a child)
- **Relationship difficulties**, dysfunctional family dynamics and conflicts
- **Unspeakable dilemma** (i.e. holding onto a 'secret' that may have repercussions and psychological consequences if released, including rejection and ostracizing – explored in Chapter 6)

Sticky leftover food

The sticky leftover food may appear as a mixed bag of psychological processes that is not much different from ignition. Both elements have the following in common: their **origins in childhood** and their **major impact on current functioning and relationships**.

The sticky leftover food looks at:

- How these early experiences **have impacted on our belief system** and **attachment to people**.
- The close relationship between **childhood 'survival' strategies** and **how distress is coped with as an adult**. Childhood and adulthood psychological coping strategies tend to be quite similar over time.

Our belief system

A pressure cooker pot is a 'container' that holds and boils food. Now, imagine that there are different layers of food piled up inside the pressure cooker pot. In the following section, we will discuss three types of beliefs (for more reading, please see Beck, 1967; Beck & Greenberg, 1984).

Sticky-sticky food: core beliefs

This food is stuck to the bottom of the pot and is difficult to get unstuck unless you actively scrub it on multiple occasions with 'heavy-duty' cleaning products and props. Even after the deep clean, some residual sticky food may still be left, or you see an imprint that will need some further work in the future. We can view the **sticky-sticky food deep in the pot** as our **core beliefs**. Core beliefs are deeply ingrained beliefs that we hold about ourselves, other people, the world, and our future (see Table 5.2). We are often not aware of our core beliefs because they are hidden and not always available to conscious awareness. In psychological therapy, you tend to stumble on them later rather than sooner; they take time to be discovered and reveal themselves. Core beliefs are useful

Table 5.2 Examples of positive and their 'counterpart' negative core beliefs

Positive core beliefs	Negative core beliefs
- I'm capable, I'm confident. - I can do this, I'm good at a lot of things.	- I'm a failure, I'm a bad person.
- I'm worthy – just as worthy as other people. - I believe in myself.	- I'm worthless, less than others – I'm inferior.
- I'm lovable, likable, I matter. - There may be people who may not like me but that's normal: not everyone will share my values.	- I'm unlovable, unwanted. - I don't matter.
- I'm fine as I am. - Everyone is different! I am different and difference is good and gives colour to the world.	- I'm different [therefore less than others].
- I deserve love and good things.	- I'm not deserving of x, y and z. - I don't deserve anything
- Others will help me. - I can choose who I will trust.	- You can't trust anyone, people will just disappoint you.
- The world is an interesting place. - I'm safe now.	- The world is unsafe.
- I can make tomorrow better. - I can see opportunities everywhere around me.	- My future is bleak.

to have because they help us make sense of the world around us quickly and efficiently. They are like shortcuts to our thinking.

Chunky and liquidy food: rules for living

If, from the very sticky food, we go up one layer, we end up with the somewhat-looser food consisting of chunks that bubble up at the surface of your pot. These looser chunks represent our **'rules for living'**. These are ways of living and daily psychological strategies that we adopt in response to our core beliefs.

For example, one of our core beliefs may be 'I am imperfect'. This is a harsh belief to deal with. But we can manage and neutralise the psychological effects of this belief by applying a rule for living that protects our feelings. We can say, 'If I work in a perfectionist and very precise manner and ensure that I am not making mistakes, then I will see myself as less imperfect/more perfect'.

Negative automatic thoughts (NATs)

NATs are the most superficial layer in our belief system and are represented by the flames element under the Pressure Cooker Model. NATs are 'surface-level' and easy-to-identify thoughts that pop up in our minds, and pretty much the first set of beliefs that we often become aware of, before we become aware of the other, more hidden beliefs in the pot (see Figure 5.2).

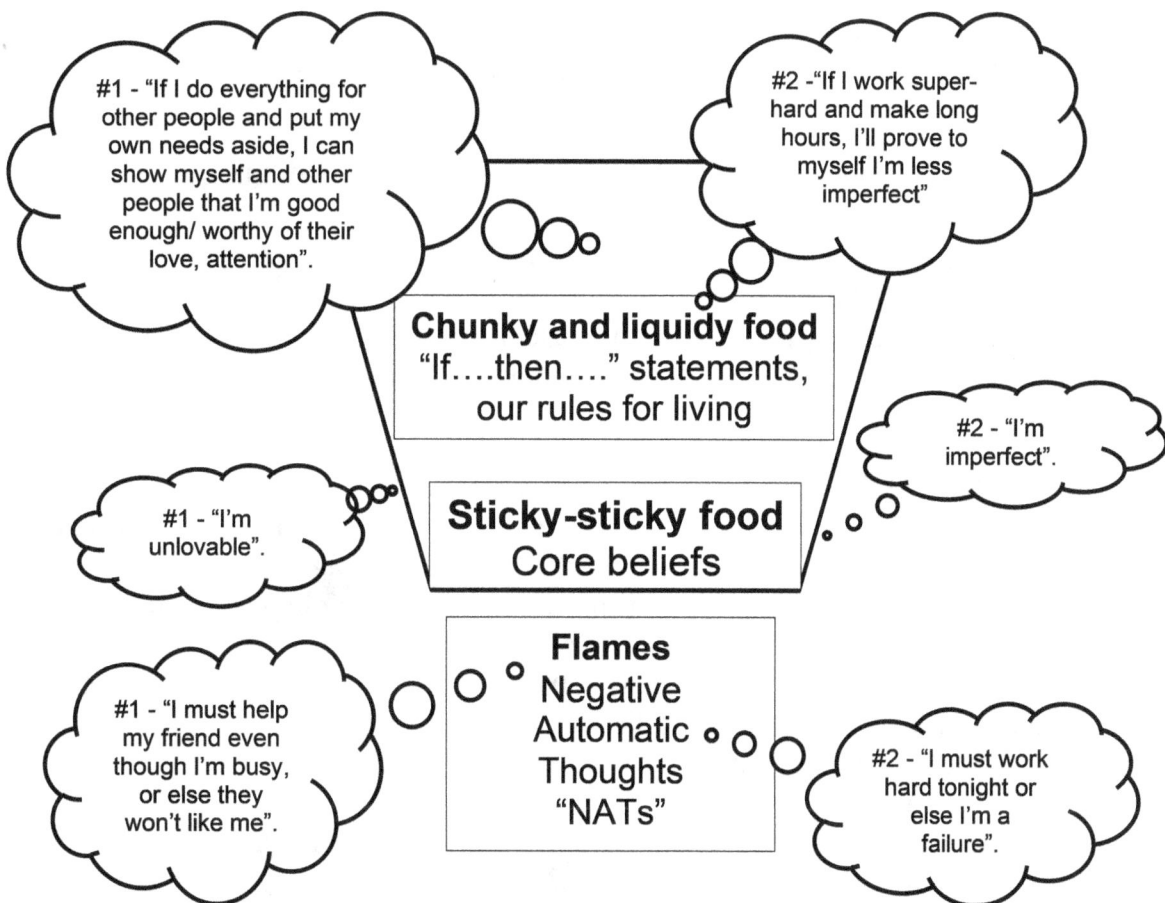

Figure 5.2 Three types of belief in the Pressure Cooker Model.

Critical incidents, our belief system, and FND

Now that we have learned about **critical incidents** and our **three-level belief system**, let us think a bit more deeply about the **connection between critical incidents** and **FND.** Do you remember that list earlier, with examples of 'biological' and 'psychosocial' critical incidents, that sparked off FND for some people? The missing link between critical incidents and the FND is . . . **our belief system**. Past and recent traumatic and stressful events, like a car accident, divorce, bereavement, relationship difficulties, illness in a loved one, house move, or job stresses, can greatly shake our belief system.

Let us suppose childhood adverse events (for example, emotional neglect and separation from a parent) have led us to believe that:

- 'I am worthless and unlovable.'
- 'I cannot trust other people because they will hurt and disappoint me [our **core beliefs**].'

Over the years, we may have developed the following **rule for living**:

- Build a **strong psychological wall**: 'If I make sure I reject people quickly before they can reject me, I will not get hurt and disappointed. I will not feel worthless or unlovable.'
- **Dissociation**: 'If I cut off my emotions, I cannot feel any hurt or disappointment. I will not feel worthless or unlovable.'

Let us imagine that years later you are in a relationship and the same thing happens: your partner neglects your emotional needs and eventually breaks off the relationship (critical incident resembling what happened in childhood). This critical event can subsequently 'shake up' your belief system and **re-trigger your core belief** of 'I'm worthless and unlovable'.

Since you . . .

- May not have had the opportunity to learn helpful strategies in your childhood – only 'the wall' and cutting off your emotions (dissociation);
- Do not really trust people anyway and are not keen on expressing your feelings to a person you trust (tight cover);
- Isolate yourself from people and activities because that is a safe option (blocked valve); or
- Work very hard to just not think about any emotions and cut them off in that way (overused valve) . . .

Where do you think all this turmoil and emotions can go?

You can see how the threshold lowers for **expressing** our **emotions in a physical manner** or **experience dissociation in a more pronounced form** by developing FND symptoms. You may ask yourself: But how does this work for critical incidents that are biological or physical, such as an accident, surgery, physical illness, injuries, or a health scare?

When a physical event (e.g. a viral infection) immediately precedes the onset of FND, we naturally think that this event must be causing FND, even if biological mechanisms have not been identified. This is your **original theory**. What if there is an **alternative theory**? Let us suppose we ask you to look at a deeper level, beyond the physical event. In particular, ask yourself how you felt around the time of the event; for example, did you feel cared for and believed? What was going on in your life around the time of the illness?

A lot of people with FND who report physical critical incidents that seemed to have sparked off the FND also report thoughts and feelings around **not having felt cared for and believed** around the same time of the physical event, either by a partner, a family member, or a healthcare professional:

- 'I did not feel cared for by hospital staff.'
- 'There was a lot of miscommunication with staff.'
- 'I was laughed at.'
- 'I felt my partner stopped caring about our relationship.'
- 'I felt uncared for by my employer.'
- 'I had an exacerbation of my physical symptoms. Staff treating me didn't believe me.'
- 'When I was admitted to the hospital, no one cared except for one person who supported me.'
- 'I was in a lot of pain and discomfort, but I was left suffering.'

Hence, on the surface, it may look like a physical incident directly sparked off the FND, but on a deeper level, the circumstances surrounding that event impacted on our belief system – in the same way this happens for more psychosocial events. The common denominator is our belief system. Always have your alternative theory ready.

Another situation where a physical critical incident can trigger FND is where people have experienced quite a few stressors for some time already. Things have been difficult for quite a while, and the person has become used to 'the new normal'. In the long list of difficult events, the accident or illness becomes 'one too many'. The mountain of stressors has grown so big that a person is unable to cope with the 'demand' using their existing coping strategies and subsequently develops FND to manage the aftermath.

Attachment

Attachment is another mechanism in which remote childhood adversity can make us vulnerable to psychological difficulties (e.g., Bowlby, 1951; Van IJzendoorn & Bakermans-Kranenburg, 2008), and eventually the development of FND later in life. When we are born, we develop a relationship (an 'attachment') to our primary caregiver(s), who consistently attends to our physical and emotional needs. The human attachment system becomes activated during times of stress. Sometimes, attachments to caregivers do not develop well for various reasons, for example, emotional neglect, abuse, and trauma. This impacts on the attachment of the child to the caregiver, which may become insecure instead of secure. Attachment is incredibly important for the following reasons:

- It provides the child with a **'secure base'** and **psychological safety** from which to venture out and explore the world. It protects and helps the child 'survive' and get their emotional and physical needs met.
- Important for the development of your **personality** and **identity** ('who you are', 'what ticks you as a person', your needs, wants, and preferences).
- The bedrock for the development of your **relationship**, **interpersonal** and **social skills**, as well as how you set **boundaries** between yourself and other people.
- Helps you develop skills to be able to **cope with difficult thoughts and emotions**, how you regulate and control emotions so that they do not linger and impact on relationships and day-to-day life, helps you find a balance between being able to do this on your own (e.g. effectively calming yourself down with strategies during times of distress), as well as through other people (e.g. speaking about and expressing your emotions to another person in a safe and trusted relationship).
- **Insecure attachment** in childhood can greatly impact on relationships formed (or not formed) in adulthood. People with insecure attachments can be supported with therapy to become capable of developing more secure attachments.

5.1 eResource alert!

Mary Ainsworth investigated attachment styles between infants and caregivers (see Ainsworth et al., 1978). Interested in learning more about the different types of attachment we can develop in childhood? Go to the eResource to read about four 'famous' attachment styles.

Our first relationships with our caregivers provide a 'template' for later relationships in adulthood. People with FND often report childhood relationships with caregivers that will have very likely impacted on their attachment style, for example a(n):

- Emotionally neglectful caregiver
- Absent caregiver
- More-than-present, 'enmeshed' caregiver
- Very strict caregiver
- Conflict-sensitive caregiver

You have already seen how adverse events in childhood during our upbringing can impact on the 'sticky leftover food' element of the Pressure Cooker Model: these life experiences influence our attachment style and shape our beliefs about ourselves, other people, the world in general, and our future.

5.2 eResource alert!

Please read this bit if you would like to find out more about how adverse experiences, attachment style, and our core beliefs may affect other psychological processes and our day-to-day life, including our thoughts, emotions, relationships, physical health, and activities.

What about attachment in FND?

Interestingly, researchers and clinicians have observed attachment problems in people with FND, with some suggesting insecure attachment as a risk factor for FND (Williams et al., 2019). In a nutshell, this is what studies on attachment in FND have found:

- Two studies reported an **avoidant attachment style,** and one found **fearful attachment** in people with FND (Holman et al., 2008; Green et al., 2017; Cuoco et al., 2021), which was **associated with psychological difficulties** (Cuoco et al., 2021).
- Quite a few studies discovered abnormal scores on attachment measures in people with dissociative seizures, indicating **insecure attachment** (Reuber et al., 2004; Green et al., 2017; Gerhardt et al., 2021; Villagrán et al., 2022).
- Jalilianhasanpour et al. (2019) found securely attached people with motor FND **more likely to improve** following a six-month period of multidisciplinary treatment.
- Significantly higher levels of attachment anxiety were detected in people with **more chronic seizures** vs those who were seizure-free (Villagrán et al., 2022).
- A fearful attachment style in people with motor FND was related to the **severity of FND,** amongst other variables (Williams et al., 2019).

Making sense of the ignition: a timeline exercise

A timeline is a great tool to help you gain insight into the relationship between life events and FND.

5.3 eResource alert!

You can make an FND timeline in different ways, but a visual format is often the most effective and sometimes mind-blowing! For some people, the timeline can suddenly reveal 'never seen before' associations between the FND and things that happened in their life. To prepare you for the timeline, the information-gathering exercise in this eResource can be helpful to get details around the FND diagnosis 'clear in your mind', including about the run-up, aftermath, and other important circumstances.

Exercise: my visual timeline of FND

5.4 eResource alert!

Figure 5.3 shows you an example timeline of a person with FND. Look at the template in the eResource and have a go at completing your own visual timeline of FND. You can ask someone who knows you well to support you with the exercise. After you complete the timeline, the guiding questions will help you check out whether you notice any patterns particularly around triggers and maintaining factors of FND.

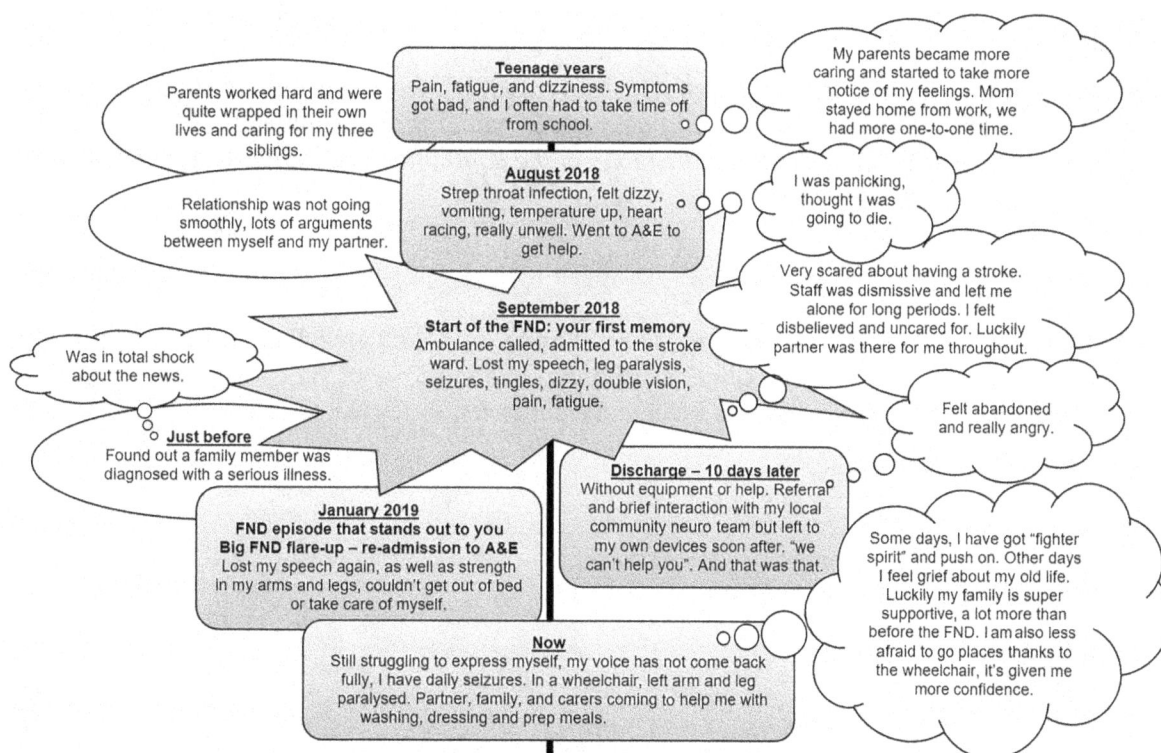

Figure 5.3 My visual timeline of FND.

References

Ainsworth, M. D. S., Blehar, M. C., Waters, E., & Wall, S. (1978). *Patterns of attachment: A psychological study of the strange situation*. Lawrence Erlbaum.

Beck, A.T. (1967). "Depression: Causes and treatment," University of Pennsylvania Press. Philadelphia.

Beck, A. T., & Greenberg, R. L. (1984). Cognitive therapy in the treatment of depression. In *Foundations of cognitive therapy: Theoretical methods and practical applications* (pp. 155–178). Boston, MA: Springer US.

Binzer, M., Andersen, P. M., & Kullgren, G. (1997). Clinical characteristics of patients with motor disability due to conversion disorder: A prospective control group study. *Journal of Neurology, Neurosurgery & Psychiatry*, *63*(1), 83–88.

Bowlby, J. (1951). *Maternal care and mental health* (Vol. 2). Geneva: World Health Organization.

Cuoco, S., Nisticò, V., Cappiello, A., Scannapieco, S., Gambini, O., Barone, P., Erro, R., & Demartini, B. (2021). Attachment styles, identification of feelings and psychiatric symptoms in functional neurological disorders. *Journal of Psychosomatic Research*, *147*, 110539.

Gerhardt, C., Hamouda, K., Irorutola, F., Rose, M., Hinkelmann, K., Buchheim, A., & Senf-Beckenbach, P. (2021). Insecure and unresolved/disorganized attachment in patients with psychogenic nonepileptic seizures. *Journal of the Academy of Consultation-Liaison Psychiatry*, *62*(3), 337–344.

Green, B., Norman, P., & Reuber, M. (2017). Attachment style, relationship quality, and psychological distress in patients with psychogenic non-epileptic seizures versus epilepsy. *Epilepsy & Behavior*, *66*, 120–126.

Holman, N., Kirkby, A., Duncan, S., & Brown, R. J. (2008). Adult attachment style and childhood interpersonal trauma in non-epileptic attack disorder. *Epilepsy Research*, *79*(1), 84–89.

Jalilianhasanpour, R., Ospina, J. P., Williams, B., Mello, J., MacLean, J., Ranford, J., Fricchione, G. L., LaFrance Jr., W. C., & Perez, D. L. (2019). Secure attachment and depression predict 6-month outcome in motor functional neurological disorders: A prospective pilot study. *Psychosomatics*, *60*(4), 365–375.

Petrochilos, P., Elmalem, M. S., Patel, D., Louissaint, H., Hayward, K., Ranu, J., & Selai, C. (2020). Outcomes of a 5-week individualised MDT outpatient (day-patient) treatment programme for functional neurological symptom disorder (FNSD). *Journal of neurology*, *267*, 2655–2666.

Reuber, M., Pukrop, R., Bauer, J., Derfuss, R., & Elger, C. E. (2004). Multidimensional assessment of personality in patients with psychogenic non-epileptic seizures. *Journal of Neurology, Neurosurgery & Psychiatry*, *75*(5), 743–748.

Van Ijzendoorn, M. H., & Bakermans-Kranenburg, M. J. (2008). The distribution of adult attachment representations in clinical groups: A meta-analytic search for patterns of attachment in 105 AAI studies. In H. Steele & M. Steele (Eds.), *Clinical applications of the adult attachment interview* (pp. 69–96). New York: The Guilford Press.

Villagrán, A., Lund, C., Duncan, R., & Lossius, M. I. (2022). The effect of attachment style on long-term outcomes in psychogenic nonepileptic seizures: Results from a prospective study. *Epilepsy & Behavior*, *135*, 108890.

Williams, B., Ospina, J. P., Jalilianhasanpour, R., Fricchione, G. L., & Perez, D. L. (2019). Fearful attachment linked to childhood abuse, alexithymia, and depression in motor functional neurological disorders. *The Journal of Neuropsychiatry and Clinical Neurosciences*, *31*(1), 65–69.

6 The FND coping triangle

Cover, valve, sticky leftover food (layer 2)

In the Chapter 5, we looked at the ignition element of the Pressure Cooker Model and learned how early childhood events can affect our belief system, emotions, attachments, and relationships with other people and, in the end, spark off the FND. Since life in general poses us with challenges, some big and some smaller, that are bound to elicit discomfort and distress in us, knowing how to handle these feelings by having a set of strategies ready will help you get through daily life. Every person, with or without FND, will learn strategies during their upbringing and in response to early experiences that will support coping with difficult thoughts and emotions.

Our **childhood coping strategies** can **bear a strong resemblance** to the coping strategies we end up using in **adulthood**. In this chapter, you will learn about an important concept: the **FND coping triangle**. This is a triangle of three pressure cooker elements: the sticky leftover food, cover, and valve. Before we delve into the FND coping triangle, let us learn a bit more about coping habits, as this will be important to help us understand where the FND coping triangle comes from.

Coping skills and habits

In psychology, **skills** and **habits** are important concepts. Check out Figure 6.1 to learn about a few well-known qualities of habits.

Psychological coping habits

A special type of habit are **psychological coping strategies**. We develop coping habits to manage difficult thoughts and feelings that come up. Coping habits create 'psychological safety' for when we experience stress and worries that are part and parcel of life. No one is exempt from stress in life: everybody experiences stress, although some people get a bigger portion of it than others.

People use many different psychological coping habits. You could say that they fall on a **coping continuum**, ranging from helpful to unhelpful. Figure 6.2 displays coping habits that are arranged around all the elements of the Pressure Cooker Model. On the left side, you will see more helpful coping habits, whereas on the right side, you will find examples of unhelpful (but sometimes very understandable) coping habits. Everyone will have their own personal story, and there is no judgement here. People have a mixture of helpful and less-helpful coping habits. There are no perfect 'copers'!

Some people find it difficult to answer the question 'How do you cope with difficult emotions?' They may be unable to come up with any helpful coping habits or simply not identify with distress. Do not worry if that is the case for you. It likely means that 'coping with emotions' is an important area to work on. In the following section, we will take a closer look at psychological coping habits.

DOI: 10.4324/9781003308973-6

Habits are behaviours based on learning processes and principles like reinforcement.

Habit formation takes time & effort Take time and consistency to develop from effortful at the beginning (requiring a lot of mental effort) to automatic later on (not thinking about it).

Learned & Unlearned Habits can be learned (for example learning to play the piano) and unlearned (for example stopping smoking, going to bed late).

Newly formed coping habits are **best practiced when relaxed** and you feel well. This way you can use the habit more easily when you are overwhelmed or upset.

Habits can become stronger ("consolidation") Habits require regular practice and repetition to make them stronger. For example, if you want to build muscle, you need to go regularly to the gym in order to grow biceps. In the same way, you need to practice your „mental muscles" regularly for relaxation strategies to work.

What are habits?

Habits are replaceable Habits may be persistent and difficult to break (e.g. not speaking about your feelings) but you can form new habits and replace an old habit with a more adaptive habit (e.g. opening up about your thoughts and feelings).

Habits and the brain The basal ganglia, an area in our brain, are important for habit learning.

Physical & Psychological Habits can be physical (e.g. learning to drive a car, ride a bike, playing the piano) and psychological (e.g. learning to manage emotions with reality grounding, or become more aware of your emotions when you dissociate).

Helpful vs Unhelpful Some habits are helpful (for example our daily showering routine), some not so (watching too much Netflix and not doing housework, biting your nails).

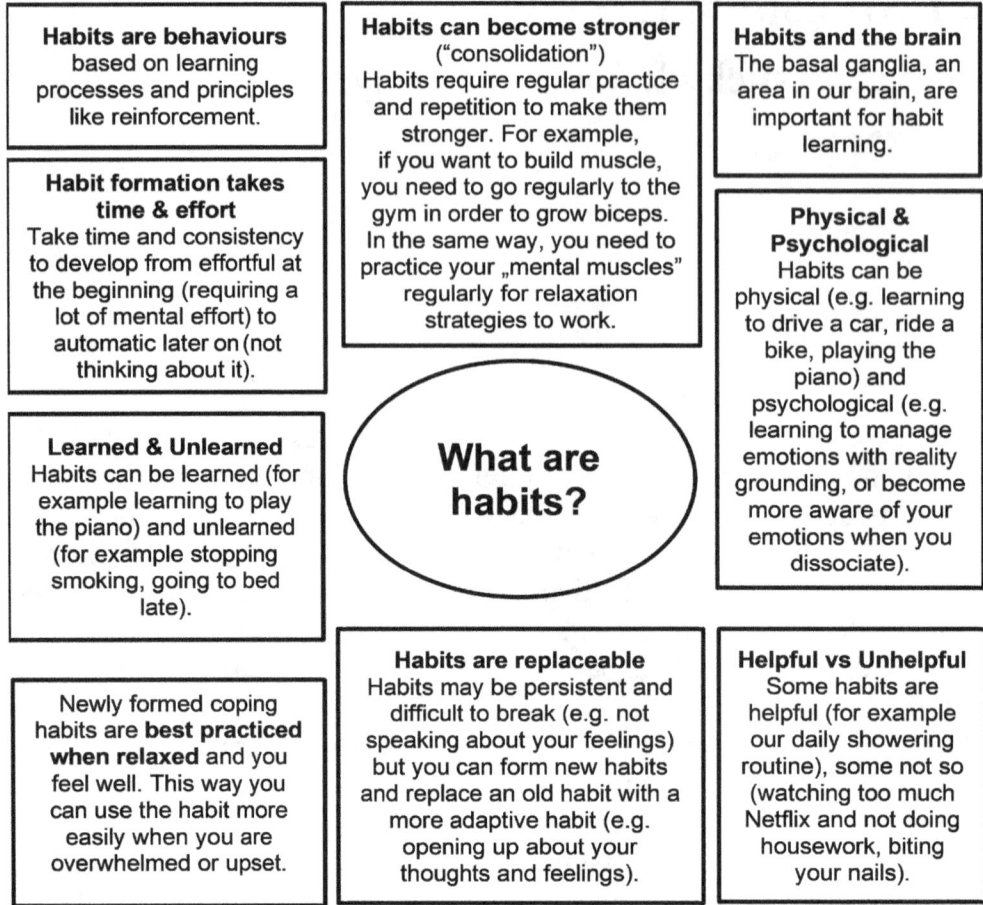

Figure 6.1 Pressure Cooker fast facts: habits.

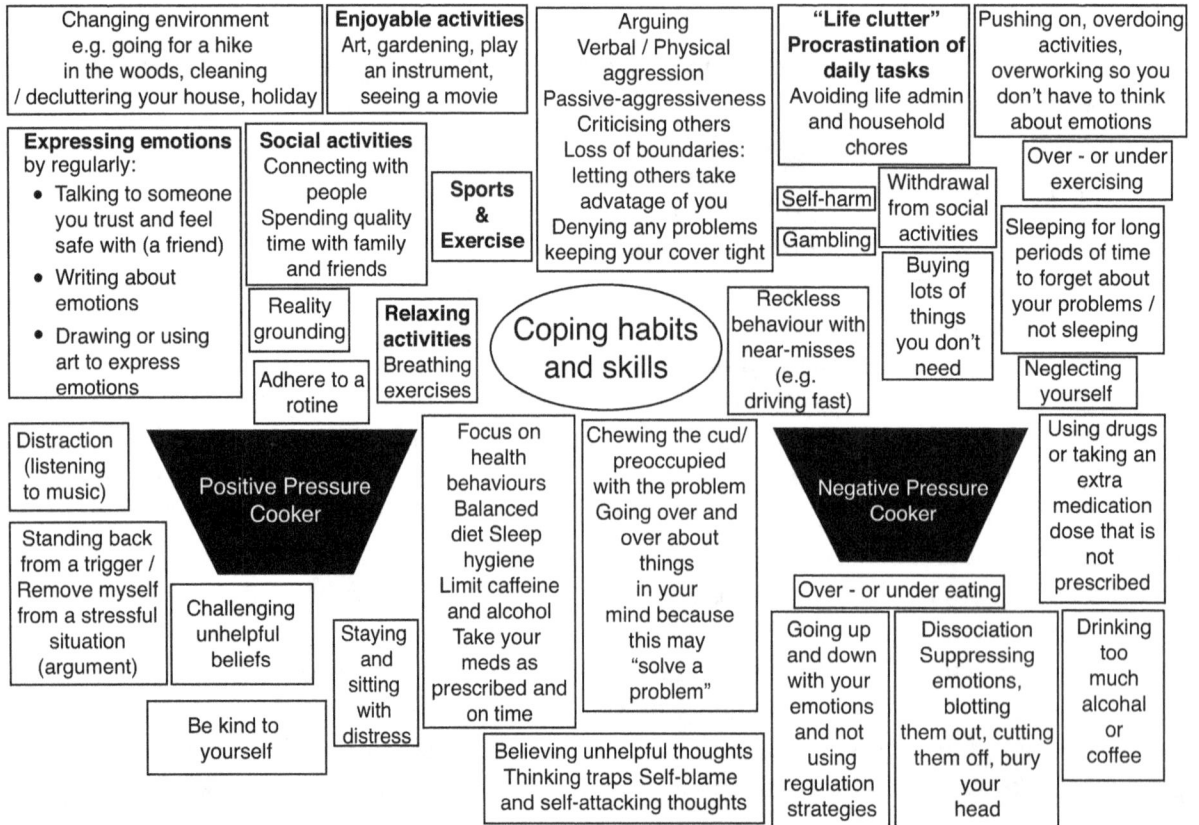

Changing environment e.g. going for a hike in the woods, cleaning / decluttering your house, holiday

Enjoyable activities Art, gardening, play an instrument, seeing a movie

Arguing Verbal / Physical aggression Passive-aggressiveness Criticising others Loss of boundaries: letting others take advantage of you Denying any problems keeping your cover tight

"Life clutter" Procrastination of daily tasks Avoiding life admin and household chores

Pushing on, overdoing activities, overworking so you don't have to think about emotions

Expressing emotions by regularly:
• Talking to someone you trust and feel safe with (a friend)
• Writing about emotions
• Drawing or using art to express emotions

Social activities Connecting with people Spending quality time with family and friends

Sports & Exercise

Self-harm

Gambling

Withdrawal from social activities

Over - or under exercising

Sleeping for long periods of time to forget about your problems / not sleeping

Reality grounding

Relaxing activities Breathing exercises

Coping habits and skills

Reckless behaviour with near-misses (e.g. driving fast)

Buying lots of things you don't need

Neglecting yourself

Adhere to a rotine

Distraction (listening to music)

Standing back from a trigger / Remove myself from a stressful situation (argument)

Positive Pressure Cooker

Challenging unhelpful beliefs

Be kind to yourself

Staying and sitting with distress

Focus on health behaviours Balanced diet Sleep hygiene Limit caffeine and alcohol Take your meds as prescribed and on time

Chewing the cud/ preoccupied with the problem Going over and over about things in your mind because this may "solve a problem"

Negative Pressure Cooker

Over - or under eating

Going up and down with your emotions and not using regulation strategies

Dissociation Suppressing emotions, blotting them out, cutting them off, bury your head

Using drugs or taking an extra medication dose that is not prescribed

Drinking too much alcohol or coffee

Believing unhelpful thoughts Thinking traps Self-blame and self-attacking thoughts

Figure 6.2 Helpful and not-so-helpful (but understandable) psychological coping habits.

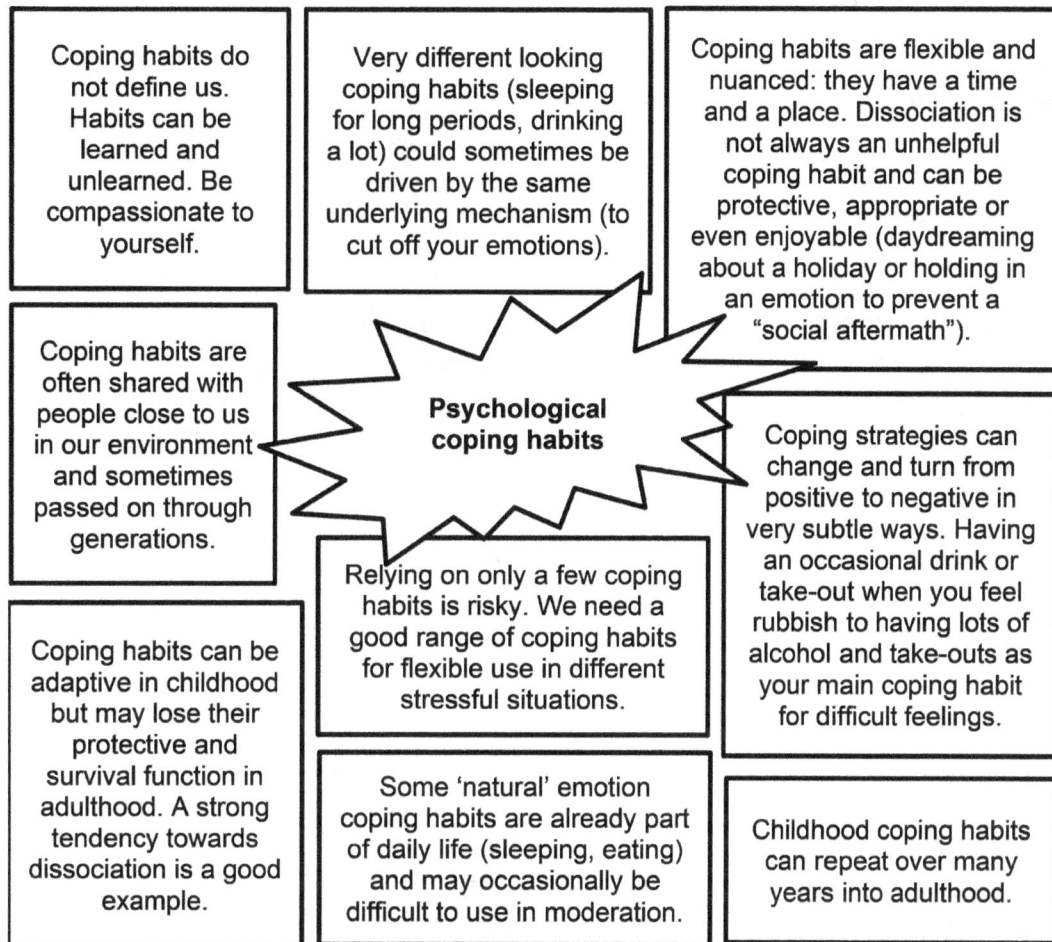

Figure 6.3 Characteristics of psychological coping habits.

6.1 eResource alert!

Figure 6.3 showed you a quick snapshot of the characteristics of psychological coping habits. Want to find out more? This eResource will provide you with an interesting piece of background reading on coping habits!

Top 10 features of helpful coping strategies

1. **Releases** a negative emotion **relatively quickly** . . .
2. And **effectively**. Gives you a better feeling afterwards . . .
3. But **does not cause physical** and **emotional harm** to yourself or to other people around you (e.g. overexertion, drugs, self-harm).
4. Gets to the **root of dealing with your difficulties** rather than operating on a 'superficial' layer.
5. You are **connecting with the coping strategy**: it is something that is nice and pleasant to use; it fits your personality (e.g. sports if you like getting active, music if you are a huge music fan and listen to it often).
6. **Long-term strategy** rather than temporary or short-term use. The coping habit has been **consolidated** over a longer period, is **well-rehearsed**, and you have derived steady and consistent benefits from it.

7. Your coping habit is **flexible**: there is a time and place for using it.
8. You use the **coping habit** 'in normal doses' and **'in moderation'**. It is not time- or energy-consuming to the point that you cannot function anymore (e.g. overexertion resulting in problems falling asleep at night because you are highly aroused).
9. **Regularly used**. Not once in a blue moon.
10. They **do not impact negatively** on your day-to-day life.

The three most common coping habits in FND (bottling emotions up, pushing on, and dissociation) make people feel **psychologically safe**. Keep in mind that psychological safety **applies to both people with and without FND in their environment**. But what does *psychological safety* truly mean? If you want to find out, it will be helpful to learn about **self-esteem**, a concept that is intricately linked to how much we **trust, have faith,** and **feel safe within ourselves**, including in relation to coping with emotions.

Sticky leftover food

Beliefs about yourself: low self-esteem

Low self-esteem is very common in people with FND. Some people report childhood adverse experiences, including rejection, trauma, abuse, emotional neglect, enmeshed 'overinvolved' caregivers, or a strict upbringing. These experiences can make us feel worthless and 'less than other people'. In a way, a person with low self-esteem does not feel psychologically safe enough to let go of all the things mentioned in Figure 6.4. If we want to build our confidence and self-esteem, we need to learn to feel and create psychological safety and security in ourselves to do exactly the things that low self-esteem stops us from doing (see Figure 6.5).

The relationship between self-esteem and FND is not straightforward. On the one hand, quite a subset of people experiences low self-esteem. On the other hand, did you know that some people report **increased self-esteem** after developing FND? This may sound paradoxical and confusing: How can you feel better about yourself after becoming unwell?

Think about the following examples:

• Feeling a lot more confident venturing out of the house and accessing the community using a wheelchair than without equipment when walking is difficult and attracts unwanted attention from other people.
• People acting kinder, caring, and more helpful can boost self-esteem and thoughts around 'I matter', 'I'm worthy', 'My opinions are valuable and taken into account', especially if this is a new experience for you and life before FND was not easy.
• People may be putting your needs ahead of their own by helping out, taking time to support you, which can make you feel better about yourself.

It is important to remember that although some people report better self-esteem after developing FND, it does not mean that symptoms are 'put on' deliberately.

6.2 eResource alert!

Find out whether you may experience low self-esteem by viewing Figure 6.4 as a 'checklist'.
Let us also help you to make a start with creating more psychological safety in yourself by finding your positive qualities with two helpful exercises on building self-esteem.

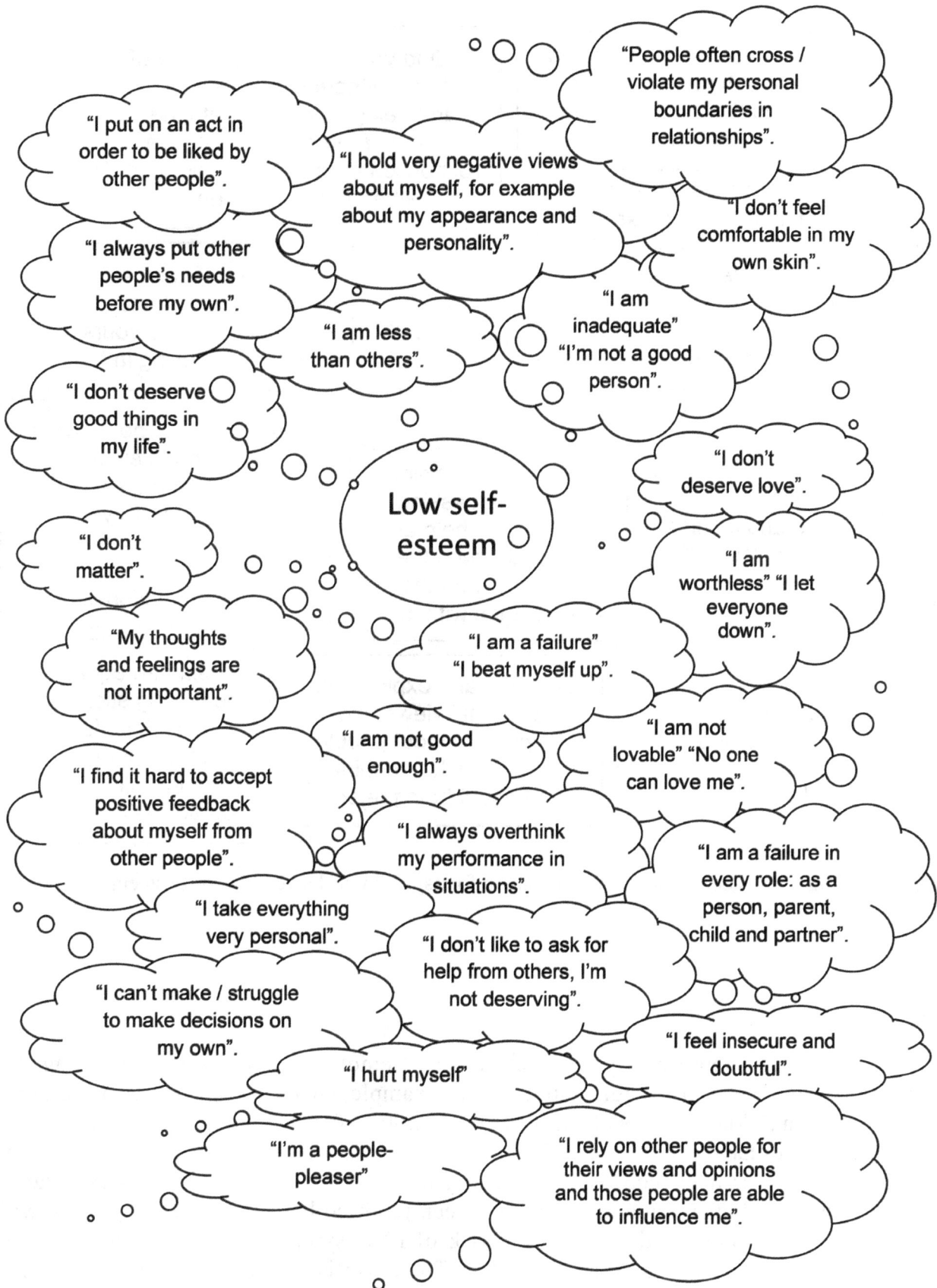

Figure 6.4 Low self-esteem 'checklist' of features.

Saying to yourself that you are worth it. Challenging and unhooking from your negative beliefs around self-worth.

Putting your own needs ahead of others' without fearing rejection and being able to tolerate the feeling of rejection or negative responses from your environment when it does happen.

Your 'self' that you express to other people (the 'you' that other people see when they meet you) is very close and in line with your 'authentic self'.

Feeling psychologically safe in yourself = Self-esteem

Cultivate self-compassion: Being kind and compassionate to yourself and truly believing in that.

Finding activities, talents and skills that make you feel secure and confident about yourself.

Make a decision without asking others to help and sitting with the discomfort that comes with it.

Guarding your boundaries even if that may cause difficult responses, risks rejection from your environment or may make you feel psychologically unsafe in relationships.

Understanding and trusting your own emotions and not second-guessing yourself – regardless of others challenging you.

Dig deep and explore your personal views and opinions without people telling you what to think or worry about being rejected.

Using an equal 'measuring stick' for yourself as for others (not using stricter rules for yourself vs others).

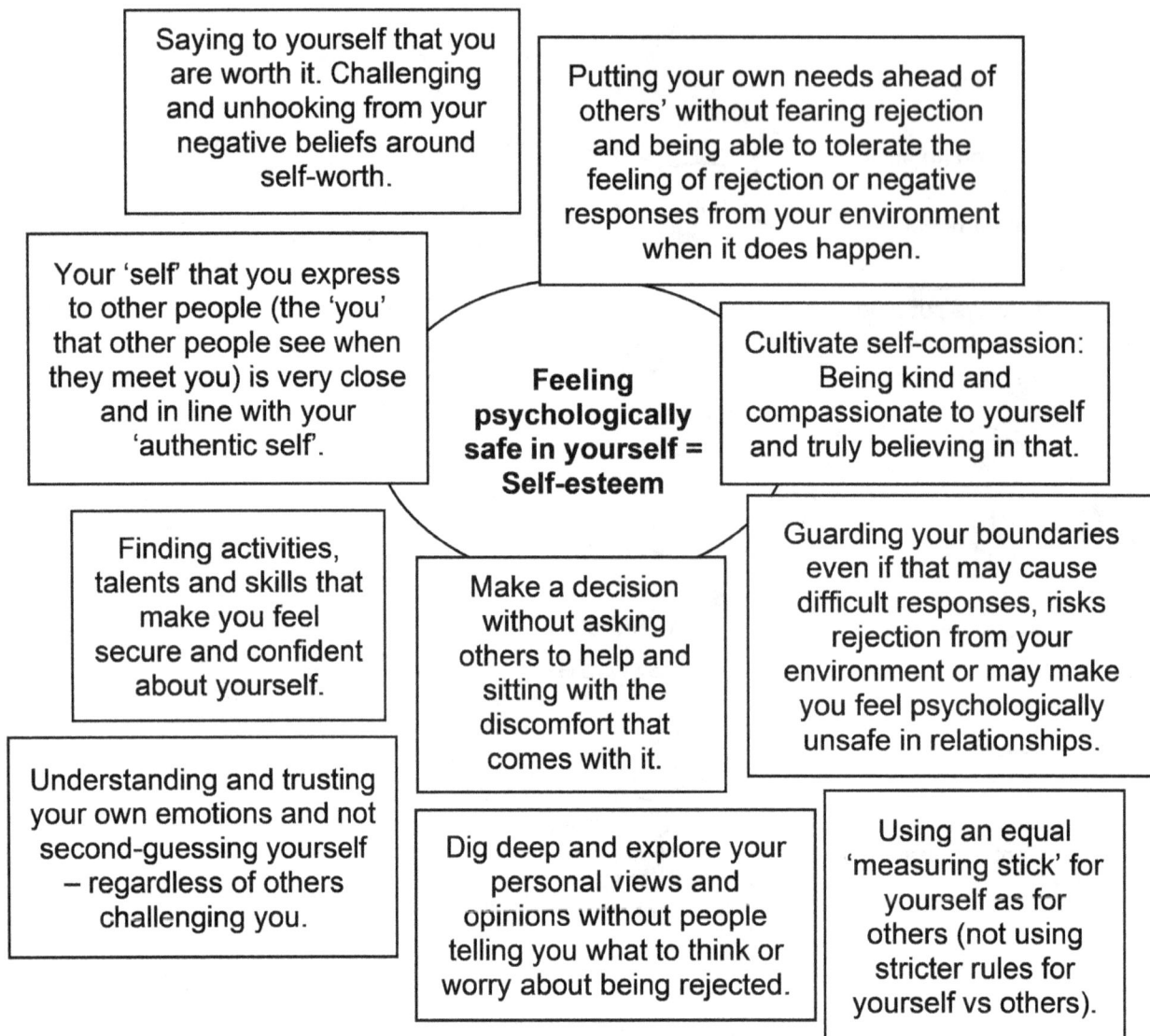

Figure 6.5 Building blocks that lay the foundation for psychological safety and self-esteem.

Cover

The cover element represents your level of verbal emotional expression, something that people with FND tend to struggle with (see, for example, Griffith et al., 1998; Wood et al., 1998; Bowman & Markand, 1999; Krawetz et al., 2001). Psychogenic nonepileptic ('dissociative') seizures have been termed a 'communication disorder' where distress is expressed via the body rather than more helpfully using language (Slocum, 2021). An association between emotional expression and FND has been reported before: the better you are with expressing your emotions, the lower your risk of FND symptoms seems to be (Bowman & Markand, 1999; Alsaadi & Marquez, 2005). The cover is intricately linked to our social environment and all about feeling safe and secure in trusted relationships to express emotions on a regular basis.

Pressure cooker fast facts: what does a tight cover look like?

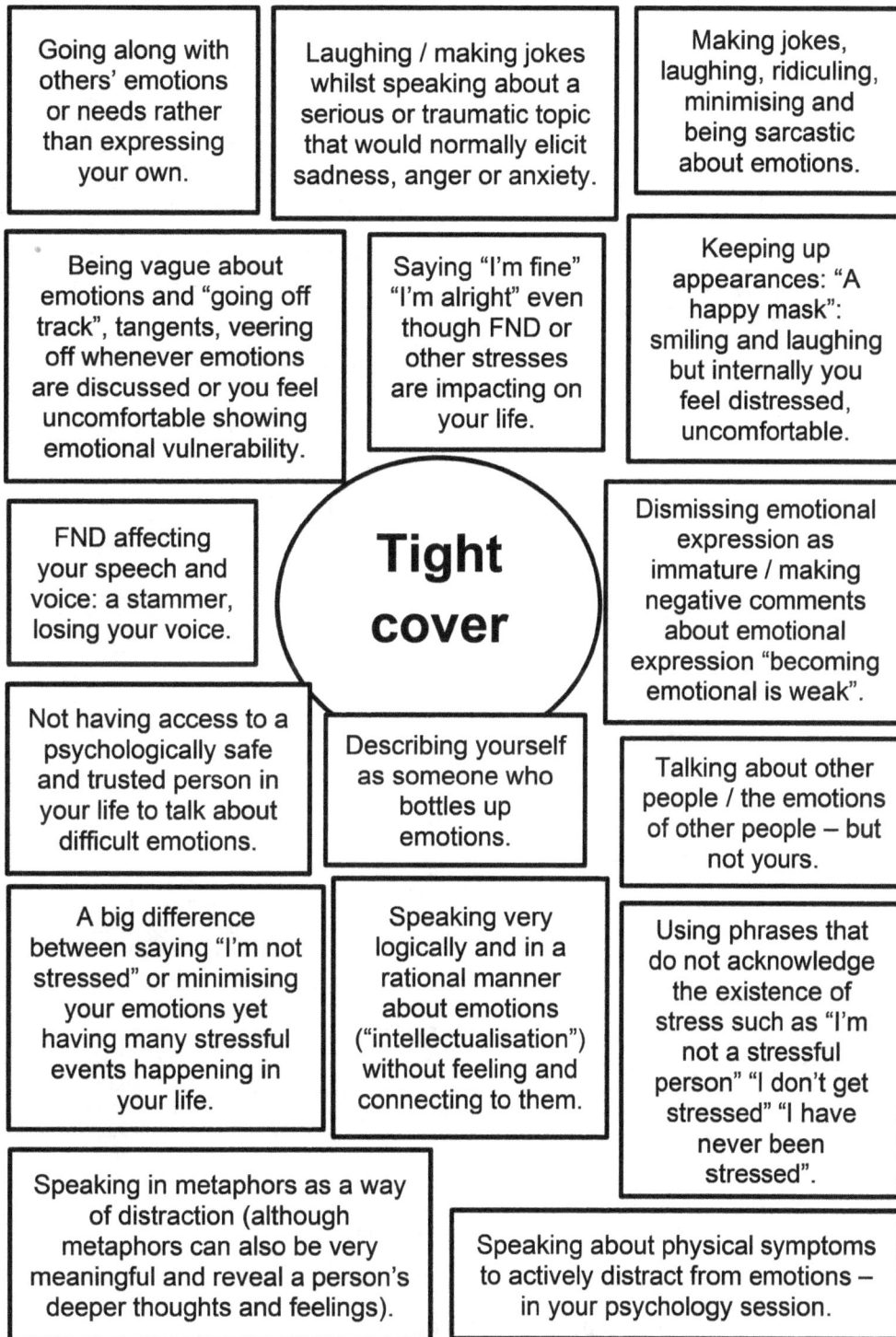

Figure 6.6 The many different manifestations of a tight cover in people with and without FND.

Pressure cooker boiling point: what keeps your cover tight?

Many people develop tight covers, both people with and without FND. However, observations from clinical practice have made it quite obvious that people with FND have a tendency to experience tight covers. In a moment, you will learn about some of the reasons that may underlie a tight cover (see Figure 6.7).

If you look at Figure 6.7 and Table 6.1, many of the reasons for a tight cover are related to interpersonal fears, rejection, and achieving psychological safety!

Family factors • General family coping style is to not express emotions. • No opportunity in the family environment to express emotions because other members are better at it/ take over. • In some families, bottling up emotions is an **ingrained family coping habit** and a family may hold **strong negative beliefs about emotions.**	**Unreleased unspeakable dilemma:** Unleashing "the secret" out "into the open" may risk upset, distress, even rejection from people close to you and damage to the family unit.	**Fear** Fear that I'll say something inappropriate or unacceptable that upsets other people and things escalate that I later regret – better to keep it closed.
	Language People may not possess the "emotion talking skill", lack emotion vocabulary and simply not know **how to put emotions into words.**	**Social anxiety** Fear of speaking to people and being judged negatively by other people. Fear of rejection if the "real" person or the "real me" is revealed.
Lack of skill You may not feel confident that you have the right skills available to you to express emotions or you do "not knowing how to", because of lack of practice in your family of origin.	**Societal pressures** "Men are not supposed to cry".	
	Invalidation of emotional expression: your direct environment (e.g. partner, family) may punish, reject, ridicule, make fun, retaliate or threaten you **with hostility or harm** if you express your emotions.	**Cultural pressures** In your family, it is culturally not appropriate to express your emotions. You "need to be in control" or else this may carry the risk of rejection.
Not having a relationship with a trusted person to speak to / or a lack of psychological safety • Because of early adverse experiences, some people may not trust others. • Lack of social network	**Speech difficulties** such as stammering or losing your voice altogether, stop you from expressing emotions. For some people, losing their voice has a symbolic meaning that literally means "I have no voice in my relationships and in the family unit".	**Fear of being a burden to other people**/ not wanting to bother people with your thoughts and feelings or upsetting them.
Coercion, domestic violence retaliation, other threats People may be victims of domestic violence and fearful or embarrassed to express this as well as their feelings, out of fear of retaliation from the perpetrator.		**Not feeling believed** You may be reluctant to open up to healthcare professionals because you feel not believed and it just confirms that it's "between my ears".
	Anger You may blow your top and damage relationships. Therefore, it may be better to hold emotions in because situations may escalate.	
Not recognising emotions & dissociation If you don't know what you feel, or how to feel your feelings and connect/experience your emotions, you may not be able to "label" and describe emotions well, and not express emotions.	**Reduced assertiveness** with low self-esteem and self-doubt: Putting other people's needs/emotions ahead of own, not speaking your truth and being your authentic self – in order not to be rejected.	**Negative beliefs, stigma & shame** about emotions and expression: "emotions are weak". Being embarrassed or ashamed about showing vulnerability to other people.

Figure 6.7 Reasons for tight covers in people with (and without) FND.

Opening up about difficult thoughts and feelings is not always easy, particularly if some of the barriers from Figure 6.7 and Table 6.1 block us from doing so. However, opening up may potentially reduce FND symptoms (see, for example, Bowman & Markand, 1999; Alsaadi & Marquez, 2005). In the following section, let us take a look at how we can work on reducing some of these barriers.

Why do we need to open the cover?

The short answer is **to make you feel better** and **prevent emotions and distress from coming out in different ways,** particularly via your body, through other less-helpful means and behaviours, or

Table 6.1 Possible underlying social and interpersonal fears that drive a tight cover

Psychological safety mechanism that maintains a tight Cover	Possible underlying social or interpersonal fear
• Unreleased unspeakable dilemma.	• Rejection / being ostracized from a social group, such as a family unit.
• Social anxiety and avoiding social situations.	• Being judged negatively by other people, for example, people thinking you look foolish.
• Holding on to societal or cultural pressures around not expressing emotions.	• Losing face and risking rejection from the group that you are part of.
• Holding on to fear of saying something unacceptable, being a burden.	• Rejection or expulsion from a social group, your family, or a cultural community.
• Believing in / holding on to stigma.	• Showing vulnerability to other people, potentially risking rejection.
• Sticking to coping habits that you know and that are acceptable in your family which feels containing and familiar.	• Invalidation and rejection by members of your family if you would use a different coping habit such as expressing your emotions.
• Focusing more on others than on yourself.	• Fear of rejection if you put your own needs ahead of others'.
• Continuing a difficult relationship where people violate your boundaries or involving domestic violence.	• Retaliation and a threat to your wellbeing, body, or livelihood from the perpetrator. Fear of not meeting another person who will treat you differently.
• Keeping your social circle restricted or opting to keep people out of your life and not have a trusted person to speak to. It is safer to be on your own.	• "Reject them before they can reject me": quickly rejecting people before they can reject and hurt you.
• Keeping yourself to yourself will protect your self-esteem and the way you view yourself.	• Not being believed by other people.

via abnormal activity levels. According to the Pressure Cooker Model, if you want to reduce the risk of FND (block the overpressure plug), opening an alternative channel (the cover) instead is a very powerful move. eResource alert 6.3 highlights some of the 'cover benefits' in more detail.

How can you open your cover?

Challenge your thoughts and feelings about emotional expression

Let us look at some **pros and cons of emotional expression** reported by people with FND and their psychologists (see Table 6.2).

It is completely understandable if you remain strongly opposed against expressing emotions, even after glancing at Table 6.2, particularly if you have held these beliefs for a long time. The 'pros and cons' table is there to gently challenge and loosen some of these beliefs, and show you that keeping your cover tight may maintain FND.

Table 6.2 Pros and cons of emotional expression

Open or close?	Pros	Cons
Opening my Cover to a person I trust in a safe relationship	• Releasing emotions may make me feel better and release the "burden". • Releasing emotions verbally may help reduce the risk of FND. • Research has demonstrated that expressing emotions can help relieve FND symptoms. • I can test out my negative beliefs about expressing emotions and find out that nothing bad will happen / people may respond positively to me / will not reject me. • In therapy sessions, expressing emotions is good for someone's psychological functioning and considered strong.	• It makes me look weak and vulnerable to the environment. • People may make fun of me and reject me. • If you put your trust into someone and you express how you feel to them, they may walk away from you, because they cannot bear the 'real me'. • Letting emotions through may be the beginning of the end: I may not be able to cope with the wave of emotions that will come flooding over me. • People never understood me and people won't understand me now, there is just no point in opening up.
Keeping my Cover tightly shut and "myself to myself"	• I'll come across as "strong" and "holding it together" to people. They won't reject me. • I don't have to worry about the aftermath: what people think of me afterwards, after "it's out" because "it stays in". • It's easier for me because it won't cause any ripple effects in my life. My life stays as it is and that feels familiar. I don't like change. • At least no one can break my trust this way.	• I won't release anything, and I will be stuck with feeling the emotion and discomfort. • Keeping myself to myself may maintain my FND symptoms. • Emotions may come out in a different way, for example drinking too much alcohol or hurting myself. • This will impact on my ability to do things in day-to-day life. • Expressing emotions may not be that bad but I won't know about it because I will not test out my belief. • If I have a secret or problem that gives me great distress and that I'm grappling with on my own, I may miss out on opportunities for others to help me / miss new insights into the problem.

Pressure cooker fast facts: assertiveness skills

Sometimes, our covers are tight because of reduced assertiveness. Figure 6.8 shows you a variety of important qualities about assertiveness skills. Read this **eResource!** 6.4 to find out about the differences between assertive, aggressive, passive-aggressive, and passive ways of responding.

Not using assertiveness skills has a lot of disadvantages. For example:

- You are **not getting** your **needs met** – neither by force nor by walking away.
- **Negative emotions stay and live in your head, not the other person's head.** We continue to carry the burden of these emotions ourselves rather than 'give this back' to the other person.
- **There is an aftermath.** If you are responding in an aggressive manner, then you may **feel guilty afterwards**, on top of the other emotions. Meanwhile, the problem still exists. Not only will you feel **'primary distress'**, or the distress that was elicited by the original problem; now you are also dealing with **'secondary distress'**, brought on by an unhelpful reaction. Aggressive responses make a manageable situation completely unmanageable. Is that worth it?
- If you are passive-aggressive, your **energy and effort are devoted to behaviours that are not serving the goal**/helping you reach your original goal. Instead, you are directing your energy to the wrong places.
- Expressing your needs, but in a diluted way and not openly (as in passive-aggressive responses), or not at all (passive response), may **make you feel worse about yourself** and **impact on your self-esteem**.
- The discomfort, distress, or upset that you feel about not expressing your true opinions may be far worse than the temporary discomfort associated with receiving an unhelpful response back from the other person, following an act of assertiveness. Ask yourself honestly: Which one is **the lesser of two evils**?
- It may also lead to other people not respecting you and **crossing more boundaries**, exploiting you or rejecting you because they are afraid to speak to you or find it unpleasant to talk to you.
- You are not speaking your truth and acting in line with **your authentic self**.

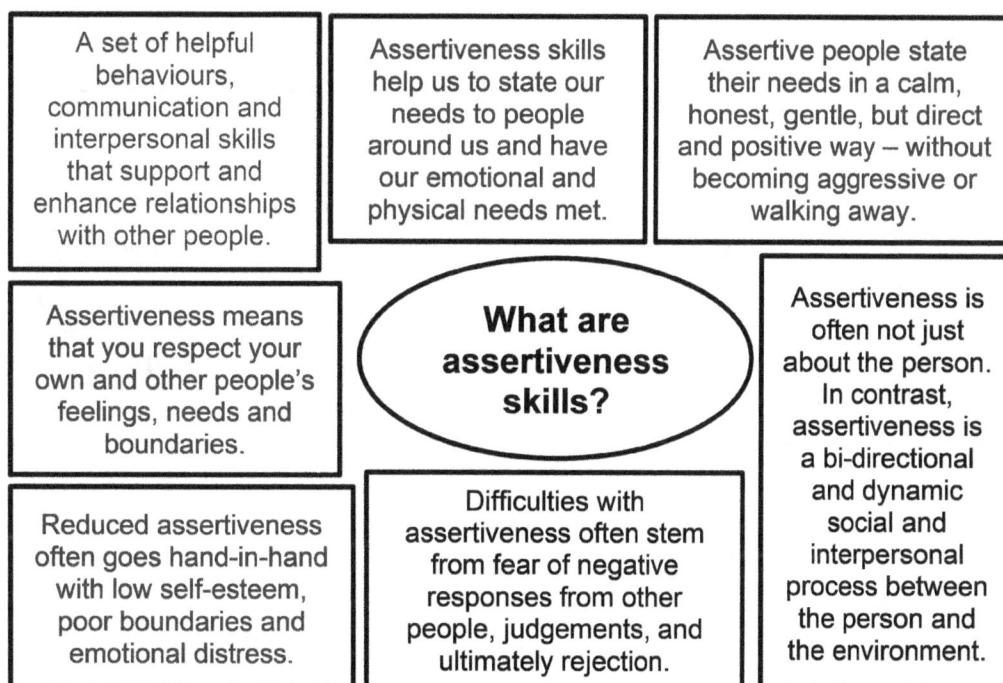

Figure 6.8 Assertiveness in a nutshell.

Assertiveness and getting the facts straight: selfish or . . . self-care? You decide!

A common misconception about assertiveness is that it is the same thing as being aggressive, rude, blunt, and disrespectful to other people. **Assertiveness is sometimes confused with anger and aggression**, but it is definitely not the same thing. Let us look at how assertiveness differs from anger and aggressiveness:

- **Feeling angry is okay.** It is even healthy to be in touch with your emotions, both positive and negative. It is better to feel angry from time to time and fully experience this emotion, than always being happy and forcing yourself to be positive 'at all costs' and perhaps denying or cutting off your true, authentic feelings.
- **Frequently feeling angry is okay too!** However, feeling angry makes you feel uncomfortable, distressed, aroused, agitated and may increase the risk of escalation to aggressive behaviours as well as worsen FND symptoms. If you find yourself feeling angry for a prolonged period, it will be good to address this for all these reasons.
- Expressing anger in an assertive way is totally acceptable. **It is self-care and not selfish.** However, expressing anger in unhelpful ways is not, for example, screaming, shouting, destroying property, drinking, cutting off all ties to people who care about you, physically attacking people, and so forth.

Some more thoughts on assertiveness

6.5 eResource alert!

Did you know that you can use the elements of the Pressure Cooker Model to ask yourself a series of questions to help increase your understanding of the psychological processes behind assertiveness?

6.6 eResource alert!

Assertiveness is a skill that can be learned and practiced. It is not something that people are miraculously born with or develop overnight. A great way of learning assertiveness skills is to actually apply them in a real-life situation using behavioural experiments. Although all the ins and outs of behavioural experiments will be discussed in detail in Chapter 7, this eResource will give you a flavour of what these experiments may look like if you want to focus on assertiveness skills.

Create your own assertiveness scenario

Think of a situation in your life that could do with a bit of assertiveness. Pre-plan what you are going to say, 'letter for letter'. Write down the steps (your detailed 'assertiveness scenario', like a movie scene played out) that you will take to express an assertive response, as well as any helpful assertiveness phrases that can assist you during that process.

Three top tips:

1. **Pre-empt the situation** to keep emotions down as much as possible. You want to apply your assertiveness skills in a calm state of mind.
2. Make sure you **convey how the other person's behaviour makes you feel** and how they impact on your psychological functioning.
3. Keep the other person's emotions in your mind, too, and **acknowledge** how the other person may feel.

'Linda, I would really like to have a brief chat with you about something that has been bothering me for a while. Would you be alright with that? It is nothing outrageous, and there is no judgement! But it is really important to me. Is that okay? [Pre-empt the situation to keep emotions down and reassure the person.] I just wanted to chat about you coming with me to my medical appointments. I am grateful for your support, but I feel I want to do this on my own from now on. When you speak on my behalf, it makes me feel frustrated and look helpless. [Convey the impact of the other person's behaviour on your feelings.] I just want to say that I can see that you care a lot and you may worry about missing any crucial info at the doctor's office. [Acknowledge the other person's feelings.] But I have got to do this on my own now. I hope you can respect that.'

Organise a role-play with a 'sensible someone' you trust

Before going into the 'real' situation, do a 'dry run' and practice your assertiveness skills during role-plays with a good friend you trust who is a sensible communicator and is able to provide you with honest and genuine feedback. The following set-up can be very powerful to this end:

- **Pick a situation and clearly describe your needs and wishes.** For example, imagine that a close family member has been making scathing comments to you about the FND. You feel distressed by the comments, but you have not expressed the impact and how you really felt to this family member, out of fear for repercussions, rejection, or an aftermath. Your need is to let the family member know about their emotional impact and perhaps educate the person on FND.
- **You play the person you would like to be assertive and state your needs with** but who you know will pose a challenge (i.e. the family member making the inappropriate comments).
- Ask your sensible, 'good communicator' friend **to model the assertiveness response** that they would use if they had encountered the person who is not meeting your needs (i.e. what exactly would they say to the family member to convey your need?).
- You could subsequently **switch roles** and practice the assertiveness response yourself.

Using your friend's feedback, plan the experiment, put your assertiveness skills into practice, and observe what happens. How did the family member respond? Was it better or worse than you expected? What did you learn? Of course, your friend is probably kind and compassionate to you. Your family member may not be that receptive at all and perhaps even become more scathing afterwards. It is good to remember that the goal of assertiveness is not always to change the person but rather for you to say what you have to say ('speak your truth') so that you have released 'the burden' and can move on, regardless of whether the person on the receiving end is transformed by the new knowledge that you share with them.

Sit with discomfort

As you develop your assertiveness skills, it is very normal to encounter **resistance**. You may have changed, but your environment must catch up with you, too, and may need time to adjust to witnessing a new 'you'! Emotional responses in your environment can vary between joy, surprise, and shock to anger, disappointment, and rejection, which may stop you from being assertive in the future! In Chapter 7, you will learn that 'sitting with discomfort' is a concept central to FND. It is also a thing in the world of assertiveness:

- Learn to tolerate your own discomfort, anxiety, anger, or guilt that may emerge when you assert your boundaries and needs.
- And do not forget to do the same when people around you do not respond well, or as you hoped for, to your new-found assertiveness.

Ride the wave of discomfort. The 'emotional aftermath' and hours of thinking following your assertion of boundaries can sometimes be worse than the act of assertiveness! Watch carefully what safety behaviours you are engaging in. Is the tension and discomfort so high that you end up 'giving in' to requests you do not want to fulfil? Do you find yourself defending and justifying your responses or choices to the other person? If this happens, do not worry, but immediately set up a new behavioural experiment to become more assertive.

Make a Pressure Cooker anti-explosion emergency plan

We cannot fully predict people's responses to your assertiveness in advance. You may get what you wish for, and you may not get the desired effect at all, but, instead, an unwanted and challenging aftermath.

When your needs are unmet and it makes you unhappy, it is always worth speaking and doing something about that.

However, before you embark on your assertiveness journey, make sure that you have pre-planned coping strategies in place that you can easily grab when things do not go as you had hoped for. Interested in learning more about what you can do when your worst-case scenario does happen? Jump ahead to this 6.7 **eResource alert!** for more information on making a 'Pressure Cooker anti-explosion emergency plan'.

Be compassionate, and please do not give up

Unfortunately, assertiveness does not develop overnight. It is a skill – like learning to play the piano. We know that developing a skill takes time, patience, effort, and a lot of rehearsals before it becomes more automatic, natural, and effective. Be kind to yourself, particularly if you did not manage to apply your new skills on your first few trials or failed to obtain the response you wished for. You may not see the results immediately, and it is not a one-off: although people may accept your assertiveness initially, the same people may 'creep back in' and pose new challenges. Even if you have been on it for a long time, the worst thing you could do is giving up on assertiveness altogether. Keep at it, and do not make your pain or hurt worse (of not having been able to express your needs the way you wanted to), by adding even more distress to it. **Is life not hard enough already?**

Dichotomous responding

Dichotomy means two opposing or contrasting options. Occasionally, when people practice with assertive responding, they can end up **responding in an 'either-or' manner**. What does that mean?

- **Response 1:** Either a person may **not respond at all** (passive, passive-aggressive, or 'bottling up', keeping the pressure cooker lid tightly sealed off).
- **Response 2:** Or the person responds **too much** (veer towards a more aggressive way of responding, 'the pressure cooker lid coming off') and not in the intended desired assertive manner, struggling to find the middle of the road.

WHAT CAN YOU DO IF YOU KEEP RESPONDING 'DICHOTOMOUSLY'
AND YOU DO NOT FEEL IN CONTROL?

People who practice with assertiveness for the first time to help break free from this dichotomous response pattern **often report losing control over (when to let out) their emotions.**

- You may feel as if assertiveness is 'beyond your control', but fear not: **it all needs time, patience, and effort**. Eventually, you will master the skill. **Do not give up** if you do not see results right away, and **do not overthink it**. Break your worry cycle (see Chapter 8 for inspiration).
- Tell yourself that learning a **new way of responding that feels quite foreign** is bound to elicit strong negative emotions. It may not feel 'like you', 'wrong', or 'aggressive', even though you are simply being assertive. The practice is to become aware of when this happens and tolerate the discomfort that comes with your new way of responding.
- **Sit with the distress for a while.** There is a fine line between *'sitting with distress'* without immediately acting on it and taking it down vs *'actively coping to bring down the emotion'*. So sit with the feelings, but do not sit for hours on your own to the point that you can no longer function in your daily life. Balance is key, and that balance is not always easy to spot!
- Say to yourself that this dichotomous response pattern and heightened emotions that come with it **will eventually stop and go away on its own after diligent practice**. Dichotomous responding can feel exhausting, and the mind and body cannot continue indefinitely.
- You are also **more in control than you think**, especially if you are able to delay or even prevent reaching the point of FND symptoms worsening or re-appearing.
- **Give yourself a pat on the back**, and do something nice for yourself for trying to change this response pattern, especially if heightened emotions do not result in more FND or a dissociative seizure. This means **you are on the right track** even though it feels unpleasant for a while. Feeling emotions, rather than cutting emotions off, is the goal.
- **It is normal to feel like this:** people have often avoided their emotions and buried their feelings deeply, sometimes for years or even decades. Your body and mind have not forgotten this unresolved hurt and pain. It is like the 'bill' of all these years of emotion avoidance still needs to be settled and is now fully presented to you: you can either pay in a lump sum or instalments. It tends to be the lump sum for quite a few people. All of a sudden, a massive wave of emotion envelopes the person in its entirety, and that feels uncomfortable for some time.
- **Beware of the 'crossover' phenomenon** (see Figure 6.9). As you are gradually overcoming the FND and losing an old coping strategy, you are slowly replacing the FND with new, more helpful coping strategies. Brand-new skills that need time to consolidate and stew for a while. During this transitional period (see the **big 'X'** where the graph intersects), it is okay to 'fall' and 'lose control' a few times. In this brittle 'crossover phase' between coping strategies, it is possible that you still experience occasional FND symptoms. **Nothing out of the ordinary, and totally expected!** Get back up and keep practicing your new strategies.

Selective assertiveness

Some people might say, 'I am not quite sure what you are getting at', I talk about my feelings all the time!', 'I have strong friendships and express my emotions', 'How come I still have FND?' 'This disproves your theory', 'I don't buy your theory on emotional expression and FND'. The Pressure Cooker Model is not the be-all and end-all of FND theory. Hopefully, most people will find some benefit, but there may be a subset of people who do not connect with the idea of emotional expression = less FND.

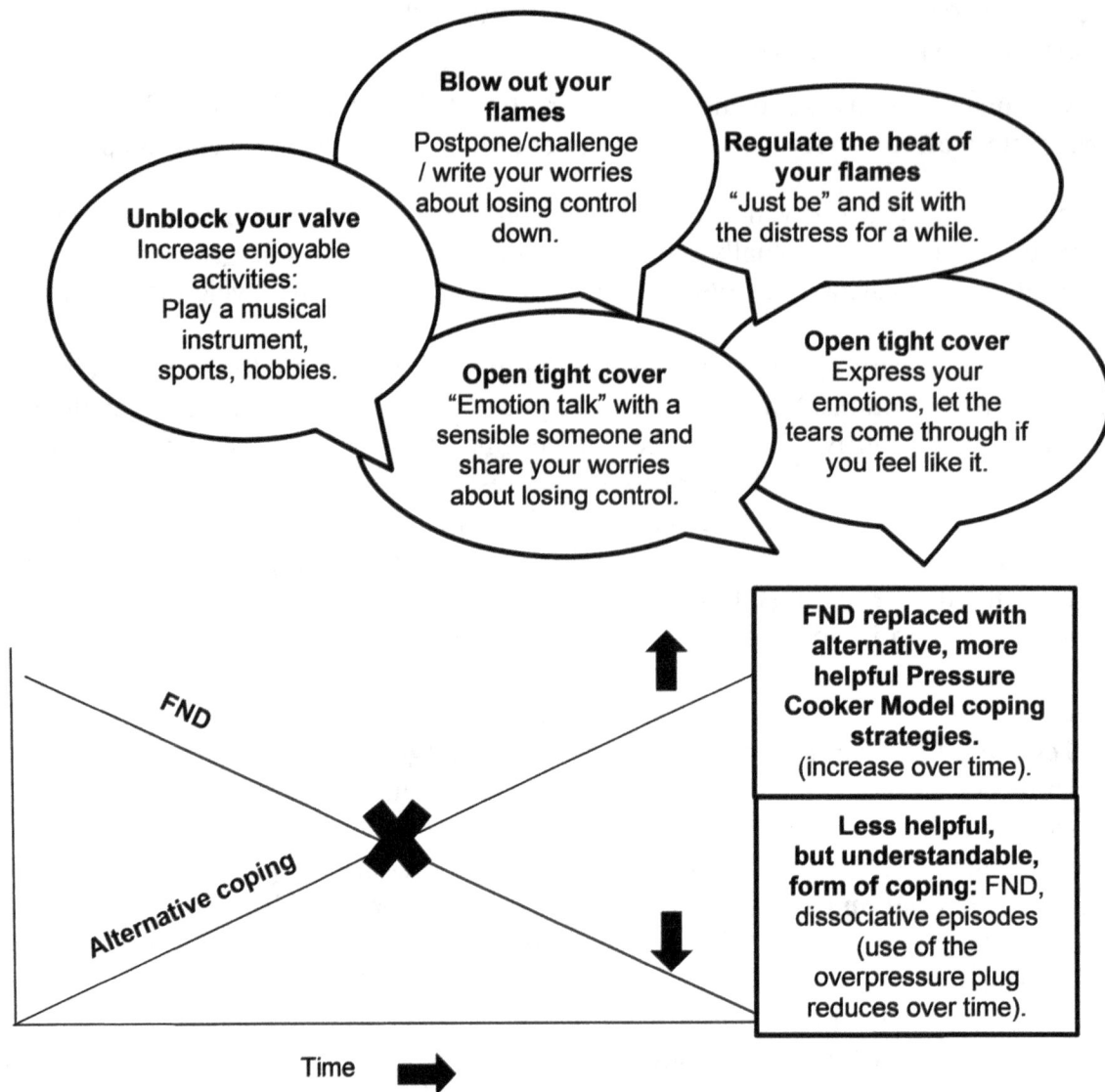

Figure 6.9 The FND crossover graph.

However, let us talk about the phenomenon of **selective assertiveness** (see Figure 6.10). This is something that people with and without FND can struggle with. *Selective assertiveness* is the process by which the person is perfectly capable of being assertive to everyone in their environment (including healthcare professionals!), **just not to the people who are important and close to them**, for example, a partner, a family member, or a friend. It is also the process by which people may freely speak about emotions and sensitive topics . . . **just not to the target people that need to hear your message**.

Being assertive and honest with our loved ones and the people that truly matter to us and we have strong emotional connections with is often the hardest thing to do as it puts us at a **potential risk of rejection** by that person. If the person will not accept your new-found assertiveness that readily, you may lose a meaningful and emotionally important relationship, and even other relationships, as well as entire social networks tied to this relationship. Remember that being assertive is not a 'social crime' but an essential part of relating, connecting, and communicating with other people. If the receiver of your assertiveness does not accept and even rejects you, then the question arises whether this relationship was healthy and good for you in the first place.

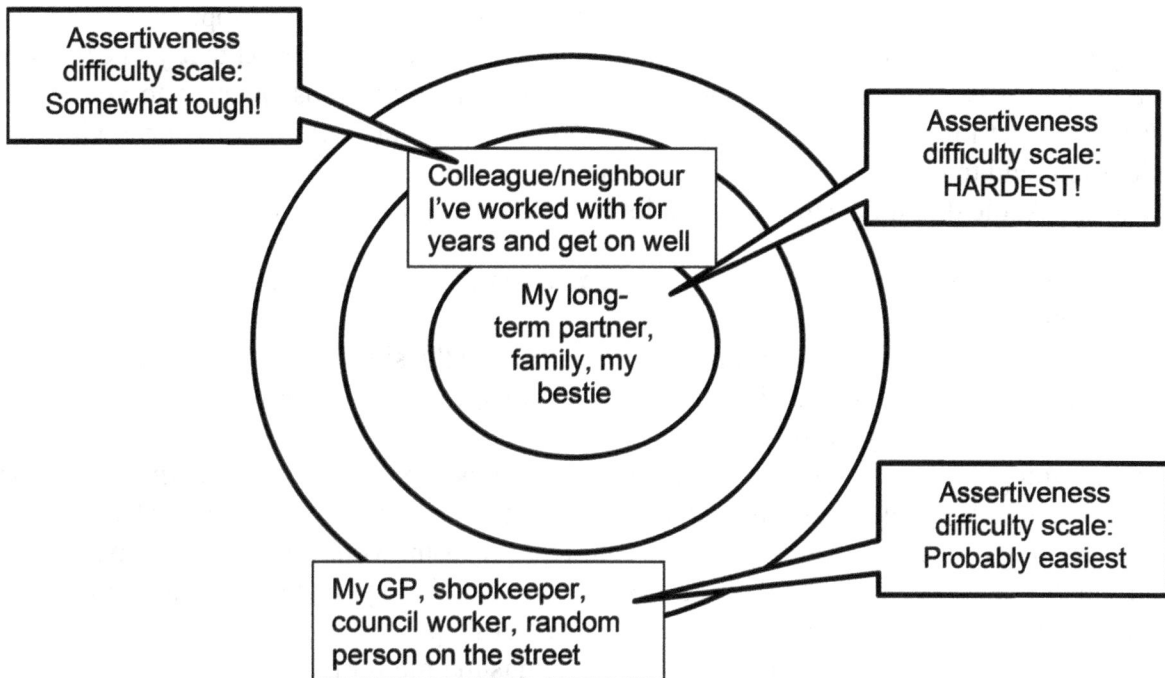

Figure 6.10 Selective assertiveness.

The unspeakable dilemma of FND: feeling trapped

Some people with FND experience an 'unspeakable dilemma' (see Griffith et al., 1998). This is often a secret, sensitive information, an unspoken wish or desire that is hidden and carried around by people, sometimes for many years, and often causing inner turmoil. What do unspeakable dilemmas look like?

- Expressing your sexual preference that is not accepted by your environment and could result in ostracizing, rejection, and abandonment.
- A secret from childhood that has not been revealed yet – often in the context of abuse.
- Past traumatic and challenging life events that you would be embarrassed or worried about if these came to light, sometimes with an active threat to your identity, social standing, and sense of social belonging.
- Current and ongoing domestic violence, coercion, abuse, or trauma in an intimate relationship.
- Feeling trapped in a relationship or a situation that you are not happy with, and not knowing how to find your way out.
- A private wish or unfulfilled desire that may not have been granted or accepted by people in your environment, or a mismatch in wishes in a relationship, for example, differing opinions around starting a family or not.
- Some people with FND would like to make gains but are not able to do so out of fear of negative reactions from their environment about the nature and realness of their symptoms. The unspeakable dilemma is associated with the person not being able to express their ambivalence about recovery.

Revealing any of these pieces of information to the people close to you may cause 'social injury' and irreversible, far-reaching social consequences that potentially risk subsequent rejection or expulsion from a personal relationship, family unit, social group, or community. This would almost 'violate' our basic human need of wanting to feel included, appreciated, and validated by other people around us. In a way, not speaking about the dilemma that you carry keeps the status quo. It is a true dilemma: not speaking causes negative consequences to yourself, but speaking about it may cause both negative consequences to yourself and to your environment. People often tend to retreat to keeping the dilemma to themselves.

The unspeakable dilemma can produce a lot of difficulties, including:

- Feeling low in mood, anxious, angry, guilty, embarrassed, and distressed about being unable to be your 'authentic self'.
- Hopelessness and helplessness around feeling trapped in the situation and not seeing a way out.
- 'Living day by day': not being able to see past the unspeakable dilemma and thinking that this will be it for the rest of your life.
- Feeling paralysed around making a choice between expressing versus not expressing, and moving forward in your life. Sometimes this can manifest symbolically in people with FND as quite literally a functional paralysis, for example, of your legs, or losing your voice ('speech paralysis').
- Continued lack of access to the tools and skills that could help you express your feelings about being trapped in the situation and ultimately plan an escape.
- And the most important issue: unspeakable dilemmas maintain FND!

Please read on further. At the end of this section, it will be discussed why carrying 'secrets' and unspeakable dilemmas can be detrimental to your physical and psychological well-being.

When there is a threat to you and emotional expression is not an option

Sometimes, people with FND do not have a trusted person whom they can speak with about difficult emotions, thoughts, and life events because there is a threat of rejection or **a threat to your person, well-being, health, and even livelihood**. Domestic violence, coercion, and other types of ongoing, as well as historic, abuse (including sexual, physical, emotional, and financial) are sometimes associated with FND symptoms, as it can serve as triggers. On the surface, the pathway from domestic violence to FND may seem far-fetched but is not unheard of in clinical practice. Let us look at some of the ways in which FND symptoms can be maintained:

- **Domestic violence and social isolation are two strongly linked concepts.** Not being able to speak about what is happening at home, not having a refuge to a trusted person who can help you (tight cover), and restrictions from the perpetrator that prevent you from engaging in enjoyable activities and accessing the community or other people (valve) all contribute to an increased risk of FND symptoms.
- FND can have a **highly protective function for the victim** and a **deterrent towards the perpetrator** seeking proximity to the victim. Some adult patients with FND, caught in a difficult relationship with an abusive partner, reported that the symptoms occasionally acted as a protective buffer against the perpetrator approaching the victim, including during intimate relations. The perpetrator may 'cut some slack' and leave the victim alone whilst they are feeling unwell, or the presence of carers may prevent further abuse. Symptoms may also elicit a more neutral or even kinder response from a person who is otherwise abusive and not caring.
- **Hospitals may be a safer place** than staying at home.
- **Dissociation** during the abuse can support the victim tolerating periods of unbearable distress and discomfort.

There are some red flags. If coercion is a problem in the relationship, the coercive partner **may meet their own needs for control** by ensuring that the person with FND is restricted from:

- Movement, 'venturing out', and ensuring that the person is unable to access the community.
- Having social contact with friends or stopping the person from meeting new people and building their own social network. The perpetrator may influence any meaningful friendships and relationships and restrict their visits to the person with FND.
- Accessing job opportunities, or even forcing the person to let go of an enjoyable job, hobbies, and interests outside the home environment, away from the partner (blocking the valve, therefore increasing the risk of more FND).
- Attending hospital appointments alone, or spending time alone with a consultant or therapist (always accompanying the person when going out together in the community).
- Having privacy: 24-hour supervision and hypervigilance, watching the person's every move.
- Keeping the person confined in the house or bed-bound, and 'taking things out of their hands', making them maximally dependent on the perpetrator.
- Taking care of medication management with a risk of under- or overmedicating the person resulting in sedation.

Eventually, these actions isolate the victim from the rest of society. Importantly, the perpetrator often **instils a sense of hopelessness** and **a lack of self-confidence**, which **maintains FND** in the victim by actively discouraging and denying them opportunities to practice strategies to become more independent.

Please note that in no way is it implied here that the victim is 'putting FND on' to protect themselves. FND symptoms are often **automatic 'defence' mechanisms** that the brain uses to protect people's feelings under highly distressing circumstances.

Why is it sometimes so hard to spot domestic violence?

Domestic violence and abuse as triggers for FND are not commonly encountered in clinical practice. However, it is conceivable that only a small minority of people will report domestic violence or abuse during sessions. There are many reasons why this tends to be 'hidden' and underreported (applicable to both people with and without FND):

- This information is sensitive in nature: victims may worry about potential retaliation and repercussions from the perpetrator after disclosure.
- The need to build a trusted and safe relationship with a person 'outside' the system, for example a healthcare professional, and the time it takes for victims to trust in the professional's actions and their sensitivity in handling the situation to protect them (not blowing someone's cover with the perpetrator finding out).
- Embarrassment about the situation, particularly 'looking like you are not in control of your life' in front of other people.
- Not being entirely sure whether you can call it domestic violence, not recognising it as such and minimising it, believing that it is normal behaviour, that you deserve it and that others may experience similar things at home.
- Not wanting to upset the system (particularly children risking losing access to a parent or other meaningful relationship) around you, and the major changes in your living circumstances.
- A victim may protect the perpetrator due to an anxious-ambivalent attachment. If a perpetrator shows kindness to the victim, then even despite abuse or violence, the victim may still find it hard to break the emotional attachment.

- The impact on family relationships when you 'let out the secret' and who might not believe you and might ostracise you. Intense fear of social rejection as often the perpetrator will have contributed to low self-esteem in the victim and will be powerful in 'keeping up appearances'. The victim may fear not being believed.
- Lack of confidence in building your own life, lacking resources to do so, being socially isolated without friends to rely on for support, and fear around the involvement of external institutions such as social services.
- Domestic violence is not always recognised as such in the clinic, as some forms of domestic violence can present as very subtle, particularly coercion.
- People with FND are particularly at risk of coercive control because they often experience symptoms and disabilities that make them dependent on other people for meeting their care needs, for example personal care, preparing meals and shopping. If tendencies towards coercive control have always been present in the relationship, then having a partner with FND may put even more control in the perpetrator's hands, under the banner of 'care'.

It is very important to seek out help when you or someone you know is the victim of domestic violence. It is against the law. Healthcare professionals are trained in picking up signs of domestic violence and can support you with referring you on to find a solution, but they need your help with this. A first port of call can be your general practitioner (family doctor), another healthcare professional you trust and have a good relationship with, or domestic abuse charities online who are excellent in supporting victims.

If you are reading this and you think this applies to you, so sorry to hear that you are in this situation. Please don't wait. There are people out there who can help you.

Pros and cons of sticking to vs releasing the unspeakable dilemma

Unspeakable dilemmas tend to be sensitive and challenging; that is exactly the reason that these dilemmas exist. They are 'unspeakable' or 'not to be spoken of' (to other people). Every unspeakable dilemma is different, including the level of social and physical threat it poses to the individual grappling with the dilemma. This book does not recommend a blanket rule on always releasing all unspeakable dilemmas at all costs. Sometimes, the consequences of releasing the dilemma out in the open is a worse fate for the person than keeping the dilemma to yourself. At other times, the timing may not be right, and one must wait with its release when, for example, more support may be available to the person or a 'rescue plan' has been developed. Once the dilemma is released, you cannot take it back if you change your mind. It is a binding decision that can have a major impact on the person's life and that of the person's environment.

However, with those caveats in mind, always remember that every human being is free and has a right to live their life without fear, abuse, violence, or any form of (social) threat. If you experience an unspeakable dilemma and you are not sure about what to do next, a 'pros and cons' table may be useful. Have a look at Table 6.3 for ideas.

6.8 eResource alert!

Still unsure about whether or how to open the cover to help you overcome FND? Do not worry! Read about the various alternative ways of expressing your emotions, plus how you can enlist the support of your social environment to help you open your cover.

Table 6.3 Pros and cons of 'sticking to' vs 'releasing' an unspeakable dilemma

Cons: Sticking to	Cons: Releasing
Risk of continued or an escalation of emotional and physical injury.	Risk of retaliation and threats including to a person's health, safety, well-being, social status, and livelihood
Risk of severe distress and psychological burden to the person.	Risk of temporary or permanent social rejection, shunning by a community and a loss of meaningful relationships.
Pros: Sticking to	**Pros: Releasing**
Personal safety.	Being able to get help and support to live life to the full, or a more meaningful and authentic life.
Not wreaking havoc or causing irreversible and permanent social damage to an existing family structure.	Sense of relief and emotional release of the burden.

Speech and language difficulties in FND ...

... can have a very **symbolic meaning** in FND because the symptoms literally prevent a person from accurately expressing their emotions. Some people experience additional functional weakness in both arms and hands, or in the dominant hand that they always use to write with, which further prevents them from verbally communicating their emotional needs.

Like many other FND symptoms, **functional speech and language difficulties are intricately linked to emotions and distress** that the person may sometimes not be able to connect with or communicate to people in the environment. Occasionally, people with FND experience **(selective) assertiveness** problems or **social anxiety** and automatically 'shut down' their physical voice in social situations as a safety behaviour to help them express or cope with distress.

Although not usually a core discipline in existing FND services, a speech and language therapist (SLT) may be part of a highly specialist neurorehabilitation team. SLTs support people with FND:

- To use their voice again after a long time of having been 'mute'.
- To use their voice in more helpful ways that stop damage to body tissues, for example the vocal folds, and prevent the progression to permanent injury.
- To apply speech/face-related relaxation and breathing exercises to release tension.
- By assessing whether speech difficulties are caused by FND or brain injury.
- By providing reassurance and 'evidence' of intact voice and speech mechanisms.
- Who tend to have speech difficulties as their most prominent, severe, or disabling symptom.

With that in mind, speech and language therapy is not automatically recommended for everyone with functional speech problems because it may **increase the attentional focus** on speech symptoms, result in **more healthcare contacts**, and have the **potential to ultimately worsen the FND**. Furthermore, if someone experiences functional speech problems as part of a wider range of FND symptoms, then **addressing the underlying psychosocial** that ties these symptoms together is probably a **more effective** approach than specifically focusing on each of the individual symptoms.

6.9 eResource alert!

If you are curious about what a speech and language therapist may focus on in FND, then this eResource may help you gain a better understanding and provide more background reading on this important role during FND rehabilitation.

Wide-open covers

Sometimes, the pendulum can swing into the other direction. Rather than experiencing a tight cover, as most people with FND probably will, **people's covers can be too open** (see Figure 6.11). What might that look like?

Here are some things to think about in relation to wide-open covers

- Some people have **not had the opportunity** to learn 'opening-up' skills and may not be adept at picking up the often-subtle social cues in their environment that help fine-tune emotional expression.
- **Reasons** include a difficult upbringing, past traumas, school bullying experiences, or neurodevelopmental difficulties and autism.
- **Oversharing your information** and overexpressing emotions with other people, especially if you have had limited opportunity to do so in the past, may make you feel more supported, safe, and secure, and the environment may respond back to you with care and validation. It can become a person's main coping strategy for distress and unmet needs.
- There is a **delicate balance to strike between opening and closing your cover**. Too tight and you risk amplifying FND symptoms. Too open and you may incur other problems with relationships, setting boundaries, and exposing vulnerabilities.

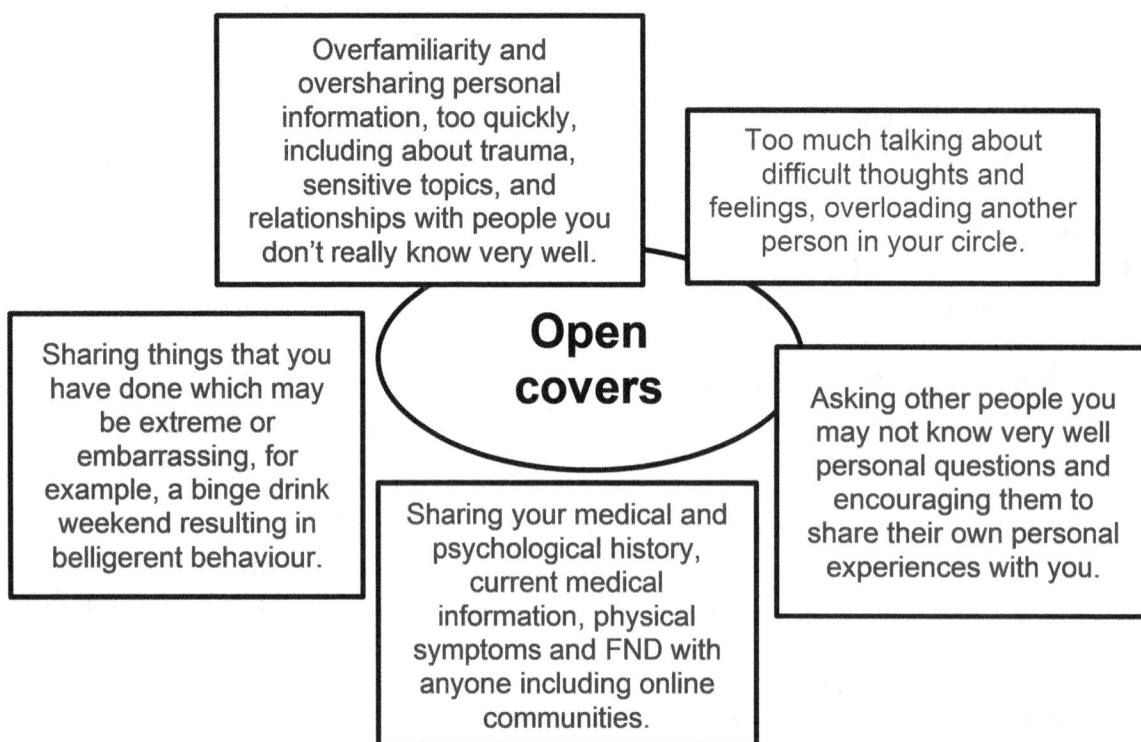

Figure 6.11 Characteristics of open covers.

- Think about **personal risks**. Oversharing makes you vulnerable to ill-intended people around you, some of whom may not have your best interests at heart. You may risk exploitation and for your information to be used in ways that you would not want.
- **Self-fulfilling prophecy.** If we think about the rejection theme in FND, oversharing information and emotional overexpression may make people reject you in the long run. For example, the other person may become tired, overburdened, or drained and starts to distance themselves from you – exactly the outcome that a lot of people fear.
- **Ultimately, a wide-open cover maintains the FND.** Talking a lot about FND and how it affects you emotionally on a daily basis feeds the FND by increasing the attentional focus on physical symptoms and keeping it going (read more about the warning light element in Chapter 8).

6.10 eResource alert!

What emotion skills, types of relationships, and qualities of social networks enable the biggest chance for helpful expression of emotions? Find out here!

Valve

The valve in the Pressure Cooker Model represents our **activity levels**. Life offers us a whole range of activities, including:

- Activities we enjoy doing and lift our moods (sports, hobbies).
- Things that help us relax and rest, like sleep, reading a good book, and 'downtime'.
- Social activities.
- Occupational activities (a job or voluntary role).
- Other meaningful activities (caring for others, being part of a religious organisation).
- And many more!

People with FND often show one out of **three activity patterns** that can maintain the FND. Let us discuss each one in turn.

Blocked valve: bust (after boom)

A blocked valve is characterised by a period of heightened activity, often over long periods of time. Suddenly, the activity levels 'bust', resulting in low or no activity. There are two versions of the bust-after-boom valve:

- **Gradual build-up.** Activity levels may have gradually and insidiously crept up over time. The subsequent 'bust' is the result of your usual but insufficiently effective coping mechanisms unable to manage the ever-increasing demand, especially if you have been highly active over long periods (the 'new normal') and your coping mechanisms have lost their effectiveness over time and started to unravel. An example is a person who has had to juggle multiple and heavy life pressures, like caring for a family, high-pressure job, illness, topped up with daily stresses that become unmanageable (see Figure 6.12).
- **Before-and-after.** There may have been continuous overactivity over prolonged periods. You fared well, until a sudden, significant, or even traumatic event happens in your life, such as an accident, relationship break-up, or job loss. Your existing coping mechanisms are ineffective to withstand the suddenly significantly increased stress and deal with the aftermath and subsequently crack under the pressure (see Figure 6.13).

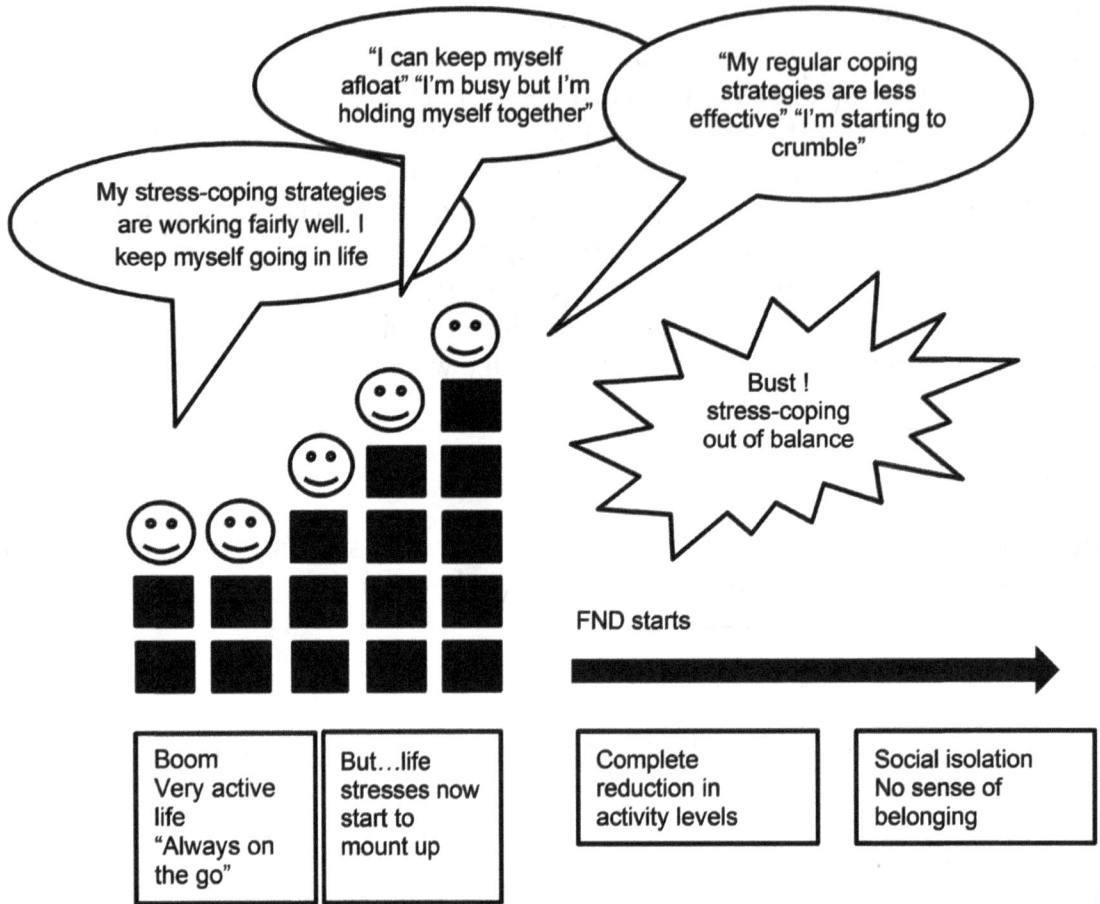

Figure 6.12 Gradual build-up scenario of the bust-after-boom valve.

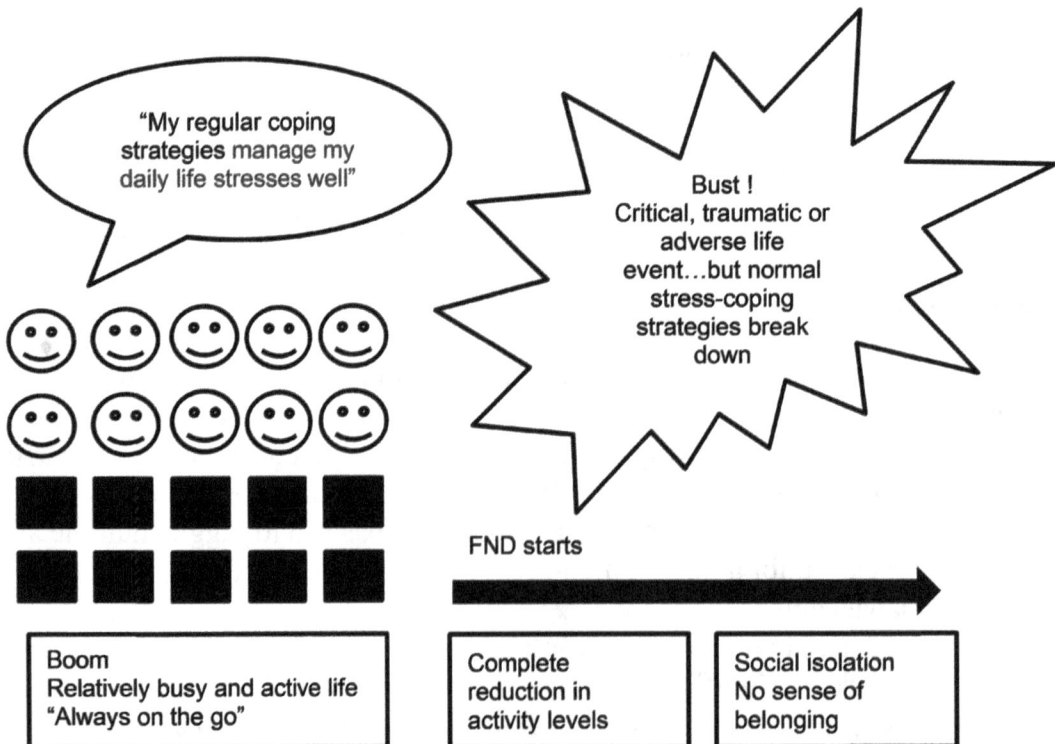

Figure 6.13 Before-and-after scenario of the bust-after-boom valve.

Sometimes people have (often unconsciously) used staying active or overactivity as **a form of avoiding difficult thoughts and feelings**. When the bust happens, suddenly all these avoided thoughts and feelings can emerge from seemingly out of nowhere and cause low mood as well as a lot of turmoil. It may feel like you have been hit by a stream of new emotions where in fact these emotions had been suppressed by the overactivity for a long time. The low mood causes thinking difficulties with your memory, concentration, and planning, and this can subsequently impact on your ability to plan your time properly and attempts at returning to your previous activity levels.

Dysregulated valve: boom-and-bust

A dysregulated valve is characterised by activity levels that follow a **'peaks and troughs'** pattern. People with a boom-and-bust profile tend to have activity levels that are consistently too high ('overactivity'), alternated with too low ('underactivity'), and somehow never manage to find an 'even keel' (see Figure 6.14).

- People may genuinely believe that booming-and-busting is an effective pattern of managing activity levels. Unsurprisingly, alternating activity levels is what life normally consists of! You are engaged with a meaningful activity that is naturally followed by a rest period for recovery from that activity (think about relaxing after a busy workday). However, the **boom-and-bust pattern** experienced by a lot of people with FND is **a magnified, long-standing, and unhealthy version** of this.

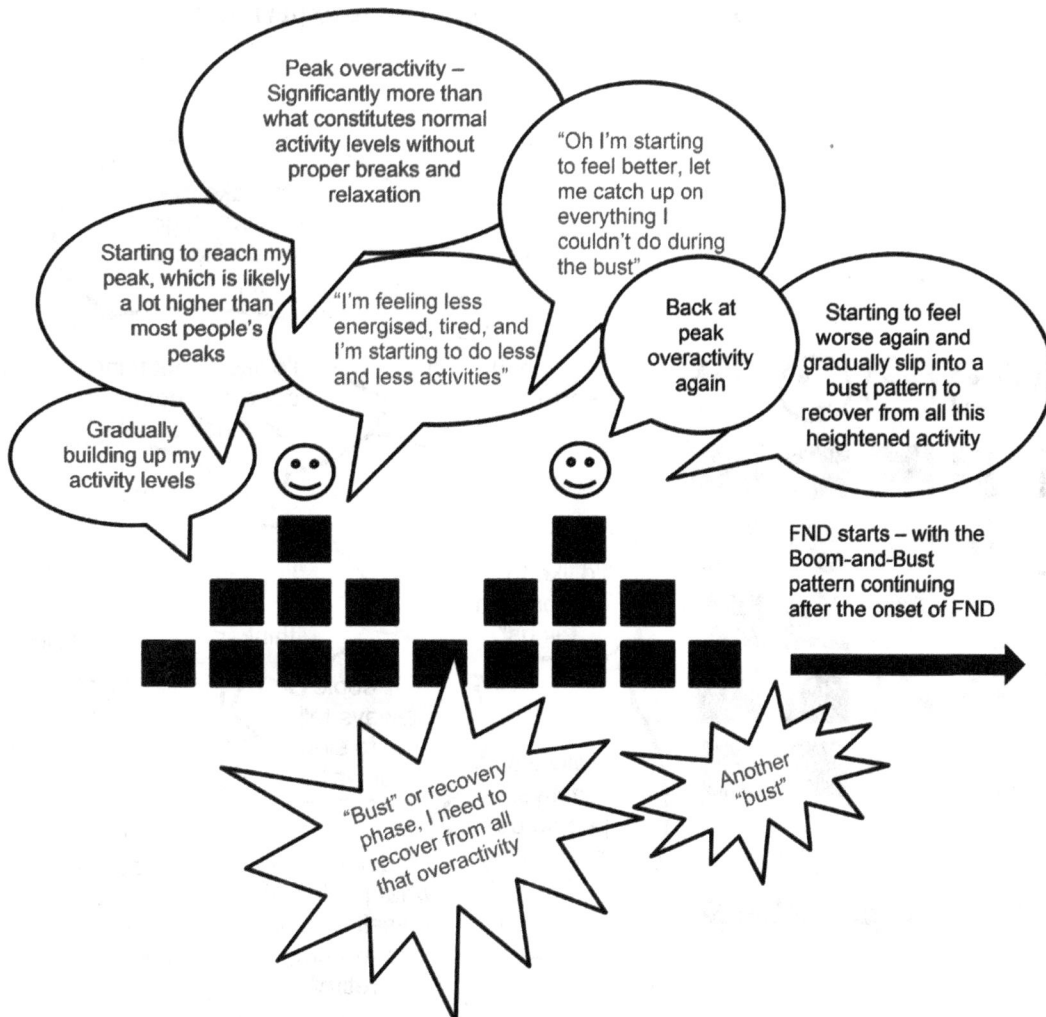

Figure 6.14 Boom-and-bust valve scenario.

- What a lot of people do not realise is that **booming-and-busting results in less efficiency and more health problems over time** than if you would adopt a paced, 'even keel' approach with **flattened peaks and troughs**, characterised by a more constant activity level with regular rest breaks as part of a healthy routine.
- **Anxiety, guilt, psychological pressure, and agitation** about not having been able to do things during the underactive 'bust' periods may drive catching up on activities during the overactive 'boom' periods.
- Some people may find it hard to stop themselves from being active, especially when they are 'on a roll'. **Achieving a state of flow** is great, but if you struggle to identify the limits of your activity levels or fail to decline activities and demands placed on you, a boom-and-bust cycle may be looming.

Overused valve: boom

The final valve pattern found in people with FND is the 'boom' valve. Figure 6.15 shows typical comments that people with boom valves often make.

Developing a boom valve is problematic for the following reasons:

- **You are not dealing with the real underlying problems:** learning to tolerate and 'ride the wave' of difficult thoughts and feelings, addressing the life problems that lead to those thoughts and feelings, dissociation, holding on to old but destructional coping habits, or problems with assertiveness. You are essentially **missing out on better life experiences**.

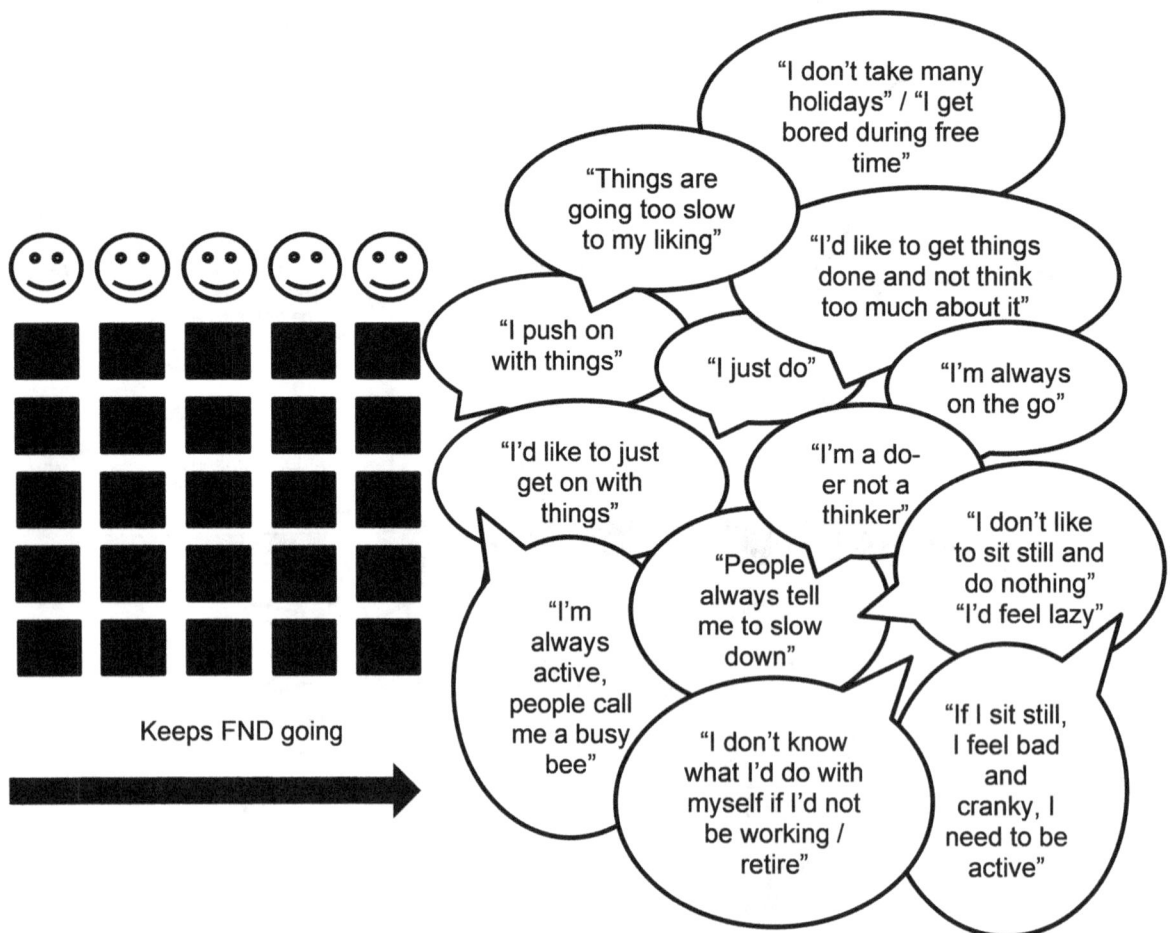

Figure 6.15 Boom valve scenario.

Table 6.4 Reasons that people with and without FND develop a tendency towards overactivity

Reason	Details
Form of dissociation & avoidance of "the difficult stuff"	Pushing on may be a form of dissociation, or "cutting off your emotions". If you are always busy and never sitting still, then you don't have to think about difficult thoughts and feelings. The moment you stop being active, the distress will kick in. Therefore, pushing on can create psychological safety.
Negative emotions about sitting still	Some people worry about falling into a deep depression if they would reduce their activity levels. The "pushing on" behaviour of other people may be driven by anxiety and worries.
Strong beliefs about sitting still	• Some people with FND entertain strong unhelpful beliefs about the opposite state of "pushing on": sitting still. They may have learned from an early age or through various life experiences that sitting still means being lazy or unmotivated. They may not allow themselves a break. • These thoughts often lead to feelings of guilt and anxiety. People may find tolerating these feelings difficult and therefore push on with activities. • Other people may have perfectionist tendencies and high expectations; they may not allow themselves to rest until the work has been finished to their high standards, resulting in a lot of pushing on.
Low self-esteem	Some people with FND and low self-esteem think "I'm not good enough". To cope with this negative belief about themselves, they may have developed a rule for living to counter that "If I work hard and do everything perfect, I can show other people that I'm good enough". Earlier we have seen how low self-esteem and reduced assertiveness go hand-in-hand. People who are not good at stating their needs and setting boundaries may end up in harmful overactivity patterns as a result of demands placed by their environment.
Sense of achievement	It can be rewarding to push on with activities. Some people only feel accomplished if they engage in high level activity. This links in with the previous point on low self-esteem.
Early coping habit and lack of awareness around alternatives	Pushing on with activities often originates in childhood. Some people are used to this coping habit and don't know any better or are unaware of other coping alternatives. Having been involved in a lot of caring activities in the past and having experienced significant carer burden can also cause someone's valve to "boom".
Lack of relaxation skill	Not knowing how to relax and not having any relaxation strategies and "me" time for yourself. This often originates in someone's childhood.
Cultural background & values	People may come from a cultural background that values "hard work" and pushing on. You may have grown up in a culture where relaxing was seen as being lazy or in some way punished whereas the opposite, pushing on, was seen as a virtue.

- Pushing on may create the **false impression** that you are finding **psychological safety** in constructive ways that produce results and achievements. However, in the end, **it is a form of avoidance** that masks difficulties that need addressing in different, more constructive, but less detrimental ways.
- Some people with a boom valve may **focus on one specific area of life** (for example, work, cleaning your house). This creates tunnel vision, a lack of variation in life, boredom, missing out on other experiences, reduction of enjoyment, and may result in you foregoing responsibilities from other important life areas and not reach other life goals.
- **Overactivity can impact on your body** and result in increased levels of fatigue, feeling drained, burnout, as well as pain and tension in your muscles from the underlying anxiety or other distress that may come with overactivity.
- The most important drawback: **a boom valve maintains FND**. Sometimes, a 'boom' valve can transform into a 'bust-after-boom' or a 'boom-and-bust' valve, particularly in people who have been pushing hard over long periods of time. Daily stresses may build up more and more, whilst people's strategies to cope with the stress demands in life gradually unravel.

6.11 eResource alert!

Read here how you can assess the state of your valve and whether it is functioning properly.

Unblocking your valve: create a sense of social belonging

In the late seventies, Professor Bruce K. Alexander, a psychologist from Simon Fraser University in Canada conducted a series of iconic addiction experiments with rats (Alexander et al., 1978; Hadaway et al., 1979). He divided rats up into subgroups that he placed in different types of cages. One cage was an impoverished environment without much mental stimulation and interesting activities to do. The other type of cage consisted of a large space, full-on 'rat heaven' colony with food, playing wheels, and opportunities for mating activities.

In the meantime, the cages also contained a drip with sweet morphine water. The rats in the impoverished environment increased the self-administration of morphine more so than did the rats in 'rat park'. It also turned out that the 'rat parkers' mostly resisted the morphine and preferred water instead. Of course, there is a lot more to 'drug addiction' than what is conveyed in this simple experiment. However, it is interesting to note that the big difference between the two cages was **the quality of the surrounding environment**. The 'rat park rats' were a happy bunch, engaged and stimulated by their environment, whereas the rats in the other cage were bored and driven to morphine.

Neuroimaging investigations point to **interesting links between our social environment and our brains** (please note that correlation does not mean causation!):

- Social network size is associated with the size of the amygdala (Bickart et al., 2011; Kanai et al., 2012), the brain's fear centre. Bickart et al. (2011) found that the larger the size of your amygdala, the bigger and more complex people's social networks.
- Social network size in people with FND was associated with the size of the brain's 'pleasure' and reward centres (nucleus accumbens), as well as the memory centres (hippocampus; Ospina et al., 2019).
- 'Online' social network size was also associated with the density of brain structures in the temporal lobes that are important for social and memory functions (Kanai et al., 2012).
- Another important finding suggests that, indeed, rejection by people is a painful experience: social rejection stimulates the same brain regions as physical pain (Kross et al., 2011).

Social isolation is often a big problem in FND. Let us go through some reasons for social isolation in FND:

- FND symptoms and disabilities may **prevent you from accessing the community** or interacting with others (e.g. functional speech difficulties), which limits opportunities for socialising and connecting.
- You may have **gradually lost friends** because of the FND. In the clinic, people with FND have reported that some of their friends do not want to deal with their symptoms, do not know how to relate to them, or may be embarrassed being seen with someone in a wheelchair or other equipment.
- Due to **adverse early experiences**, you may find it difficult to interact, trust, or make contact with people. You may feel **low in confidence** around interacting with people.
- **Psychological conditions** such as social anxiety, agoraphobia, and depression may stop you from seeking out social company due to anxiety or low motivation.
- **Coercive control**, for example, a family member or partner who prevents you from going out and socialise with others, due to their own insecurities and need for control.

Social isolation leads to a reduced sense of belonging. Sense of social belonging is associated with the thoughts, feelings, and behaviours displayed in Figure 6.16.

There are many forms of community and social groups that can generate a sense of belonging, for example, a sports team, hobbies, church and other religious groups, volunteering networks, but also your family, friendships, neighbourhood, town, or culture.

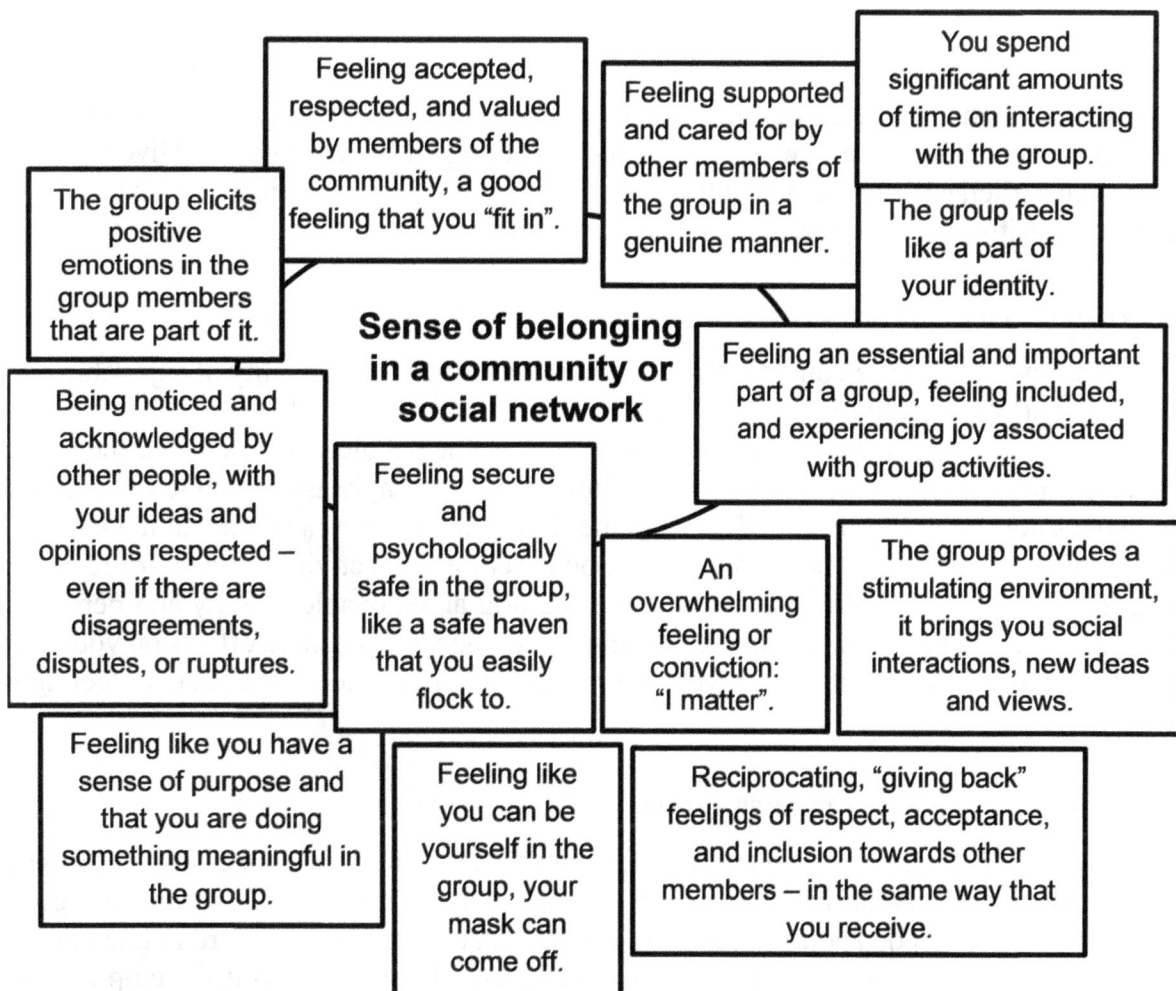

Figure 6.16 Characteristics of a healthy sense of social belonging to a group or community.

Sometimes there is a mismatch between being part of the social group and feeling that you truly belong to that group. Being part of a group does not automatically mean a sense of social belonging. Just existing in a group, 'coasting along', attending group events, and even actively participating without the feeling of emotional and social connection to that group are all signs of a reduced sense of belonging.

Sense of belonging is a very important concept in FND. Not only does a feeling of belonging to a group lift your mood and improve your psychological as well as physical well-being; a closely knit, cohesive, and psychologically safe group can also help disconfirm any unfounded negative beliefs that you hold about yourself.

A significant group of people with FND report long-standing experiences of rejection, social exclusion, being singled out, and systemic re-traumatisation in childhood and adulthood. These rejection experiences fuel unhelpful beliefs and emotions ('I don't matter', 'I'm different', 'I'm less than other people', 'People are untrustworthy', 'The world is unsafe'). A group that creates a sense of belonging, acceptance, and psychological safety can be a powerful antidote ('I matter', 'I am fine as I am', 'I am a good person', 'Other people are trustworthy and will help me').

6.12 eResource alert!

If you feel socially isolated, read about what you can do to increase your social network size and create a sense of social belonging.

Behavioural activation: increase your positive experiences

Behavioural activation is the act of finding enjoyable activities in your life to lift your mood. This is not just about picking up a new interest or re-connecting with an old hobby. Given what you have learned earlier, it is important that the enjoyable activities create a sense of social belonging, acceptance, positive experiences, and connectedness to people.

MOOD–ACTIVITY LINK

There is a strong link between our mood and the number as well as the quality of enjoyable activities in our life ('mood–activity link'; see Figure 6.17).

It is often unclear which came first: chicken or egg? Some people with FND find their moods plummeting after developing FND. For others, low mood is strongly associated with the onset of FND. It does not matter how it started; what matters more is what we can do about it. One powerful technique to break the link is to slowly re-introduce enjoyable activities into your life. Despite feeling low in energy and 'down in the dumps', starting an enjoyable activity and persevering with it, regardless of how you feel inside, will eventually generate positive effects on your mood. You just need to persist with it, even if you do not see immediate effects: the positive feeling will follow.

BOILING SOUP IN THE PRESSURE COOKER: CHANGING THE FLAVOUR

Do you remember the ignition element from Chapter 5? This Pressure Cooker Model element is often associated with past difficult and adverse circumstances in childhood. Maybe you feel that there is nothing you can do about the ignition. It is true that time moves forward in one direction; we cannot go back in time and change events. However, what we can do is develop an understanding of the vulnerabilities that contributed to the emergence of FND symptoms, as we have

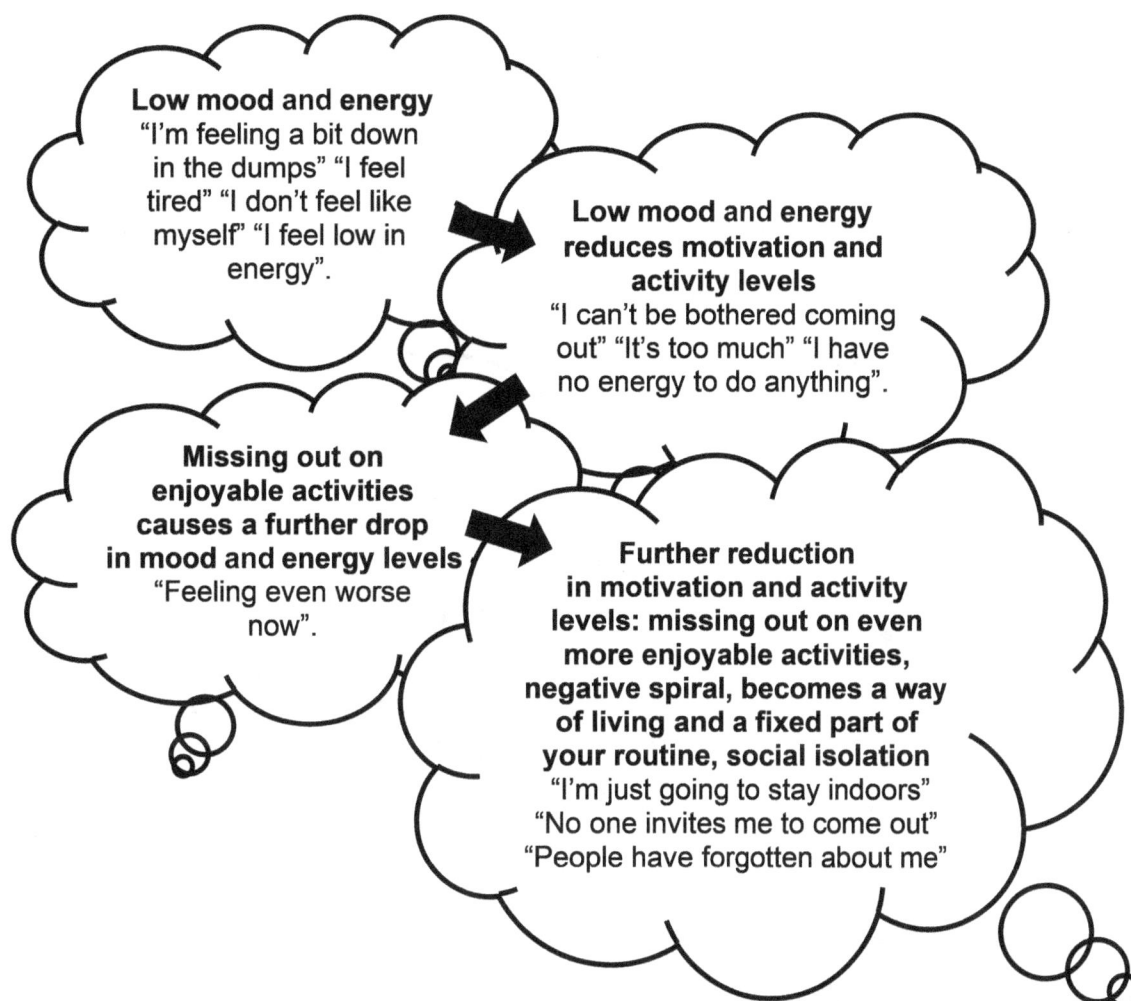

Figure 6.17 Mood–activity link.

done in Chapter 5. Another technique is to **change our relationship to these adverse life events**. How can we do that?

Imagine the following situation: You have experienced childhood adversity and several difficult life events in adulthood. Those experiences have changed you as a person. Let us suppose that these experiences make the contents inside your 'pressure cooker soup' unpleasantly salty or bitter. Understandably, you report a lot of unhelpful core beliefs about yourself, other people, the world, and your future.

Now imagine that you find a way of making the soup less salty and bitter. Adding condiments, herbs, spices, sour cream, sugar, and perhaps some roux to the boiling pot could improve the soup contents. After boiling the soup for a while, you notice that the soup has taken on a better flavour. It is less salty, not as bitter, and just tastes a lot more pleasant. It is actually edible, and you are starting to enjoy the soup!

In this metaphor, adding the condiments represents **adding enjoyable activities** that give you **a sense of achievement, give you positive emotions, and are pleasurable**. The soup is like your life experiences: the salty and bitter bits are still in the pot, just as our adverse life experiences are still in our memories and part of our past life. There was no way of removing these bits from the soup with any means, in the same way as we cannot turn back time.

However, with the addition of new ingredients, you managed to change the flavour of the soup into a more palatable experience. In the same way, **adding more positive and enjoyable**

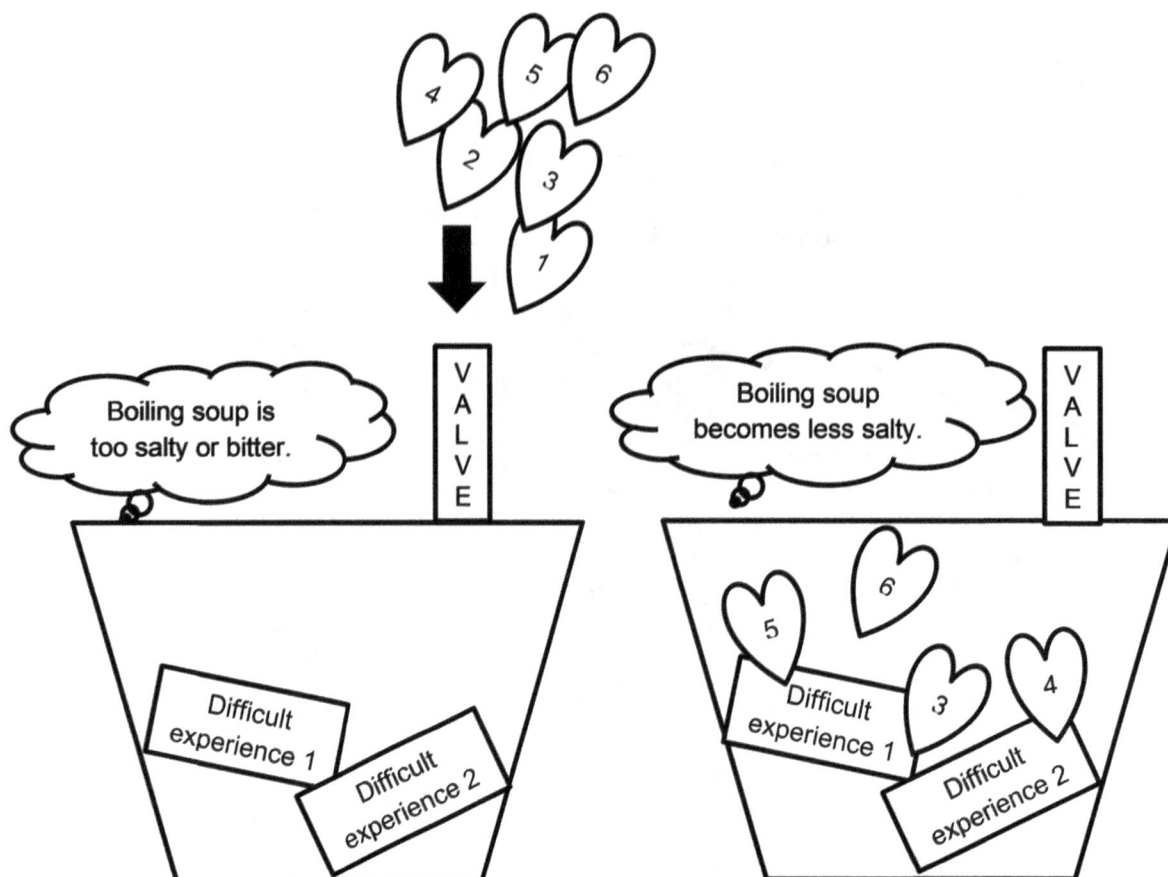

Figure 6.18 Relationship between enjoyable and difficult experiences in the Pressure Cooker Model.

experiences (sweet flavouring) to a salty and bitter soup (adverse experiences) **can neutralise difficult rejection experiences without necessarily removing them**. You will still have memories of the past; however, the more enjoyable experiences you add into your life, the more you dilute and change your relationship to these adverse experiences. You are building a 'buffer' of positive experiences that soften the blow of difficult memories. Figure 6.18 displays that process in visual form.

Slowing down!

The following section is a helpful read for people who would like **to regulate their valve to stop booming and busting,** or those that are always on the go and would like to learn how **to alleviate their valves to reduce the boom**.

Assess the situation

- **Are you a busy bee . . . or avoiding?**

Some people are just natural 'busy bees' and enjoy being active. There is nothing wrong with that! The purpose is not to change your personality from a busy bee into something that you are not.

However, if you are a person with FND who enjoys being busy, you are encouraged to think about another layer to increased activity levels.

To become more aware of this 'extra layer', ask yourself an honest question: Do my increased activity levels serve an extra purpose? Am I avoiding distress or sitting with emotions by always being active?

- **Explore underlying reasons**

Flick back to Table 6.4. Do any of the reasons for overactivity speak to you? Pick your main reason, as this will guide you in choosing your target area. For example:

- Building your self-esteem.
- Challenge strong beliefs about activity rooted in past life experiences.
- Finding alternative ways to obtain a sense of achievement, psychological safety, and cope with emotions.
- Learning how to relax.
- Behavioural experiments to learn to sit with distress.
- Assertiveness training.
- Beware of cultural considerations.
- And so forth.

- **Make fair comparisons**

How does your definition of slowing down compare to the definition that other people hold? Make multiple enquiries with people in and outside your family environment to make a fair judgement on what constitutes normal and acceptable activity levels.

What you can do yourself

- **Make a psychological commitment to stop**

Think about the consequences of continuing 'the boom' any further:

- Less efficiency and productivity compared to paced activity schedules
- Fatigue
- Depression and guilt during the bust
- Longer-lasting bust phases over time
- A complete bust.

Is it worth pushing on?

- **Something's got to give: prioritize**

For other people, overactivity is born out of necessity – it is a need: life consists of so many activities, tasks, demands, and responsibilities that you hardly have time to 'breathe' and are pushed from one thing to the next without feeling in control.

If that is you, determine what could go from your schedule to allow sufficient rest breaks. Prioritise what is most important to you. There are only 24 hours in a day, and we sleep about 7 to 8 hours.

You could prioritise attending to your basic needs first: get enough sleep, time to eat and take care of yourself (you need to look out for you!). Whatever is left timewise: consider ways that you can cut out less urgent tasks so that you can prioritise activities that need your focus right now. If overactivity is making you feel unwell and is a likely contributor to FND, then making changes is a priority.

- **Rest up!**

Build in sufficient and regular rest periods. Allow yourself time to do what you prefer and enjoy. Rest does not always equal an enjoyable activity; it can also be rest from any activity.

Some people have no idea of what to 'do' in order to rest and feel compelled to 'do something constructive' at all costs. How about binge-watch a series, take a long bath, spend quality time with your partner, an old hobby that released a lot of tension for you? If you are really stuck for ideas, brainstorm options with a loved one.

- **Create and stick to a routine**

A routine can be a powerful way of regulating our activity levels. Routines can create psychological containment and prevent over- and under-activity. Be realistic and pace yourself. A good rule of thumb is, 'little and often' instead of 'a lot all at once'. It will pay off in the end: you gain more time and efficiency by stopping booming and busting.

What your social environment can do to support you:

- **Ask a friend or family member for help**

Sitting with distress does not mean sitting with distress on your own all the time. Think about opening your cover and express your feelings to someone else you trust to help with alleviating the valve.

- **Collaborate with an ally to both reduce activity levels**

Be mindful of people in your close environment who may also not have mastered the skill of slowing down. Collaborate and learn to slow down together, hold each other accountable.

- **Respect your boundaries and learn to say 'no'**

Ensure that you have sufficient 'me' time and make that clear to your environment. People around us can, purposefully or inadvertently, encroach on 'me' time by neglecting to honour your relaxation breaks. Learn to decline activities and demands placed on you, as well as tolerating the feelings that come with it.

Monitor your process of slowing down

- **Watch out for subtle safety behaviours creeping in.**

For example, allowing yourself to have a movie night but doing dishes or other chores in the background.

- **Unhelpful thoughts and emotions.**

When people start to slow down, they may suddenly experience a flurry of difficult thoughts and feelings (often guilt and anxiety) about not being active enough, or emotions that were suppressed with activity all this time.

- **Dos.** Expect that this is bound to happen. Try tolerating and sitting with the discomfort: 'just be' without immediately taking action to bring down the feelings. You can also challenge unhelpful thoughts around resting, not deserving to 'sit still', and the boom-and-bust cycle. Would you think the same way about a good friend in a similar situation? Explore this 6.13 **eResource** for inspiration.
- **Don'ts.** Ensure that you are not quickly distracting yourself with new activities to cope with the difficult thoughts and feelings, since these can act as psychological safety behaviours.

• Self-compassion

Oftentimes, being kind to ourselves is the hardest challenge of all. You are deserving of rest breaks, allowing necessary restoration of your body – irrespective of how you have been brought up or whatever life experiences you have been through.

If you are also a carer for another person, then self-compassion is even more important, as attending to your own needs first ensures you having enough energy to be the best possible carer for another person.

Final thoughts

Some people with FND say:

> I know people who have always bottled emotions up (i.e. tight cover) and worked long hours without many hobbies and rest breaks (i.e. overactive valve) – how come they don't have FND?

Good question!

There is (still) a good balance between 'stress/difficult life events' and 'effective coping strategies'

It is true that a lot of people in society consistently use these coping strategies and somehow do not seem to experience any FND. People can fare well in life for a long time, sometimes for decades since early childhood, until a big life event becomes 'one too many'. The usual coping strategies that served you well in the past just cannot properly do the job anymore and are unable to manage the upsurge in emotion, stress, discomfort, or whatever you prefer to call the unpleasant state of being that difficult life events tend to create. It is like the balance between 'stress/difficult life events' and 'effective coping strategies' has tipped over and the coping system shuts down leading to an increased risk of developing FND.

Same process, different manifestations

It is also important to know that some people with this specific configuration of coping strategies may not develop FND but then go on to develop other coping strategies that may bring down the distress or discomfort quickly and effectively, in the same way as FND, but are less helpful, for instance, drinking, overeating, or deliberate self-harm. This is not to say that FND falls in the same category as these other strategies. It simply means that you have to look at the underlying 'process'. What do these strategies have in common? They all reduce discomfort (Flick back to Figure 2.30 at the end of Chapter 2).

Both the individual and the environment equally contribute to FND

Also keep in mind that for FND to emerge, a whole lot of other factors play a role, including what people around you do, act, feel, and believe. Check out the Pressure Cooker Model for each element that is important in FND.

There is so much more to FND than just the Pressure Cooker Model, but do remember that sticking to this formula will help you take your first steps on your way to FND recovery:

- **Opening the cover** (regularly expressing difficult thoughts and feelings in psychologically safe relationships)
- **Regulating the valve** (returning to normal activity levels in your life)
- **Blocks the overpressure plug** (reduces the risk for FND symptoms to emerge)

References

Alexander, B. K., Coambs, R. B., & Hadaway, P. F. (1978). The effect of housing and gender on morphine self-administration in rats. *Psychopharmacology*, *58*(2), 175–179.

Alsaadi, T. M., & Marquez, A. V. (2005). Psychogenic nonepileptic seizures. *American Family Physician*, *72*(5), 849–856.

Bickart, K. C., Wright, C. I., Dautoff, R. J., Dickerson, B. C., & Barrett, L. F. (2011). Amygdala volume and social network size in humans. *Nature Neuroscience*, *14*(2), 163–164.

Bowman, E. S., & Markand, O. N. (1999). The contribution of life events to pseudoseizure occurrence in adults. *Bulletin of the Menninger Clinic*, *63*(1), 70.

Griffith, J. L., Polles, A., & Griffith, M. E. (1998). Pseudoseizures, families, and unspeakable dilemmas. *Psychosomatics*, *39*(2), 144–153.

Hadaway, P. F., Alexander, B. K., Coambs, R. B., & Beyerstein, B. (1979). The effect of housing and gender on preference for morphine-sucrose solutions in rats. *Psychopharmacology*, *66*(1), 87–91.

Kanai, R., Bahrami, B., Roylance, R., & Rees, G. (2012). Online social network size is reflected in human brain structure. *Proceedings of the Royal Society B: Biological Sciences*, *279*(1732), 1327–1334.

Krawetz, P., Fleisher, W., Pillay, N., Staley, D., Arnett, J., & Maher, J. (2001). Family functioning in subjects with pseudoseizures and epilepsy. *The Journal of Nervous and Mental Disease*, *189*(1), 38–43.

Kross, E., Berman, M. G., Mischel, W., Smith, E. E., & Wager, T. D. (2011). Social rejection shares somatosensory representations with physical pain. *Proceedings of the National Academy of Sciences*, *108*(15), 6270–6275.

Ospina, J. P., Larson, A. G., Jalilianhasanpour, R., Williams, B., Diez, I., Dhand, A., Dickerson, B. C., & Perez, D. L. (2019). Individual differences in social network size linked to nucleus accumbens and hippocampal volumes in functional neurological disorder: A pilot study. *Journal of Affective Disorders*, *258*, 50–54.

Slocum, R. B. (2021). Breaking the spell: narrative medicine applications for psychogenic nonepileptic seizures (PNES). *Seizure*, *86*, 96–101.

Wood, B. L., McDaniel, S., Burchfiel, K., & Erba, G. (1998). Factors distinguishing families of patients with psychogenic seizures from families of patients with epilepsy. *Epilepsia*, *39*(4), 432–437.

7 The FND maintenance cycle

Fuel, flames, heat, overpressure plug (layer 3)

If you are a person with FND, a family member, a friend, or a healthcare professional who has only just started to learn about FND, you may be wondering about how emotions suddenly can turn into FND. What are the exact steps between emotions and FND, and can we pinpoint to any clear, underlying mechanisms? What sorts of things keep the FND going? And more importantly, what can you do to stop FND from happening?

So many questions – welcome to Chapter 7! We have arrived at the 'heart' of the Pressure Cooker Model. You will learn about a process called **'internal regulation'**, which is the way a person copes with difficult thoughts and feelings on their own or by themselves without relying on another person. Chapter 9 will explore the **'external regulation'** mechanisms of FND, or the way a person and their environment both cope with difficult thoughts and feelings together, by relying on each other. Feel free to jump ahead if you would like to get an idea of the difference between these two types of coping mechanism in FND.

In Chapter 5, you learned **how the FND started** with the ignition. The chapters that follow teach you everything about **what keeps the FND going**. Chapter 6 focused on the FND coping triangle and the way that the sticky leftover food, cover, and valve work together as an understandable but unhelpful combination of coping strategies that increase the risk of FND. However, that is not the whole story of FND. Chapter 7 will teach you about another group of elements, called the **Pressure Cooker chain reaction**, consisting of the overpressure plug, fuel, flames, and heat.

Do not worry if this all feels too overwhelming. Chapter 7 will guide you through each element, step by step. Shall we make a start with the overpressure plug, the most important element of the chain? Off we go!

The Overpressure Plug

FND is an umbrella term that covers every neurological symptom that exists and a person can experience in their body. FND symptoms are inconsistent with a neurological, medical, or organic cause and explanation, in contrast to, for example, a stroke, hypoxic brain injury, multiple sclerosis, or dementia. The overpressure plug is an element of the Pressure Cooker Model that represents all your FND symptoms. FND symptoms often show high levels of variability, varying day by day and from person to person. Some people's FND starts with one type of symptom (seizures) and changes over time into an entirely different type of symptom (paralysis), whereas other people start with one symptom but gradually end up with a large constellation of different FND symptoms that cover the entire neurological system.

Clearly, every person experiences their own unique mixture of symptoms, and because of that, FND can be a really confusing condition to understand. To help you make better sense of the symptoms, it may be beneficial to keep in mind the five general categories of FND symptoms (displayed in Figure 7.1): **motor, sensory, cognitive**, and **awareness** symptoms. Since **speech and language problems**, a specific subcategory of motor symptoms, are incredibly common in FND and often have a symbolic meaning in FND; they deserve a special box of their own.

DOI: 10.4324/9781003308973-7

Functional Motor Symptoms
- Weakness, not being able to move your body or limbs, legs giving way, knee buckling
- Tremor or "shakes", tics
- Functional dystonia or "spasms", for example your foot in an unusual position
- Functional gait or walking problems (like slow walking, not able to stand or walk at all)
- Functional jerks and twitches, or "myoclonus".
- Functional bladder and bowel symptoms.

Functional Sensory Symptoms
- Loss of sensation, not being able to feel your legs or arms, or feeling the base underneath your feet
- Tingles
- Numbness
- Functional visual loss or blurred/double vision
- Hypersensitivity/ too much or altered sensation

Functional Speech and Language Symptoms
- A stammer, halting speech, repeating words, or parts of words.
- Problems with pronouncing and articulating the words due to functional facial or tongue weakness, including slurred speech.
- Generating distorted sounds or mumbling your words.
- 'Telegraphic' speech using simple grammatical structures - sometimes accompanied by developmental speech errors seen in children.
- Soft, whispering voice or losing your voice altogether and not being able to produce any speech.
- Word finding difficulties.
- Speaking in a foreign accent.
- In addition, functional swallowing difficulties can appear.

FND Overpressure Plug

Functional Seizure ("Awareness") Symptoms
- Dissociative or non-epileptic seizures, blackouts, drop attacks, vacant episodes.
- Fight/Flight: seizures involving lots of movement.
- Freeze: seizures with immobility and lying still.

Functional Cognitive Symptoms
- Problems with your memory, concentration, planning
- Word finding difficulties
- Brain fog
- Dizziness
- Foreign accent syndrome

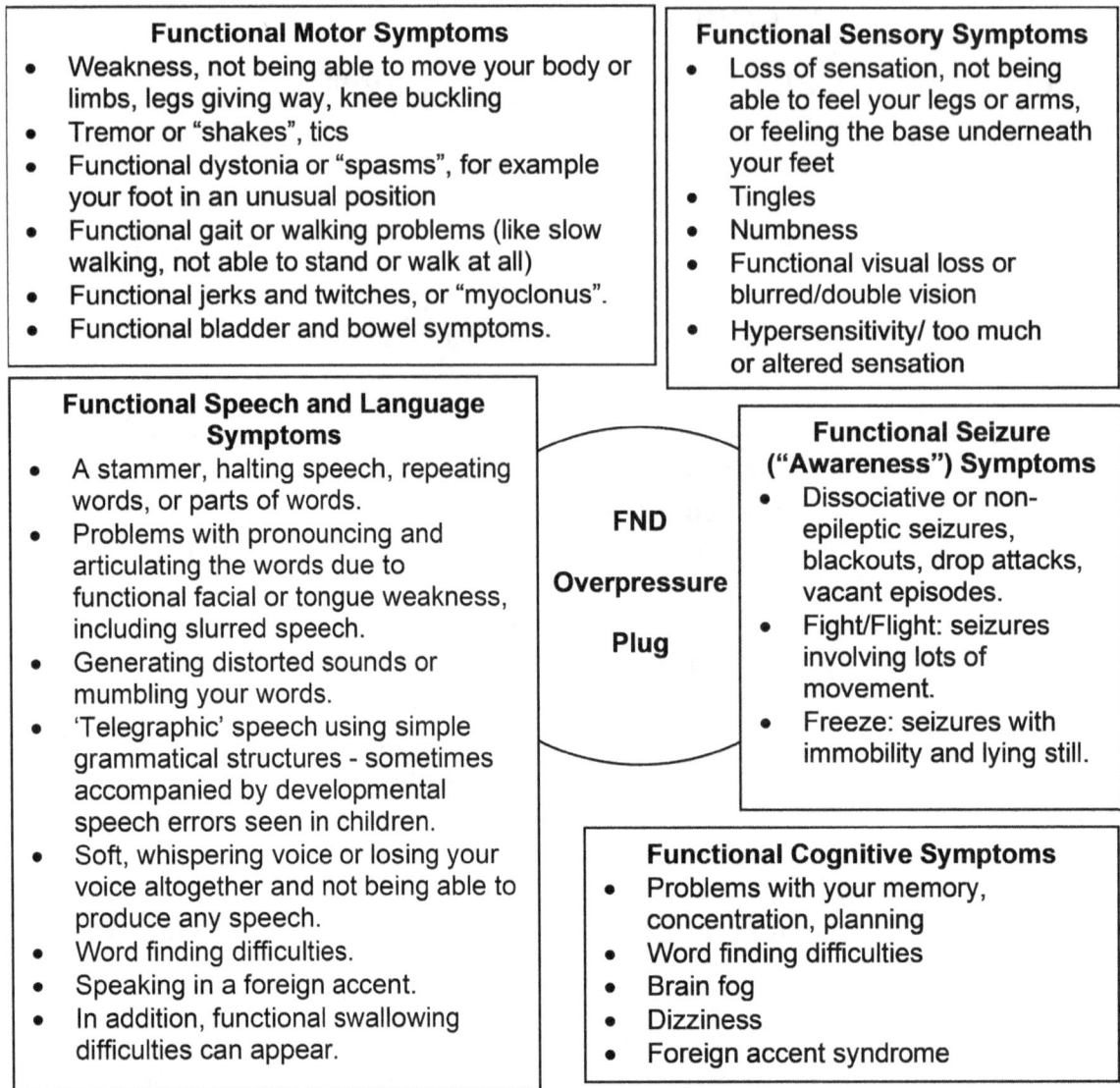

Figure 7.1 The five categories of FND symptoms.

7.1 eResource alert!

Find out what criteria and investigations are used to diagnose FND.

Figure 7.2 displays the most common symptoms that were found in a sample of people with FND who were at the very beginning of an intensive neurorehabilitation treatment programme. As you can see, the symptoms covered all the five areas of FND from Figure 7.1. Did you know that, for some people with FND, the symptoms can take on a **psychological or symbolic meaning**? (See Table 7.1.)

Who gets FND?

A better question to ask is: Who doesn't get FND? The short answer is, everyone can develop FND symptoms, and no one is exempt:

- **Any age and gender**, including, but not limited to, children, teenagers, young and middle-aged adults, senior citizens, men, and women.

Figure 7.2 -
The ten most frequent symptoms in people with FND

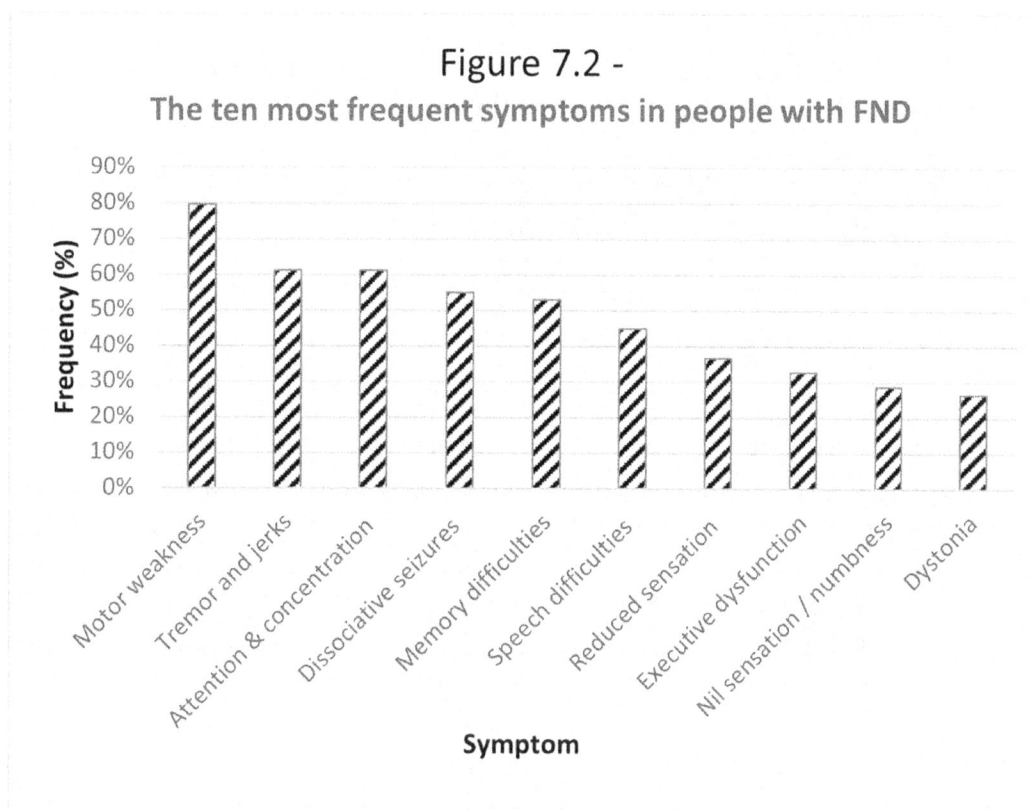

Figure 7.2 Most frequently reported FND symptoms in an inpatient neurorehabilitation sample.

Table 7.1 The symbolic meaning of FND symptoms

FND symptom	Psychological or symbolic meaning
Lower limb weakness and falls literally cause people to not feel their physical base.	Lack of feeling steady in yourself, often with a lack of a psychological secure base in your relationships.
Functional speech problems, stammering and loss of your voice.	Symbolic for not having a voice in relationships, the family setting and parallel to reduced assertiveness.
Tremor and shakes.	Can be an expression of underlying anxiety, you are "literally shaking".
Reduced or loss of physical sensation, inability to "feel" or altered sensations.	Not being in touch with, connecting or sensing emotions. The lack of physical sensation mirrors the lack of emotional sensation.
Immobility and physical paralysis in your limbs.	Feeling trapped and psychologically immobilised in a personal situation.
Some people experience speech and movement features that are characterised by hesitation and minimal progress over time, almost as if two opposing forces prevent the person from progressing further in speech and physiotherapy.	Can be an expression of fears of the unknown or "life consequences" after recovery. The person is often keen to recover but fears prevent the person from recovering, often unconsciously.

- **All cognitive and language abilities**, including people with learning disabilities, or cognitive difficulties due to brain injury or epilepsy.
- Any form of **employment** and **educational background**.
- People from across the world and of all **cultural, ethnic, and socio-economic** backgrounds.
- People in all forms of **relationships**, including married, single, divorced, widowed, and those with a relationship status that is complex or not clearly defined.

You may notice perhaps a higher risk for developing FND in some groups of people than in others. This is anecdotal evidence based on years of clinical experience:

- Both women and men can develop FND, although **women are more often seen in the clinic**. This could be due to a **higher risk**, but also to **historic and systemic influences**. In the past, FND was considered a 'women's condition'. The word 'hysteria' (an older pejorative but now disused term for FND) comes from the Greek word for *uterus*. This loaded historical context will shape healthcare professionals' own perceptions and 'viewing lens' of FND as a predominantly female condition. Societal pressures on men experiencing psychological difficulties associated with FND can lead to a higher threshold for men to access services, whereas this threshold is lower for women, potentially leading to earlier and better recognition of FND in women than men.
- In the FND clinic, there is probably a **trend towards younger women in their late teens and early to mid-20s** to experience **dissociative seizures** – occasionally with a background of complex trauma and, not unusual, a range of other physical health conditions, like Ehlers–Danlos, POTS, fibromyalgia, and chronic fatigue syndrome. In people with a complex trauma background, thinking about **'the underlying process'** behind the FND symptoms is a useful approach. FND is often one manifestation of underlying distress or discomfort (even if people are not aware of it) amidst other coping strategies that are very understandable and need our compassion but are less helpful in daily life and for achieving future goals.
- People who have experienced or witnessed a traumatic, frightening, dangerous, or threatening event (for example, an accident, assault, or combat stress) and subsequently develop **post-traumatic stress disorder**. Dissociation, a central concept in FND, is common and an understandable, protective mechanism against difficult memories, thoughts, and feelings in PTSD.
- Some **pregnant or post-partum women** may develop FND. This may be associated with a complex trauma background in their own childhood, the pregnancy, or a (trauma) trigger that coincidentally happens whilst pregnant. The news and experience of the pregnancy may retrigger a constellation of difficult thoughts, feelings, attachment issues, and 'psychological unsafety' that culminate in FND. Interestingly, men can also develop FND in the context of a new birth.
- **Healthcare professionals**, professional and family **carers**, as well as non-healthcare workers with exposure to physical or psychological health conditions.
- People who already have a physical illness themselves like **epilepsy** or **spinal issues** (jump ahead to Chapter 8 to explore possible reasons for this association), as well as people on the **autism spectrum** (FND and autism share overlapping features; check out Figure 7.3 to learn more). Please note that for the majority of people with both of these conditions, FND tends to develop a lot later in life than autism where features are present since childhood.

For both groups the symptoms impact on **social, work,** and **important areas of life**.	**Difficulties with social interactions** (think about someone with FND in the context of social anxiety or complex trauma, and **social isolation.**	**Sensory sensitivities** to noise, light, touch, smells, requiring ear defenders or sunglasses for example.

Overlapping features between FND and autism

Preferring things to be the **same and predictable, and struggling with change** (think about people with FND who have experienced complex / childhood trauma and grew up under unpredictable circumstances).	**Repetitive movements** (think about a tremor in FND) and **speech problems**, including not speaking at all.	Difficulties with **experiencing and managing emotions** including not being able to identify and label what you feel. Problems with understanding and maintaining **relationships**.

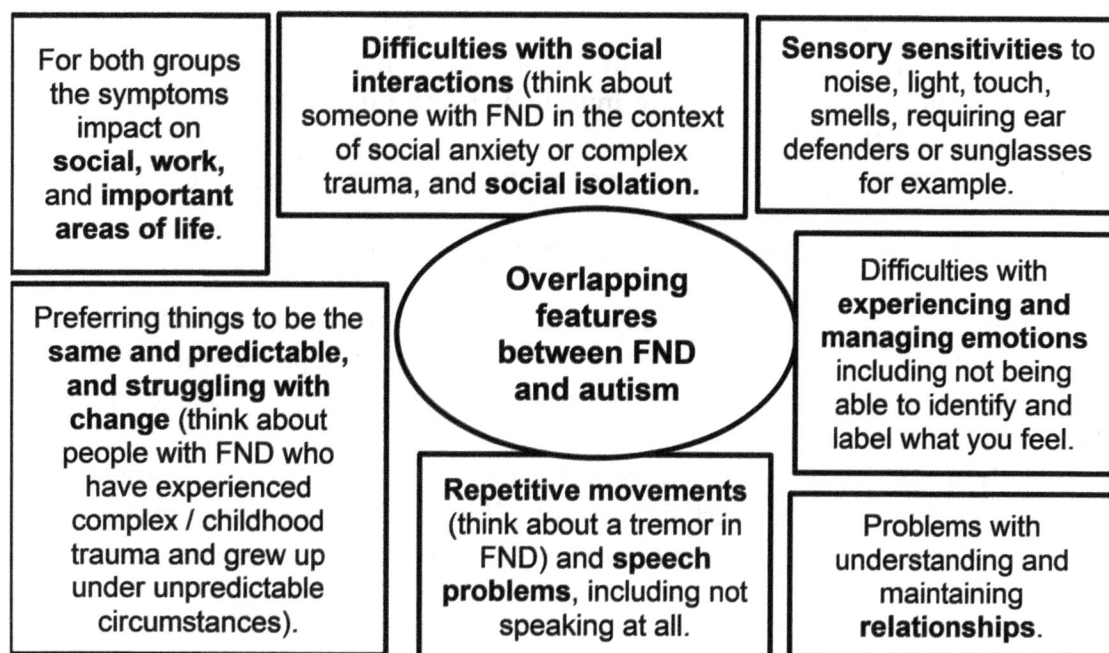

Figure 7.3 Overlapping features between FND and autism.

7.2 eResource alert!

A lot of myths and misunderstandings on FND float about. Let us increase your understanding of what FND is, and what it clearly is not, using a series of statements and explanations.

It is important to remember that the overpressure plug element conveys a lot more than just FND symptoms. The Pressure Cooker Model postulates that the **interpersonal dynamic between people with and without FND** equally contributes to the emergence and maintenance of FND. Whether you have FND or not, we all have an inner Pressure Cooker Model. Therefore, it makes sense that, **in people without FND** who regularly interact with the person with FND, **the overpressure plug also has meaning: their very own responses to FND.** Jump ahead to Chapters 9 and 10 if you would like to explore this further.

In the next section, you will learn more about another important concept in the Pressure Cooker Model: the **FND after-effects**.

FND after-effects

FND symptoms in themselves can be really hard to deal with on a daily basis. But did you know that the '**FND after-effects**' can be equally bothersome? FND after-effects are symptoms that do not necessarily fall into the 'official' diagnostic category of FND but are nevertheless frequently associated with – **most often but not always!** – the aftermath of FND.

What are some specific examples of FND after-effects?

- **Overwhelming fatigue** and the feeling of exhaustion after a dissociative episode. FND symptoms take a lot of energy from people. It is no surprise that your batteries feel like running on empty.

- **Disorientation**, amnesia, not knowing who and where you are, or what just happened.
- Painful muscle **cramps, spasms, and aches** because your limb has been in an uncomfortable position for a long time, or post-seizure muscle pain from the movements that some people experience as part of the seizure.
- **Wounds and injuries** to your body sustained during a dissociative episode.

Let us delve a little bit more into **fatigue** and **pain** next. Before we start, a few comments:

- Although fatigue and pain are two big topics in themselves that deserve their own discussion space that would go beyond the scope of this book, these symptoms cannot *not* be mentioned either! If you want to learn about FND, it is important to also gather knowledge about these two most often reported co-occurring symptoms in FND.
- It is probably useful to know that triggers, treatments, and theoretical approaches towards FND, fatigue, and pain tend to overlap. Therefore, if you experience symptoms that go beyond the FND, the strategies explored in this book may help your other symptoms too.

Fatigue

The vast majority of people with FND experience fatigue (see Figure 7.4).

Fatigue in FND shows up in many different ways, shapes, and forms:

- Fatigue may encompass **physical**, **mental**, **cognitive**, or **all three**.
- Fatigue can **pre-date**, **co-exist**, and **amplify the FND**. A subgroup of people with FND has a diagnosis of chronic fatigue syndrome.

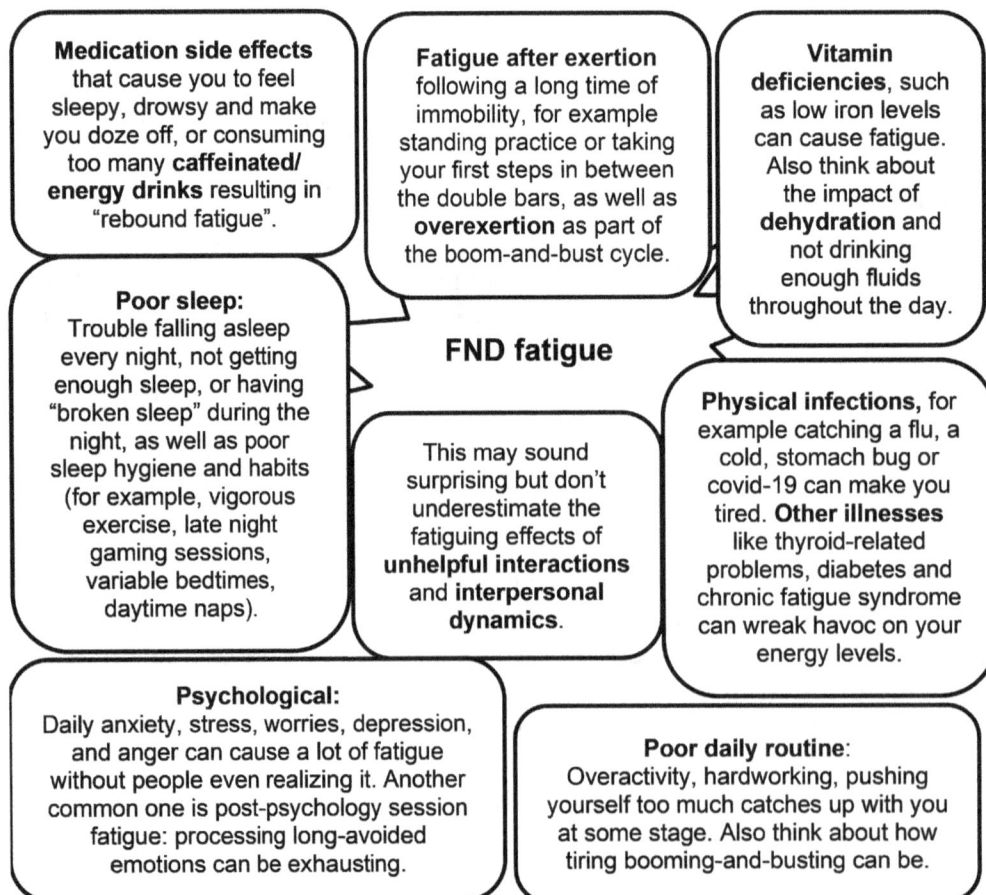

Figure 7.4 Reasons for fatigue in FND.

- For some people, fatigue may always be present with **'good days and bad days'**.
- For others, fatigue may be **temporary** and only emerges following an FND episode and then disappears again after the person has recovered.
- Fatigue episodes **vary widely** between people, with some falling asleep for a few hours afterwards, while other people may not be able to come out of bed for days due to extreme tiredness.

Inadvertently, and often completely outside people's awareness, fatigue can serve an important function: **cutting off or reducing difficult emotions**. When you feel extreme tiredness and fall asleep after a dissociative episode, you cannot feel anxiety and any other unpleasant emotion or internal arousal to the same degree, if at all. Both the seizure and 'post-seizure fatigue' do a good job at removing something unpleasant and providing relief, increasing future risk of seizures. Your body and mind, often unconsciously, have learned that this is an effective, quick, and long-lasting strategy to deal with difficult feelings.

Pain

Let us talk about another important FND after-effect. Pain is reported by nearly everyone, and unfortunately, it is rather unusual to hear if a person with FND does not experience pain. Pain, a normal response to injury and illness, can be a warning signal that indicates something is not entirely going well for your body and warrants your attention. What might be some of the reasons for FND-associated pain?

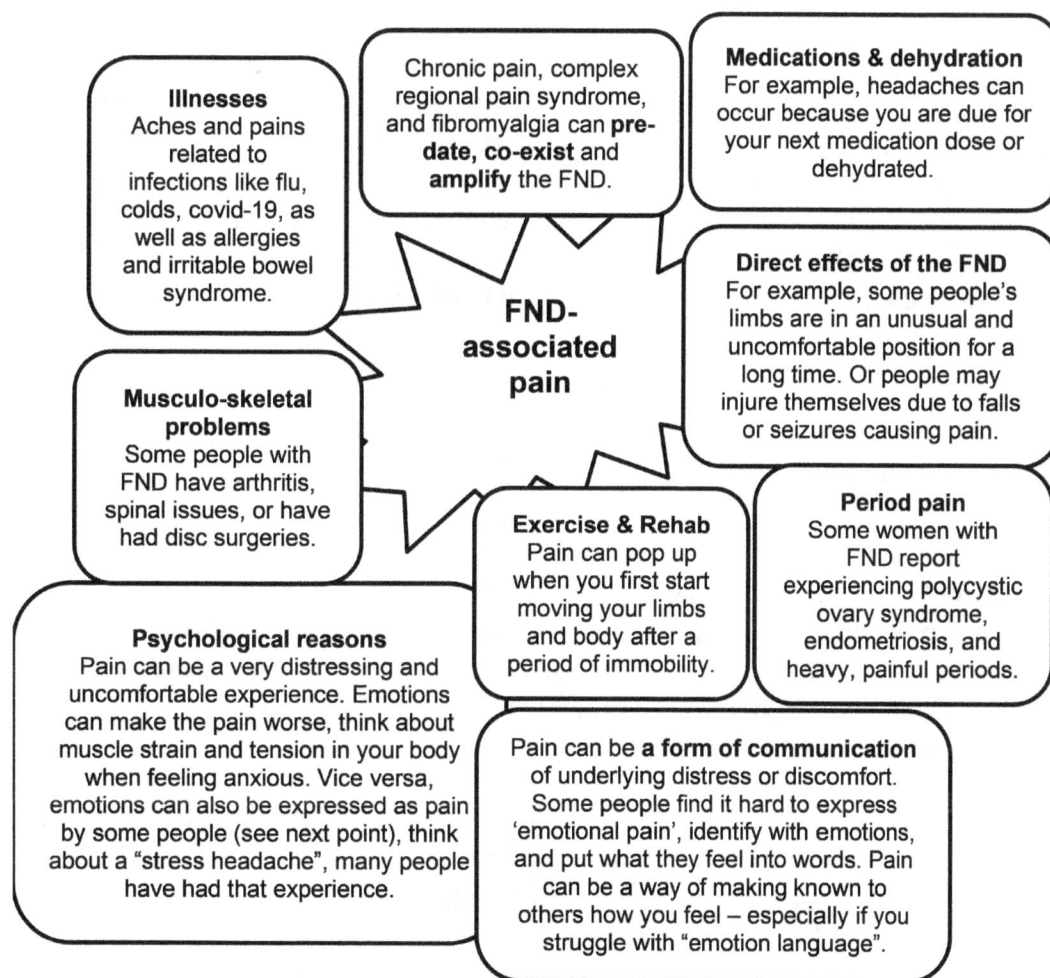

Figure 7.5 Reasons for pain in FND.

What does pain look like, and how can it affect people with FND and their lives?

- Can affect **every part** of the body.
- **Localised** in one or a few body parts or experienced as a **'whole-body ache'**.
- Pain can **'come and go'** in some people, while for others, it is **chronic and enduring**. For some people, pain flare-ups are associated with things happening in their relationships and environment.
- Pain can also **'travel' around the body** and be **'unpredictable'**: it does not always show up in the same places over time or can start in one location, then spread or 'grow' bigger over time.
- People report **various types of pain**: stabbing, pounding, burning, or shooting pains.
- Pain can be experienced across the entire spectrum of **severity**, from mild to extreme intensity.
- Pain can have a **massive impact on your daily life**, including poor sleep, struggling to take care of yourself, difficulties with memory and concentration, reduced emotional well-being, problems with relationships and employment.
- **Pain medications** can cause a host of additional problems: worse dissociation, people finding ways to self-medicate, or create a dependency.
- Pain can become a factor that **slows down** and **even halts neurorehabilitation**.
- On the upside, people with FND **can recover from pain**, often going hand in hand with FND recovery.

Pain is always real and genuine

Pain patterns across the body may not always correspond with what would be expected based on how the body and neurological system are built. Please note that this does not mean the pain is not real, genuine, or put on. You cannot look into someone's head or feel someone else's pain if you are not that person. What the person experiences and reports is, by definition, real and should not be challenged. It is not the lived experience that is questioned. Actually, nothing is doubted here!

Like FND, pain is best viewed through **a biopsychosocial lens**. Pain has a multitude of layers that impact on a person's lived pain experience. Although psychology is probably not everyone's preferred topic, neglecting to pay attention to psychosocial factors risks missing out on helpful strategies. In fact, all FND after-effects cause an impact on the responses of the environment to the person with FND. Environmental responses are explored in detail in Chapters 9 and 10.

Fuel

Think back about a time when you wanted to make a flame or ignite something. For example, at a campfire, kitchen hob, or New Year's Eve fireworks. Table 7.2 displays some fuel options for you.

As Table 7.2 demonstrates, we have plenty of choice to make flames. Do you see the variety? Now, imagine that in the same way as we can use multiple fuel types to help us cook, we also have multiple fuel types that can make FND symptoms worse or provoke an FND episode. Imagine that **every type of fuel represents a different trigger for FND**. In this section, you will go through a range of common triggers that have sparked off FND symptoms and are often reported by people with FND, their family, friends, and healthcare professionals.

It is useful to look at triggers in FND for many reasons:

- **Knowledge is power.** If we find an association between a trigger and FND symptoms, then addressing that trigger can help you manage and recover from FND.
- People with FND often do not feel in control of the FND, causing high levels of anxiety, depression, anger, and feelings of 'overwhelm' – compounding already-existing anxiety and distress. It is like the FND completely rules and controls a person's life. Searching for triggers **may give you back a sense of control**.

Table 7.2 Different types of fuel

Type of fuel	Type of equipment
Electricity	Electric hob
Paraffin	Paraffin burner
Magnetism	Induction hob
Diesel oil	Diesel burner
Wooden logs	Wood burner
Gas	Gas hob
Charcoal	Open fire

- Fingers are frequently pointed at the person with FND as 'the problem'. However, we know from clinical experience that interpersonal triggers often contribute to FND. Finding out about interpersonal triggers is useful; it helps the environment gain more clarity on why we need to shift the responsibility away from the individual to the 'family or relationship unit with FND'. **It takes the psychological pressure off the person experiencing the FND symptoms and invokes the environment to do their bit to control triggers.**
- Some triggers are part of an existing and treatable psychological problem with evidence-based therapy protocols, for example, PTSD, social anxiety, or panic disorder. The level of threat and anxiety that people experience in the context of these conditions can be incredibly high. Discovering and learning about how these threatening triggers cause FND **will help you feel and function better.**
- **Identifying and treating triggers sets you up for an FND-free future.** Knowing what has worked well in the past will help reduce or prevent future setbacks and increase your sense of control.

7.3 eResource alert!

Although they might superficially look quite similar, this eResource will highlight the differences between the fuel and ignition elements of the Pressure Cooker Model.

Triggers for FND can be viewed as representing **different levels of human needs**. The term 'human needs' sounds quite vague and abstract, but it often revolves around the following ideas (printed in bold lettering):

Most ideas in Table 7.3 seem to be **associated with other people**. There is something about human needs that is **intricately interwoven** with the existence of other human beings. In CBT-style therapy approaches, it is common to look at key beliefs, the often more superficial

Table 7.3 Examples of human needs

Wants and wishes	Upcoming feelings	Necessity
To connect to other people and have friendships, have a good social support system, a varied life with new experiences, a happy and healthy family.	To feel cared for, believed, important, needed by 'heard', listened to, others, or noticed	To be respected and valued by other people, to sleep well, having appropriate clothing on without being cold, to live in a warm house, take care of your health and body, to breathe.
Needs	**Desires**	**A right that you are entitled to**
A need to be comforted by another person when feeling sad. A need to have certainty and predictability in your life. A need to feel closer to family, children or a partner, or the opposite, a need to feel more space from others.	A desire to feel peace in a family situation, to help and support other people, to be healthy, to think better about yourself, to grow and develop your skills/ knowledge about an area of interest	To feel secure and safe without threats in your relationships, at work, where you live
Aspirations, goals, objectives	**An urge for something**	**Longing, craving, yearning**
To learn to scuba-dive, explore an underground cave, spread your wings into the world by travelling	Food, drink, water, connect with another person, or the opposite: disconnect from someone.	For closer relationships, a union with another person, a fruitful career

thoughts and feelings that maintain a psychological condition. There are very good reasons to do so; not in the least, this time-limited approach is backed by a strong evidence base that helps guide and treat a person with overcoming the symptoms. However, there are often more 'hidden' human needs that drive these conditions in people with and without FND (see Table 7.4).

Sometimes, these hidden needs are unmet by the people in our environment. Exploring unmet human needs shines a bright light on underlying psychological or social factors that may contribute to FND:

- Needs are attached to inner, sometimes **strong beliefs** that we hold **about ourselves, other people, and the world in general**. For example, if you experience low self-esteem, this may influence your need for perhaps more validation from other people as you do not really trust yourself.
- **Current unmet needs can reveal something about a person's past.** Basic physical and emotional needs may not have been consistently met or neglected in childhood as well as in health-care settings. In daily life, these past adverse experiences can 'retrigger' a person with FND at a much deeper, unconscious level without the person even realising it.

Table 7.4 Relationships between key beliefs and human needs

Psychological condition	Superficial thoughts, key beliefs, and feelings	Hidden human need
Panic and health anxiety	Fear of stroke, heart attack, seizures, fainting, serious illness, or afflictions	A need for self-preservation and existence to keep reaching life goals, spend quality time with loved ones.
Generalised anxiety	Worries about different topics including health, safety, daily tasks, demands, relationships	A need for certainty, predictability, control and to feel safe amongst people and in the world.
Social anxiety	Social fears, feeling embarrassed, self-conscious	A need to feel accepted and not rejected by other people
Complex trauma	Attachment anxiety, fear of rejection, abandonment.	A need to feel safe and secure in human relationships.

- **Explain strong responses** to what seems like a superficial issue (which it is not). In the same way, it is important in FND to look beyond the first set of triggers that may be visible to the eye and look for more indirect, hidden, deeper layers: like peeling down the layers of an onion until you get to the core.
- Human needs are often part of a complex social web and an interpersonal dynamic between people meeting each other's needs (or not). Commonly reported unmet needs in FND involve **not feeling understood, heard, listened to, accepted, cared for, equally treated, or validated by other people.**

Maslow's hierarchy: a useful concept for thinking about FND triggers?

Triggers for FND can come in different shapes and sizes. Occasionally, this feels overwhelming, daunting, and confusing, both for the person with FND as well as for family, friends, and healthcare professionals. What if we can think of a system that can organise these triggers a little better?

Have you heard of 'Maslow's hierarchy of needs', a well-known **'pyramid' of human needs,** created by the American psychologist Abraham Maslow? The pyramid consists of several layers (Maslow, 1943). On the lowest level of the pyramid, human needs are basic and revolve around having shelter, sufficient sleep, air to breathe, food to sustain yourself, clothing to protect yourself from cold.

If your needs at this most basic level of the pyramid are not sufficiently or consistently met by other people or you are not able to meet those needs yourself, for example, because you struggle to eat or are chronically sleep-deprived, the needs on the next levels above will be more difficult to hold in mind and perhaps not always a priority, for example, when thinking about meeting our human needs for connecting with people in friendships or increasing our sense of self-esteem; you clearly have more basic unfulfilled needs to think of that require your full attention at the

"Self-actualization"
Having realised your life goals and dreams, you are 'living life to the absolute full' with your needs met

Interpersonal "external" triggers
Family arguments / dynamics
Long-term bullying experiences at school or work without appropriate support and solutions
Emotional needs not met by family or partner
Severe social isolation
Academic or work pressures

Esteem needs
Self-esteem, being noticed, respected, recognition

Environmental PTSD triggers
Memories and flashbacks from traumatic / near-death accidents, injuries, assaults,
Encounters of interpersonal or domestic violence

"Re-triggers"
An interaction with a healthcare professional re-triggers older unconscious memories of not feeling cared for, believed or abandoned

Love and belonging needs
Friendships, romantic relationships, intimacy, family, sense of belonging and connection to a group or a community, social support system

Psychological "internally generated" triggers
Worries, health anxiety

Social anxiety triggers
Social situations causing a fear of negative judgements, embarrassment and feeling self-conscious in social groups

Safety needs
Security, safety from threats, employment, health, property

Bodily symptom triggers
Funny sensations, dizziness, nausea, heart racing, feeling sweaty

Physiological needs
Food, shelter, sleep, clothing, water, air

"Multi-triggers"
Any combination of these triggers, most often a physical/ bodily trigger with an interpersonal trigger

Environmental "non-PTSD" triggers
Complex psychosocial issues such as living in an unsafe neighbourhood, difficult housing and living circumstances sometimes (not always) with financial hardship; court cases and legal issues

Physical triggers
Noise from alarms, light or smell sensitivity, sudden unexpected movements in the environment

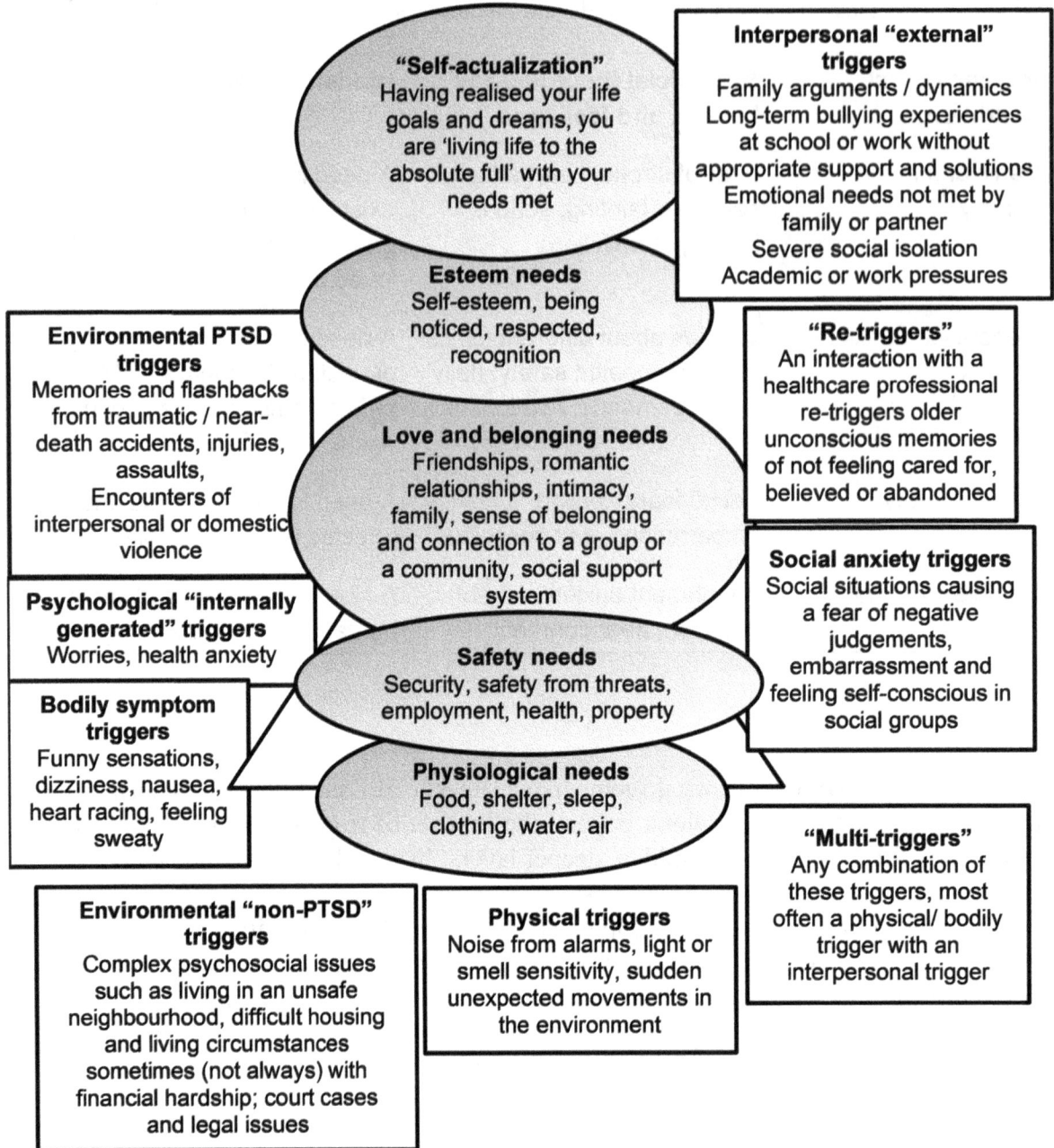

Figure 7.6 Maslow's hierarchy applied to FND triggers.

minute. To meet these 'higher-level' needs more fully, it can be helpful to have dealt appropriately with the lower levels in order to move up on the pyramid.

Let us look at Figure 7.6 to explore how FND triggers can be organised according to Maslow's pyramid of human needs.

7.4 eResource alert!

Read this comprehensive eResource to learn more about the wide range of triggers reported by and encountered in people with FND. Each FND trigger will be explained in great detail, with real-life examples to guide your thinking and understanding, as well as with a description of the mechanisms that explain the pathway 'from trigger to FND'.

Identifying the underlying human needs behind FND triggers is incredibly important:

- **FND is a multi-layered condition.** Looking at human needs may help increase someone's awareness, knowledge, understanding, and clarity of what factors are driving the FND. Knowledge about your condition can be psychologically very containing in itself, reduce difficult emotions you experience as a result, and take away any confusion you may have.
- **Helps you consider the potential core of the FND symptoms.** Without investigating and addressing the core of the problem, FND symptoms may keep going and interfere with activities in daily life and your mood – without you knowing why and being able to manage it appropriately.

Sometimes, 'a spade is just a spade'. We do not always have to dig further and obsessively look for the hidden human need behind every FND trigger. If symptoms persist, however, despite many prior attempts to treat the FND, then exploring underlying human needs may provide another avenue for intervention.

Perhaps you have not identified the triggers for your FND symptoms yet. Do not worry! And even if you are sure that you have identified all your triggers, it may still be worth to read this section further, particularly if FND symptoms keep persisting:

- **People with FND can experience multiple triggers and might not be aware**, particularly if the FND keeps persisting: one person can experience different triggers for different episodes and symptoms. By learning more about the nature of FND triggers, you can uncover whether you may experience more than one trigger and address them all.
- **Some triggers may 'hide behind' the triggers that we have already identified.** A good example is noise or heat, which is a commonly reported physical trigger of FND. When exploring these triggers in more detail during psychological therapy sessions, it may transpire that something strongly connected to those physical triggers, such as an event involving other people, or an argument that produced a negative emotion or an unpleasant state of being, is what triggered off the FND symptom rather than the physical trigger itself.

7.5 eResource alert!

Read how you and your family, friends, loved ones, and healthcare professionals can find the fuel and discover FND triggers using a specially designed tool called the **structured FND diary**. This eResource contains some more background information on what led up to the development of the tool, clear instructions on how to complete the diary, templates for you and the people in your environment to give it a good go, diary examples, helpful exercises, as well as hopefully some useful tips and tricks on what to look out for in your diary entries. Why not have a go at it?

Find your fuel: exploring FND-free periods

People with FND are often asked the question 'Do you know what makes your FND better or worse?' In practice, this question does not always provide clarity, as often people have no idea. Discovering triggers for FND is the reason the person visits a clinic!

In addition to the structured FND diary, another informative way to explore your triggers is to picture a time in your mind when you were FND-free: **What were the specific characteristics of these FND-free life periods?** Ask yourself whether there was ever a time or situation in your life when:

- Your FND symptoms seem to have disappeared altogether (and then came back)?
- Frequency, duration, severity, or intensity of the symptoms changed for the better: you did not seem to have as many, shorter, less severe, or subdued FND symptoms. Holidays are often a good point for reflection.

7.6 eResource alert!

Let us guide you through an exploration of what your Pressure Cooker Model may have looked like during an FND-free period. Find out, by reviewing each element, what you might need to pay attention to in your own situation.

FND trigger management: learn strategies to help with removing your fuel

Physical triggers

People with FND often report physical triggers for FND, such as heat, noise, smells, or light. What may be the underlying mechanism? In response to a physical trigger, a person may experience an array of bodily symptoms (e.g., dizziness, a funny turn, nausea, tingles, and many more) that are subsequently misinterpreted by our bodies and minds as a sign that a feared FND symptom is about to follow (also known as a 'catastrophic misinterpretation'). It may seem impossible to avoid physical triggers: they pop up everywhere and are hard to escape! Is there anything you can do about physical triggers?

INCREASE YOUR AWARENESS INTO THE PHYSICAL TRIGGER AND FND CONNECTION

One strategy is to try to **identify what happens in between the physical trigger and the FND symptom.** Physical triggers do not just miraculously provoke FND. We need to carefully inspect the links in the chain. Often, the link is **a thought or a feeling.**

Do you feel discomfort, distress, or a worrying thought passing through your mind? A very common thought is, 'I am going to have a seizure' (or a stroke, heart attack, lose control, dissociative seizure). Thoughts are not always easy to spot because, often, thoughts are quick and automatic under these circumstances. A useful question to ask yourself to find out about any thoughts is the following: Given the bodily symptoms that I feel in response to the physical trigger, what would be the worst thing that could happen to me?

LET GO OF PROTECTIVE EQUIPMENT ALTOGETHER IF YOU CAN

People with physical triggers may avoid places and situations in which these triggers appear or wear protective equipment, such as sunglasses, earpieces, ear defenders, or continuous music in one ear. Although completely understandable, avoiding places and wearing equipment to help you cope with physical triggers will likely maintain your FND symptoms, as it **does not address the underlying problem.** You will also **miss out on interactions** with other people, social opportunities, and positive sensory experiences which **increase social isolation** and your risk of **low mood.**

INCREASE THE PHYSICAL TRIGGER AND FND LAG

The time between a physical trigger and the FND symptom may be ultrashort. For some people, the FND emerges instantly, whereas others may have a bit longer before the FND fully takes over. Either way, try to practice with increasing the time between the physical trigger and the FND. Easier said than done (and please do not give up too quickly!), but **(1) raising your awareness** into what may be happening in your body and mind **and (2) psychologically tolerating and 'riding the discomfort'** as long as you are able to in that moment when you encounter a physical trigger **are the first steps**. People with and without FND have found the following strategies useful for tolerating discomfort, especially at the beginning of treatment, to help 'take the edge of things'.

BREAK THE HABIT: RESPONSE PREVENTION AND REPLACEMENT

Sometimes, an FND symptom in response to a physical trigger has become **an automatic habit** that our brain and mind have learned over time, highly 'practiced' through experience. To break the link between physical triggers and FND, a good strategy is **exposure** to the physical trigger **on multiple occasions** or **for a prolonged period** (taking off ear defenders or sunglasses to expose yourself to sound or light) while simultaneously trying to withhold the response (the FND) or replacing it with an alternative response instead (naming different movies for every letter of the alphabet). By exposing yourself for a longer period to the physical trigger without it being followed by the FND, you will be able to eventually break the habit. **Be aware that this takes time and practice; it is not an overnight solution.**

REALITY GROUNDING

If you do not experience any uncomfortable thoughts, feelings, or sensations in response to the physical trigger **but you still get FND**, then it may be possible that you are not sufficiently in touch with your body and mind, dissociating quickly from whatever is happening following the physical trigger. Reality grounding techniques can teach you to become **more aware of your emotions** and are also a great **'replacement coping strategy'**.

TELL YOUR ENVIRONMENT TO 'STAND BACK'

Your environment needs to tolerate its own discomfort too! The Pressure Cooker Model believes that, to some extent, FND is the product of interpersonal processes between the individual and the environment.

Adopting this radical viewpoint means that we cannot just overload the person with FND with the responsibility of learning strategies and changing their response pattern on their own. On the contrary, the **responsibility for recovery equally lies with the environment**.

In the case of dissociative episodes, particularly those happening in public places where noises can be a big problem, the environment often steps in 'to help' and reassure the person. Although this is well-intended, these caring responses feed into the FND symptoms through reinforcement. The person's FND symptoms, **as well as the environment's discomfort at witnessing the symptoms, reduce (a.k.a. 'reciprocal reinforcement')**.

As a result, the environment inadvertently prolongs and maintains the episode. The environment is often **recommended to stand back** and not engage by touching, patting, reassuring, holding hands, speaking kind and compassionate words: all the things that we want to do when we see someone in distress or unwell with symptoms, right?

This is a hard one, and sometimes far more difficult for the people in your environment. Standing back often **feels harsh and punitive** to people with and without FND. However, if you look at the available research and clinical treatment practices, you will find that this is **counterintuitively** one of the most powerful strategies that effectively achieves breaking the link between the physical trigger and the FND.

There are **several issues** with the strategies we just explored:

- Tend to be **superficial** and **'scratch the surface'** more than that they hit at the core of the problem: addressing your beliefs, emotions, and interactions at a deeper level. Although useful temporarily, perhaps not so much on a longer-term basis. Read more about dissociation and reality grounding in the (Pressure Cooker Model) 'heat element' section later in Chapter 7.
- Some of these strategies can also **serve as a form of distraction** and **do not properly test out your beliefs**, creating a sense of dependency. The end goal of treatment is for you to feel comfortable and embrace your life without the pressure of 'I need to use my strategies quickly or else my FND symptoms will spiral out of control'. Later in Chapter 7, you will learn about a more sophisticated strategy that requires quite a bit of practice but can produce longer-lasting results: setting up a behavioural experiment adapted specifically for people with and without FND.
- **Paying attention to your body**, one of the biggest maintaining factors of FND, **may 'feed' into symptoms**. Toeing the line between 'too little' and 'too much' attention is not an easy feat. Jump ahead to Chapter 8 (section 'Warning light') for more details.
- The environment succumbs and is **unable to cope with their own discomfort** of withholding reassurance. Later in Chapter 7 (again in the section on 'heat'), you will learn more about the 'standing back' technique and how you and the people close to you can best apply this in your day-to-day life to help you overcome FND. Chapters 9 and 10 will be useful for acquainting yourself with a concept vital in FND: 'reciprocal reinforcement'.

ONE FINAL NOTE ON PHYSICAL TRIGGERS AND AUTISM

A subset of people with FND is also on the autism spectrum and may report feeling overwhelmed and overstimulated in busy places, like a city centre or shopping mall. Overstimulation and sensory sensitivities made worse by the environment can lead to FND symptoms. Please note that in those specific circumstances, **saying no** to visiting busy environments **is not a form of avoidance but self-care**. A person may opt to shop at quieter times or with ear defenders/plugs.

Look further: interpersonal triggers

7.7 eResource alert!

Peter is a young gentleman with a functional tremor. Learn how interpersonal triggers from Peter's environment contribute to the FND and, most importantly, what the Pressure Cooker Model can do to alleviate some of these difficulties.

Let us explore a special type of FND trigger that deserves extra mention. **Interpersonal triggers** are strongly associated with other people, relationships, interactions, interpersonal communication, unmet needs, and just generally, with the social world around us. Interpersonal triggers were associated with dissociative seizures in 90% of people in one study (Bowman & Markand, 1999). To help you better understand their nature, let us pit interpersonal triggers directly against more obvious and intuitive triggers, for example, physical, trauma-related, and bodily symptom triggers (see Table 7.5).

Table 7.5 Differences between primary and secondary triggers in FND

Primary	Secondary
"Every trigger that is not interpersonal"	**"Interpersonal triggers"**
Example: dissociative seizure in response to feeling dizzy, 'electric' sensations in the body and feeling sweaty and heart racing.	**Example:** functional leg weakness in response to an argument with a family member.
Obvious, clear, and **more on the surface** – does not take much time to discover and becomes clear fairly early onwards in the therapy process. Called primary because often the first and sometimes only focus of treatment.	**Hidden** – take time to find out about, for example through a therapy journey. Called secondary because often not the initial focus of treatment.
People are often **highly aware** of this type of trigger, with full conscious access.	People are often **less or not at all aware** of interpersonal triggers, they tend to be outside our awareness, or with less conscious access.
FND symptoms **reactive to environmental changes**, for example lighting, noise, sudden movements, smells, strange feeling in the body.	FND symptoms **reactive to an unmet need** such as wanting to feel accepted, noticed, validated, acknowledged.
Direct and clear – the link between physical triggers and FND tends to be clear and straightforward.	**Indirect and murky** – the link between interpersonal triggers and FND is often unclear and not straightforward at all.
Often **connected to basic emotions** such as anxiety, sadness, and anger.	**Often connected to low mood, depression and social emotions** (for example, embarrassment, shame, guilt, envy, jealousy) and negative beliefs about other people around us (called "attachment anxiety" or an "interpersonal fear" of abandonment and rejection).
Discussion of primary triggers **do not tend to generate feelings of shame, embarrassment, or anger**, to the same level as interpersonal triggers may do. People will feel believed and validated by the therapist when discussing these triggers.	**Can generate a lot of shame, embarrassment and anger** when explored in therapy and people are asked about, sometimes leading people to 'not feeling believed'. Requires a very strong therapeutic relationship between the person with FND and their therapist, to unearth these interpersonal triggers.

Some more facts you need to know about interpersonal triggers

INTERPERSONAL EVENTS: SOMETIMES THE MISSING LINK?

Occasionally, the link between physical triggers and FND is all about an underlying interpersonal event or a relationship. What does that mean? On the surface, a physical trigger (noise of an alarm) that everybody automatically assumes is causing the FND symptoms to appear or worsen, no matter how unlikely, may not be the main driver for FND, after all! Rather, an interpersonal event **that happened earlier, immediately before, simultaneously,** or **closely around the physical event** is the culprit for the FND – and not the physical event itself. By temporal association, the physical event puts everybody on the wrong track, often unconsciously and outside people's awareness.

SOME PEOPLE EXPERIENCE BOTH PHYSICAL AND INTERPERSONAL TRIGGERS

In other situations, the **same FND symptoms can be elicited by two different triggers**. A classic example of this **two-trigger situation** happens in dissociative seizures. A subset of episodes is triggered by a physical event (trigger #1, a smell that re-triggers a traumatic memory or flashback), whereas another subset of episodes is clearly interpersonal in nature (trigger #2, a preceding family argument). Although the end result is the same (a dissociative seizure), the starting point is entirely different, and both sets of triggers may need different types of treatment.

IF YOU WANT REAL AND LONG-LASTING CHANGE, EXPLORE INTERPERSONAL
RATHER THAN PRIMARY TRIGGERS

Primary triggers are always a useful starting point in therapy and, in some situations, the only target of treatment. Primary and obvious triggers often **act as a gateway door** to the discovery of secondary and hidden interpersonal triggers, especially when the professional relationship with your therapist gradually strengthens and deepens over time and you feel more comfortable and psychologically safe to disclose this often-sensitive information to your therapist. Like an onion, FND treatment is often about peeling off superficial layers one by one before you finally get to the core of the problem.

WHAT ARE SOME EXAMPLES OF INTERPERSONAL TRIGGERS?

People with FND report many types of interpersonal triggers, both in the research literature as well as in the clinic (see Figure 7.7).

A SPECIAL TYPE OF INTERPERSONAL TRIGGER: DOMESTIC VIOLENCE

Although as an interpersonal trigger, domestic violence is at the extreme end; it is not unheard of. Unfortunately, some people with FND may be in a coercive or abusive relationship. If you would like to refresh your memory about how domestic violence may maintain FND, flick back to Chapter 6.

What can you do about interpersonal triggers?

1. Normalise

Witnessing other people getting care and support from a parent or professional, feeling short-changed.		An upcoming basic human need for feeling psychological safety, human connection and wanting to get close to someone, with the FND facilitating that process.	Cultural triggers like an expectation for you to care for your family / or excel in your work or study performance – even though you are exhausted and not able to keep up and meet your family's demands.
Arguments and strife with a partner or in the family environment.	Family or partner placing heavy demands on a person & the FND protects the person.		
Perceived or real psychological pressure from another person, e.g. family member, spouse or healthcare professional.	Conflict between your family's expectations (going into a specific field or job) vs your deepest personal wishes (not wanting to do that job but completely something else that would not be accepted).		Sibling rivalry
Contact about a crime perpetrated against the victim. (Imminent) release of the perpetrator that has been incarcerated and has hurt or threatened you in the past.	Coercive control and other domestic violence with the FND having a protective effect or helping the person to manage and survive difficult circumstances.		Feeling emotionally neglected by a partner, parent or professional.

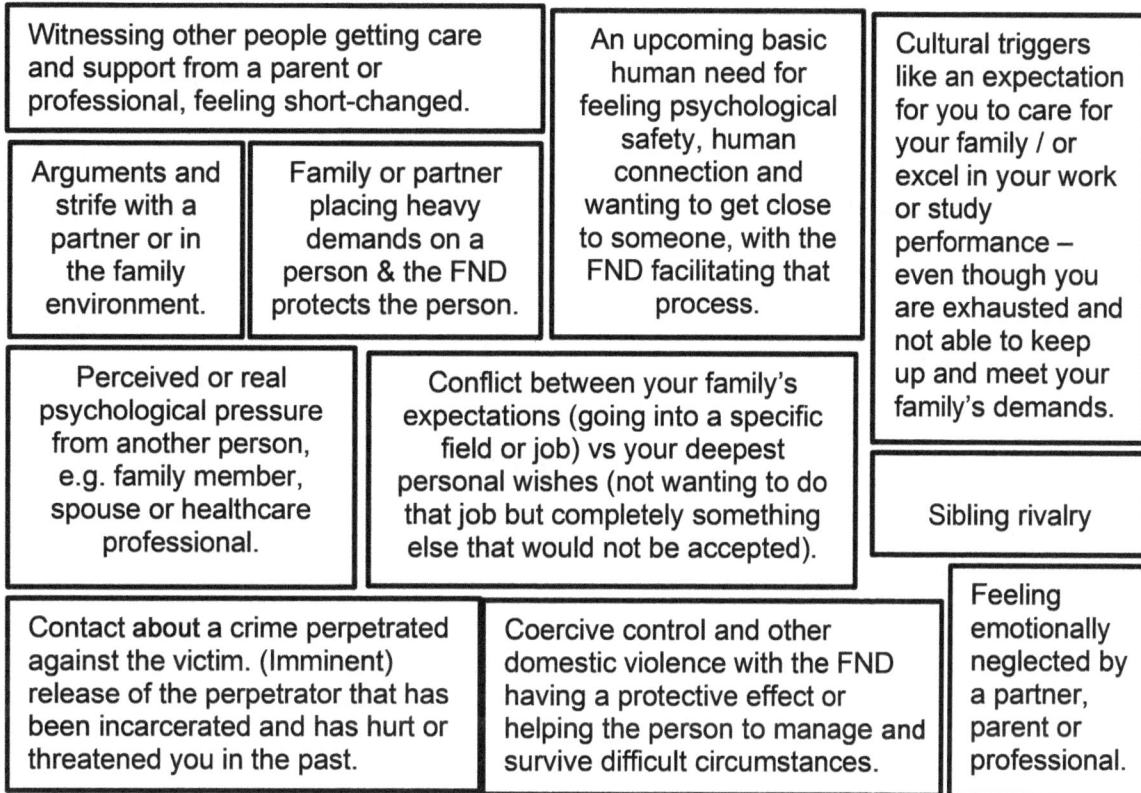

Figure 7.7 Examples of interpersonal triggers that maintain FND.

We do not live in a social vacuum: all of us possess interpersonal triggers, whether you have FND or not. It is a normal and integral part of our human experience; we get 'triggered' by the people around us! Think, for example, about a good friend who has something that you would really love but do not have:

- Fantastic, new three-bedroom house
- Fancy car
- Relationship with a caring partner, children, or a cohesive family
- Big social group of brilliant friends, an invite to the party of the year
- Health
- Great figure
- Happiness in life
- A passion that motivates them to get up and work hard for it
- Talent in sport
- Your parents still alive
- Work promotion or a big salary
- Being able to pay the bills without getting stressed every single month
- Dream holiday on a remote bounty island that you are not able to afford
- And the list is endless!

In response to your friend's success and your not-yet-success or loss, you may feel anger, jealousy, envy, embarrassment, shame, low mood, or anxiety about your own situation. Learn to accept that we get triggered regularly, sometimes more consciously than at other times. But the fact is, as social beings, we constantly get triggered by other social beings.

2. What do people around you do . . . or not do?

A good way to obtain clues about interpersonal triggers is to carefully check in what ways the environment tends to respond to the FND.

Examples of **positive reinforcement** (rewarding things that are 'added' right after FND symptoms emerge or worsen and generally make you feel better or relieved):

- Expressions of concern
- Compassion
- Things dropped to quickly jump into action
- Reassurance
- Kindness
- Care: people taking far better care of you, people who normally do not care suddenly caring
- Physical or emotional support
- Goods (cup of tea, snacks)
- More regular check-ups

Examples of **negative reinforcement** (unpleasant things that are 'removed' right after FND symptoms emerge or worsen and generally make you feel better or relieved):

- Argument stops immediately.
- Chores, tasks, or activities are dropped.
- An anxiety-provoking exam or meeting does not have to be attended anymore.
- 'Being let off the hook' for something you dread.
- Anxiety, distress, discomfort or any unpleasant internal state of being.

3. What does the person with FND do . . . or not do?

Make no mistake: reinforcement learning pertains to everyone, whether you have FND or not. In your quest for solutions to address your interpersonal triggers, do not forget that 'the other part' of the interpersonal dynamic also contributes to FND **in equal ways** and needs to be involved in the recovery process too. To get an idea of the multitude of potential reinforcement processes that can take place during one dissociative episode, imagine the following (very common) scenario:

> Every time a discussion becomes heated between him and his partner, Edward feels the psychological pressure rising inside himself. He experiences a dissociative seizure, followed by a long recovery 'sleep' afterwards. During the episode, his partner reassures Edward and stays with him at all times.

Negative reinforcement

- Edward feels a near-instant relief from the psychological pressure.
- During the long recovery sleep, Edward cannot feel any psychological pressure temporarily.
- Argument stops immediately.
- Sensitive topic that the argument was about now does not need discussing. Edward is 'let off the hook' for the unforeseeable future as he is in recovery.
- Simultaneously, his partner feels a big relief at seeing the seizure settle over time. The seizure eventually stops and takes something distressing and uncomfortable away from Edward's partner. His partner has now learned that reassurance and looking after Edward helps manage the seizure quickly and effectively.

Positive reinforcement

- Quarrelling partner turns into a kind, caring, and compassionate human being.
- Staying vigilant and in close proximity beside Edward.
- Bringing him snacks and a cup of hot chocolate.
- The couple stays in, spends some quality time together with no further seizures.
- Partner's self-confidence in managing Edward's seizures grows steadily.

After reading about all these reinforcement processes, ask yourself whether it is a good idea to exclusively focus on the person with FND? Chapters 9 and 10 will explore more deeply how this interpersonal pattern of responding to each other **not only maintains the FND** over time but can also **cause people to respond in more unhelpful and even aversive ways** in the long run. These chapters will support you with seeking dialogue, discovering, and resolving any unhelpful interpersonal dynamics that may drive the FND symptoms. Note how it is purposefully stated: *'the FND symptoms'* and not *'your FND symptoms'*. The FND is viewed, in part, **as a manifestation of an underlying systemic problem** that both yourself and whoever is in your environment actively contribute to. In order to achieve full recovery from the FND, all of you need to be on board, not just the person who carries and experiences the FND symptoms! One of the Pressure Cooker Model's unofficial assumptions is the following core idea:

Where there are people, there is dynamics!

4. Spot any differences

Think about a time **you did not experience the FND ('the baseline' or 'pre-FND')** and compare this with the **current period with FND** in your life. Now zoom in and compare the psychosocial and interpersonal characteristics of each time period. Useful questions to ask for both periods are:

- What were my relationships and interpersonal communications with people like, generally positive or negative? Think about a partner, family, friends, healthcare professionals, work colleagues, other meaningful people in your life.
- Did I feel a sense of social belonging to a group, community, and people in general?
- What social activities were you engaged in? Were they enjoyable? Did you feel it helped release daily life stresses?
- Can you say anything about the level of support you received from people? What was your perception? Did you feel supported, especially during the trickier times in your life?
- What beliefs and feelings can you describe? Happy, sad, angry, fearful, including fears around losing attachments to people? Did you feel noticed, cared for, accepted, a sense of mattering to other people, treated with respect, in compassionate ways?

Look at your answers. Can you spot any differences between the two time periods? Which situation is connected to better and more pleasant psychosocial circumstances? For more ideas on how to complete this exercise, please check the **eResource** (7.7) that describes Peter, a young man with a functional tremor associated with interpersonal triggers.

5. Check out Maslow's hierarchy

Remember Figure 7.6, that big pyramid, and Table 7.3, which displayed **our basic human needs**? Briefly flick back to these sections to investigate whether the FND could have something to do with **an underlying unmet need(s)** that you and people in your environment may feel presently? Think of needs around connecting with other people, belonging to a social group, to matter, to be noticed and feel cared for, as well as a need to express distress to other people that cannot be expressed verbally at the minute.

6. The 'R' word

Rejection is a big theme in FND and often happens, or has happened, on multiple levels in a person's life history, including by healthcare professionals, parental caregivers, school peers, partners, other family members – and the list goes on. Could any of the symptoms be **connected to the fear of rejection and people walking out, and is the FND somehow protective against rejection and abandonment?**

7. Remove yourself from a long-standing and challenging interpersonal situation

Sometimes, an interpersonal trigger requires you **to remove or distance yourself, either permanently or temporarily, to manage the FND**. Think about the following examples:

- **Constant arguments and strife** without the opportunity to carry a constructive conversation with no one ever listening to you and your needs.
- Perhaps resulting in an **unsafe** and **risky situation**, including domestic violence.
- The **trigger cannot be removed that easily**, for example, a disruptive neighbour in a house that you have lived in for a long time, or emotionally unsettled people you live in one household with, but a lack of finances prevents you from moving out.
- There is an expectation that you drop everything in your life in service of another person: caring for a family member in crisis.

All this does not automatically mean that the 'blame' lies with you or the other person. Interpersonal triggers are always part of a wider dynamic. It simply means that **preserving some physical and emotional distance may be the healthy option**, particularly when emotions are heightened and stop you from functioning in day-to-day life or pursuing your own life goals. That said, take care of two things in particular:

- Distance is great, but it is not recommended to continuously avoid these interpersonal situations at all cost or always leave when things heat up too much. Sometimes, you need to teach yourself **to sit with the distress** or **practice assertiveness techniques** to prevent FND.
- For some people, taking your distance emotionally without leaving a tricky psychosocial situation physically equals dissociation, exactly the problem that needs to be addressed in FND!

KEY POINTS ON INTERPERSONAL TRIGGERS

- Physical triggers are often not the full story in FND.
- It is important to consider deeper emotional and psychosocial reasons that contribute to FND.
- Physical and interpersonal triggers are not mutually exclusive: they often co-exist together within one individual.
- If strategies that tackle the physical trigger are found to be ineffective or the FND persists for unknown reasons, check for the existence of interpersonal triggers.
- Look out for underlying unmet basic human needs and feelings around rejection and feeling cared for.
- Especially for interpersonal triggers, it is vital that people with and without FND gain awareness about their own contributions and work together during their recovery process.
- And always remember: **where there are people, there is dynamics!**

DISCLAIMER

It is possible that some people, after reading the section on interpersonal triggers, feel frustrated and instantly jump to the conclusion: 'What if people think I am doing this to gain attention?' 'What if people think I am faking and putting the symptoms on?' This is certainly not the view that is adopted here. We all experience needs that are not met in the moment by other people. Think for a moment about the following words: *'unmet need'* and *'not met by other people'*. In Peter's story, what do you think Peter's unmet need may be? In what ways is this need not met by other people *in between the fits when Peter feels relatively well*? You could hardly reframe this as 'attention-seeking'. It is a pressing need that both Peter and his environment have not been able to fulfil yet. Reflect for a moment on your own situation, and try to explore whether you have any unmet needs that may be associated with FND.

PTSD environmental triggers

Some people develop FND following traumatic events that are associated with an immediate threat to their or other people's life, body, and well-being, for example, a car accident, an assault, natural disaster, or being in combat. The condition that can develop after being exposed to these circumstances is called 'post-traumatic stress disorder', or PTSD. Did you know that:

- FND symptoms can be directly related to PTSD triggers.
- People who experience FND and acute PTSD following a traumatic event may need a different type of treatment than people without PTSD or those with complex PTSD – which is different from more acute PTSD.

People with PTSD report a combination of three symptoms:

- **Re-experiencing** the traumatic event, for example, through flashbacks, memories, or frightening nightmares.
- **Avoidance** and numbness, including dissociation.
- **Hyperarousal.** Being on the outlook for danger or cues, being on edge, and feeling the physical symptoms of anxiety.

Sometimes, reminders of the trauma can cause FND:

> John was involved in a fire at his home. He escaped without many injuries, but the experience was harrowing for him, and he developed both PTSD and FND afterwards. The FND consisted of John experiencing dissociative episodes and a functional tremor. He was also sleeping for long periods of time and missing entire days. In one of the therapy sessions with his psychologist, John reported that his FND symptoms worsened when he recently watched a television programme that featured a fire, as well as 'small random things' that reminded him of the fire at home and that set off an overwhelmingly unpleasant feeling, like smells of people having barbeques outside in the hot weather, hearing sirens, or seeing someone with the same colour T-shirt that one of his friends wore at the time of the fire.

For John, reminders of the trauma as well as seemingly innocuous things in his environment had taken on a threatening meaning that transported John instantly back to a traumatic situation, causing an overwhelming feeling of distress, and subsequently resulting in an FND episode.

If you experience both PTSD and FND, the Pressure Cooker Model can help you with understanding the relationship between PTSD and FND, as well as developing coping strategies that may prepare you for more comprehensive trauma therapy, such as trauma-focused CBT or EMDR (Eye Movement Desensitization and Reprocessing therapy). As you have seen in

Chapters 6 and 7, people with FND (and, similarly, those with PTSD) often use coping strategies that are understandable but just not always helpful, in particular, dissociation, keeping yourself to yourself, pushing on, or dropping all enjoyable activities.

Multi-triggers

A subset of people with FND experiences the same FND symptom, but brought on by multiple triggers. A classic example is the combination of a **bodily trigger** and an **interpersonal trigger** for dissociative episodes:

> Doreen experiences dissociative episodes. Immediately before an episode, she feels hot, sweaty, and uncomfortable. Given these warning signs, Doreen knows, 'I'm going to have another seizure!' and subsequently experiences a dissociative episode where she falls on the floor and shakes her arms and legs for about 20 minutes. Since a few weeks, Doreen's husband has been noticing an increase in her dissociative episodes whenever they have an argument. The episode stops the argument immediately, and Doreen's husband holds her hand, makes sure she does not injure herself, and reassures her with kind words until she comes out of the episode.

Doreen's episodes seem to be triggered by two types of fuel: **bodily triggers** (feeling hot, sweaty, and uncomfortable) and **interpersonal triggers** (arguments with her husband).

Different triggers often require different interventions. In Doreen's situation, the bodily triggers can definitely benefit from a CBT-informed psychological approach that is often used for panic disorder (a little later in Chapter 7, as well as bits from Chapter 8, will give you some ideas, so stay tuned). The interpersonal triggers are probably better addressed with an approach that involves both Doreen and her husband, for example, exploring the reasons for the couple's arguments or helping Doreen become more assertive if that is identified as the key problem. Only treating the bodily triggers will clearly not be sufficient because Doreen's FND would continue to be sparked off by the interpersonal triggers in her marriage. Importantly, both types of trigger can be treated by looking at the couple's two Pressure Cooker Models. Chapter 10 will show you how.

Re-triggers

Let us suppose that you start to feel unwell and your FND is becoming worse, but you cannot exactly put your finger on why you are feeling this way. Try to think about a time when you felt like this before, particularly in an interpersonal situation or a social interaction that happened in the past or even in childhood. Is it possible that you may have been re-triggered by past experiences? Uncovering re-triggers often takes time because they are not that obvious and may be protected by strong defence mechanisms.

> The other day, Deborah visited her GP. She had developed a new symptom and was worried that her FND was getting worse. The worries kept her up all night. The GP prescribed her a cream. When Deborah expressed her worries about the symptom, the GP told her 'not to worry, it is minor' and ushered her out of the clinic. Within a few minutes, Deborah stood outside. Deborah felt 'not listened to', 'not cared for', and 'not believed'. She started to feel confused, dizzy, and overwhelmed, with an uncomfortable feeling that grew stronger by the minute. Before she knew it, Deborah had a dissociative episode in the waiting room.

When talking through this example with her psychologist, Deborah explained that in childhood, she had been through difficult bullying experiences at school. She expressed her worries to her parents, but they dismissed her concerns and told Deborah 'to toughen up', stand up to the bullies, and just continue attending school. Deborah did not feel listened to and felt that her parents did

Table 7.6 The relationship between Deborah's present and past life experiences

Present life experience	Past life experience
Going to the GP	Going to her parents
Expressing worry and anxiety (FND symptom) to a person who can help (GP)	Expressing worry and anxiety (being bullied) to a person who can help (parents)
Being dismissed "not to worry, it is minor"	Parents dismissing concerns about bullying "toughen up and stand up to bullies"
Ushered out of the clinic	Being heavily encouraged to attend school, 'ushered out of the family home'
Not feeling listened to, not feeling believed	Not feeling listened to, not feeling believed
Feeling overwhelmed and coping with dissociation (dissociative episode)	Feeling overwhelmed and coping with dissociation (daydreaming and cutting off emotions)

not believe her. In the classroom, she often felt confused, dizzy, and 'out of it'. Deborah learned to 'survive' her difficult school experiences by daydreaming a lot and cutting off her emotions.

THE VERTICAL MIRROR IN FND

It is always useful to look back at how our past relationships fared, because features from our old relationships may re-emerge in our current relationships (not necessarily through fault of our own), **particularly parent–child relationships** and **including our relationships with healthcare workers**. Our current relationships can act as a **vertical mirror** reflecting our past relationships.

Uncovering re-triggers may feel a bit like playing detective because re-triggers tend to be more hidden and less conscious, and they may not be noticed as easily or quickly, as, for example, more obvious bodily triggers. Re-triggers are far more common in FND than people think. If anything, people without FND will also experience re-triggers from time to time, with the difference that they will not result in FND, but they may still cause a person to feel anxious, low in mood, angry, distressed, upset, or overwhelmed.

INCREASING SELF-AWARENESS INTO RE-TRIGGERS

Try to raise your awareness into what your re-triggers could be. You can do this by asking yourself the following questions, particularly if you are starting to feel discomfort or overwhelmed during an interpersonal interaction but you cannot quite put your finger on it:

- Do I feel listened to by the other person?
- Do I feel believed?
- Do I feel respected, noticed, validated by the other person?
- In the past, have I felt like this before?
- Could there be a link between how I felt then and how I am feeling now?
- Is there something similar about those past and present situations that make me feel this way?

- Do my FND symptoms worsen when I do not feel listened to, believed, or respected?
- Ask yourself: Do I feel 'heard' or 'hurt'?

Bodily symptoms

PANIC ATTACKS

Bodily symptoms that tend to come up quite suddenly, 'out of the blue', within a brief space of time, and quickly go from 0 to 100 may indicate a panic attack. The panic cycle starts with a bodily symptom (the fuel) that is 'misinterpreted' as something very scary or as a catastrophe (a.k.a. a 'catastrophic misinterpretation', your flames; see Figure 7.8).

Experiencing these beliefs understandably causes high levels of anxiety, fright, or terror (your 'flames' and 'heat': who wouldn't feel this way?). This anxiety now causes new bodily symptoms and feeds into the old ones that you were already experiencing, creating a panic loop. In order to cope with the feelings, people engage in all sorts of **safety behaviours**. For example:

- Quickly escaping the room.
- Holding on to something like a table or another piece of furniture.
- Opening all the windows in a room for fresh air.
- Counting down.
- Playing a game on your phone for distraction.
- Breathing exercises.
- Taking a pill to calm yourself down.
- Calling an ambulance or visiting the emergency department.
- Blowing air in a plastic bag.

Although totally understandable, instead of helping you beat the panic attack, all these safety behaviours keep the panic loop alive and kicking. In people with FND, the panic attack often ends with a dissociative episode (see the Pressure Cooker Model in Figure 7.9).

Once people with FND have experienced a panic attack that was followed by a dissociative episode or a motor symptom, such as losing strength in your limbs, the fear for having the catastrophe (stroke, heart attack, falling, the **original type 1 worries**) will often be replaced by a 'secondary' fear of another dissociative episode, also called **type 2 worries**. The flames become about the misinterpretation of bodily symptoms as a sign that you are going to experience a dissociative episode and not the 'primary' or past fear of, let us say, having a stroke.

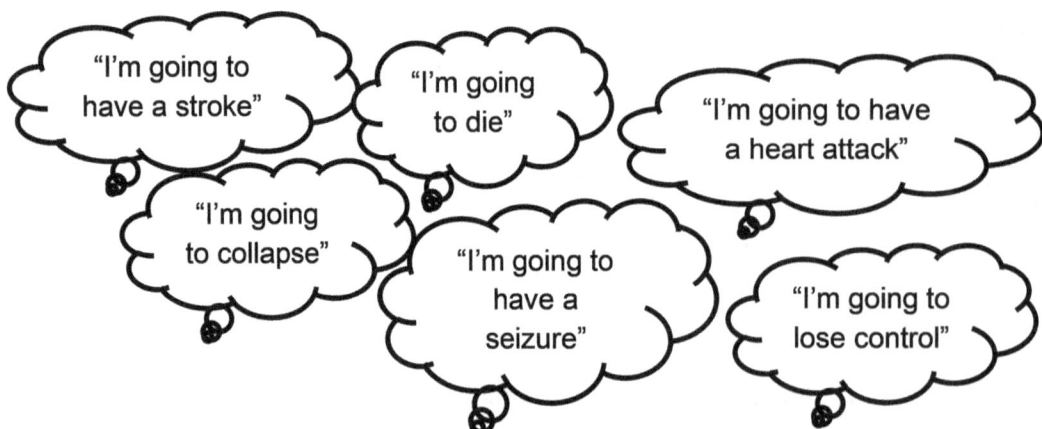

Figure 7.8 Commonly encountered beliefs in panic attacks.

Kitchen
Every time I experience an attack, people rush to support and reassure me.

Cover
Not being able to express the intense feelings you are experiencing.

Overpressure Plug
The build-up of discomfort and intensity level is so high: result is a dissociative episode or losing strength in my limbs.

Valve
Avoid exercise and going out in case you will have a heart attack.

Self-focused attention
High internal focus on the symptoms and how to cope with them in the moment.

The Pressure Cooker Model of Panic

Pot
More of the symptoms in your body, feeling hot and tingling, heart racing, sweaty palms Holding on to equipment to prevent fainting.

Ignition
Previous history of panic attacks and dissociative episodes

Flames
"Catastrophic misinterpretation"
Type 1 worry: "I'm going to have a stroke / heart attack / fall down / faint / lose control/ die"
Type 2 worry: "I'm going to have a seizure"
Highly uncomfortable state

Heat
This state of discomfort develops over a brief period and is highly unpleasant, "from 0 to 100"

Fuel
Feeling hot and tingling in your body, heart racing, sweaty palms

Sticky leftover food
Low self-confidence in managing panic / FND attacks.

Safety features
Good insight into how panic is related to FND.

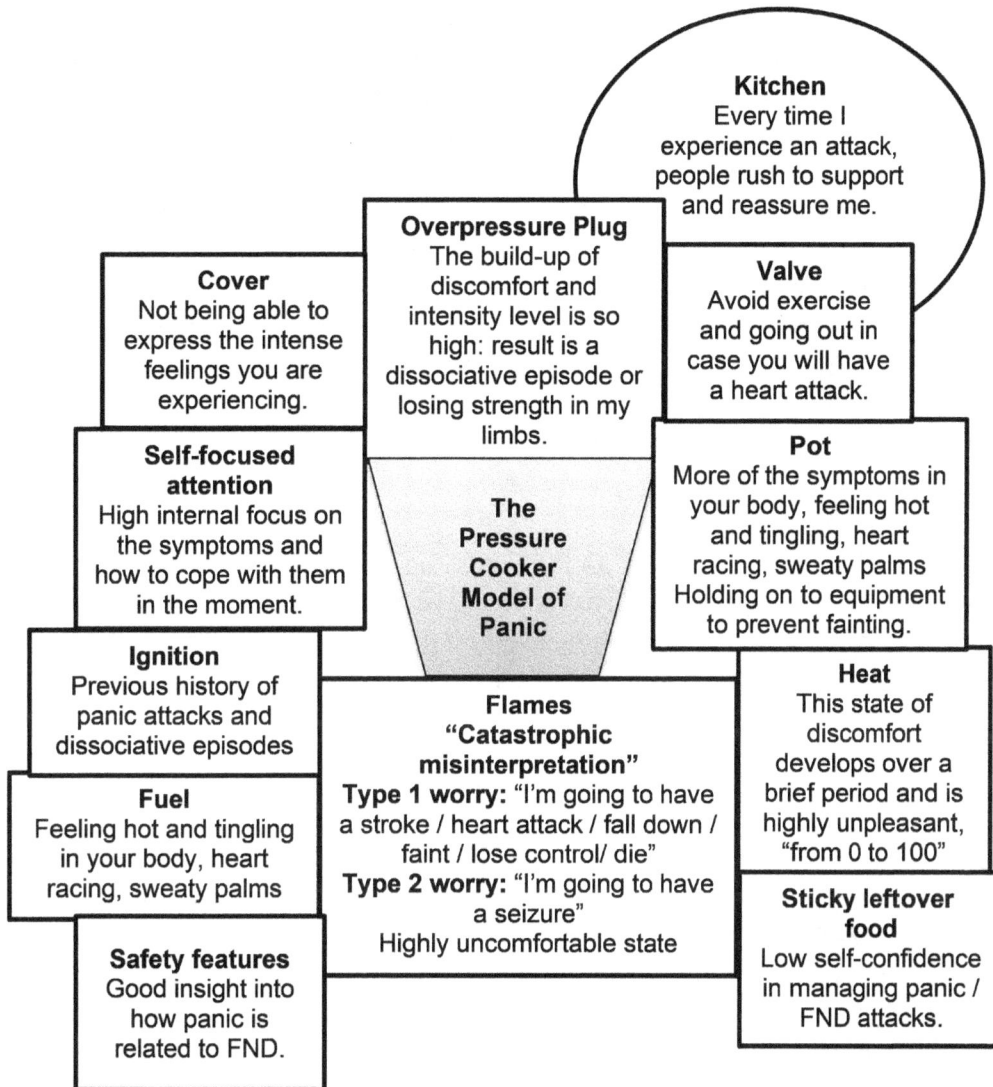

Figure 7.9 How panicky beliefs and feelings can lead to FND.

Some people with FND report multiple dissociative episodes after each other in close succession. After a person has just experienced a dissociative episode, they may go into another one. In this situation, the physical symptoms that you have just experienced may provoke more worries and panic feelings around 'I'm going to have another seizure', which then becomes a self-fulfilling prophecy and indeed results in another dissociative episode.

Complex psychosocial circumstances as triggers for FND

People with FND sometimes revealed challenging living circumstances that were 'full of complexity', characterised by a web of tangled, complicated relationships and sometimes unpleasant daily interactions. If the FND appears, or becomes, worse when the person is *in the environment (for example, at home)* but the symptoms disappear, or are milder in nature, when *out of the environment (for example, in hospital)*, that could be an important sign that the environment has a lot of bearing on maintaining the FND.

• FND could be an **internal regulation mechanism** for the person in a difficult psychosocial situation. This means that FND is a coping habit for the inner turmoil that, for example, not setting your boundaries or not being assertive during a challenging family interaction may create in the person. The FND helps relieve the psychological pressure from the person.

- The FND could also act as a protective factor and a deterrent against people in the environment to finally stop putting pressure on the person with FND **(external regulation mechanism)**, for example, in situations where the person is expected to meet high care needs of another person (beyond what is deemed 'normal' and 'acceptable' in society) or in domestic violence situations. It is important to note that this is not 'put on' or done deliberately but the brain's protection mechanism that kicks in.
- Often, for people in those difficult psychosocial circumstances, the FND helps both internally and externally regulate 'psychological pressure' (see Chapters 9 and 10).

7.8 eResource alert!

Learn more about the characteristics and the specific difficulties of people with FND who live under challenging life or complex psychosocial circumstances. This eResource will also show you an example of a treatment plan based on the Pressure Cooker Model that can help resolve some of these difficult circumstances and the FND.

Flames

The flames element represents our thoughts and feelings. In Chapter 5, you already took a good look at our intricate belief system. You may remember that we have three different 'thought' layers: **core beliefs, rules for living**, and **negative automatic thoughts (a.k.a. NATs)**. Let us delve a bit more deeply into the **contents of these beliefs** and learn what **emotions** look like for people with FND. Please note that **environmental beliefs** that are held by the people close to you will be discussed in Chapters 9 and 10.

Illness beliefs in FND

Quite a lot of researchers have done comprehensive investigations into the **illness beliefs** of people with FND (Stone et al., 2010; Ludwig et al., 2015; Whitehead et al., 2015) (Figure 7.10).

Illness beliefs are normal, understandable, and can even be uplifting, almost like a coping strategy. Viewing yourself as a 'warrior' and a 'fighter' may benefit your rehab for sure. However, holding strong illness beliefs can cause problems, too, and unhelpfully influence your feelings and behaviours. Think about the following scenarios:

- If you believe that FND is 'lifelong', 'incurable', and 'part of me', you may lose hope, not attempt rehab with a view towards full recovery, or stop looking for treatment altogether because you feel there is no point. Acceptance is good but less helpful when there is hope for full recovery.
- If you view FND as strongly caused by physical factors or brain damage, then you may miss out on potentially effective psychological, couples, or family treatment that could turn your life around.
- If you think of FND as a confusing enigma beyond your control with unknown triggers, you are likely to feel **scared, depressed, and overwhelmed** – stopping you in your tracks towards recovery.
- Illness beliefs can adversely impact on physical symptoms and, what is worse, **fuel more FND**. Think for a moment how confusion about symptoms or thoughts around experiencing brain changes contribute to higher anxiety levels, which in turn cause additional physical effects on the body.

FND is part of me and my life, I have learned to live and adapt to my symptoms. I will have to try to make the best of it, despite my symptoms.

I'm an FND warrior, a fighter, FND is not going to take me down.

FND is an irreversible diagnosis and incurable, I will carry this for the rest of my life.

I don't think the FND will improve. My body may not ever return to normal, my life will not be the same as before because of my symptoms

I have no idea where my symptoms / the FND that I am experiencing comes from. It is a source of confusion to me.

FND is caused by physical factors and not by psychological factors like stress or worry. In my case, FND was caused by a bacterial infection/ accident/ injury that I recently experienced

Illness beliefs in FND

FND symptoms have changed my life upside down and left a major impact on my life, including family, relationships, and work.

The FND makes me feel low in mood, anxious about the future and angry about the system that has let me down.

Stress can be powerful but I don't believe that psychological issues can create the severe physical symptoms I have – I don't even have stress. I can get dissociative episodes when I'm in a happy mood.

I tried everything to manage and treat my seizures but this feels beyond my control and unmanageable.

FND symptoms are caused by damage to the nervous system. The messages from my brain are not being passed on to my legs. My brain is disconnected from my body.

FND is a chronic and unpredictable illness, my symptoms wax and wane, there are peaks and troughs.

FND symptoms greatly concern me, especially every time I notice a new symptom.

It is best to rest and stay in bed or I might damage my joints, muscles and get too fatigued.

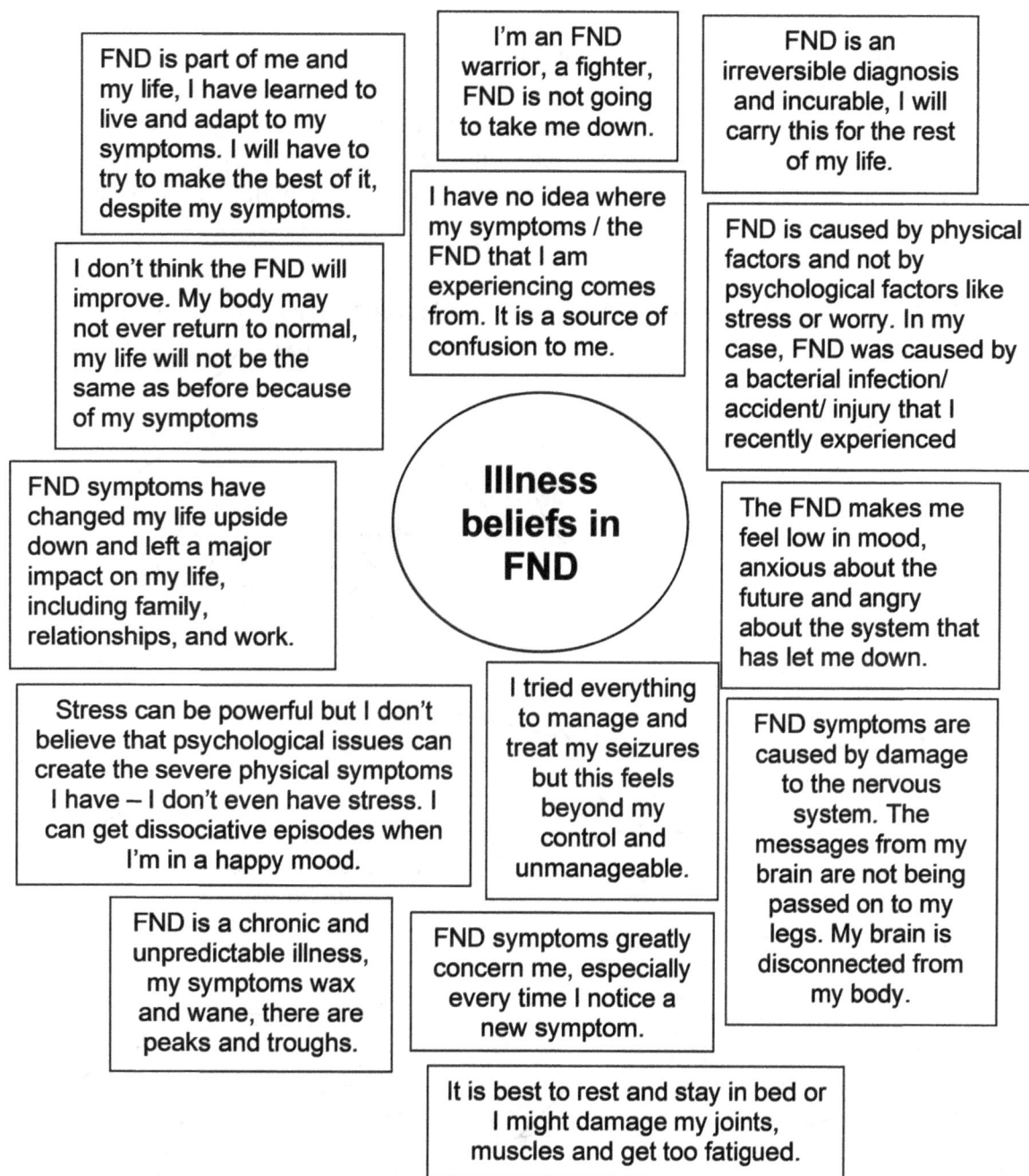

Figure 7.10 Some examples of illness beliefs in people with FND.

Beliefs about other people: not being believed

Although the field has come a long way in raising insight and awareness on FND, '10 out of 10' people with FND still report not feeling believed by healthcare professionals. Unfortunately, thoughts about not being believed by the system are very much mirrored in reality. That means that the system around you may indeed not always believe you and even openly express this to you by calling you 'attention-seeking', 'manipulative', and 'faking it'. It would be counterproductive to challenge these thoughts! What are some things that we can do in this situation?

Find out what the meaning is of not being believed: downward-arrow it

It is important to find out why this 'belief about not being believed' by others is so meaningful and hard-hitting to most people. What is it about not being believed that is important to us, and what basic human need might this belief touch upon? Let us use an accelerated version of the **downward arrow technique** to help you unlock the deeper meaning behind this powerful thought (see Figure 7.11).

When you carefully analyse the chain of thoughts between **'not feeling believed by others'** and **'I don't matter'**, you can see how the idea of not feeling believed by others closely relates to core basic human needs around 'wanting to matter'. Not feeling believed seems synonymous

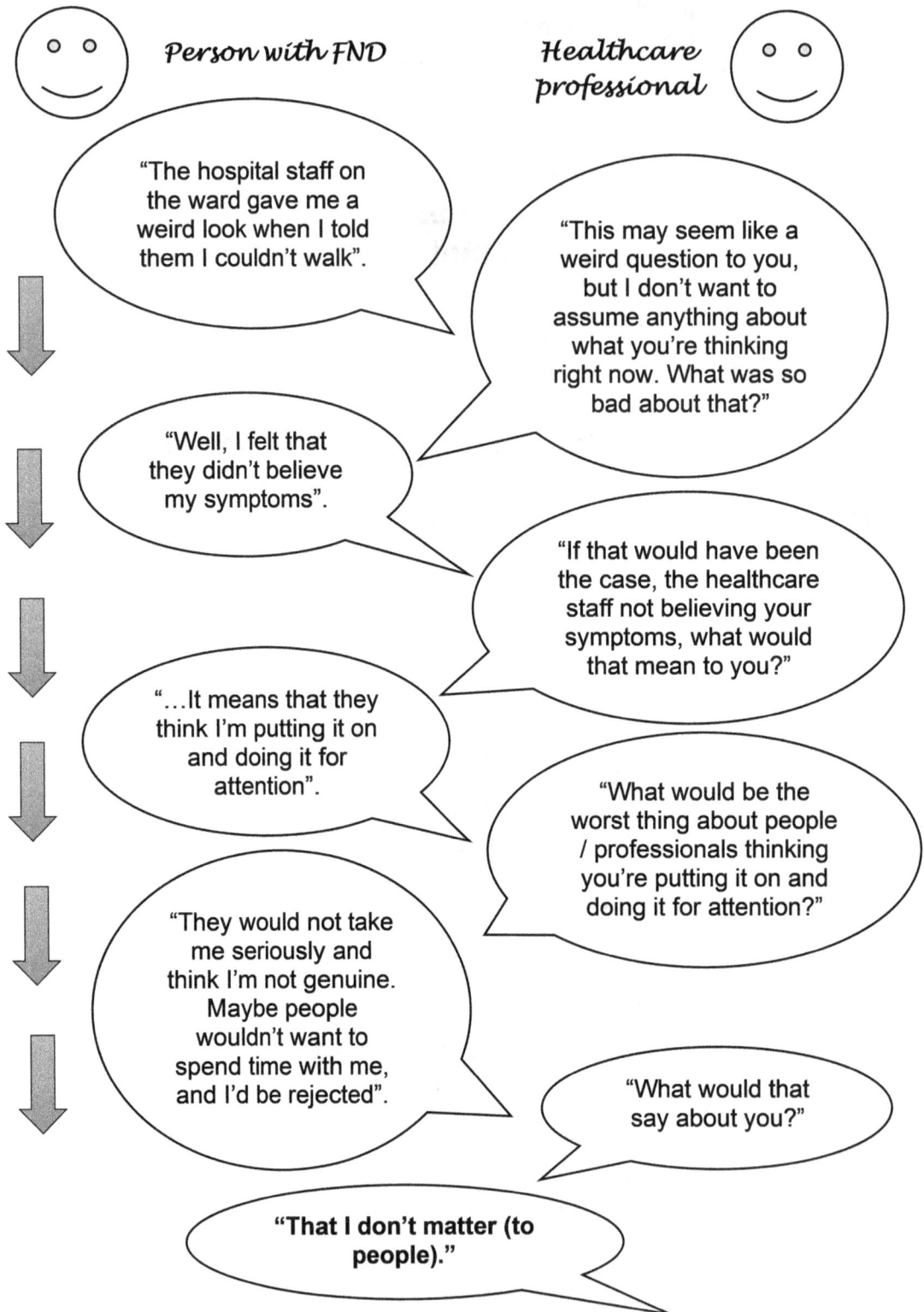

Figure 7.11 Downward arrow technique in FND.

to not mattering, or in other words, not feeling accepted, noticed, validated, cared for, a sense of belonging, and on an even par to other people.

Understand the nature of the impact of the belief about not being believed: re-triggering

Do you remember the section on re-triggers earlier? It is very important to keep in mind that some people are especially vulnerable to visual, auditory, and emotional cues in conversations with healthcare professionals that may indicate 'I'm not believed'. These interpersonal processes often take place quickly, nonverbally, and unconsciously. You may feel an emotion or a level of discomfort that you cannot quite put into words and don't know where this suddenly comes from.

Why is this relevant? Some people with FND describe a difficult upbringing with experiences of trauma and abuse that involved disbelief by key members (often a parent) in the family at crucial points in their life when they most needed a believing person for validation and protection. Fast-forward to the future: imagine that the same family member or a healthcare professional does not believe the FND symptoms. Again, the person is transported back to a familiar experience of disbelief. Given their early experiences of not being believed, it makes sense that the person feels unwell and invalidated. The worst thing about this 'belief about not being believed' is that it can quickly create emotional turmoil that makes the FND worse. Raising your insight and conscious awareness into this re-triggering process is half the battle.

Double standards?

A lot of people with FND experience low self-esteem. You can define *self-esteem* as a 'belief in yourself'. There is often a stark difference in worry between 'belief in yourself' and the perception of being 'believed by others'. Sometimes, we put more value into the beliefs that other people hold about us than we hold about ourselves. Some people have a double standard in favour of others' perceptions about them. If that is the case for you, please feel free to go back to Chapter 6 and complete some of the self-esteem exercises in the 6.2 **eResource**. Rather than working on the 'belief about being believed by others', it may be more helpful to strengthen positive beliefs about yourself so that the impact of other people's beliefs on you lessens.

Distancing yourself from the thought: the bubbles in your pressure cooker soup

IMAGINE . . .

Imagine that you are preparing to make a tomato soup in a big pot. The contents of the soup start to boil quite vigorously, and bubbles start to form on the surface. Our thoughts are like the bubbles that come and go. We are simply standing next to the pot and looking into the boiling contents, watching the bubbles that come and go.

VISUALISE THE THOUGHT

Think about a recent event that made you not feel believed. It could be an interaction you had with a healthcare provider. Visualise the thought of not feeling believed as one of the bubbles in the soup.

SIMPLY WATCH AND OBSERVE

When the bubble (thought: 'I'm not feeling believed') shows up, sometimes it just shows up and then disappears again in the soup. At other times, the bubble grows a bit bigger. When the bubble (thought of not feeling believed) stays on the surface and grows for a while (remains in our mind), we can start to feel different emotions.

SIT WITH THE DISCOMFORT FOR A WHILE

It is okay to feel things; that is no problem. This is a good time to sit with the discomfort and practice with lengthening the time before it may turn into a dissociative episode (for example). Breathe in deeply and breathe out. Focus on the breath and not the bubbles (thoughts), because soon the bubbles will disappear again. Watch as the bubble (thought of not feeling believed) disappears. In time, just like the bubbles in the soup, our thoughts move on.

SOME WISDOMS ABOUT THIS TECHNIQUE

- You are not actively challenging or rejecting the thought. You are simply observing the thought without interacting with it or putting a negative label on it.
- With this technique, the idea is not to make the thought disappear but to reduce the impact of the thought of not feeling believed on your feelings.
- Sometimes, whatever we do, we cannot change someone's thoughts and feelings. What is most important is that you know that your symptoms are real and genuine.
- Accept that some people will continue to not believe you, and ask yourself, 'Would that change anything about the way I look at myself or impact my daily life?' If it does change things for you, review whether it is worth letting this thought impact on you. Are other people's views about you more important than your own views about you?
- Be very careful not to dissociate during this exercise; there is a fine balance to strike.

7.9 eResource alert!

Did you know that you can challenge your thoughts and feelings about not being believed using the Pressure Cooker Model? Try out this exercise to find out more!

An investigation

Sometimes our beliefs about somebody else's beliefs about us may be false because of our previous experiences. We may also be at risk of misinterpreting cues that make us draw conclusions in a hasty manner. Research has shown that people with FND may have a tendency to 'jump to conclusions' (Pareés et al., 2012). It is important to take this view into account.

Joel has FND and has been admitted for a period of neurorehabilitation in an inpatient programme. Joel lost strength in his legs and needs support with personal care and toileting in the morning before attending his sessions. He is in a bay which he shares with three other male patients. Joel notices that every day he has been left last to be cared for in the bay by the nursing team. One day, he commented on this. One of the staff said, 'I will get to you soon, Joel, we are very busy', and then scurried off to help one of the other patients. This made Joel feel upset and rejected. His FND symptoms started to worsen too. Joel feels that the nurses do not believe his symptoms and, even if they do, that they are not taking his symptoms seriously.

In the psychological therapy session, Joel was upset. The psychologist suggested that they go on a little investigation together and speak to the charge nurse and the ward doctor to explore what was happening for everyone.

Influence the system: start a dialogue and educate on systemic re-traumatisation

With the support of his psychologist, Joel explained the reason that he felt upset and low in mood. Joel explained to the doctor and nurse that being left last in the bay re-triggered difficult childhood experiences of emotional parental neglect. The staff acknowledged Joel's hurt and how this led to not feeling believed by the staff's actions. They felt sorry hearing about Joel's early childhood experiences and their continued impact on interactions. The doctor and nurse learned something new and commended Joel for being so open and educating them about systemic re-traumatisation.

Challenging thoughts: could there be an alternative explanation?

The staff decided that they also wanted to break down the reasons for Joel being left last to be cared for, as there were practical reasons. The results of this conversation revealed that Joel was left last in the bay because he was in a bay with patients who were very disabled, highly dependent on the environment for their care needs, and using a hoist with assistance of two staff to receive care. Relatively speaking, from the hospital staff's point of view, Joel's physical care needs were less heavy than those of the other three, as he only needed supervision. Other patients' medical needs were also more pressing, including measuring high blood pressure that required close monitoring in the context of their conditions.

The ward doctor explained that being left last in the bay was actually a good thing for Joel and it showed that his physical health and care needs were less heavy. The nurse added that she felt that she could give Joel more psychological support by leaving him last. Otherwise, if she had tended to Joel earlier, it would have been stressful for her. Now they could have a nice chat together, as she enjoyed talking to Joel. What Joel interpreted as a rejection and not being believed or cared for turned out to be a very different situation.

After this discussion, Joel felt heard and not hurt.

Pick your battles

Not being believed can be detrimental for your psychological health and amplify FND symptoms. As humans, we all want to be believed by other people. We want our thoughts and feelings acknowledged and validated by others. However, in our reality, this may not always be an option.

Consider the height of the Covid-19 pandemic in 2020. Not all people believed that our hospitals were flooded with Covid-19 patients, even though staff were making long hours to care for people and keep the hospital work afloat. Footage even emerged of empty hospital corridors providing 'proof' to the world that it was all a sham. Hospital workers on extremely busy brain injury wards with a constant flow of newly admitted and discharged patients witnessed with their own eyes that our hospitals were more than overwhelmed, accompanied by occasional Covid-19 outbreaks, and with sickness absence rates going through the roof.

Hospital workers can say all these things, but no one is forced to believe any of it. In fact, there will be people in this world who did not and will not ever believe that hospitals were overwhelmed, no matter how many pieces of evidence are provided to the contrary. You could stage a protest or start a campaign to actively convince people of the realness of hospital overwhelm due to Covid-19 and the effects it had on the entire healthcare system. But you know what probably the best advice to you would be? Pick your battles!

In the same way, ask yourself whether constantly proving and defending yourself to other people that your FND is genuine and not fake is worth the effort, your precious time, or your brain space. Is, perhaps, leaving as is and not fighting disbelief not a more attractive option? There is certainly a place for raising awareness and education on FND – the more, the better.

However, this piece of advice is simply for when you have exhausted all your options and you find yourself feeling unhappy, let us say, with the responses from your family or other people in your direct environment.

Lots of the preceding text has to do with how psychologically secure you feel in yourself ('self-esteem') to tolerate the discomfort that comes with not being believed by other people.

Beliefs about other people: not feeling cared for

Feeling cared for is a basic human need. It is the essence of being human and the foundation for maintaining relationships (see Figure 7.12).

We are hardwired with a need to care for others, and feel cared for by others, since the day we are born. Did you know that there is a **neuroscientific basis for caring**?

- **Empathy**, the ability to stand in someone else's shoes, a concept strongly connected to caring and showing compassion for others, is supported by specific areas in our brain called the **frontal lobes**.

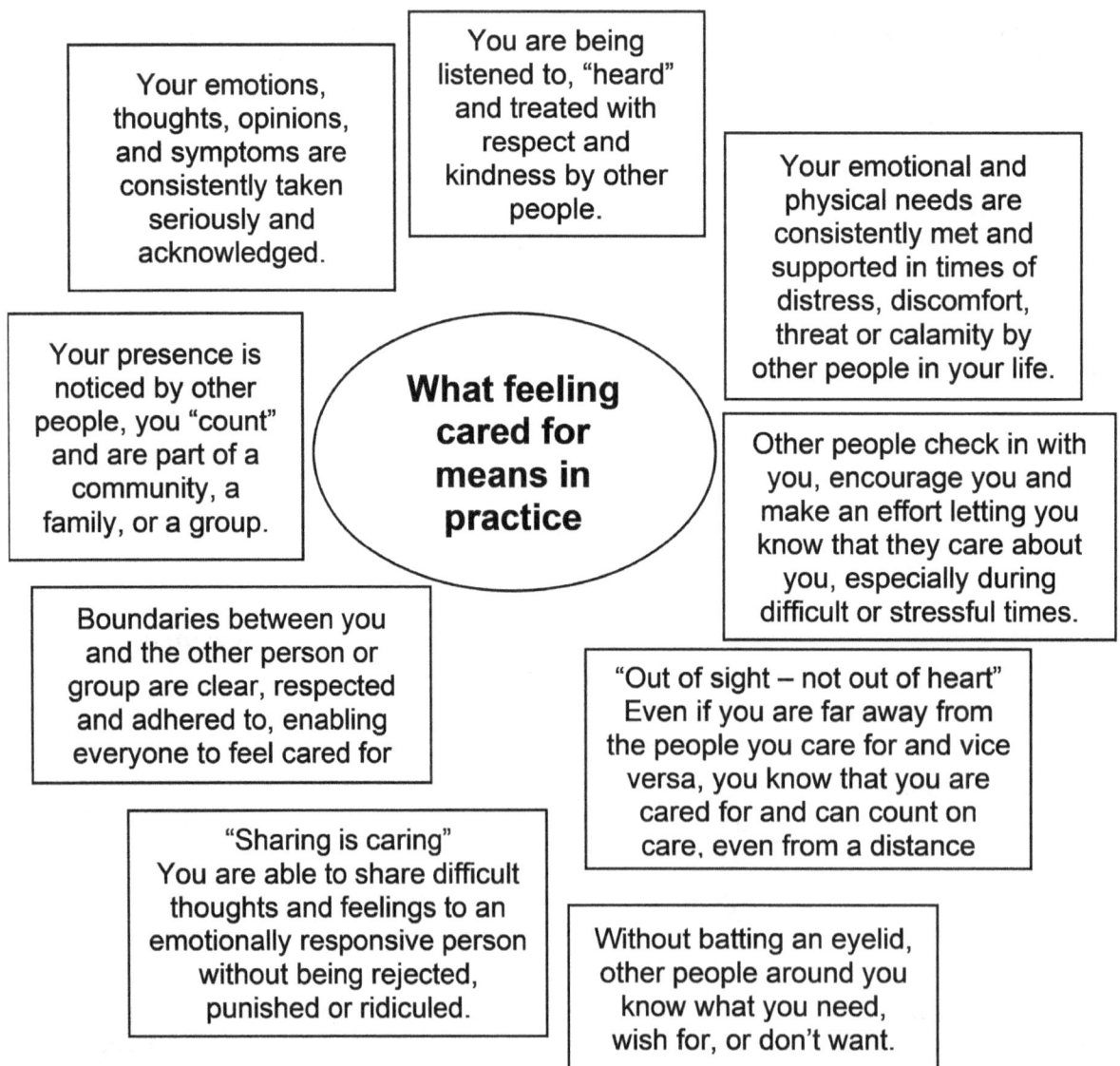

Your emotions, thoughts, opinions, and symptoms are consistently taken seriously and acknowledged.

You are being listened to, "heard" and treated with respect and kindness by other people.

Your emotional and physical needs are consistently met and supported in times of distress, discomfort, threat or calamity by other people in your life.

Your presence is noticed by other people, you "count" and are part of a community, a family, or a group.

What feeling cared for means in practice

Other people check in with you, encourage you and make an effort letting you know that they care about you, especially during difficult or stressful times.

Boundaries between you and the other person or group are clear, respected and adhered to, enabling everyone to feel cared for

"Out of sight – not out of heart" Even if you are far away from the people you care for and vice versa, you know that you are cared for and can count on care, even from a distance

"Sharing is caring" You are able to share difficult thoughts and feelings to an emotionally responsive person without being rejected, punished or ridiculed.

Without batting an eyelid, other people around you know what you need, wish for, or don't want.

Figure 7.12 Characteristics of feeling cared for by another person in relationships.

- People with injuries to the **orbitofrontal** and **ventromedial prefrontal cortex** experience problems with empathy and keeping other people's needs, wishes, and preferences in mind (Stone et al., 1998; Shamay-Tsoory et al., 2005; Decety, 2015).
- **Altruism**, an unselfish concern for the well-being of other people, characterised by acts of putting other people's needs ahead of your own, has been associated with the activation of brain regions, for example, the posterior superior temporal cortex (Tankersley et al., 2007).
- Caring for another person has its neurobiological benefits for the receiver **and the giver**. An interesting study (Inagaki & Eisenberger, 2012) scanned the females of 20 romantic couples in an MRI machine. Their partners were not scanned but were near and received electric shocks. Caregiving, providing social support, and socially connecting with the other person were associated with activation in brain regions called the ventral striatum and septal area. Importantly, activation in the amygdala, the fear centre of the brain, reduced!
- **Rejection**, the opposite of feeling cared for, but rather feeling uncared for ('emotional pain'), causes activation in the same brain areas important for physical pain, namely, the somatosensory cortex and the insula (Kross et al., 2011).
- Children who have not been cared for in their early years developed **decreased brain metabolism** in the brainstem, frontal, and temporal areas, including the amygdala and hippocampus – important for our fear response and memory functions (Chugani et al., 2001).

Not feeling cared for is **one of the most powerful beliefs and experiences** that both people with and without FND report. However, people with FND spontaneously generate these beliefs **so often** during therapy sessions that it is hard to ignore and not notice. It suggests that **care beliefs have an important meaning** and warrant further exploration, particularly in terms of their impact on FND.

In present times, these not-feeling-cared-for beliefs tend to emerge in the context of negative healthcare experiences, as well as with unhelpful dynamics in personal or family relationships. But that is not the full story. **In past times**, people with FND often report having been exposed to unhelpful care experiences where emotional/physical needs were not always fully met in childhood and/or throughout their adult life (see Chapter 5). Explore this **eResource** 7.10 to learn more about early family life experiences, what care might have looked like in these environments, and how this all impacts on our current beliefs of care. **Please note that this applies to people with and without FND.**

Difficult care experiences often stop a person from accessing appropriate 'care role models' and 'care learning opportunities' to fulfil important psychological needs:

- **Cope with emotions** and **apply self-care** during times of stress and adversity.
- **Emotionally connect** with other people and **form healthy** as well as **high-quality relationships.**
- **Set appropriate boundaries** in personal, family, and more distant relationships.
- **Express emotions** to another person you trust and feel psychologically safe with.
- Be able to **appropriately read and identify emotions**, as well as **put yourself in someone else's shoes** and pick up on emotional needs of other people.

Psychological safety behaviours around care

People who have not had the experience of feeling cared for, or had very unusual, out-of-the-ordinary, and even traumatic care experiences, may **develop alternative strategies to feel cared for** in order to meet that basic human need. In response to challenging childhood, teenage, and/or adult care experiences (including in the healthcare setting), people with and without FND will develop **psychological safety behaviours** that will help them **feel safe, secure, and cared for** by other people. Sometimes, people develop totally understandable but problematic **care and help-seeking behaviours** (see the 7.11 **eResource** for more details).

At other times, FND takes on that role of providing psychological safety and security automatically and inadvertently. For example, a dissociative episode can help a person cope with an unpleasant emotion, internal state, or arousal, by bringing this down quickly and effectively. In this situation, FND takes something unpleasant away, and that feels like a relief – a very understandable form of coping.

Although in the short term, any of these behaviours can indeed provide psychological safety, in the long run, these behaviours will 'come at a price':

- Impact on our emotions, day-to-day life, time, and future goals.
- Result in the social consequences that we are most fearful about and **make us feel 'psychologically unsafe' rather than safe** (rejection and abandonment).

To recap

- Feeling cared for, and to care for another being, is a **basic human need**.
- **All of us, FND or no FND, engage in care and help-seeking behaviours**; it is **normal** and the essence of the human experience.
- Whether you have FND or not, **wanting to feel cared for is not unique to FND**.
- Even if we do not realise, **unconsciously**, that we experience this care need in the depths of our minds and hearts.
- Psychological safety behaviours around care are often **automatic and protective**, reframed as normal responses to abnormal circumstances or **survival strategies**, and **maintained by both the individual and the environment**.

7.12 eResource alert!

Some people feel sad, disappointed, frustrated, or even angry about having developed psychological safety-seeking behaviours, particularly those that greatly impact on day-to-day functioning, and struggle to be kind to themselves. If that is you, please have a look at the compassionate phrases in this **eResource** that you might connect with and find helpful. The phrases are meant to encourage you to take on a different, kinder perspective.

Re-triggering experiences

Let us read Jesse's story:

Jesse had been admitted to an inpatient programme to receive support with dissociative episodes and with his feelings 'quickly going up and down'. Jesse arrived on the ward and was put in a large bay with other men. In the first few weeks, Jesse fared well and was making some gains in rehab. After some time, however, Jesse's dissociative episodes gradually became worse and started happening in public places with lots of patients and staff present. In therapy, Jesse brought up that he felt ignored, disrespected, and mistreated, mostly by the staff as well as by a few patients. He reported that the staff would be overly nice to his neighbours in the bay and take time to chat with them but give Jesse short responses. Although Jesse struggled to identify his emotions, he looked angry and hurt. Jesse's psychologist thought that these observations were crucial to understanding the triggers for dissociative episodes. Initially, Jesse did not understand why the psychologist brought up these experiences: 'Can we just move on from this and continue with proper therapy?' 'I don't want to spend time talking about these people anymore.' The psychologist gently asked Jesse for permission to explore and formulate these interpersonal triggers further, to which he agreed even though he was confused.

After several sessions, it transpired that Jesse had felt like this many times before in early child-hood. Since a young age, Jesse, and his siblings, had been neglected by his parents. With the psychologist's help, Jesse made the link between his early childhood experiences and his current experiences in the bay which re-triggered feelings that had been buried for a long time.

Jesse's Pressure Cooker chain reaction

Using the details from his story, let us make a start by exploring Jesse's Pressure Cooker chain reaction (Figure 7.13), which shows you the strong relationships between:

- Jesse's interpersonal 're-triggers' **(check the fuel box in Figure 7.13).**
- His re-triggered emotions around not feeling cared for **(do the same for flames; check the box).**
- The level and intensity of these feelings **(heat box).**
- How this all leads up to dissociative episodes **(overpressure plug on top of the Pressure Cooker Model).**

Do you see how Jesse's background of emotional neglect made him more vulnerable to pick up on cues in his environment that signalled 'I may be neglected and not cared for' once again?

However, that is not the whole Pressure Cooker Model story for Jesse. You may remember that, in Chapter 6, you learned about the **cover** and the **valve**. To truly understand Jesse's Pressure

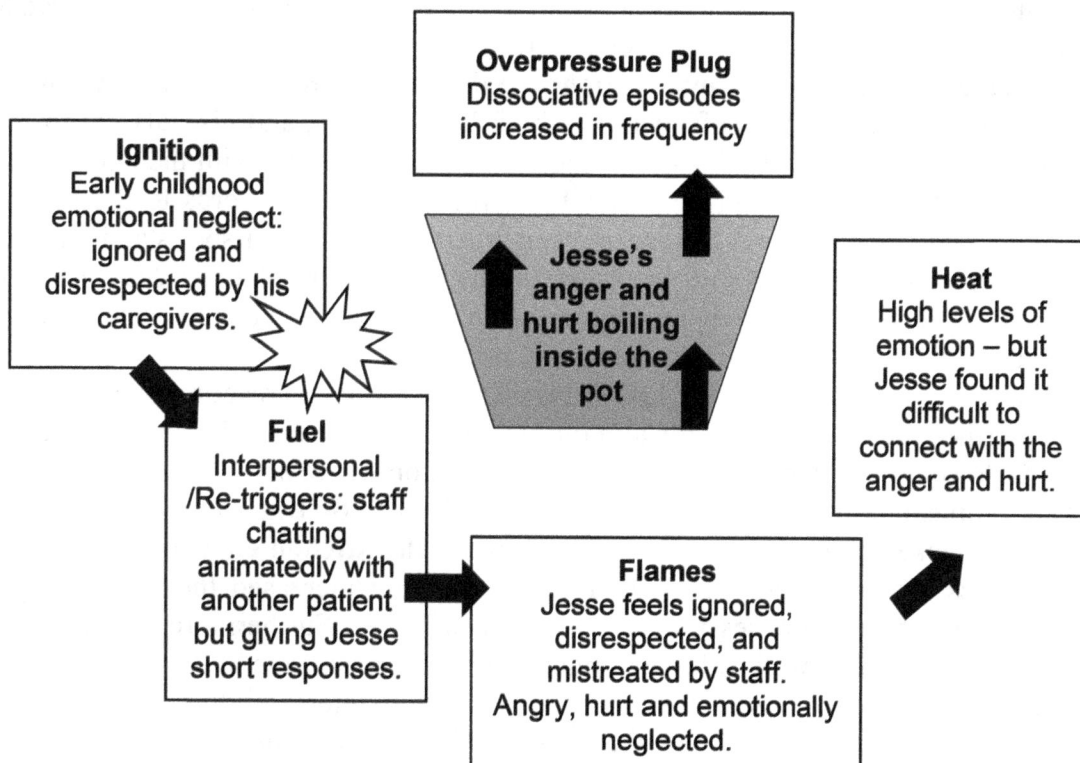

Figure 7.13 Making a start with Jesse's Pressure Cooker chain reaction.

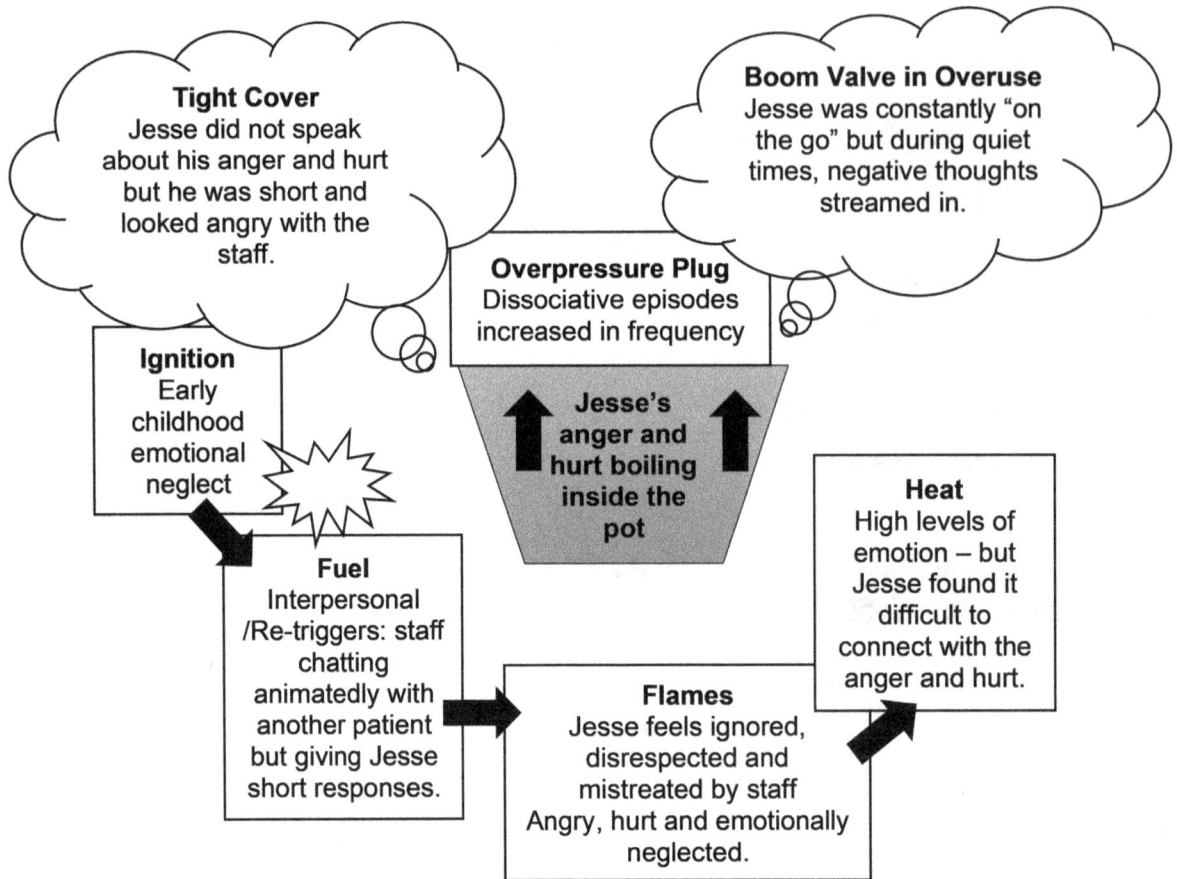

Figure 7.14 A more comprehensive Pressure Cooker chain reaction for Jesse.

Cooker chain reaction and how this eventually led to more dissociative episodes, we need to take these two elements into account as well (see Figure 7.14).

You may have seen that Jesse's **cover is tight** (he did not express his anger in words, did not speak to anyone or the specific staff member about how he felt), and his **valve is in overuse** (he pushed himself with a lot of activities because he struggled sitting with the hurt). These two channels for emotional expression (**channel 1**, expressing anger in words to the people who made Jesse feel hurt, and **channel 2**, releasing anger using enjoyable or sports activities that are not over-the-top active and 'blows off the steam' of his anger) were blocked. Jesse had no other option than to express his hurt through his body (overpressure plug), the only channel he was left with. This is where the dissociative episodes came from.

One of the advantages of completing Jesse's Pressure Cooker chain reaction is how Figure 7.14 not only describes what is going on for him during a dissociative episode but, even better, also how it points to solutions! Table 7.7 describes some ideas on where and how Jesse can intervene in the chain. **You can do this, too, and soon will learn how to do this yourself!**

We have not spoken about another important element: **the kitchen environment**. The staff's caring responses fed into Jesse's dissociative episodes and increased their frequency. Jesse started missing out on therapy sessions and spent days in bed. Furthermore, the large number of dissociative episodes, as well as Jesse's anger and his short answers in between the episodes, made staff ignore and reject Jesse more often and not want to interact with him. Jesse was stuck in a **'self-fulfilling prophecy loop'**: the very thing that he tried to avoid (being ignored, rejected, and not feeling cared for by people) started to become reality: **he was ignored, rejected, and not cared for.**

Table 7.7 Possible strategies to help Jesse overcome the dissociative episodes

Pressure Cooker Element	Example strategies
Ignition & Fuel	• Jesse's insight was raised into the relationship between his early childhood adverse experiences and how his current experiences can re-trigger feelings of rejection, emotional neglect and hurt that resembled his past experiences.
Flames	• Jesse learned to identify, label, and connect with his emotions. This increased awareness helped Jesse to gain better control over his emotions and responses to re-triggering events.
Heat	• Reality grounding exercises and behavioural experiments supported Jesse to sit with his emotions a bit longer without immediately experiencing a dissociative episode.
Open the Cover	• Jesse practiced with expressing his feelings in psychological therapy with a non-judgemental therapist and one-to-one chats with staff without worrying about rejection or hurt.
Alleviating/unblocking the Valve	• Jesse learned to slow down and release his anger through his beautiful drawing activities. • He went for daily short bursts on his exercise bike – instead of using the bike for hours at a time and subsequently feeling too exhausted to do anything afterwards apart from sleep. • Jesse participated in regular exercise group with other peers, enjoying interactions and creating a sense of social belonging.

7.13 eResource alert!

Did you know that the self-fulfilling prophecy loop that we just explored can show up in other areas of people's lives too? A very understandable fear reported by people with and without FND is the **fear of an FND setback** in the future, especially after a period of steady progress and in the face of discharge from services. Learn about the biological, psychological, and social factors that contribute to this common fear and how to reduce your risk of an actual setback by looking at the Pressure Cooker Model and developing your own 'stay well plan'.

A big unspoken fear: the fear of the unknown and recovery from FND

People with FND and their families experience many types of fears, but there was one type of fear that consistently stood out in therapy sessions, time after time, in nearly every person with FND.

A special category of fears in FND revolves around **fears of the unknown, recovery, and relapse**. This fear can be defined as a high anxiety or feeling of discomfort about the idea of recovering from FND. The fear of the unknown that often accompanies progress and recovery in

FND is a real, genuine fear and something that truly needs attention and support during neurorehabilitation. Why is it so important to discuss this fear? Why not just leave it and accept as is?

To some degree, the **fear of the unknown is a normal part of recovery**. If it was not there, that would even be strange! Have you ever experienced a change in another life area? Think about a house move, change in schools, family circumstances, new job, break-up, and so forth. Some changes can be exciting and fear-inducing at the same time!

So it is normal to feel fear, a funny feeling, or discomfort about what is coming after the FND. That said, **copious amounts of fear around the unknown and recovery**:

- Can wreak havoc on progress and slow down or prevent actual recovery from FND.
- Serve as a psychological safety behaviour and maintain or even generate new FND symptoms.
- May mean that there are things and maintaining factors you have not yet worked on but deserve extra attention.
- Stop you from working on challenges that you need the most help with.
- Could risk you and your family missing out on a better quality of life or venturing out in new, unexplored territories in life, following your dreams, preferences, and wishes.
- Put your life on hold, in a state of paralysis, and sometimes, quite literally stop people from moving.

Please note that **this does not mean that you are on purpose, blocking recovery**. On the contrary, because of the fear of recovery, people may inadvertently engage in thoughts, feelings, and actions that operate on a far more unconscious level and do not help recovery. Not fully accessible to conscious awareness, people often do not even realise that these psychological processes are unfolding at the back of their minds. It is like **the brain protects the person** against experiencing these overwhelming feelings more consciously.

Before you continue reading this section, it is really important to emphasise that the **fear of recovery is not about a conscious effort to block recovery** or something that you have full control over and, like flicking a switch, can just change in the moment. **It is also not the case that 'you are not trying hard enough'**. It is rather the opposite: time after time, people try very hard to recover. People frequently describe an inner battle characterised by ambivalence and choice paralysis: a simultaneous **push towards getting better** vs a **pull away from recovery** and keeping the status quo.

7.14 eResource alert!

So what is the fear of recovery about, then? Times of transitioning towards more independence can stir up conscious and unconscious thoughts and fears of 'life after FND' revolving around overwhelming demands, psychological pressures, and a return to the same pre-FND life that contributed to FND in the first place. Read this **eResource** to find out about some important aspects of this special category of fear in FND.

Fear of recovery is often about social consequences

WALKING . . . BUT WHERE TO?

This fear is **not necessarily about recovering from the FND symptoms itself** ('I want to walk'), as people with FND often express that there is nothing more they would like than to get rid of the symptoms, since the FND clearly stands in the way of living a full life. Fear of recovery is more about the social consequences attached to FND recovery and what will happen to relationships and interpersonal processes once recovered from FND. 'I want to walk . . . that is awesome . . . but where would I walk to if I do not have a social support network, friends, family, a job, hobbies, interests, a vision for the future?'

SOCIAL POSITIVES VS SOCIAL LOSSES

The fear of recovery tends to revolve around the idea of 'social positives' and 'social losses', which are not at all obvious or easy to spot. Although FND is debilitating and stops people from living life to the full, as counterintuitive as this sounds, people with FND have also reported **positive 'personal' influences** on:

- Identity
- Self-esteem
- Sense of psychological safety
- Day-to-day independence
- Stable and predictable life routines

As well as positive 'social' consequences on:

- Quality of relationships
- Communication and interactions in the family home
- Responses from other people
- A sense of social belonging and inclusion into a caring and validating community
- Positive social perceptions from others
- A sense of control over psychosocial circumstances and family dynamics that was not present before
- Reduced social demands, expectations, psychological pressure, and responsibilities
- Reduced social isolation and an improved social life in general that started since the development of FND.

For lack of a better word, you could call these **social positives or 'gain'**. Please note that gain is 100% not the same thing as 'purposefully getting something out of the FND' or 'putting on symptoms'. The term simply refers to a positive consequence on social life that a person noticed ever since the FND.

A social loss in the context of FND recovery is the exact opposite. People have reported that, by recovering from FND, something precious was lost in the recovery process that somehow was connecting the person more strongly with the social world and the people around them in positive ways. The fear of recovery is often associated with the prospect of letting go or risking the loss of social positives.

SOCIAL POSITIVES VS SOCIAL LOSSES: AN EXAMPLE WITH CATCHING A FLU

The idea that a health condition has attached social positives and losses is not new at all. A good example is getting the flu. Can you think back to a time that you experienced a flu and were mostly bed-bound? Perhaps you had a doting partner or family member that looked out for you and measured your temperature, brought you salty chicken soup, tea with honey, sweet-tasting cough syrup, a box set of DVDs for you to watch, hot compresses on your head, a bunch of comfy pillows and extra blankets to make you feel more comfortable. Maybe your loved one held your hand when your head was pounding with pain, which softened the blow. Possibly, your manager at work told you to take as much time as you needed to recuperate from your bout of flu. You did not have to attend this horrible meeting that had been planned for ages and you were not exactly looking forward to. Perhaps there was a chore at home that you were excused from participating in because, clearly, you were feeling ill.

Think for a moment about how this situation might have felt for you. Being ill and having the flu is no walk in the park, and you could do without the headaches, stuffed nose, and coughing episodes; however, the support, care, doting, checking in, the fact that you were noticed by someone who had your best interests at heart may have felt quite nice and validating. You mattered to this person.

Some people may have never had this experience and were not doted on or cared for but rather experienced the opposite circumstances. For people who have been 'devoid of being doted on' and have not had their emotional and physical care needs consistently met in the past by an attachment figure (like a parent, a partner, or a family member), the doting experiences associated with a bout of flu sickness may feel qualitatively very different. The feeling of being doted on may far outweigh the feeling of discomfort that a condition such as flu may impose on the person.

This does not mean that this applies to you. However, **being ill comes with social positives**, and **recovering from illness comes with social losses**. It will depend on the individual person to what extent these social positives and losses will be balanced or whether the balance tips over into one over the other direction.

Before continuing, let us debunk a myth, the big pink elephant in the room. In no way does this mean that FND is disingenuous, put on, or simulated, and that people with FND have FND because they want attention from other people and that it is the only reason FND exists. That would be an incredibly narrow-minded view of FND. **It simply means that any condition – including FND – is more than just an illness. We cannot ignore the social context that a health condition is embedded in, including FND.** Another way of looking at this situation is to imagine that social positives and losses do not revolve around FND but an organic condition like epilepsy, the type that causes abnormal electrical storms in the brain. Do this for a moment; replace 'FND' with 'epilepsy'. What do you conclude?

You may conclude that the social positives and losses in those conditions are quite similar to the ones described in FND. The bottom line of this exercise is to show you that (physical, neurological, psychological) **illnesses or conditions do not exist in a social vacuum** but, rather, are **always tied to social consequences** and **psychosocial processes**. In some people, these social factors may play a larger role in their condition than for other people.

7.15 eResource alert!

Check out some common social positives and social losses reported by people with and without FND in their environment. If you would like to look more closely at social positives and social losses in your own situation, then completing the **eResource** exercise will help you obtain a better understanding and insight.

Fears of the unknown and recovery: wider social factors

Although the focus of the discussion around social positives and social losses was mostly on the person experiencing the FND, please note that **wider social factors, beyond the individual level, are equally at play here**. This is not just about the person with FND! Think about what the idea of social positives and losses means for the family system around you should you recover. Once you recover from FND, family and personal relationships may destabilise because, in some (not all) situations, the FND has been 'holding the family unit together'. As the individual is progressing on the path towards recovery, relationships undergo qualitative changes or may not be as close-knit as before. A parent or partner may lose a meaningful identity as a carer and proximity to the person with FND. Social positives and losses are not just experienced by the person carrying the FND symptoms but just as well by people in their environment. Chapters 9 and 10 will delve more deeply into these social aspects of FND.

Another important issue in relation to the fear of recovery is the present state of FND healthcare services . . . or rather their scarcity. Recovery from FND can be tricky if no help is available, with services not specialised in treating the condition, discharging the person, providing limited involvement, excruciatingly long waiting lists, or not having a contingency plan for re-referral to services if someone experiences an FND setback. The wider social setting clearly has a major impact on the fear of recovery.

How the fear of recovery can maintain FND: another self-fulfilling prophecy

Do you remember our discussions about the **self-fulfilling prophecy about rejection** in Jesse's story earlier in Chapter 7? The 7.13 **eResource** further explored how **another self-fulfilling prophecy loop** can take place around the **fear of an FND setback**. Having a strong fear of future setbacks can result in thoughts, feelings, and behaviours that contribute to an actual setback. Did you know that something similar can happen with the fear of recovery? (See Figure 7.15.) The fear of recovery can actually feed into FND symptoms and, **via a self-fulfilling prophecy loop, stall actual recovery from FND**. Look at the Pressure Cooker Model that follows.

7.16 eResource alert!

The period before discharge from a service is often fraught with fears of the unknown that are not always obvious or spoken about. Even if people are unable to use language to express these fears more explicitly, a person's behaviours and symptoms can suggest, sometimes in more subtle ways, that perhaps these fears are at play, either consciously or more subconsciously. Before we look at some examples, please note that this list is not meant to catch people out or blame people in any way.

A note for people who do not feel the fear of recovery

You might not identify with any of this at all and say:

- 'I don't feel fearful about the future. You are putting words into my mouth.'
- 'I look forward to my recovery and cannot wait to do all the things that I want to do but cannot do as a result of the FND.'
- 'I don't have a fear of recovery, and I do not feel believed by you saying that.'
- 'How could you even suggest that I do not want to recover because of fear?'

It is always possible that you do not experience any fear of recovery or the unknown. However, it is also important to keep in mind that sometimes people with FND are unaware of negative emotions, because of high levels of dissociation, which is often a key feature in FND, **and may not be in touch with emotions, including the fear of recovery**. How could you find out? Several clues may indicate an underlying fear of recovery without you 'experiencing' the emotion:

- **Plans . . . without action.** Some people formulate a lot of plans and activities that could help them move towards recovery from FND. People know exactly what to do and what skills to

Kitchen
Worsening FND symptoms cause more rejection in my environment: *"She's putting more symptoms on, you see?"* But also protection against the environment: no psychological pressure, not having to cope with unrealistic demands, some preserved relationships and perceptions of me, my illness being "seen".

Tight cover
Unspeakable dilemma: embarrassed to speak about my fears with anyone. Keeping this to myself and isolating from other people.

Overpressure Plug
Old habits kick in: My fears feel intolerable and uncontrollable: Dissociation and FND symptoms worsen, I'm switching off from the problems.

Blocked Valve
Standing at cross-roads and pondering about what to do next activity-wise: Not knowing what meaningful activities I'll be able to fill my days with when recovering further and not able to take steps to explore this as I feel frozen with fear. Procrastinating, status quo / staying the way I am feels containing and familiar.

Warning light
FND symptoms worsen as my fears about recovery are building up. Focusing more on the symptoms

Fear of recovery and the unknown

Ignition
Past rejection experiences (e.g., bullied, singled out by parent).

Sticky left-over food
Dissociation as an early childhood coping habit.

Pot
Sleepless nights, the fears keep me awake at night, feeling shaky and having to rely more on equipment again, visiting my GP.

Fuel
Making some progress in rehab / treatment. People in my social circle and at work giving me puzzled looks and openly questioning the FND.

Fear of recovering further: what will I tell people about how I recovered?

Fear that people will think I've put the symptoms on. Will my family and friends understand the change and how will they respond?

Fear about losing my identity and about what's next in my life.

Fear of rejection and being shunned by people.

Fear of people putting pressure on me now that I'm getting better.

Questioning my recovery, being hard on myself. Overthinking and worries.

Fear of being unable to cope with new demands.

Fear of relationships turning back to the (unhelpful) way they were before.

Fear of people not recognizing that I'm still recovering and expecting the world of me.

The fear of recovery-o-meter indicating high heat

Fear of people not seeing my hidden disabilities, especially psychological.

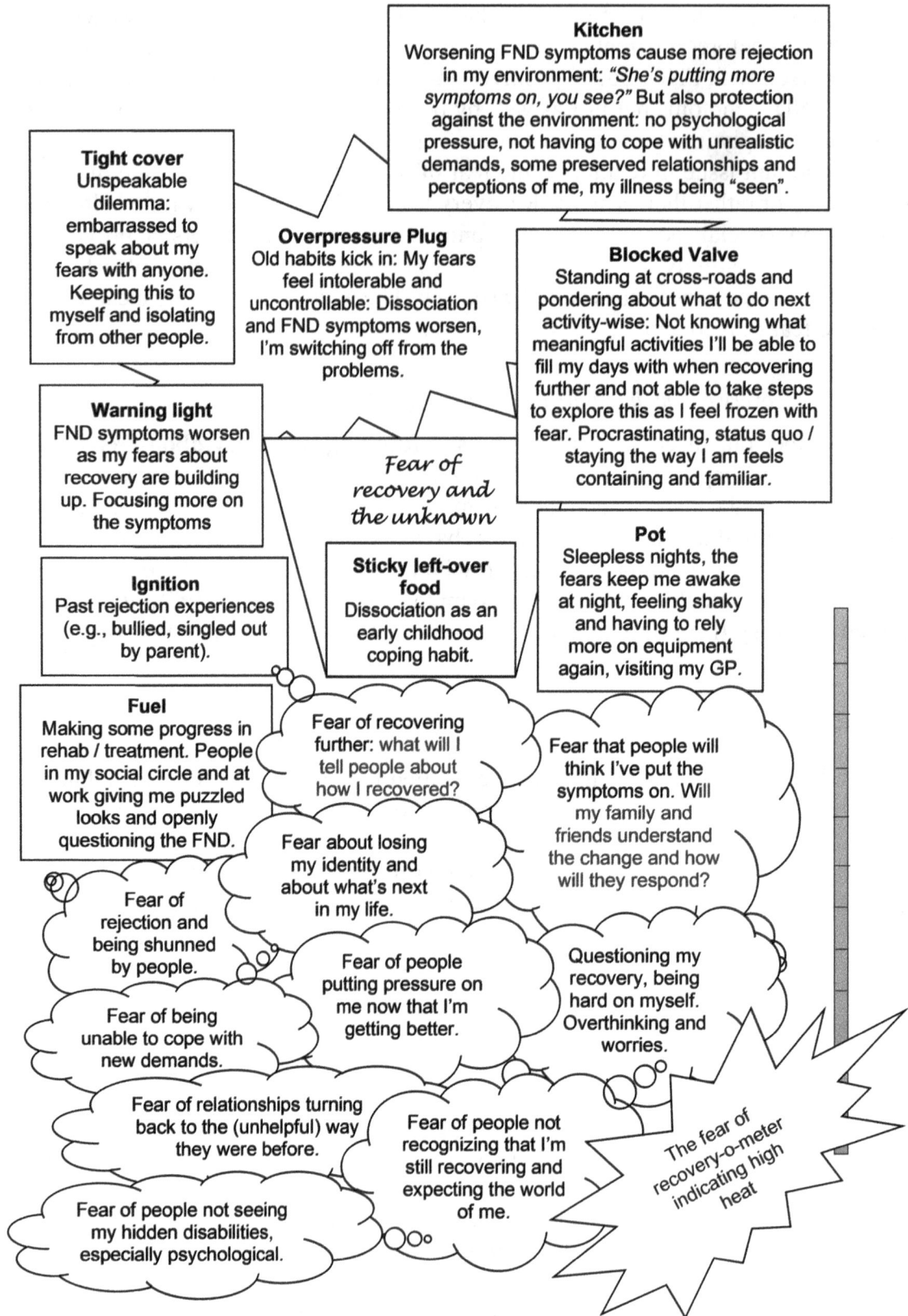

Figure 7.15 How the fear of recovery can lead to actual problems with recovering from FND symptoms.

practice. However, **putting these well-formed plans into action is often the roadblock**. There is **a huge abyss** between plans on one side and concrete steps to act on these plans on the other side. It can be difficult under any circumstances to follow up on plans, but you can imagine that if you experience an unconscious fear of recovery on top of that, plans may stay plans.

- A person's **extent of progress towards therapy goals** can be another manifestation of recovery fears. Despite putting their very best efforts into the rehabilitation, some people may:

  - Not reach their goals.
  - 'Just about' reach goals.
  - 'Just not' meet their goals.
  - Only set modest goals with limited progress over time.
  - Vague goals that are hard to execute and pin down.

  Goal setting that is moving you slowly on your pathway to recovery **can reveal an underlying fear of recovery**. It is like your mind wants to recover but your body is stopping you from doing so.

- **Accepting the 'new normal'.** Some people have had FND for a long time and found their own way of dealing with disabilities, often having been left to fend for themselves in the context of unresponsive healthcare services. Despite the disabilities, people feel fairly accepting of the 'new normal' and do not think much about the future. People may have given up hope on recovery, but life with FND is doable with good routines and a support network in place. It makes sense that a person's mind has stopped entertaining the possibility of recovery. As a psychological 'protection' mechanism, people may say to themselves that their current situation is good enough. If a person would bring into conscious awareness other, darker thoughts and emotions about recovery ('It is not good enough', 'I do not even know where to begin', 'I am stuck', 'I have been abandoned by services') but there are not many treatment options available to help with achieving goals, then it may feel better altogether to not connect with these thoughts and emotions in the first place. Not thinking about that reality will save a lot of pain and hurt.

7.17 eResource alert!

The fear of the unknown and recovery from FND is one of the most debilitating fears reported in treatment. You may remember the **'unspeakable dilemma'** from Chapter 6. The fear of recovery, particularly around the interpersonal and social consequences of recovery from FND, can be like an unspeakable dilemma. It is often a **deep-seated** and **less conscious fear** that remains **hidden and unexpressed** and is sometimes associated with **embarrassment, guilt, and shame**.

People with FND may sometimes avoid thinking about the future. The fear of recovery wants us to exactly do that. But the more we avoid and run from the problem or future, the worse it gets. Have you ever experienced a toothache? You may initially just want to avoid it and try not to pay too much attention. However, once a toothache comes knocking on your door, it tends to hang about only to become worse over time, if left untreated. Days or weeks go by and you find yourself in an even more painful situation. You may even need a root canal to fix the issues. In the same way, people with FND can sometimes find themselves in a status quo that feels familiar and psychologically containing; however, the longer you wait, the harder it becomes to think about change and the more entrenched we become in our thoughts, habits, and equipment.

Luckily, there is a lot that you and your family can do to get rid of the fear of recovery! Read this comprehensive **eResource** to assess your personal situation, practice strategies, and tackle your fear of recovery once and for all. This **eResource** will review a wide range of techniques with you. As with all strategies in this book, and in line with the Pressure Cooker Model ethos, the exercises probably work best if you can **invite a trustworthy** and **supportive 'FND ally'** to do this work with you.

Let us start off with a relatively easy tool that quite a few people with FND reported as helpful and enjoyable in their own journey of beating the fear of recovery: visualising the future with **the FND mood board exercise**. Have you ever seen a mood board? It is a **visual representation** of your **life without FND**. Mood boards are particularly useful for people who like to be creative with different materials.

It is also very important to note that **mood boards are not just intended for people with FND**. Your loved ones and the people close to you will often have been impacted by the FND too. This can result in their own lives having come to a standstill or altered in some way, for example, not seeing friends as often, changing jobs, not pursuing certain interests, dropping hobbies or life goals. All these circumstances lead to further problems, including low mood, frustration, and feelings of hopelessness.

To help you and your partner, family, and friends on the way, check the **eResource** for an example of an FND mood board and other ideas on what your mood boards could contain (including searching for mood board inspiration on the internet).

Watch the process rather than content

Any of the techniques described earlier can help you act against the fear of recovery and 'grab the bull by the horns' by actively visualising your future. By doing this, you give yourself a better chance of 'moving' out of a stuck position. For example, when you start a mood board, treat it as your initial version that you will chop and change along the way. Start brainstorming ideas for each life area, and do not pay attention to how realistic the ideas are. Let your creative juices initially flow without putting any constraints on it and shooting down any ideas. You can always do that later! Use a 'funnelling' process to prune your options to more tangible and realistic activities, goals, and plans.

The goal of these 'fear of recovery' exercises is not just **to generate the desired product ('FND recovery')** but maybe even more so **to engage our brain with the process**, with something that has not recently crossed our minds. A lot of people are so consumed with day-to-day management of disabilities that the thought of what is next after FND has not been entertained, for understandable reasons.

As you are engaging with these exercises, track your thoughts and feelings: What is happening? Is it anxiety-provoking? Uncomfortable? Unpleasant? If you struggle with labelling or describing emotions, as many people with FND experience, do you notice anything in your body that could give you a clue of the underlying emotion, for example, heart palpitations, sweating, a tremor, or any FND symptoms that are getting worse? Do not worry: as much as this may feel uncomfortable, this is good news. It means that you are pushing a pressure point that needs tackling.

Bridging the gap: what to do if you are too scared or uncomfortable to act

Some people may not be able to think about anything to do with what life might look like after recovery and struggle to engage with ideas around the future. Other people may be a little bit further in their recovery journey and have lots of ideas and plans but stumble against making concrete inroads. No actions are undertaken, and ideas remain ideas. You feel stuck between a rock and a hard place and perhaps psychologically paralysed between choices: neither situation feels comfortable, and you know that things are bound to be challenging whether you 'choose' the rock or go for the hard place. The rock may be a familiar but uncomfortable challenge (the FND and the major impact it can have on daily life), whereas the hard place (moving towards recovery) is unfamiliar and uncharted territory. These are well-known issues for people with a fear of recovery. If you find it difficult to act on your plans, there are a few things that you could do to help the situation:

- **Be kind and compassionate to yourself!** You are engaging with the idea of finding out what recovery might look like for you.
- **Don't give up hope.** Looking at the chasm between where you are now and where you would like to be can be daunting and filled with hopelessness. Do not stare too long into that abyss, but start thinking about how you could build a bridge from where you are now to where you would like to be. Start with a simple bridge.
- **Think of it as a process or a journey, not the ultimate goal.** The goal of all these exercises you just did is to experience what it must feel like thinking more deeply about what recovery entails. The goal is not to ensure that you have neatly completed all your exercises and you are now ready to roll on with recovery from FND.
- For some people, **a seed needs to be planted first** before they can truly engage with recovery more fully. And that is totally okay. Forget about it and come back after a while; re-engage with the ideas you have worked through just now, then leave it again if it becomes too overwhelming. Again, this is a process, not the end goal.
- Sometimes it may help to **do a 'mini version' of what FND recovery** must feel like. Suppose you are holidaying on a beautiful beach, for example, a lovely beach on the East Coast of the United States of America. The beach is next to the Atlantic Ocean, which is ice-cold. You could lunge yourself into the ocean and become startled and shaken by the cold wave that just enveloped you or, knowing that the ocean is cold, decide to dip in your toes first to test the temperature of the water. If you feel confident, you may progress to walking into the ocean a little further until the water reaches your waist. Perhaps then you feel brave to fully immerse yourself and go for a brief swim.

People with FND sometimes view recovery as taking the plunge into a big, cold, and daunting ocean. However, in the same way as getting slowly used to the freezing water, all steps towards FND recovery will more likely succeed if these are small, 'a little bit every day', and gradual, rather than radical with huge leaps. Without dipping your toes first, you are less likely to move forwards. Have a think about how you can dip your toes in your own recovery journey.

- If you are a bit further into the process but you struggle to get past the 'essentials and necessities' of life (e.g. preparing a meal, making sure that you are taking your medications, doing groceries, keeping your house clean and tidy), look beyond the basics.

Imagine that you are about to move into a new place. You need essential furniture, like a sofa, dinner table, a television or laptop to watch movies on, cutlery, plates and cups, a kettle to boil water for your tea, a wardrobe, and a bed to sleep in. These pieces of furniture will make the place liveable, but not necessarily cosy and warm.

In order to make your house more of a 'home', you could add more 'colour' to your house by hanging family pictures and paintings on the wall, books and candles, funky towels, sending some invites for people to come over for dinner parties and social gatherings.

The point of this exercise is that we can stick with the basics of life and basic furniture to keep us going. But to make our life colourful with meaning, we really need to hang the decorations ourselves! **Ask yourself: How can I live, not just exist?** How can I make new memories?

A final word on the fear of recovery

If you have tried these techniques and they are not working for you, do not worry, and do not give up hope! Recovery fears are often **strongly tied to interpersonal dynamics** that people have with other people in their environment. What sorts of things can you think about?

- **People** putting **psychological pressure** on you to recover fully or quickly.
- **High expectations and assumptions** about your completed recovery from people in your environment, for example, to jump straight back into 'normal life' like it used to be pre-FND. Picking your life up where you left it 'like nothing ever happened'.
- **Demands placed** on you **by other people**, 'too quick, too soon', for example, not seeing the need for a phased return to a job, or to try a voluntary or part-time role first as a stepping stone to a paid and full-time role.
- Your environment not being able to see your **ongoing rehab** or the **invisible disabilities** that may still be lingering in the background. A common example pertains to people who regain their physical abilities but are still working through the psychosocial bits of the FND, which are more hidden and get overlooked quite often ('you walk and talk' = 'you are better!'). Physical disabilities generally tend to recover faster than psychosocial difficulties because it takes a longer time to undo unhelpful thoughts, feelings, behaviours, and relationship patterns.

It is important to know that the **fear of recovery is very much about the interpersonal dynamics between people.** That is why inviting your direct environment into your rehab process is essential. To learn more about this topic, jump ahead to Chapters 9 and 10.

A special type of thoughts: cognitive abilities

You could argue that our thinking skills (also called 'cognition' or 'cognitive' skills, from the Latin word 'cognoscere', which means 'to know, to learn, or knowledge') belong to a specific category of thoughts.

Cognitive symptoms can be the **main presenting issue in FND**, for example, a severe memory problem but otherwise quite good walking and speech abilities. Most often, though, people's **cognitive difficulties will co-exist with other FND symptoms.** For example, a person with loss of power and sensation in the legs may have brain fog and some memory problems, but the leg issues are the most bothersome to the person in day-to-day life.

7.18 eResource alert!

Let us look a bit more closely at the different cognitive abilities that our brains support. This **eResource** will help you understand two important cognitive skills that people with FND often experience problems with: How does memory work? And what does the term 'executive functions' really mean? Attention skills will be discussed in a lot more detail later in Chapter 8, so watch this space!

What type of cognitive problems do you see in people with FND?

Cognitive problems can be psychologically driven or brain injury–related (i.e. resulting from a permanent loss of neurons [brain cells]; think about dementia, stroke, or a knock/blow to the brain) or be a combination of both in a subset of people with FND. There is often a wide spectrum of thinking difficulties reported by people with FND, including:

- **Orientation in time, place, and person.** Knowing what time of day it is, the name of the day, what month and year, where you are, and who you are, for example, after coming out of a dissociative seizure.
- **Attention.** Struggling to focus on conversations, following a storyline in a movie on television, being unable to concentrate on reading a book.
- **Memory.** Problems with recognising the names and faces of people around you, or the names of places and household objects, recalling past conversations, important events (e.g. weddings), or time periods in your life.
- **Prospective memory.** Forgetting to take your medications on time, remembering to be (on time) somewhere, for example, a future doctor's appointment.
- **Language.** Not being able to come up with the correct word, making speech errors.
- **Executive functions.** Difficulties with organising your life, planning ahead or doing multiple things at the same time. Forgetting the sequence of personal and domestic care activities, for example, how to dress yourself, make a cup of tea, or prepare a warm meal for dinner.
- Problems with **visual, spatial, and navigation skills**, like wayfinding on familiar and unfamiliar routes.

It is really important to find out what the underlying reasons may be . . .

Cognitive problems do not just come out of nowhere for people with FND. A lot of factors can impact on someone's cognitive functioning and could plausibly explain your memory and thinking difficulties (see Figure 7.16).

What can I do about cognitive problems in FND?

First things first: it is important to establish the reason(s) for your thinking difficulties. A multidisciplinary assessment by professionals that look at your brain, neuropsychological functions, and overall health is a very useful starting point. You may be asked to participate in a neuropsychological assessment and a brain imaging investigation, which can shine a light on the possible reasons for your cognitive problems.

Once the reason has become a bit clearer, and depending on the underlying reason, there are a variety of approaches that you can take to cope with your cognitive problems. The following list of strategies is not exhaustive but has offered support to people who, as part of the FND, experienced cognitive difficulties:

- **Addressing any underlying psychological difficulties may ameliorate thinking difficulties.** For some people, this may be low mood. Luckily, we can reverse mood-related thinking problems by helping a person keep their mood lifted and plan in enjoyable activities or connect socially with a community ('unblock the valve'; see Chapter 6). For other people, working on their worries, panicky feelings, anger, trauma, interpersonal relationships, communication, or stabilising their emotions to keep them at an even keel, could greatly help improve memory and concentration (see Chapters 7 to 10 for strategies).
- **Learning to manage dissociative episodes** will prevent memory, orientation, and 'brain fog' difficulties that follow afterwards for a subset of people. It is less helpful to re-orient the person after an episode, because this risks feeding into the episode. You will learn more on that topic later in Chapter 7.

Emotions. Low mood, feeling anxious or angry; lots of worries; panicky feelings, any strong and intense emotions.

Dissociative episodes can result in post-episode amnesia, confusion and disorientation about who and where you are, and what just happened.

Prior brain injury (e.g. stroke or bleed to the brain, concussion, inflammation of the brain or the layers that protect your brain). Epileptic seizures, in contrast to non-epileptic seizures, cause abnormal brain activity and occasionally can cause injuries to some parts of the brain, particularly the regions important for memory.

Traumatic experiences and PTSD can cause 'fragmented' memories and cause dissociation which impacts on our thinking skills.

Interpersonal triggers – for example, suppressing memories around the distress and topics from arguments.

Other physical illnesses, for example like flus, colds, covid-19, as well as diabetes (hypo's). Sleep apnoea can cause issues with the brain and impact on oxygen levels.

Feeling tired, chronic **fatigue** syndrome, **poor sleep** (hygiene).

Chronic **pain**, fibromyalgia, as well as specific heavy pain medications can cause memory and thinking issues.

Focusing a lot on your symptoms – we only have a limited store of attention: that is attention not going to the things that you may need to focus on.

Lack of vitamins, not eating enough **nutrients** or being **dehydrated**.

Factors in FND that impact on cognitive symptoms, our thinking abilities

Medications – some medications make us drowsy, help to cut off emotions and impact on our attentional functions. **Polypharmacy** (when people take lots of medications) can also influence our thinking skills.

Sometimes, memory problems can help us to **communicate** how we feel to the people around us, especially when we don't have the words available to express ourselves.

Normal ageing processes – as we grow older, our thinking skills may become less efficient over time. This is completely normal and expected. (our speed of thinking tends to 'deteriorate' already in our thirties!).

Past or current **substance misuse** issues (e.g. alcohol, cannabis) and/or **overdoses**.

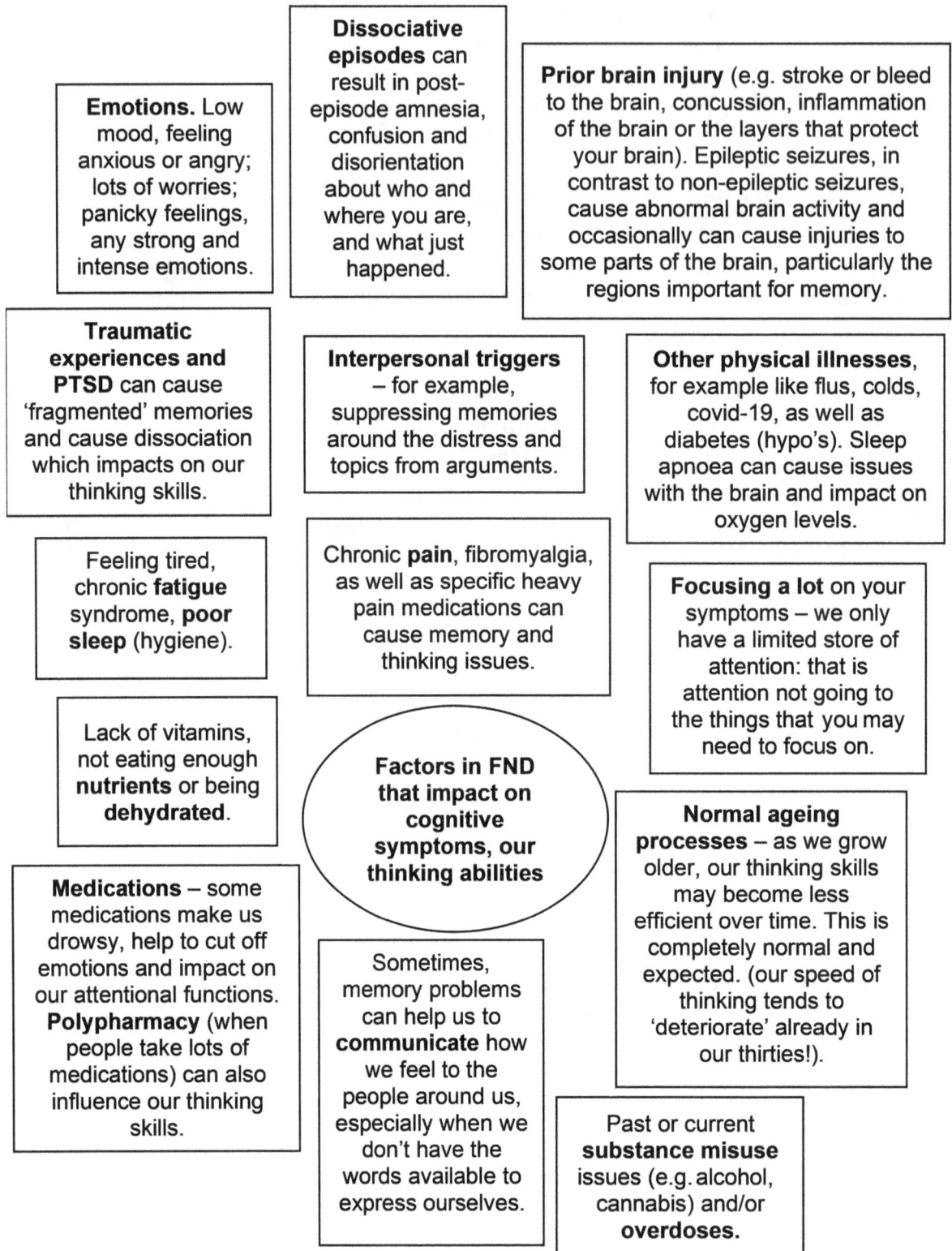

Figure 7.16 Reasons for cognitive difficulties reported in people with FND.

If you have a brain injury and FND, then **cognitive rehabilitation techniques** could benefit you, for example, using a diary, phone, alarms, tick lists, rehearsal techniques, using imagery or establishing a daily routine to help prompt your memory, and a whole host of other mnemonic and organisation techniques.

- Cognitive neurorehabilitation is probably a less-helpful avenue for thinking difficulties that are strongly associated with psychological or interpersonal factors, because the use of these strategies could maintain a person's thinking problems and illness beliefs without addressing the underlying drivers.
- **Regular reviews** of your physical state: any co-existing physical illnesses, your medications, diet, and fluid intake – including alcohol, caffeinated beverages, and illicit substances – by a medical and multidisciplinary team can be really helpful to determine any 'culprits' that impact on your thinking skills.
- A deeper dive into **strategies to help you with pain, fatigue, and sleep symptoms** can have a positive knock-on effect on thinking skills.
- **Normalise.** Some people are 'worried well'. A person may notice a thinking problem and instantly worry about dementia or another serious condition but are subsequently found to have a healthy memory. **Reassure yourself:** memory 'failures' are common in everyday life (a word on the tip of your tongue, searching for your glasses whilst they have been on your head all this time, going into a room but forgetting the reason why). Worried-well people often view their memory problems as far worse than they are in reality.
- And **do not focus** or **try to worry excessively** about your thinking difficulties, especially if multiple investigations have shown these to be normal. It only takes up headspace. Choose wisely on where to allocate your precious attentional resources to! (See Chapter 8 for techniques on how to manage your worries.)
- Finally, the Pressure Cooker Model emphasises **psychosocial contributions** to difficulties in people with FND. The same holds true for **cognitive problems**, which **can be maintained by the social environment**. Although often coming from a good heart and a place of care, some partners and family members may be highly focused on a person's memory, take a lot of work out of the person's hands where in fact the person could do a few tasks independently, and not afford them the opportunities to properly test out whether memory and thinking abilities are really that poor or maybe better than initially thought. The problem is that you will not find out if everyone is doing everything for you.

In addition, these social experiences do not help with building trust and confidence in a person's own cognitive abilities – no matter how well-intended. It is also important to know that **memory suppression** can be an **effective and protective coping mechanism** to forget about difficult events, interactions, arguments, and other unpleasant interpersonal dynamics in the social environment.

Social anxiety

Social anxiety disorder affects quite a substantial subset of people with FND – **it is a lot more common than people think**. People with social anxiety fear the negative judgements and social rejection from other people. What are some prominent features of social anxiety? Figure 7.17 shows you all the important components of social anxiety (based on the social anxiety model of Clark & Wells, 1995) and highlights the strong association with FND.

Treatment of social anxiety is based on addressing each of these components with your therapist. It goes beyond the scope of this book to discuss social anxiety treatment in detail; however, one of the later sections of Chapter 7 will discuss an essential part of CBT for social anxiety: 'behavioural experiments'. Stay tuned!

Feeling self-conscious, shame, or embarrassment in a social situation, which results in your attention focused inwards.
In FND, attention is also often focused inwards, particularly on physical symptoms and the body.

Fears of being judged negatively and rejected by other people, for example people thinking you're stupid, crazy, boring or silly.
In FND: worries about how you walk, looking 'drunk', or looking 'weird' with your shakes.

Worries that other people will see the physical features of your anxiety (e.g. becoming red and blushing of your face, stammering, the shakes)
In FND: the physical symptoms of anxiety can be expressed in shakes (functional tremors)

Safety behaviours are ways or strategies that help you cope with and endure the social situation, including avoiding or escaping the situation, not making eye contact.
Common safety behaviours in FND: can be your mind 'switching off' or dissociating each time you are in a social situation, to cut off feelings of high anxiety, as well as the wheelchair (people don't have to make direct eye contact and can quickly speed off in a power chair)

Social anxiety in FND

There may be a clear link between FND and social fears/ situations: Every time the person enters a social situation the shakes become worse and amplified. The shakes are an 'amplified' physical symptom of anxiety: Where some anxious people may get shivers, a person with FND may experience a much stronger level of shivers in the form of shakes. (the fight-or-flight response in maximum overdrive - please see Chapter 8).

Anxiety is the key emotion in social anxiety. **However, in FND: anxiety may not be recognised or identified as such.** This is because people with FND are not always in touch with their emotions because of dissociation or alexithymia (not being able to describe your emotions well).

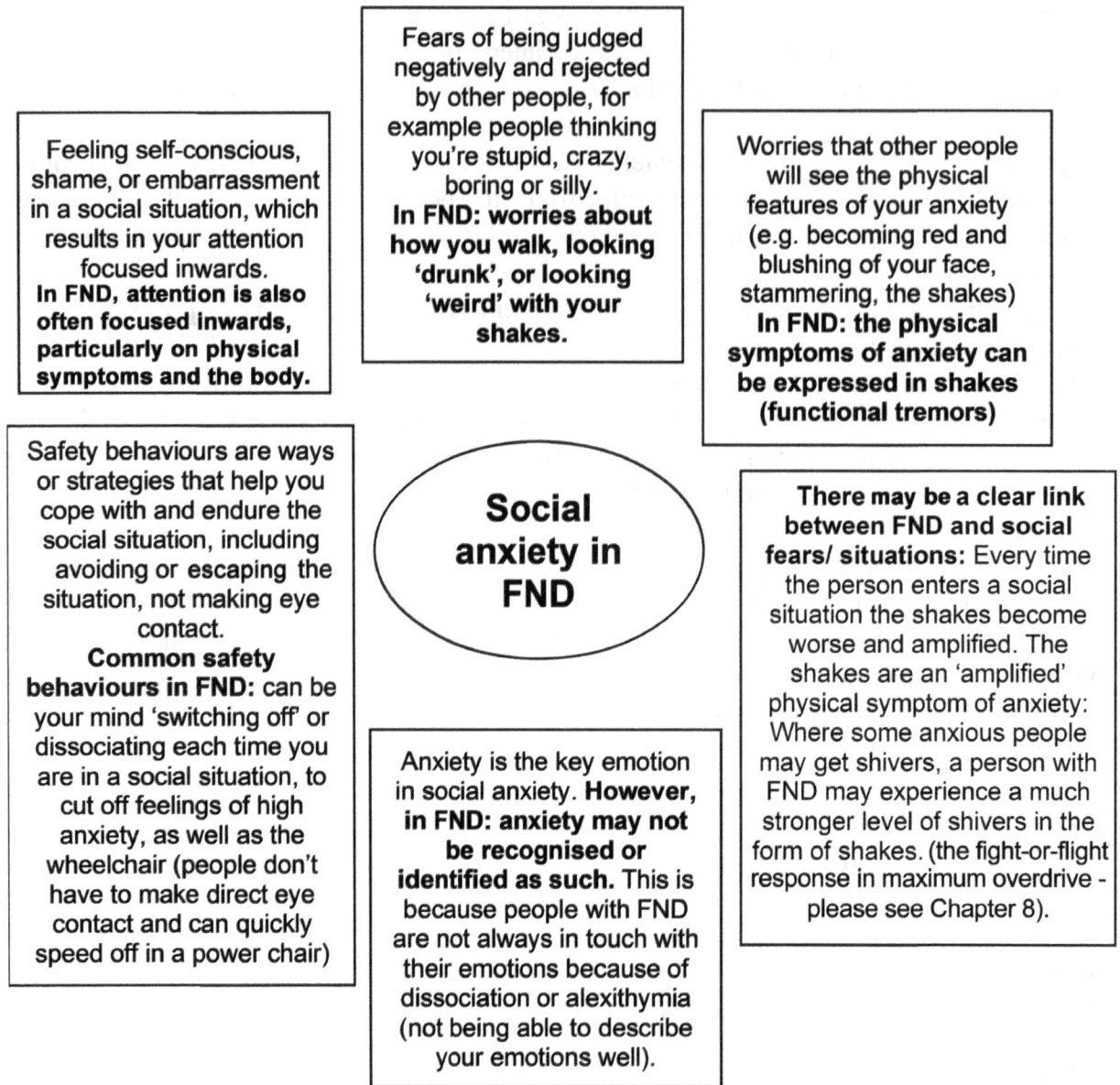

Figure 7.17 Relationship between social anxiety features and FND symptoms.

The flames in the Pressure Cooker Model: delving a little deeper into the world of emotions

The topic of emotions is big and, occasionally, very controversial and tense in FND. People frequently report not feeling believed or taken seriously by healthcare professionals when a link between FND symptoms and emotions is tentatively suggested. This section is not meant to force you to accept 'stress' as the reason for FND or convince you to fully believe in the FND–emotion link using some sort of psychological trickery. Emotions are complex phenomena and often a source of confusion, particularly around the process of how emotions 'convert' into FND. The following section focuses on emotion education and helping you understand the basics of emotions. You are free to think and feel whatever you wish after reading this section, and perhaps you feel differently after reading the blurb on emotions. Let us go on a journey together and learn more about emotions!

There are many different types of emotions

'Basic' emotions

In a classic research study, Ekman and Friesen (1971) discovered that human emotions are universal: different cultures across the world recognise and experience similar emotions. There are often six basic emotions identified: fear, sadness, happiness, anger, surprise, and disgust. We are born with these emotions and hard-wired to feel and experience them.

Table 7.8 Examples and characteristics of basic emotions

Basic emotion	Why do you feel the emotion?	Body language	What you do or not do
Fear	Something threatening in your environment or in your thoughts about the future, causes you to worry.	Heart pounding, increased breathing, heart rate and blood pressure, stomach butterflies or knot, tense muscles, feeling sweaty and hot.	Avoidance, escape behaviours, including freezing, fleeing, or fawn.
Sadness	Losses, death, abandonment, rejection by other people.	Fatigue, slower-than-usual movements and thinking processes, lack or increased appetite and sleep.	Reduction or withdrawal from social and enjoyable activities, self-neglect.
Happiness	Feeling of joy in response to a beautiful, pleasant, or amusing event, achievements, and connection with other people.	Laughter, feeling high energy, uplifted, tingling and warm.	Approach rather than withdraw, jumping for joy.
Anger	Something negative has been done to you, or something/someone is blocking a goal in your life. Believing that you have been treated in an unfair manner by another person.	Increased heart rate, feeling warm, sweaty, or hot, reddening face, tensed up muscles, clenched jaw or fists.	Urge to fight or hit out, you want to attack something or someone. Verbal expressions involve shouting and screaming.
Surprise	Sudden, unexpected events, sounds and movements. Surprise increases attention and helps to decide whether something is dangerous or not.	Wide open eyes, raised eyebrows, jaw drop, gasp of air.	Moving a step away from the thing that surprises you, to gauge what's happening.
Disgust	Triggered by unpleasant sensations, bodily products, decaying foods, as well as people's actions, ideas, or looks (=social disgust).	Nausea, gastro-intestinal symptoms	Turning away from the thing that causes disgust.

'Social' emotions

Another important category of emotion that people with FND report are social emotions (see Table 7.9). These are also called 'interpersonal' emotions because:

- We tend to feel these emotions in relation to the presence or absence of other people.
- They emerge in the context of relationships and interpersonal interactions.
- We can experience them when recalling or thinking about events that involved other people.

Table 7.9 Examples of social emotions and circumstances in which they emerge

Social emotion	Why and when do people feel them
Shame	You have done something / or something has been done to you that is socially not acceptable. You judge yourself in a negative manner and believe that other people view you in the same way. "I'm a bad / worthless person". As a result, you blush, hide yourself, keep a low profile away from a social group. You may slump your shoulders and look down.
Embarrassment	Stems from when a perceived or real characteristic, feature or quality related to you as a person is (or threatens to be) revealed or witnessed by other people, may make us look less appealing, attractive, likeable, or undermine the way we would like to come across to other people.
Guilt	You believe, or, have done something unacceptable to another person, wronged the person in some way, and this requires behaviours that "repair" the guilt, some sort of compensation.
Envy	A desire to have what another person has, but you don't have. Another person has something that you would like, desire, long or crave for (e.g. a nice job, car, relationship, family) and this thing makes them appear better, more desirable or attractive in comparison to you – an unfair advantage as perceived by yourself. Impetus to work more, harder or in different ways to obtain what the other person has.
Jealousy	Quite similar to envy – but often the opposite way around: another person may threaten to take away or make you lose something desirable or prized that you may already possess (e.g. another person is heavily pursuing your partner on the dancefloor). Can result in expressing hostility or irritability to the other person, intimidation, or violence.
Resentment	Your perception of having been treated unfairly, mistreated, having been wronged, insulted or disadvantaged in some way by another person.
Schadenfreude	Enjoying, feeling better about yourself, deriving pleasure about another person's hurt, pain or misfortune.
Pride	You possess a quality, a thing or have achieved something that is judged or perceived by yourself as well as by other people as praiseworthy and positive. Pride sets you apart from other people, as more positive, with an advantage for you in comparison to others.
Contempt	Feeling superior over others. Contempt helps you to feel powerful, accompanied by a smug, disapproving facial expression, eyerolls.
(Attachment-anxiety)	(Fear of rejection, abandonment, or the possibility of not being cared for by a person important to you).

As you will probably have noticed, emotions are multi-layered and often associated with specific triggers, beliefs, behaviours, physical features, and the wider social environment.

Secondary emotions

We can distinguish primary from secondary emotions. Think about the following scenarios: you just gave a presentation, and you were visibly anxious and stressed. People clearly noticed and, afterwards, provided you with a cup of water, asked how you were, and checked in with you. The fact that people noticed made you feel embarrassed about your performance being perceived in a negative manner by other people. Another example may be a scenario where you became angry and threatening towards other people. After the anger subsided a bit, you felt ashamed that you 'flew off the handle' in front of others. In both situations, the person initially expressed a primary emotion (anxiety or anger). Once these primary emotions lessened, the person became aware of a new, secondary (and social) emotion in response to the original emotion. Emotions are complex!

Emotions come in different levels of intensity and strength

Emotions have different levels of intensity and 'heat' levels. For example, both 'frustration' and 'rage' fall into the anger category. However, the emotion of frustration feels milder than the more potent emotion of rage. We can see emotions resting on a gliding scale. Table 7.10 shows the different levels of emotion. Keep in mind that this is just an example. Different people may have different ideas about the strength of emotions.

Table 7.10 The gliding scale of emotions

Happiness	Anxiety	Value	Anger	Sadness
Ecstatic	Terrified	10	Rage, Outraged	Devastated
Overjoyed	Scared	9	Mad, Incensed, Ballistic	Heartbroken
Gleeful Beaming	Fearful	8	Furious, Infuriated, Livid	Miserable
Merry Upbeat	Perturbed	7	Bristling, Seething	Despair Desolated
Cheerful Joyful	Anxious	6	Angry, Irate, Aggravated	Dejected Sorrowful Dispirited
Happy Blissful	Apprehensive	5	Steaming	Mournful
Delighted Chuffed	Nervous	4	Frustrated	Sad Despondent
Pleased Glad	Stressed	3	Irritated	Gloomy Disheartened
Content	Worrisome	2	Irked, Worked up	Down in the dumps Downcast
Satisfied	Unsettled	1	Annoyed, Sulky, Crabby, Grumpy, Cranky	Low in mood Forlorn

Emotions have neural underpinnings and are associated with different brain areas

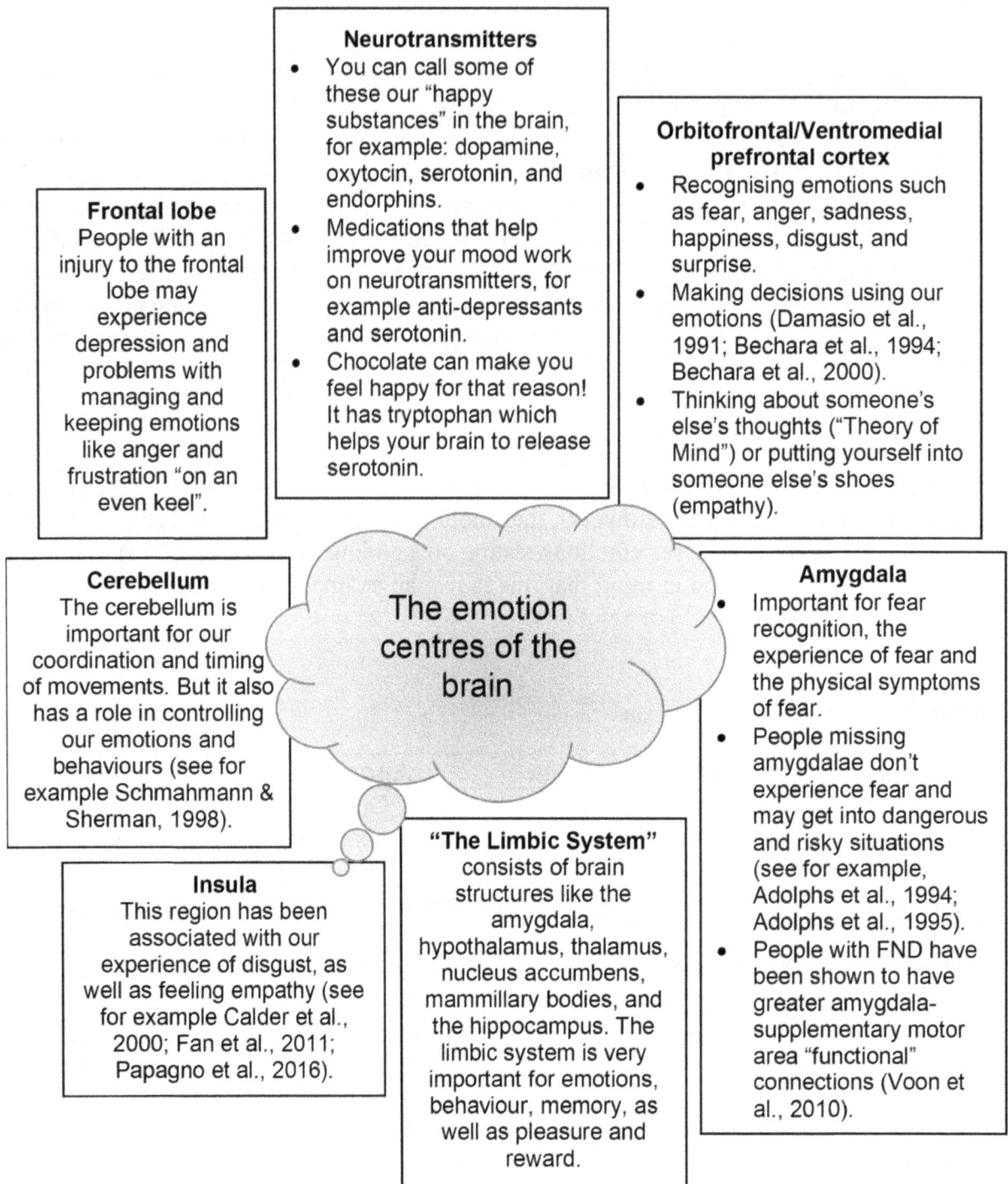

Neurotransmitters
- You can call some of these our "happy substances" in the brain, for example: dopamine, oxytocin, serotonin, and endorphins.
- Medications that help improve your mood work on neurotransmitters, for example anti-depressants and serotonin.
- Chocolate can make you feel happy for that reason! It has tryptophan which helps your brain to release serotonin.

Orbitofrontal/Ventromedial prefrontal cortex
- Recognising emotions such as fear, anger, sadness, happiness, disgust, and surprise.
- Making decisions using our emotions (Damasio et al., 1991; Bechara et al., 1994; Bechara et al., 2000).
- Thinking about someone's else's thoughts ("Theory of Mind") or putting yourself into someone else's shoes (empathy).

Frontal lobe
People with an injury to the frontal lobe may experience depression and problems with managing and keeping emotions like anger and frustration "on an even keel".

Cerebellum
The cerebellum is important for our coordination and timing of movements. But it also has a role in controlling our emotions and behaviours (see for example Schmahmann & Sherman, 1998).

The emotion centres of the brain

Amygdala
- Important for fear recognition, the experience of fear and the physical symptoms of fear.
- People missing amygdalae don't experience fear and may get into dangerous and risky situations (see for example, Adolphs et al., 1994; Adolphs et al., 1995).
- People with FND have been shown to have greater amygdala-supplementary motor area "functional" connections (Voon et al., 2010).

Insula
This region has been associated with our experience of disgust, as well as feeling empathy (see for example Calder et al., 2000; Fan et al., 2011; Papagno et al., 2016).

"The Limbic System"
consists of brain structures like the amygdala, hypothalamus, thalamus, nucleus accumbens, mammillary bodies, and the hippocampus. The limbic system is very important for emotions, behaviour, memory, as well as pleasure and reward.

Figure 7.18 Brain regions and neural circuitry involved in emotions.

Emotions impact on our attention

Who does not remember feeling nervous before a school exam, attending a job interview, or giving a presentation? Too little or too much anxiety can wreak havoc on your motivation and performance. However, our brains need a little bit of anxiety to sharpen the senses and reach peak performance.

The Stroop task (1935) is a famous neuropsychological test that measures your attention and concentration abilities and how good you are at suppressing an automatic response. A typical Stroop task often consists of two parts.

On part 1, a person is asked to read the names of colour words. A list of words denoting different colours (for example, the words 'blue', 'red', or 'green') are printed in black ink. Your job is to read out loud the words as quickly and as accurately as you possibly can.

RED	GREEN	BLUE	RED
BLUE	RED	GREEN	RED

On part 2, a person is presented with a sheet of colour words. This time, however, they are asked to name the colour of the ink the words are printed in, rather than read the colour word. Why don't you try it for yourself with the following two lines?

RED	GREEN	BLUE	RED
BLUE	RED	GREEN	RED

How was this experience for you? You may have noticed that the second part of the Stroop test is a lot harder than part 1. In day-to-day life, we are far more likely to read words in a book, a blog, or a newspaper and less likely to name ink colours. But on the Stroop task, our brains must actively override our very well-rehearsed skill of word reading with the far less well-practiced skill of naming ink colours. The frontal lobes of our brains need to put in a lot more effort and will take much longer to process these words than the words from part 1.

A variant on the Stroop task is called the 'emotional Stroop task', which contains words that elicit often strong emotions in people:

DEATH	ILLNESS	DANGER	ACCIDENT
ATTACK	SCREAM	TUMOUR	BULLYING

Due to the strong emotional responses these words provoke in most people and their ability to capture our attention, naming the ink colours of these emotional words will be markedly slowed down in comparison to emotionally more neutral words (like 'table', 'lemon', or 'book').

Attention–emotion tasks in people with FND and dissociation

Neuropsychological researchers have found that emotionally charged materials, like facial emotional expressions, greatly impact on the attentional skills of people with FND (see Table 7.11). Highly relevant findings, particularly if you think about the frequently encountered issues around mood, anxiety, and interpersonal triggers in people with FND.

Table 7.11 Attention–emotion interactions in people with FND and dissociation

Scientific research findings in FND	Type of FND	Type of task	Authors
Attentional bias towards angry faces, suggesting an increased vigilance and sensitivity towards faces characterised by a 'social threat'.	Dissociative seizures	Emotional Stroop task (pictorial version).	Bakvis et al. (2009a) Bakvis et al. (2009b)
Attentional bias towards emotional faces.	Dissociative seizures	Emotional Stroop task (pictorial version).	Pick et al. (2018)
Difficulties disengaging from emotional information conveyed in facial expressions on a reaction time task.	Dissociative seizures	Emotional Task Switching experiment	Gul & Ahmad (2014)
Attentional bias shifted away from emotional (particularly sad) faces.	Motor-type FND	Dot Probe task	Marotta et al. (2020)
"Body-related" interpretation bias of ambiguous information viewed as negative/illness-related.	People with FND	Interpretative bias task	Keynejad et al. (2020)
People with high dissociative tendencies showed more attentional problems than those with low dissociative tendencies.	People with high vs low dissociative tendencies	Normal Stroop task	Freyd et al. (1999)

Emotions have different functions

Did you know that we are born to feel emotions? They serve different purposes, and we are lucky to have them (see Figure 7.19).

To warn and make us aware of something important
- For example, you may feel angry about a comment that someone made to you and crossed a social boundary.
- Your anger tells you that something wasn't quite right in that conversation.

To communicate a message to other people
For example, low mood, tearfulness, and withdrawal from social activities may prompt others around us to reach out, care for us, validate our feelings and sympathise– all basic human needs.

Emotions can help us make changes to our unhelpful behaviours
We may feel guilty about having shouted at someone and saying hurtful things during an argument. Feeling guilty may help us change our behaviour and stop arguing / trying to repair "the damage".

Emotions motivate us to reach goals
- Have you ever had a tight deadline? Anxiety may have helped you to give yourself "an extra push" to help you reach the deadline. Without anxiety, you may not have made it!
- Too little anxiety may not have been enough to make you work a bit harder. Too much anxiety would have made you worried and unproductive.
- You may feel jealousy or envy witnessing someone who has something that you would like to obtain but don't have (a good grade on a test). These social emotions may motivate you to work harder to obtain the same thing.

Survival and Protection
Emotions help us to survive and protect us from harm. For example, experiencing fear prepares us to fight, flee, or freeze in response to a threat on time.

Emotions can improve our thinking skills and help us to make decisions
- You may feel anxious about giving a presentation at work or a difficult conversation with a friend. A little bit of anxiety can help you focus your attention better, it "sharpens our senses".
- Emotions can also help us remember. Have you ever watched TV and saw a historic or world event, such as a (natural) disaster, first Covid-19 lockdown, or the passing of a famous person or celebrity? Do you remember where you where and what you were doing at the time when you received the news? These "flashbulb memories" are mediated by emotions.

Figure 7.19 The different functions of emotions.

Describing emotions using physical features People with FND may report an uncomfortable physical state but not realise these are emotions.

They may experience problems with recognising and labelling the emotion that they feel ("feeling tired" or "lacking energy" but the underlying emotion it points to is sadness.

Emotion labels may be mixed up because they feel the same in the body: someone may feel anxiety but labels this as anger instead.

A dissociative episode is often **a safety behaviour that brings down a negative emotion** or uncomfortable state very quickly and effectively.

The **emotion does not fit with the thoughts**. Saying you feel angry, but you report worries (fitting better with anxiety or fear) rather than hostile thoughts that more likely indicate anger.

Feeling a negative emotion…about a negative emotion Feeling shame, embarrassment, or guilt in response to feeling a certain emotion (for example, feeling guilty about feeling angry).

The huge variety of emotion problems in FND People with FND can experience different emotions including anxiety about health, social situations, traumatic events, "the future", relationships, as well as low mood.

A subset of people with FND may experience **strong and intense emotions** ("emotion dysregulation"), where their emotions go up and down quickly, or increase from 0 to 100 within a short space of time.

Some people experience **"dissociation" and may not be in touch with their emotions** / not report feeling any emotions at all. They may not be able to tolerate or sit with strong emotions.

"La belle indifference" / Emotion may not appear consistent with what's happening in their life situation. Other people may come across as happy and smiling even though they are very disabled by the FND.

Emotions that are cut off **may not be recognised or mis-labelled**: someone may label their emotion as "non-existent" but visibly look anxious, for example showing sweaty palms, shakes, a red face, and report nausea (all indicators of anxiety).

People may also occasionally report **a mixture of different emotions** all at the same time ("feeling overwhelmed") but may not be able to pinpoint to the individual emotions.

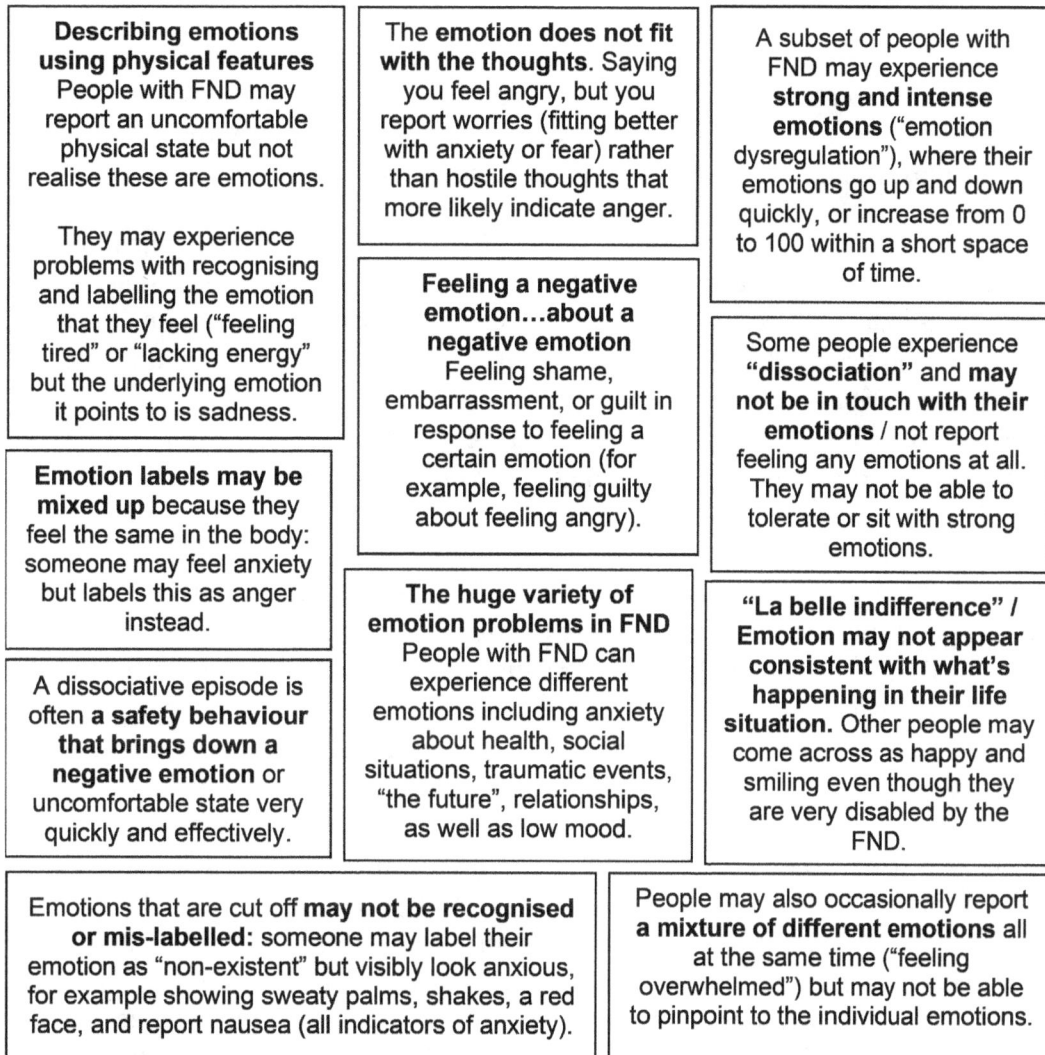

Figure 7.20 Pressure Cooker fast facts: common problems with emotions in FND.

7.19 eResource alert!

Understanding and learning about emotions is one thing. It is equally important to practice with 'experiencing' the emotions. Look at the four emotion exercises that may help you reconnect and get more in touch with your emotions. Please note, as with many of the exercises in this book, the emotion exercises are not just for people with FND! The Pressure Cooker Model views FND as a problem shared between the person and their environment, and oftentimes, family and partners will also share similar emotion coping strategies. Not everyone is aware of this either. So if you are a family member, partner, friend, or healthcare professional, come have a go at the exercises yourself!

Emotional release: tips and tricks

It is important to know that the 7.19 **eResource emotion exercises** can make you feel worse. That is not a reason to not do them! As our awareness into our emotional world is gradually growing, there may be a chance that people will start 'connecting, 'feeling', and 'experiencing' emotions, especially after a long time of dissociation and avoidance. In a paradoxical way, experiencing and releasing emotions is actually a good thing in FND, even though you may feel worse. This is often temporary and necessary, as you need to learn for your emotions to find their way out via the 'usual' channel of verbally and emotionally expressing them, if we want to reduce the risk of FND. Remember, there is a strong link between bottling emotions up and FND.

If you are in the process of reconnecting with your emotions and you are finding it hard, read some of the following suggestions to support you on your journey from 'dis-association' (cutting emotions off) to 'association' (connecting and relating to emotions):

- People can feel self-conscious, embarrassed, and frustrated about crying, tearfulness, and emotional release. Do not be hard on yourself and remove all self-attacking statements that you hold about emotional release. It is healthy and necessary for our 'mental healthcare'. Just like we need to eat and drink on a daily basis to sustain ourselves, we also need to take care of our psychological functioning.
- Emotions may have been pent up for many years, even for decades in some people. The floodgates may open, and that is okay. You may find yourself expressing a lot of emotions at the same time.
- Accept that it may hurt for a while and that it may be unpleasant. Of course it is! People with FND may have cut off emotions for a long time. Think along the lines of 'better yesterday than today'. The earlier I go through the motions of these pent-up emotions, the sooner this period will end.
- Do not try to fight it or frantically look for quick-fix strategies to cope or to 'get it over and done with' (and basically use strategies that make you avoid the emotions again, for example, by distracting yourself continuously to 'not feel' the emotions). Just let the emotions flow out and sit with them. Sometimes the strategy is that there is no strategy but 'to be'.
- 'Have a good cry', but if you find yourself feeling overwhelmingly tearful, paralysed with emotion, it has been going on for a prolonged period of time, and it is impacting on your day-to-day functioning (for example, not seeing friends, not doing your daily household tasks, feeling exhausted, and experiencing long sleeping episodes), consider this a good moment to start implementing strategies that help you actively manage the emotions to try to get unstuck from this position of tearfulness, for example, distraction, doing a physical activity, meeting a friend, doing a household chore. There is a fine line between using distraction all the time to not sit with distress vs not using distraction and sit with the distress but the distress impacting too much on your daily activities. It needs to be in manageable doses for you.
- Some people experience 'secondary' worries and anxiety when they experience prolonged episodes of tearfulness and strong, intense emotions around 'will this ever get better?' Remember that if you have cut off emotions for a long time, your mind may need that space to process, experience, and express emotions again. Give it time.
- Try labelling the emotions. What is it that you feel? What are we dealing with right now? Use some of the emotion detective strategies that were just discussed. Can any of these techniques help you make sense of what you feel?
- Find a person whom you are close to, have a psychologically safe relationship with, and who is a friend who has your best interests at heart, to talk things through.
- Do not try to jump as soon as possible to strategies that 'intellectualise' your emotions: make endless lists, keep logs, diaries, or anything that uses a logical approach to your emotional experience – yes, even the emotion detective exercises! Although on the surface, completing exercises or making lists can help you with making sense of your emotions, there is a risk that the exercises may be a subtle form of avoidance: a form of avoiding to 'feel' and 'experience' emotions.
- A helpful way to become more aware of whether you are 'intellectualising' is to use a diary and jot down whenever you are engaged in using strategies. Are there a lot of them? Is it helpful? Does it make you feel better in the long term, or does it only help in the short term? Be careful: the diary itself can become a form of intellectualizing!
- It is always good practice to check your intentions behind using any emotion coping strategy: Is it helpful or hurtful? Are you trying to 'associate' with or 'dis-associate' from feeling emotions?

Behavioural experiments: breaking the flames–overpressure plug link

A **behavioural experiment** is a carefully planned activity that you undertake to test out a belief that causes you to feel unwell and impacts on your day-to-day functioning and the FND. Common beliefs that people with FND have put to the test in behavioural experiments include "I'm going to have a dissociative episode", "I'll be judged poorly by other people, "I'm going to lose control", "I won't cope / will fall without equipment", "I'll have another panic attack" and so on. A person who strongly believes that they will have a dissociative episode in public and stays indoors all the time may decide to do a behavioural experiment and (1) not avoid stepping outdoors by visiting a corner shop and (2) use reality grounding / breathing techniques to cope with dissociation in the moment and, in this way, test out whether their belief of having a dissociative episode comes true or not. The 'unwell bit' covers the emotion and subsequent FND symptoms. This emotion can be the feeling of anxiety, panic, or dread. However, experiments in the context of FND symptoms can be done with other emotions, too, for example, low mood, anger, and even social emotions, such as guilt, shame, and embarrassment. Even if you are unable to label the emotion or cannot identify what it is that you feel (other than that whatever you are feeling feels unpleasant), do not worry: you can still do an experiment on the distressing feeling or an internal state that is making you uncomfortable and is associated with FND. Behavioural experiments work particularly well for people who experience:

- **Dissociative episodes** that come up quickly or suddenly without any warning, in an 'out-of-the-blue' manner, as part of a panic cycle, and that, within a split second, lead to FND.
- Dissociative episodes **in public places with people** in the context of social anxiety.
- An **initial 'prodrome'** characterised by an unpleasant state, arousal, or emotion that gradually builds up and eventually culminates into FND.
- Dissociative episodes **with and without loss of awareness**, responsiveness, or shakes.
- **Episodes of temporary motor weakness** that last a bit longer (sometimes hard to distinguish from dissociative episodes; in the end, all these FND subtypes are a form of dissociation).

In the next section, let us discuss a variety of reasons for the usefulness of behavioural experiments in tackling FND.

Practice with tolerating intense feelings

Some people with FND episodes struggle with tolerating an intense feeling or unpleasant internal state that comes up. This is often linked with worsening motor FND symptoms or a dissociative episode. **The goal of a behavioural experiment is to learn that you can tolerate feeling unwell and still manage and control your FND symptoms.** The experiment aims to help you tolerate the feeling for a longer period of time without you experiencing an FND symptom and eventually break the link between our beliefs and feelings (flames) and the FND (overpressure plug). In the end, you will be able to experience the feeling without the FND emerging.

Helps to connect with the outside world and stop depression

People with FND episodes may be worried about leaving the house because of worries about having an episode in public and not being able to manage. As a result, people may stay indoors for long periods of time and miss out on enjoyable social activities. The lack of interaction and socialising, a basic human need, in turn, can cause someone to feel low in mood – in addition to feeling anxious. Staying indoors can also affect our physical health as you receive less of the 'sunshine' vitamin D.

Increases confidence and self-efficacy

Doing regular behavioural experiments on the FND helps build confidence, self-esteem, and a sense of achievement and mastery. It increases your 'store of evidence' about your ability to manage the FND on your own. A series of successful behavioural experiments can also provide reassurance and confidence for the people around you, for example, family members who may have been very anxious around you as you are gaining more independence, venturing out more, or letting go of equipment. Behavioural experiments benefit everybody!

Safety behaviours

Before we move on to discussing behavioural experiments, it is important to learn a little bit more about the concept of (psychological) safety behaviours. A successful behavioural experiment often involves dropping safety behaviours.

Quick recap: what are safety behaviours again?

A safety behaviour is a coping strategy that takes down strong, intense feelings; a negative emotion; arousal; an unpleasant internal state; or an event in the environment that causes all these feelings, in a quick and effective manner. This provides relief and achieves a state of psychological safety. To refresh your memory, flick back to Chapter 3 to read about operant conditioning and reinforcement learning principles.

Big question: is FND a safety behaviour?

You could say that FND and dissociation are a special type of psychological safety behaviour. It is the main safety behaviour in people with FND that aims **to help achieve a state of psychological safety and security**. For example, a dissociative episode quickly brings down the emotion or uncomfortable state, providing relief from the discomfort that the emotion and trigger causes. Your mind and body will remember next time that 'FND was a helpful strategy to bring down this uncomfortable state': the FND is reinforced and has a bigger chance to show up again in the future. This does not mean that the FND is put on, fake, or conscious or you are doing this to yourself. On the contrary, psychological safety behaviours such as FND are often an **automatic response** that emerges quickly and can happen **outside or with reduced awareness**. Furthermore, one of the assumptions of the Pressure Cooker Model is that **safety behaviours** serve bidirectional social functions and **are always maintained by our environment**. That means that the environment plays an important role in their persistence. Chapter 9 will explore this in more detail.

Not having FND does not preclude you from experiencing some of the same issues experienced by people with FND and that are listed in Table 7.12, including a tight cover or blocked valve. And what about learning to tolerate the uncertainty of FND recovery in your loved one or patient and how this may impact on your own thoughts, feelings, and self-esteem, or sitting with the discomfort of witnessing a dissociative episode? In the spirit of the Pressure Cooker Model that emphasises psychosocial processes and relationships, if you are a family member or healthcare worker, please read further, as this is just as applicable to you! Safety behaviours from family members and healthcare staff will be discussed elsewhere, mostly in Chapters 9 and 10, since **people without FND are not exempt from safety behaviours**!

Table 7.12 Common reasons for doing behavioural experiments in people with FND

What is the behavioural experiment for in FND? What is the ultimate goal?	Common safety behaviours that people need to learn to let go off or drop using behavioural experiments.
• To reduce dissociation and be able to tolerate an unpleasant feeling or internal state that happens before an FND symptom emerges or worsens.	• Dissociative seizures. • Switching off/vacant episodes. • Motor-type FND symptoms like a sudden, or gradually worsening existing, functional weakness.
• To tolerate an unpleasant feeling or internal state that emerges when your loved one with FND 'has an episode' / is venturing out more / regaining their independence.	Excessive caring or hypervigilant monitoring of your every step by a family member or a partner.
• To walk/transfer independently and unaided.(if psychological reasons, like anxiety, are holding you back from progressing in walking practice).	Gradually step down/ rely less on equipment and people.
• To manage the fear of falling.	Holding onto equipment (crutches, wheelchair), pieces of furniture and people. Avoidance: not going outdoors or accessing the community without equipment or people.
• Tight Covers: to experiment with emotional expression and help you sit with the discomfort of doing so.	Not open up about difficult thoughts and feelings because you fear rejection/feel embarrassed (or any of the reasons for a tight Cover explored in chapter 6).
• Boom Valves: to reduce overactivity for people who are "always on the go" with the main goal of avoiding or cutting off from emotions.	Overactivity to avoid sitting with difficult thoughts and emotions.
• Blocked Valves: to increase activity for people who have reduced activity levels, particularly meaningful, enjoyable, relaxation and social – often as part of depression and physical disabilities.	Avoidance by not engaging with hobbies, social activities, staying indoors and not connecting with communities outside FND, long sleeping episodes.
• To reduce social anxiety that maintains FND.	• FND symptoms like 'switching off', seizures or sudden weakness can be safety behaviours, as can be: • 'Standard' social anxiety safety behaviours such as not making eye contact, avoidance or escape of social situations, not saying much in conversations.
• To cope with the feelings of guilt and anxiety that may come up when stating your true and authentic needs.	Safety behaviours include saying yes to everything, withholding your views, not stating needs at all, or putting other people's needs ahead of your own.
• To tolerate the uncertainty of a potential feared outcome in the future and learn to sit with worries without derailing your daily life.	Safety behaviours may be a wide variety of 'worry processes', for example worrying a lot in advance on purpose or think about all the feared outcomes and worst-case scenarios to help stave off a feared outcome.

Safety behaviours make your world small

Although safety behaviours work well in the short term (they do an effective job in reducing a difficult emotion or an unpleasant internal state), they unfortunately restrict your life in the long term and stop you from living life to the full. If your safety behaviour is staying indoors because you worry about having a dissociative episode outside the confines of your home, then you will miss out on the world, including fun, positive, social, and enjoyable experiences. Importantly, the world will miss out on you, too, and your wonderful personality.

Safety behaviours can cause physical, psychological, and social harm

- Switching off may **impact on day-to-day functioning** and **put us in danger**, for example, whilst showering or taking a bath, cooking in the kitchen, doing your ironing, driving in a car, or operating machinery such as do-it-yourself tools. Some dissociative episodes that are accompanied by a lot of movement have the potential to result in **falls** and **potential serious injuries** to the head and limbs. This is often termed *accidental self-injury*.
- Safety behaviours can be **exhausting**; they cost us a lot of mental energy, effort, and time. We can free up headspace with much more enjoyable, productive, and constructive endeavours by not engaging with safety behaviours.
- Recuperating for hours, days, or weeks following a dissociative episode (post-seizure fatigue and pain) may greatly **impact on our jobs, social interactions, and relationships**. In some people who experience boom-and-bust cycles, the recovery phase may become longer and longer over time.
- They **can look odd** and **attract more unwanted attention**. People may not want to spend time or even reject you because of your safety behaviours. This is often exactly what we do not want and try to avoid at all cost: **social rejection**. There it is again: the **self-fulfilling prophecy** that was discussed earlier.
- For these reasons, safety behaviours are often **not the most optimal ways of regulating or coping with difficult feelings**. Alternative strategies, for example, learning to tolerate the discomfort better or talking about your feelings, have a better 'pay-off' schedule in terms of longer-term consequences on our life. Obviously, this is not to say that it makes it easy to just drop safety behaviours, but it may help you put things in perspective: Is this a coping habit that is worth working on as it has more disadvantages than advantages?

Safety behaviours maintain your difficulties

Safety behaviours **prevent us from working on the root cause of the problem that is driving the FND** and risks getting you stuck in a cycle. We do not give our minds and bodies the opportunity to properly test out our unhelpful beliefs to find out that we will actually manage just fine and the discomfort will reduce over time. For example, if you stay indoors all the time because you worry about experiencing a seizure in your local shopping centre, you will never find out that, with newly learned strategies, you will be okay and the seizure may not happen in the first place!

Tackling your safety behaviours can make a real change in your life and on the FND

Engaging in safety behaviours can have a **knock-on effect on the other maintaining factors in FND**. For example, not testing out unhelpful beliefs around letting go of equipment you may not need, or having a seizure outdoors, may cause more unhelpful thoughts and worries about the FND (flames), keep the increased focus on FND symptoms (warning light), and adversely impact on enjoyable activity levels and connecting with communities (valve), as well as relationships (kitchen). Safety behaviours can wreak a lot of havoc.

7.20 eResource alert!

Read here to learn about some tangible and possibly relatable examples of safety behaviours in the day-to-day life of a person who experiences social anxiety.

So how does FND as a safety behaviour work?

Look at Figure 7.21. The y-axis represents a person's level of discomfort, distress, arousal, or unpleasant emotion. The x-axis signifies the length of time that someone's mind and body experience and try to tolerate an uncomfortable or unbearable internal state. Let us call that state of discomfort the 'prodrome'. A prodrome is not yet a full-blown FND episode but characterised by early warning signs (e.g. a funny feeling, strange sensation). During that prodrome, the person feels unwell and often predicts or 'knows' that worse symptoms may happen soon. Ultimately, a prodrome has a higher chance of developing into FND.

Now, imagine that the three 'FND explosion figures' in the graph represent three people who experience varying lengths of a prodrome but are 'FND-free', until the prodrome starts to shift into full-blown FND symptoms, for example, a dissociative episode or a period of functional weakness.

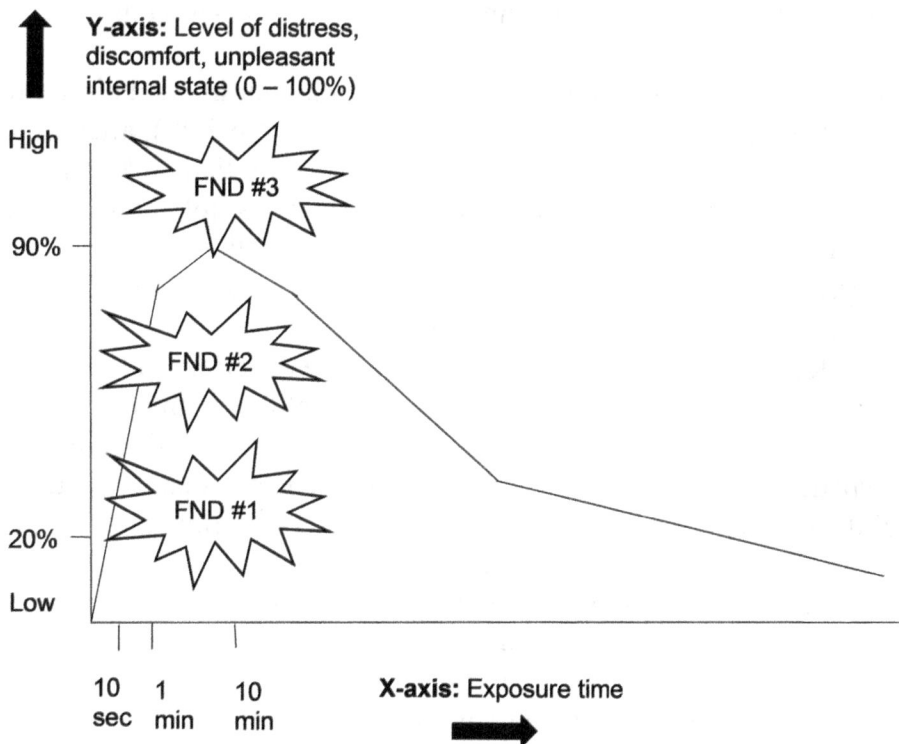

Figure 7.21 Exposure graph #1.

Person 1 experiences the shortest prodrome (10 seconds) before it unfolds into a full-on FND episode. Person 2 experiences the prodrome for 1 minute before FND symptoms significantly worsen. Person 3 has the longest prodrome, lasting for 10 minutes before experiencing a full-blown FND attack. The goal of behavioural experiments in FND is to help you:

- Tolerate the prodrome, arousal, or a state of distress as long as you possibly can before it transforms into a full-blown FND episode. Please note that in the beginning phase of practicing behavioural experiments, the goal may not necessarily be 'to prevent an FND episode from happening' but rather 'to prolong the time before the FND episode finally happens' and therefore prolong the prodrome.
- Fully tolerate the prodrome without it shifting into an FND episode or worsening FND symptoms.
- Nip the prodrome in the bud as soon as the first signs start to appear.

When the person learns to tolerate the feeling of discomfort without 'resorting' to FND, as more time passes, their level of distress gradually and automatically reduces over time. That is a natural response. If the person escapes the situation prematurely 'with FND' (at 10 seconds, 1 minute, 10 minutes, or any time period), the person will not be able to witness and experience the marked reduction in distress or discomfort over time. That experience is withheld from them, and the person will not learn that they are able to tolerate the unpleasant state over time as long as they 'stay with it and ride the wave'.

The problem with escape

Look at Figure 7.22. This is another 'exposure graph' which displays what happens when we engage in a series of behavioural experiments to help tackle FND. Imagine that you are a bit further into the process of experimenting and you are managing to tolerate the increasingly uncomfortable prodrome without experiencing full-blown FND symptoms (but you are still not feeling well).

During our first behavioural experiment (the steepest line), our internal discomfort will rise up strongly within a short space of time and peak (90%; see Figure 7.22), after which it gradually and slowly reduces over time. That reduction in distress may initially take a long time. Eventually, you will feel this reduction, but you need to be patient whilst tolerating a highly uncomfortable state for a chunk of time. Not a nice feeling, but ultimately the key to success.

Leaving the experiment earlier than you planned, in the peak discomfort phase, does not enable you to learn that, over time, if you had been able to 'sit it out' a bit longer or more frequently, no matter how uncomfortable and distressing, you would have experienced the drop in distress and eventually it would tail off and you would be shaken but feel fine in the end.

Although engaging in one experiment and 'surviving' the distress curve once is great, we need multiple repetitions and 'practice rounds' to strengthen and consolidate these experiences. We need to build our evidence base and prove to ourselves that, time after time, we are indeed able to tolerate the discomfort. Only then can you convince, and feel secure in, yourself of your ability to manage the FND. Doing only one or two behavioural experiments can also provide people a false sense of security that 'you have made it' where in fact you are still unsure and reeling from the idea of doing another experiment. We need to fully test out our beliefs around our ability to tolerate the discomfort, until we get bored with it rather than distressed and uncomfortable.

The higher the frequency of behavioural experiments, the more often and longer we expose our body and mind to the discomfort, anxiety, distress, arousal, or some other unpleasant internal

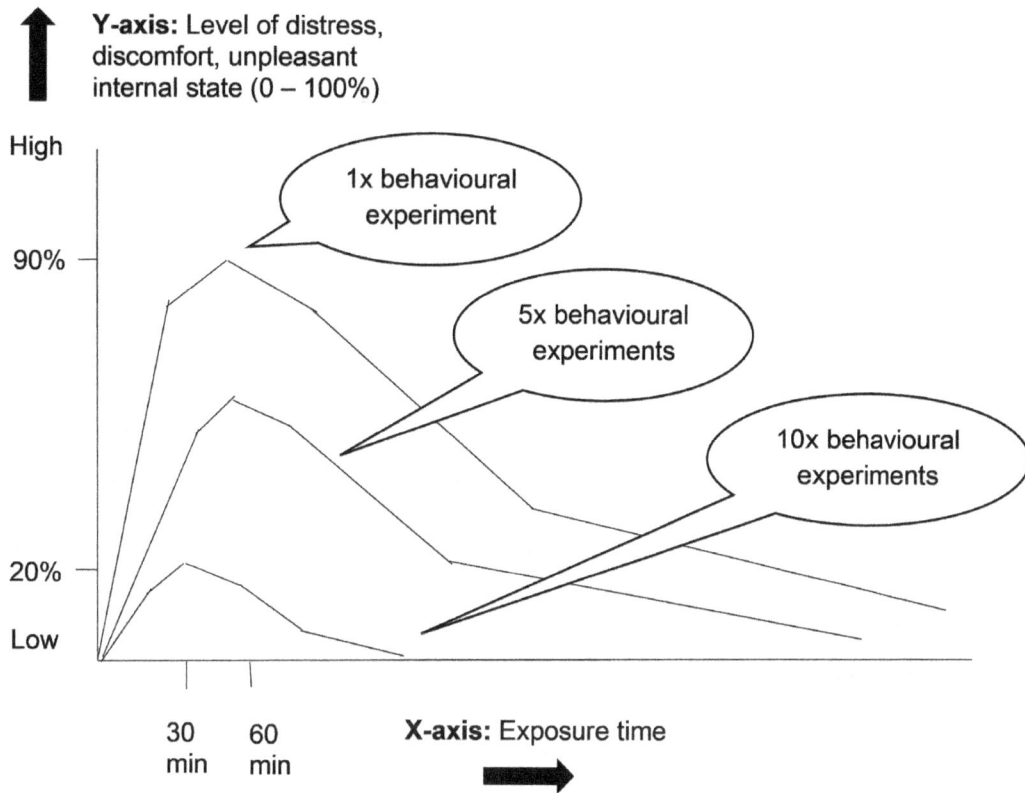

Figure 7.22 Exposure graph #2.

state, the less of it we will experience over time. This means that during behavioural experiment 10, we will not reach the high peak of discomfort that we experienced the first time around (at 90%). The peak after ten behavioural experiments will likely rise to only a low level of discomfort (in Figure 7.22, for example, only 20%) and tail off more quickly (after 30 minutes instead of 1 hour), in comparison to the first behavioural experiment. With every learning experience, you flatten the curve.

Managing high distress

Exposure therapy works best if you 'expose' yourself to some degree to unpleasant feelings. We have seen that if you bow out before your mind and body have had a chance to experience some reduction in the discomfort or arousal, you will not learn that your unpleasant experiences will eventually go away. Escaping prematurely will not give you that opportunity. As uncomfortable as it may feel, you will have to get through it and sit with the discomfort as long as you possibly can. It may or may not culminate into worse FND symptoms or a dissociative episode. The longer you can stretch the time between early warning signs to full-blown FND, the better. Even if it results in the outcome you did not want (FND), if you are able to stretch the time, that is a win already. That said, we know that **exposure therapy can be really emotionally uncomfortable**, to the point that you think you are about to combust and lose control. You may find yourself becoming very emotional before, during, and after the experiment. This is not unexpected and will be temporary.

In short, there are different phases of FND episodes (and this will mostly apply to people who experience dissociative episodes, or those people with time-limited periods of functional paralysis, basically symptoms that 'come and go'):

1. **Early warning phase** – this is the prodrome with early warning signs which are not yet the full-blown FND episode.

2. **Active FND phase** – you are past the prodrome and now experience a fully fledged FND episode.
3. **Post-FND phase** – the FND episode is tailing off and eventually stops. You are in a phase where you do not experience active FND symptoms anymore but are not yet feeling 'your old self'.

Depending on where you are in this chain of events, you will benefit from different types of techniques. The 'heat' element section later in Chapter 7 will help you manage the symptoms with strategies for every phase.

Keep in mind that people sometimes can also become emotional as their insight and awareness increase into what they may have missed out on in their life by tightly having held on to their safety behaviours. This realisation can be really painful, especially if people have been in a difficult situation for a long time. Another reason that behavioural experiments elicit distress (on top of the main reason that you are doing it) is replaying memories of your 'performance' and giving yourself negative feedback about how you performed. Some people attack themselves with negative statements and lack self-compassion. No matter how your behavioural experiment went, **give yourself kudos for attempting one**. The goal is important, **but the process and your journey may sometimes be even more important and revealing**.

7.21 eResource alert!

Curious to find out how to set up a behavioural experiment? To ease you into this process, read the story about Eve's journey of FND, as well as the role that her family played in maintaining the symptoms and, importantly, what Eve and her family did to beat the FND! To support you and your family in the best way possible, a bunch of top tips and useful strategies for creating your own behavioural experiments, whether you have FND or no FND, will also be outlined. The Pressure Cooker Model believes that FND is shared by the person and the environment; therefore, this is essential reading for people with and without FND.

7.22 eResource alert!

Behavioural experiments can be a very powerful tool to overcome FND symptoms. But did you know that, in addition to behavioural experiments, there are a few other CBT-based techniques that you and your family could use to tackle FND? Take a look!

Heat

The heat element represents the **strength, intensity, and 'how much'** we feel of an emotion (or an internal state, if you find it difficult to identify emotions). You can view the heat element as **a temperature regulator** for our flames (emotions) found on a gas hob with a dial that can be turned up to high heat or turned down to low heat.

People with FND generally experience one (or multiple) of three temperature settings (see Figures 7.23 and 7.24 below).

+10

0

-10

Extreme heat volcano: +10
High heat, dial is turned up to "extremely high".
You feel a lot of the emotion, and it all feels unbearable.

Freezing iceberg or ice block: -10
Low heat, dial is turned down to "extremely low".
You don't feel any emotions at all, they have been cut off.

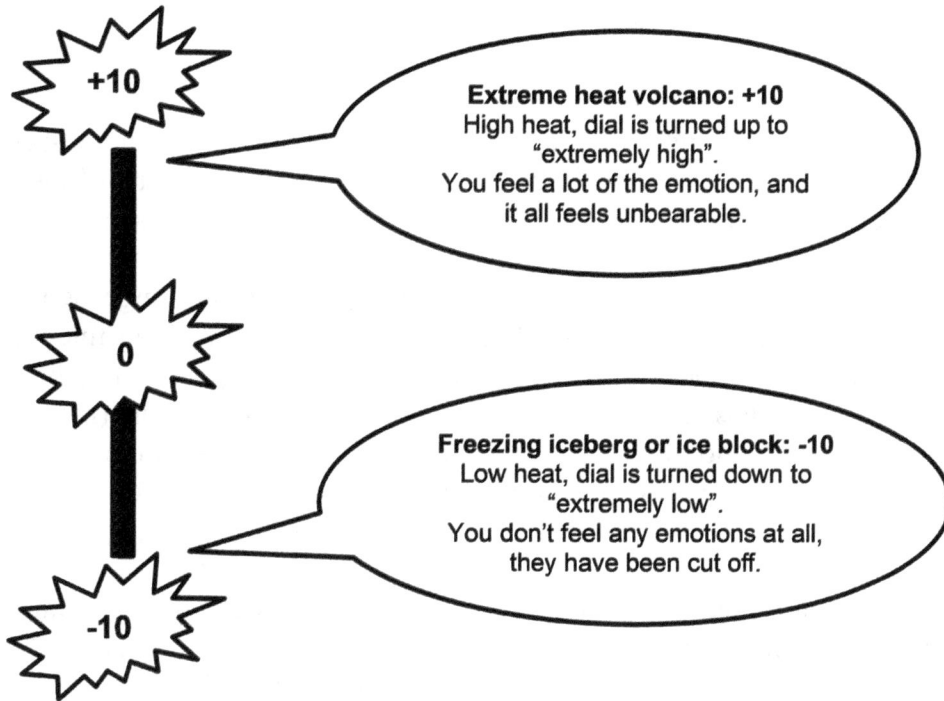

Figure 7.23 An example of an emotion thermometer.

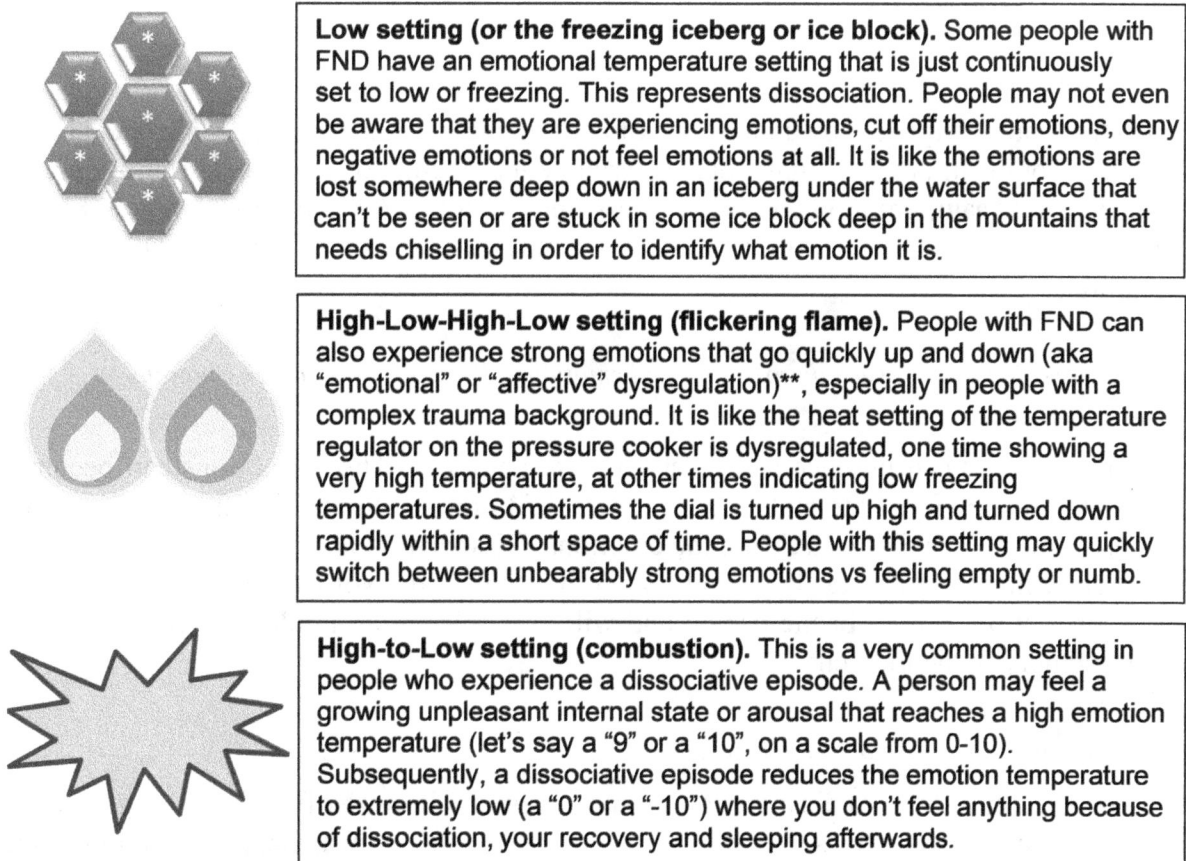

Low setting (or the freezing iceberg or ice block). Some people with FND have an emotional temperature setting that is just continuously set to low or freezing. This represents dissociation. People may not even be aware that they are experiencing emotions, cut off their emotions, deny negative emotions or not feel emotions at all. It is like the emotions are lost somewhere deep down in an iceberg under the water surface that can't be seen or are stuck in some ice block deep in the mountains that needs chiselling in order to identify what emotion it is.

High-Low-High-Low setting (flickering flame). People with FND can also experience strong emotions that go quickly up and down (aka "emotional" or "affective" dysregulation)**, especially in people with a complex trauma background. It is like the heat setting of the temperature regulator on the pressure cooker is dysregulated, one time showing a very high temperature, at other times indicating low freezing temperatures. Sometimes the dial is turned up high and turned down rapidly within a short space of time. People with this setting may quickly switch between unbearably strong emotions vs feeling empty or numb.

High-to-Low setting (combustion). This is a very common setting in people who experience a dissociative episode. A person may feel a growing unpleasant internal state or arousal that reaches a high emotion temperature (let's say a "9" or a "10", on a scale from 0-10). Subsequently, a dissociative episode reduces the emotion temperature to extremely low (a "0" or a "-10") where you don't feel anything because of dissociation, your recovery and sleeping afterwards.

Figure 7.24 Different settings of the heat element in the Pressure Cooker Model.

Note: If you would like to learn more about the idea of 'emotional dysregulation' in people with FND, then for scientific references, please read the work of Uliaszek et al. (2012), Brown et al. (2013), and Williams et al. (2018), who investigated emotional dysregulation mostly in people with dissociative seizures.

Pressure cooker fast facts: dissociation

Dissociation: what is it?

As humans, we experience thoughts, feelings, sensations, and memories and possess a personal identity, all intricately linked to our body. In day-to-day life, all these parts of the human mind and body are nicely tied together and make us 'me'. You could view dissociation as a psychological process that temporarily disconnects these links between our thoughts, feelings, sensations, memories, identity, and body. Somehow, all these parts are no longer working together like a well-oiled machine. This can manifest as some of the parts working fine but other parts not so much. For example, a person experiencing a dissociative episode may be quite mobile but report a loss of awareness for their thoughts, feelings, and sensations (mind switched off during the episode, 'feeling nothing', lack of awareness of pain, and accidental self-injury), as well as loss of memory for the episode (forgetting what just happened, not being able to recall what led up to the episode) and their identity and whereabouts (not knowing who or where they are afterwards).

Although dissociation is common in people with FND, the phenomenon is certainly not something unique to FND! From time to time, we all experience 'low-level dissociation', the type that does not impact greatly on our daily lives. Have you ever daydreamed about a nice holiday or got absorbed into an interesting book, totally forgetting the time and your surroundings? How about 'motorway hypnosis', where you ended up at a restaurant to meet up for a meal with friends without truly remembering your car journey?

What triggers dissociation?

Dissociation can be triggered by a multitude of natural phenomena, events, people, and activities in your environment: smells, sights, noises, arguments, interactions, physical sensations, traumatic memories, pain, emotions, worries, stress, and so forth. Anything that triggers FND, by definition, can trigger dissociation, as these are highly similar concepts and FND is a form of dissociation.

What is the relationship between dissociation and emotions? What happens to our emotions when we dissociate?

Certain experiences can produce some very intense emotions. These emotions can become so strong that they may feel 'intolerable' or 'unbearable' to the individual. To manage these strong emotions, some people dissociate from the emotions. Dissociation is a coping strategy that helps cut off your emotions temporarily so that you do not feel them. Not letting emotions through is psychologically protective for the person and will help tolerate an intolerable emotion, experience, or memory in the moment.

Do some people dissociate more than others?

There are different levels to dissociation. Some people do it more often, have longer periods, and experience stronger levels than others, much in the same way as people with dissociative episodes which vary in frequency, length, and severity. Clinicians who believe that someone may be dissociating will review the person by looking at their behaviours, language, and emotional life. You may be asked to complete questionnaires to find out your level of dissociation, for example, the Dissociative Experiences Scale (Carlson & Putnam, 1993; Van Ijzendoorn & Schuengel, 1996), or a tally chart to establish the frequency of the dissociative episodes.

Does dissociation originate in childhood? Can it repeat into adulthood?

Dissociation often has its origins in childhood and can repeat across many years, even decades, to become your main coping strategy for distress. It is important to understand that dissociation very likely had a protective function in childhood. For example, if you experienced trauma in childhood or grew up in a harsh and punitive environment, then dissociating from your emotions was a sensible and adaptive strategy to use and helped you survive in those difficult circumstances. It was the brain's automatic protection mechanism to tolerate some very intense and unbearable feelings. You could say dissociation was a normal response to an abnormal situation and the best thing that the person under those circumstances could have used to protect their emotions.

However, these same coping strategies that were protective in early childhood may later lose their usefulness because dissociation can be bothersome for your day-to-day functioning. Think about people wandering off at night and risking untoward events (e.g. accidents, running into strangers with malevolent intentions) or experiencing a dissociative episode that causes accidental self-injury and losing chunks of precious time. In addition, when people have relied on dissociation as their main coping strategy, they may lose touch with their emotions over time and may not know how they 'feel', what emotions look like, or recognise emotions. Some people become embarrassed and harsh on themselves for having developed these strategies. It is important to feel self-compassion: people figured out the best possible strategy to use under challenging circumstances. We need to see these people as 'survivors' using survival techniques.

What happens to a person's attention when they dissociate?

Dissociation affects our attentional abilities; it could be viewed as the opposite of 'paying attention and being focused'. Remember the Stroop task earlier? Freyd et al. (1998) found that people with high levels of dissociation demonstrated worse attention on the Stroop task than did people experiencing lower levels of dissociation. That said, even though attention may be impacted, the brain appears to be very hard at work when dissociating. Think, for example, about someone suppressing painful memories that requires some strong metaphorical 'psychological brakes' to keep the memories pushed away and out of conscious awareness (and therefore must rely on sturdy attention and inhibition abilities).

The link between dissociation and attention is good news because that means we can help improve a person's dissociative tendencies by manipulating attention with strategies. Reality grounding techniques for dissociation are based on this idea; they help your mind become more attentive and 'touch base' with the world around you again.

Are there any biological and physical factors that can make you prone to dissociation?

Most definitely! Some medications can make you vulnerable towards dissociation, for example, opiates, painkillers, and some anxiety medication. You should also think about the influence of other substances on dissociation, including alcohol and drugs, as well as lack of sleep (Selvi et al., 2015). Please also note that

- Sleeping or working for long periods,
- Being a physically active 'busy bee' and keeping yourself busy at every moment of the day,
- Visiting the gym for an intensive work-out every moment you can, and
- Fatigue following a dissociative episode . . .

can (but don't have to) be physical manifestations of someone, often unconsciously, trying to cut off and forget about their emotions. To some extent, we all use these activities as coping strategies during times of stress and heightened emotion. However, if used in excess, then dissociation could be the culprit.

Is dissociation dangerous? Are there any risks to dissociation?

It depends on the way we look at it. Dissociation does not cause brain injury. However, dissociation carries risks, especially high levels of dissociation. Imagine that you are dealing with very strong, intolerable emotions and you go through long and frequent periods of dissociation. Can you think of how this may impact on your day-to-day life? There may be risks in the kitchen; you may struggle with keeping focused on cooking a meal, mismanage your medications and take the wrong dose. Some people with more extreme forms of dissociation may wander off for hours, lose their way, and get in danger. Dissociation may pose difficulties if you are a parent and caring for young children, as well as when driving a car.

Can dizziness be a form of dissociation?

Physical sensations such as dizziness can also point to dissociation. Figure 7.25 shows a Venn diagram between the two concepts. As you can see, dissociation and dizziness are not the same, but there is quite some overlap between the two phenomena. Dizziness and nausea can also be the physical manifestations of anxiety and panic as part of the fight-flight-freeze response. It should be noted that dizziness in a person with FND is not always a form of dissociation **and can be caused by other physical reasons**, such as dehydration or a medical condition. It is important to always work closely with a medical team, as life-threatening causes of dizziness, other than dissociation, can be otherwise missed.

What sorts of language, phrases, and verbal expressions do people use that can suggest dissociation?

People who experience stronger levels of dissociation may express phrases and words that suggest its presence. Look at the following expressions from people with FND who experience dissociation (see Figure 7.26 on the next page/below for common examples of 'dissociation' language).

Dissociation comes in all forms, shapes, and sizes

What does dissociation look like, and how does dissociation manifest in terms of our behaviours? We can consider dissociation to be on a spectrum of severity and impact on day-to-day life (see Figure 7.27).

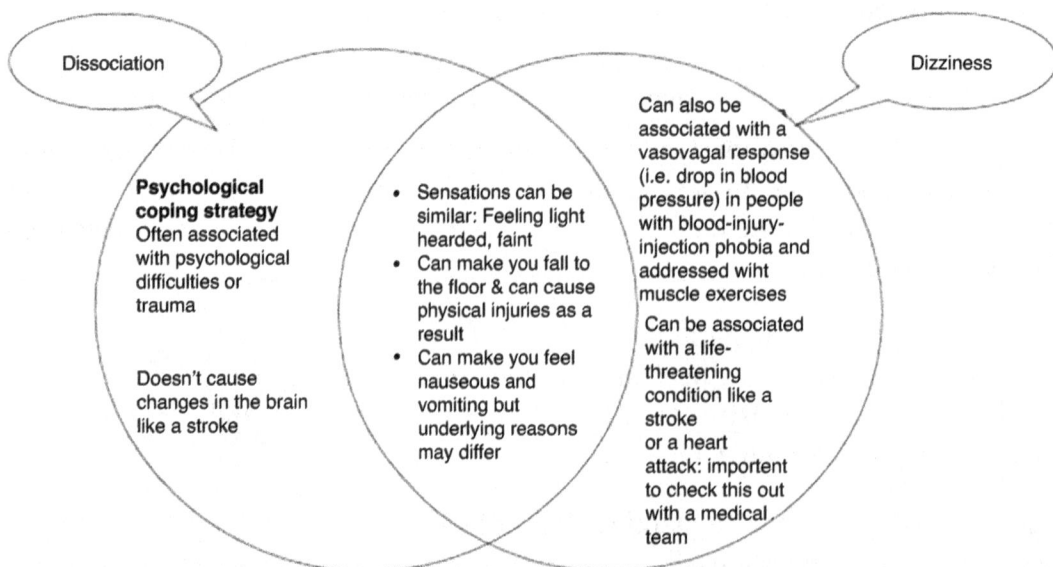

Figure 7.25 The relationship and differences between dissociation and dizziness in FND.

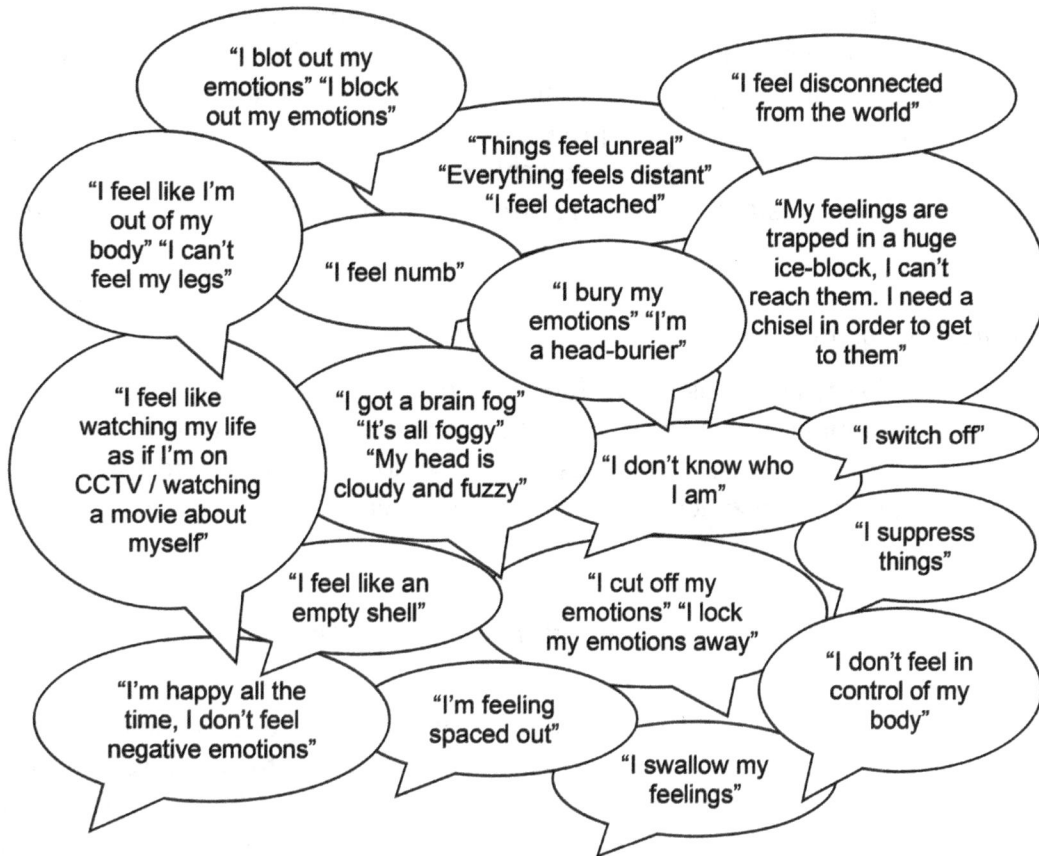

Figure 7.26 Examples of 'dissociation' language.

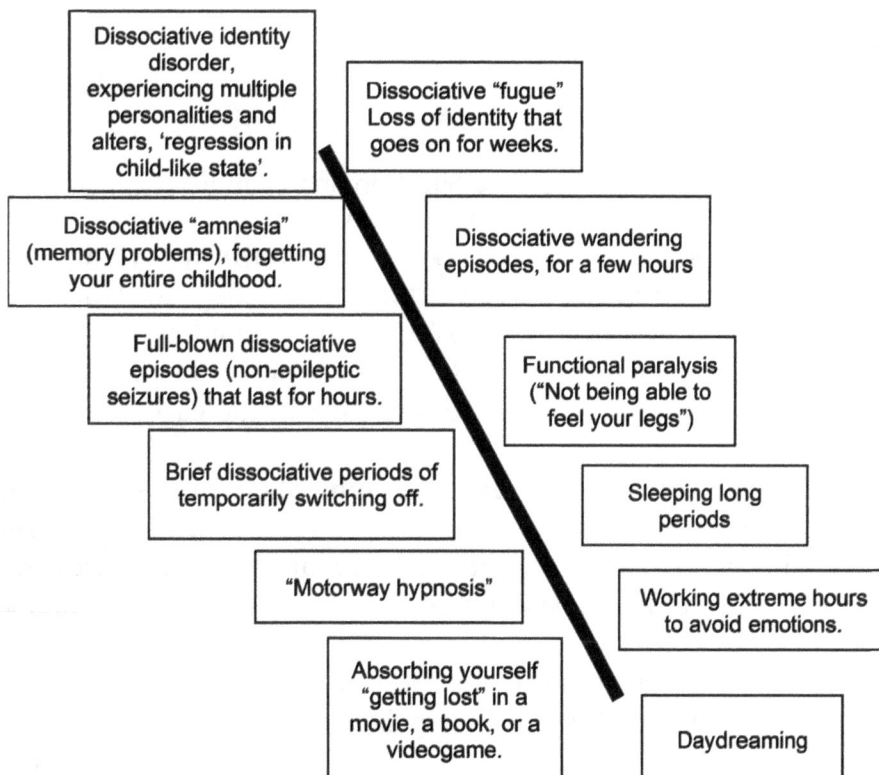

Figure 7.27 Spectrum of dissociation.

Dissociative seizures and functional symptoms that affect your motor system can be regarded as more elaborate and complex forms of dissociation because of their impact on daily life and the risks they can carry. It is important to remember that none of these manifestations of dissociation are viewed as 'bad' or 'maladaptive'. We need to consider these forms of dissociation, especially the examples at the top, as normal coping responses to abnormal situations and life circumstances, or understandable coping strategies in response to intense and intolerable emotions.

What are the functions of dissociation?

Did you know that dissociation has social functions too? Someone with a dissociative episode may express and communicate their distress to the environment in that way, as they do not have access to other coping strategies, such as expressing emotions verbally to a person they feel safe with. Dissociation may also act as a deterrent to the environment, for example, to stop an argument.

Is dissociation always 'pathological', suggesting that there is something wrong with me?

Not at all! Dissociation can be 'functional'. That means, in some situations, it may actually be adaptive and useful to dissociate. Imagine being in a situation where someone is shouting at you and you know that it will not be easy to simply escape or gently extract yourself from the situation that you are in. Temporarily shutting off your emotions while the shouty person is doing their thing is helpful. There is no reason whatsoever to warrant being fully aware of your emotions whilst you are on the receiving end of a screaming tirade.

Mild levels of dissociation do not stand in the way of our day-to-day life and can even be a fun experience, such as daydreaming about our next holiday. However, if dissociation becomes so intense that it starts to interfere with functioning in daily life, for example, our relationships, social circle, work, shopping, taking care of ourselves, and it poses risks to us, then it is probably a good idea to start addressing dissociation.

The pressure build-up stages of FND

It is important to distinguish different pressure build-up phases in FND because:

- **Each phase of FND requires a qualitatively distinct approach to manage symptoms.** Strategies that are effective in the early warning phase may not work that well in the active or post-FND phase. For example, using reality grounding strategies in the active phase of a dissociative episode when you have fallen down, lost awareness of your surroundings, and are shaking may be less helpful than in the early warning or post-FND phases.
- Another example is **the role that the environment plays in FND management**. During the early warning phase, it may be helpful to receive a nudge or support from a friend 'to start using your reality grounding techniques now'. However, physical and verbal support in the active and post-FND phases can be less helpful and keep the FND going.
- **Identifying early warning signs is important** because it can help stop a gradually worsening episode or symptom in its tracks. By recognising the signs early, you may be able to intervene quickly and keep yourself safe from FND. Full-blown FND episodes carry risks and inconveniences, including a risk of accidental self-injury, where you could hurt yourself, lost quality

The time between feeling an unpleasant, overwhelming feeling and developing FND can be very quick for some people, for example when you experience a sudden dissociative episode.

Other people may progress more gradually to experiencing worsening FND symptoms, for example, functional leg weakness that develops into full-blown left-sided paralysis over several days.

The period between the feeling and experiencing sudden or worsening FND symptoms can be broken down into a series of stages.

Let's call them the Pressure Build-up stages of FND.

FND
Dissociative episode /
tremor or leg
weakness worsens

"I feel overwhelmed"

FND
Dissociative episode /
tremor or leg
weakness worsens

Warning signs

Three stages of Pressure Build-up of FND:

1. Early warning phase
2. Active FND phase
3. Post-FND phase

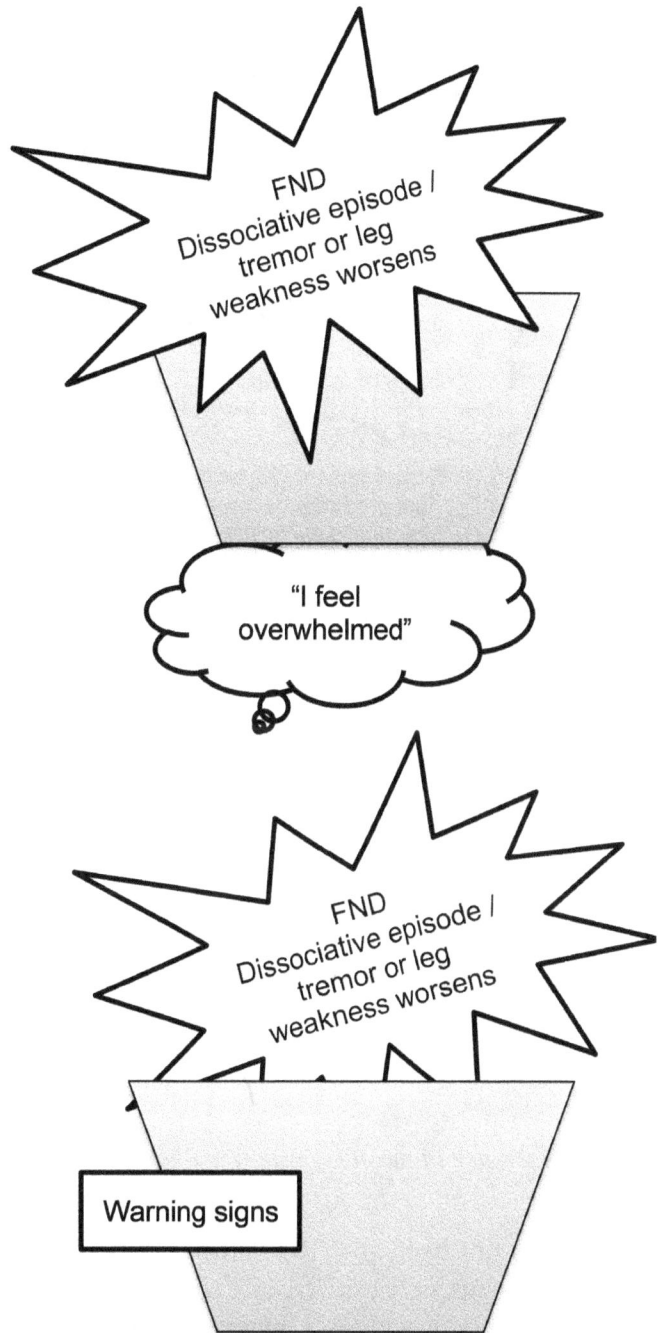

Figure 7.28 The pressure build-up phases in FND.

time and personal experiences, for example, having to take sick days at work, cancelling a dinner with a friend, impact on family relationships.

Early warning phase

Some people report FND warning signs or a 'prodrome' (see Figure 7.29 for examples): psychological and physical phenomena that signal an impending dissociative seizure or worsening FND symptom. Warning signs do not cause the FND but give you an inkling that more, stronger, or new symptoms are imminent. A prodrome can further develop into a full-blown FND episode (the 'active FND phase').

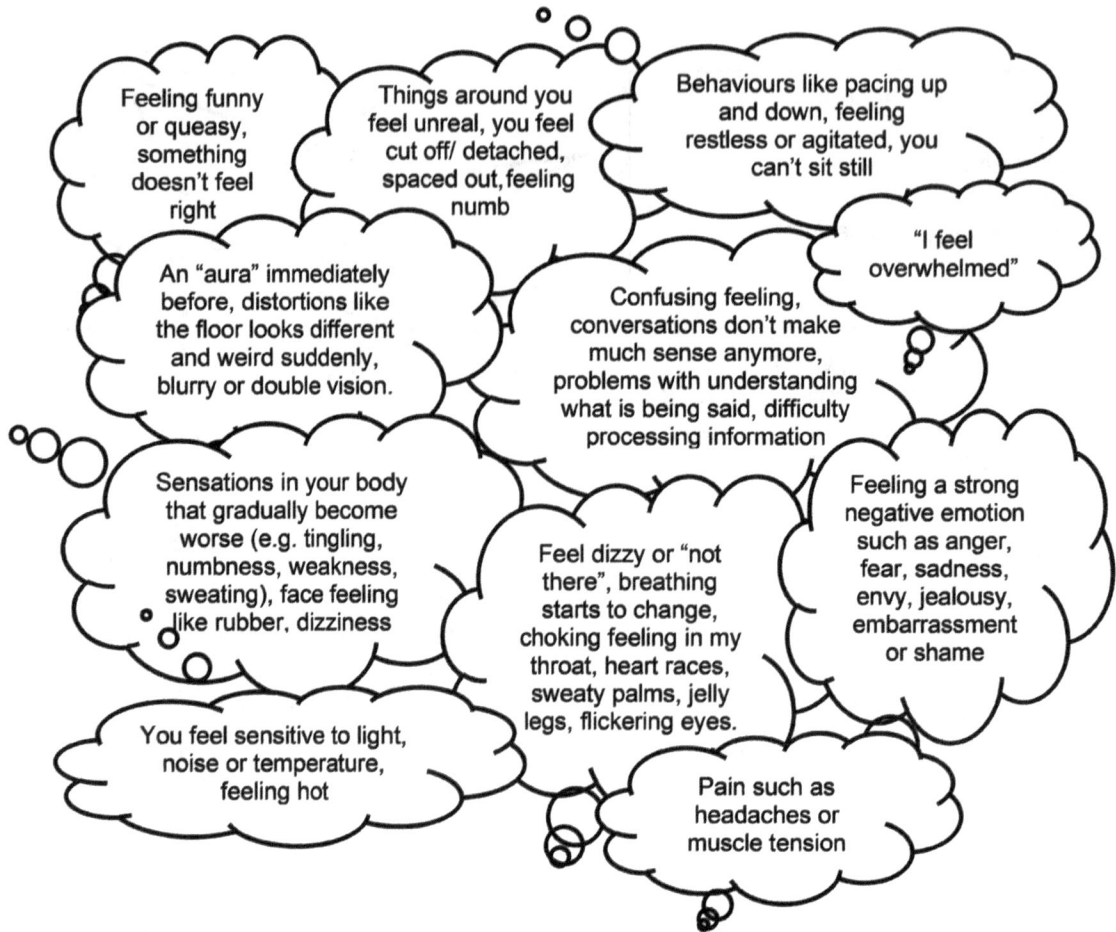

Figure 7.29 Physical and psychological warning signs reported by people with FND.

Strategies for use in the early warning phase of FND. Strategy #1: educate yourself and raise your awareness into warning signs

If you have not been able to identify any warning signs yet, do not worry! Sometimes, an FND episode happens very quickly and reaches an extreme intensity. The FND symptoms can feel disconcerting, distressing, and uncomfortable and 'mask' these often-subtle warning signs. It may initially feel like searching for a needle in a haystack.

Let us think of a way to help you learn to recognise your own warning signs. Every person with FND has a set of warning signs – some may be more accessible to your conscious awareness than others. Early warning signs are often associated with physical and psychological processes that happen in our body and mind.

Have a look at Figure 7.29 again, keep it in mind, and raise your awareness on what might be happening in your body and mind in the early stages of FND whenever you start to experience the first signs of discomfort and that tell you that an episode is about to happen or that your symptoms may worsen soon. Ask people around you who know you well, like a partner, family member, or a healthcare professional, what they have noticed, to support you with uncovering your warning signs. Because FND is accompanied with changes in awareness and dissociation, the people around you could sometimes be one of the best sources of information in your quest for early warning signs.

Strategy #2: simply direct your attention to the warning signs – without judgement

When you start to feel uncomfortable, take a moment to stop and notice whether you can discern any warning signs. At this stage, only notice without describing anything in words, predicting, or judging what may be happening next. All you do is noticing, sensing, and perceiving.

- What **sensations and perceptions** do you feel or see in your body and mind (for example, a funny feeling in your stomach, arousal, sensitivity to light, heart pounding).
- If you can, what **emotions and thoughts** may come up (for example, racing thoughts, an over-whelming feeling that you cannot describe).
- What is **happening around you** and whether things start to **feel unreal**, strange, or distant.
- What your body and mind want you to do, what **urges** you are feeling in the moment (escape a situation, bring down the uncomfortable state you are feeling as quickly as possible).

The key is **to pay attention without judging** ('Oh no, it is happening again, I'm going to have an episode', 'My legs are getting weaker, that means trouble', 'This must mean I am heading towards a relapse' – these are all judgements).

Strategy #3: describe these warning signs in words

Now, try to describe the experience of these sensations and perceptions without immediately jumping to the worst-case scenario, predicting the worst to happen (an FND episode), or judging yourself if you struggle to put in words what you notice and feel:

- 'I can feel tingles on my face, around my mouth, and on my arms.'
- 'The tingles feel like I have been touched by electricity.;
- 'My chest feels really tight.'
- 'My legs feel weak, like they are about to give way.'
- 'My body feels warm and sweaty.'
- 'I'm getting confused.'
- 'I feel emotional.'
- 'I feel something, but I cannot quite describe it in words just that it does not feel right and it is unpleasant.'
- 'My thoughts are racing at full speed.'
- 'Everything around me feels distant.'
- 'I feel like I'm getting into the zone.'
- 'I'm getting spaced out. Things look blurry around me. There are visual changes.'
- 'I feel I want to escape/quickly bring down this uncomfortable feeling.'
- 'I feel tingles, and I am getting confused, but this does not mean I am 100% going to have an episode or that the FND is going to get worse.'
- 'I feel emotionally uncomfortable, but from a logical point of view, I know that these tingles are not harmful to me.'
- 'This is the fight-flight-or-freeze response, a normal biological response that every human being is born with.'
- 'I am going to absorb myself into this experience of how these tingles feel and not divert my attention from them.'
- 'I will not put any label or judgement on the symptoms.'

Strategy #4: put the plug back on FND with reality grounding techniques
to control early warning signs

A dissociative episode with reduced or loss of attentional awareness can be viewed as a withdrawal or disconnection from reality. Luckily, techniques have been developed to help 'ground' a person quickly 'back into reality' (hence the name 'reality grounding' to describe these strategies). Reality grounding techniques are often organised around our five senses. Many people with FND use and will be aware of reality grounding techniques. Please read this 7.23 **eResource** if you would like some inspiration for reality grounding.

Although well-practiced reality grounding strategies can be of great help, some people with FND dismiss these techniques as not very beneficial to managing their FND symptoms. What could possibly be the reasons for the ineffectiveness in some people?

DO NOT SWING THE PENDULUM TO DISSOCIATION

Although reality grounding techniques are intended to help you with 'finding your way back into reality' (the opposite of dissociation, which is withdrawing from reality to help you not feel an emotion or internal state), reality grounding can come with a drawback: the intolerable or unpleasant emotions that you were previously cutting off from may now 'come through' again and become too intense to handle, particularly if you just started practicing these techniques or have not got other well-rehearsed coping strategies at your disposal yet. For people with FND, feeling this type of high heat again can risk a dissociative episode or another FND symptom.

A further potential issue with reality grounding is that some techniques could have the potential to elicit strange, unusual, and funny sensations that your brain and mind may misinterpret as an impending sign of another FND episode, particularly in people who experience panic-like episodes with anxiety and high arousal states.

REALITY GROUNDING CAN BECOME A SAFETY BEHAVIOUR

Take a look at the reality grounding techniques in the 7.23 **eResource**. If the header of that section was changed from 'reality grounding' to 'distraction' techniques, would that be any different? The point is that these same techniques can simultaneously serve multiple functions: reality grounding (coming back into reality, which opens up the window for a person to feel the emotion) and distraction (actually distract or shift a person's focus away from feeling the emotion, at least to some degree). Using these techniques as a distraction from emotions or an uncomfortable state can turn them into safety behaviours, in the same way as FND symptoms.

REALITY GROUNDING IS A SHORT-TERM SOLUTION

Although reality grounding techniques can be effective, it will be difficult to maintain the use of these strategies on a continuous basis. You cannot use reality grounding all day long, as it is impractical, it impedes on day-to-day activities, and paying attention to as many stimuli in your environment as possible can feel overwhelming rather than calming for the mind. Our brains generally do not pay 100% attention to reality at all times.

REALITY GROUNDING TENDS TO BE A SUPERFICIAL PATCH

Reality grounding techniques often do not address the origins or root causes of dissociative tendencies; they serve as a short-term patch. For some people with FND, reality grounding provides sufficient support to manage FND symptoms on a daily basis, and they may not feel it necessary to further explore what may be underlying their dissociation. However, dissociative features often have roots in childhood experiences. In addition, many people experience more hidden and less conscious interpersonal triggers for FND that reality grounding techniques may not be able to fully treat.

REALITY GROUNDING REQUIRES YOU TO GROW YOUR MENTAL MUSCLE

People sometimes say, 'I tried using the reality grounding strategies in situation X, but they do not work for me', 'Yes, tried that, and that, and that – it all didn't work for me, nothing works', and then dismiss these strategies as ineffective. It is important to practice these strategies regularly on a daily basis, whether you feel good or poorly. When you go to the gym to train your 'physical' muscles because you want to grow your biceps, you cannot just go once a month, because you will not achieve your goal. It works in the same way for your 'mental' muscle. When a time arrives that requires you to apply reality grounding (for example, the first signs of an FND episode have emerged), having already practiced the strategies will have made them more automatic and will help you quickly access them.

Strategy #5: use distraction with physical and psychological activities to control early warning signs

The time period between emotions 'transforming' into FND can be very quick, sometimes in a matter of seconds for some people with dissociative seizures. How can we deal with that?

When there is a lot of emotional turmoil and overwhelming feelings or arousal in your mind and brain, sometimes the best thing is to 'break' this high level of psychological activity directly with either a **physical** or **psychological counter-activity**. The point of this is to:

- **Break the link** between the (1) emotion or unpleasant feelings and (2) subsequent FND.
- **Prolong the time** between the emotion before it 'converts' into FND, where each time you practice applying your activity, that period becomes longer and longer until no FND emerges.

Here are some 'counter-activities' that can work:

- **Physical activity that elicits a strong positive emotion (afterwards)**, such as:
  - A gym visit.
  - Using your resistance bands.
  - Any exercises or stretches that your physiotherapist has prescribed you.
  - Doing your household chores and life admin.
  - Giving yourself a pampering session.
  - Doing something creative.
  - Gardening.
  - A change of scenery by walking into a different room at home or a journey outdoors may be helpful.
  - Actively use all your five senses to absorb your environment: smelling pine trees, hearing birds chirp, looking at colours of a wildflower patch.
  - Do something for someone else: prepare or help out with cooking an exquisite meal for someone you care about, help someone with an activity they find difficult (e.g. homework).

- Get social and connect. Call or spend time with a friend. Focus all your attention towards supporting them with a problem they experience. Do a family or social group activity together with other people.

- **Get absorbed in a psychological activity** that uses your brain's full attentional resources for a longer period of time and is not related to FND:

  - Working a big puzzle or a 'brain teaser' game.
  - Counting to 100.
  - Naming a movie, song, food, flower, plant for every letter of the alphabet.
  - Watching an enjoyable movie, a funny show, or listening to the radio.
  - Reading an exhilarating or suspenseful book.
  - Doing a complicated DIY project.
  - Something piecemeal, like diamond painting or crocheting.

Distraction with physical activities can sometimes be problematic for people with FND:

- Some people who experience a lot of disabilities may not be physically able to access these activities quickly, especially during times where a quick distraction is needed before it proceeds to a dissociative episode.
- A new connection between an emotion and the activity can form that may be unhelpful. For example, if you often experience overwhelming emotions and each time this happens a loved one quickly gives you a hug and reassurance, you risk not learning to self-regulate the overwhelming state yourself.
- In addition, pushing on or distracting yourself for prolonged periods of time can become a form of dissociation (i.e. safety behaviour) – exactly the state of mind that we do not want to reach. Balance is the key here.

Strategy #6: ask the environment for help to manage early warning signs, but only as a nudge

Ask someone close to you or a nice person to help you kick-start your own FND management. Helpful questions and comments your environment can use when the first signs of FND start appearing:

- 'It may probably be a good time to use your reality grounding strategies.'
- 'Let us start off together, and then you take over the lead.'
- 'Let us take a deep breath first and make an action plan to help you stop these symptoms. What helped you in the past? Shall we try this again?'
- 'I noticed your legs giving way earlier, but let us not jump to conclusions immediately. This does not mean you will experience a setback of your symptoms. Let us take stock of the situation first: What strategies can you use now in this moment?'
- 'Let us watch and wait rather than act hastily on what might not even come.'
- 'Even if your symptoms worsen, we have strategies at our disposal that we can try to use to make you feel better.'

The following thoughts, feelings, and actions of people around you would be less helpful to stave off early warning signs:

- 'Stop all presses – let us dial an ambulance immediately!'
- 'Make an appointment with your GP first thing tomorrow.'
- 'Let us go online and learn everything we can about this new symptom.'
- Panic as well as any rash and impulsive decisions to do everything to stop the FND in its tracks.
- Taking a person's independence away by doing everything for them.
- Becoming hypervigilant and constantly focusing on the symptoms.
- Always spending time or hanging around the person (24-hour supervision) to ensure they will not experience a setback or, if they do, be on standby, at the expense of your own activities.
- Being aware of making a new but possibly unhelpful connection between early warning signs and consistent reassurance from another person. If this person is not present, you still need to be able to self-regulate early warning signs. It is important to regularly practice strategies on your own too.

Strategy #7: breathing exercises – blow out hot flames

Ask yourself:

- Am I breathing normally?
- Am I holding my breath?
- Is my breathing pattern in any way contributing to the feelings of discomfort?
- Could I be hyperventilating?

Hyperventilation is common in people who feel high levels of anxiety and arousal (whether you have FND or not). It is an unhelpful pattern of breathing characterised by a fast pace of shallow and quick breathing. Hyperventilation leads to a reduction of a gas in your bloodstream called 'carbon dioxide' and can provoke light-headedness, dizziness, and fainting. Sometimes, these symptoms may:

- Overlap with the common warning signs of FND.
- Contribute to a stronger subjective state of dissociation in people with FND who may already experience higher-than-usual levels of dissociation.

It is therefore important to stop hyperventilation in its tracks. So do not forget to breathe! Need some inspiration? Try any of the following quick exercises that people with FND have reported as very useful in their FND recovery journey. The exercises are short and easy to remember, particularly helpful if you are feeling unwell and are unable to think straight.

BREATHING EXERCISE #1

A great way to generate deep and prolonged breaths is to breathe in for 4 seconds (1, 2, 3, 4), hold at the top for 2 seconds (1, 2), and breathe out for a slightly longer period of 6 seconds (1, 2, 3, 4, 5, 6), and repeat a few times (you can vary the amount of seconds in each breathing stage that you feel comfortable with, this is not a prescriptive, fixed rule). This should help you manage your breathing better. Initially, it can be very powerful to do this with an FND ally.

BREATHING EXERCISE #2 (RE-BREATHING TECHNIQUE)

Another technique is to cover your nose and mouth with both of your hands, like a makeshift oxygen mask. Gently breathe in and out whilst you hold your hands in the mask position. You will be breathing in your own exhaled air.

BREATHING EXERCISE #3 (BOX BREATHING)

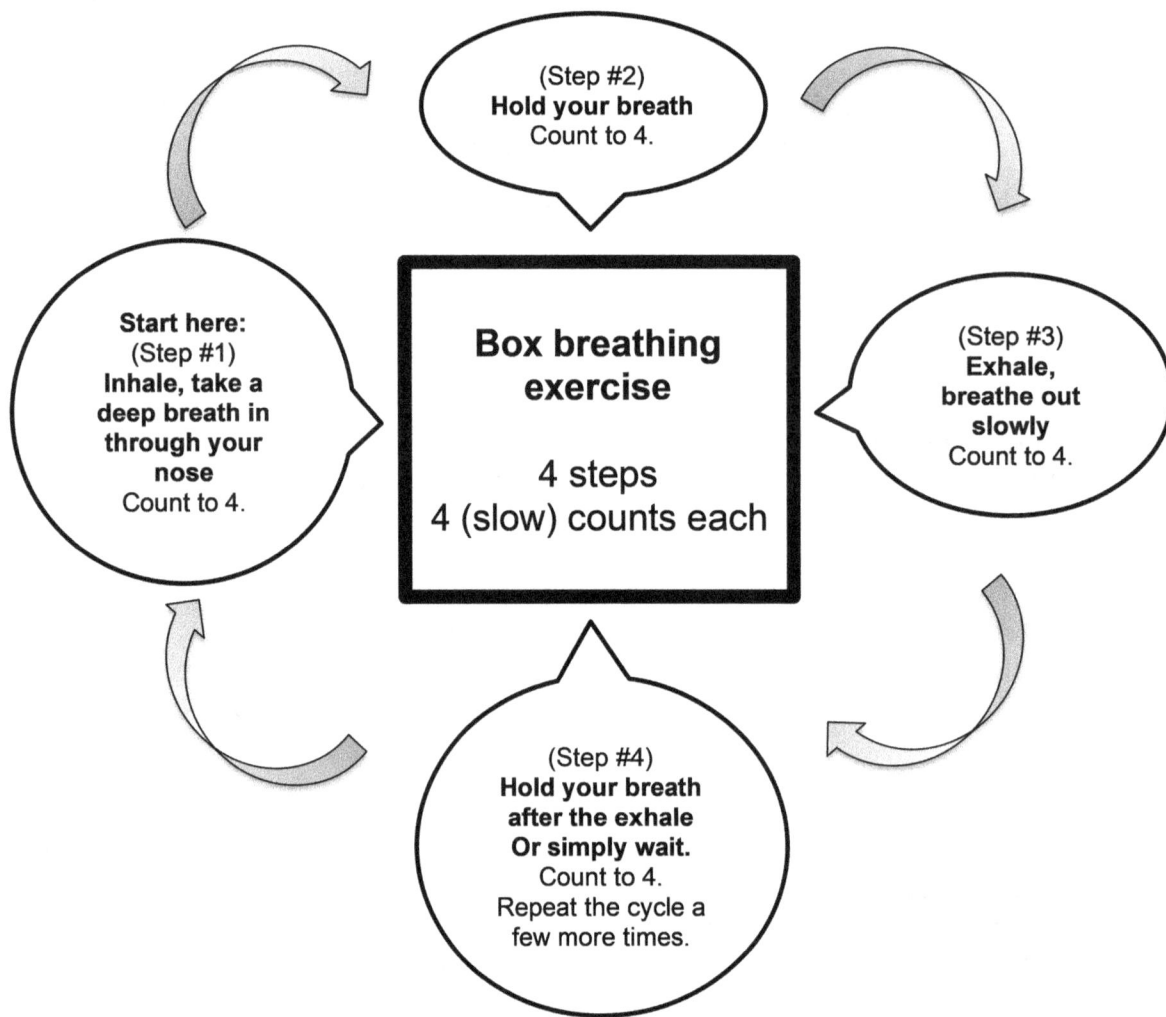

Figure 7.30 Box breathing technique.

Strategy #8: use the 20/30-minute rule to give your brain some breathing space

Sometimes, the best strategy is to immediately take yourself physically out of the situation that is causing you the high distress or arousal. Think, for example, about a big argument that does not lead to any constructive conversations in that moment (if you are bed-bound because of the FND, ask people to leave you alone for some time, including carers). Twenty to thirty minutes is the time that your brain needs, at the very least, to properly calm down before it is ready to engage in clear thinking processes. Be aware that 'escaping' each time things get heated is not a long-term solution. Make sure that after a cooling-off period, you address whatever issues led up to the distress.

Strategy #9: relinquish control of the FND

The previous techniques are all active strategies which require you to put mental effort into controlling the episode. People with FND tend to find these useful and effective in helping to manage symptoms. However, a subset of people will not derive any benefit from, let us say, reality grounding techniques.

What about doing something radical and counter-intuitive – the total opposite? This may sound like a recipe for trouble, and you may wonder whether this is the same thing as 'giving up' or 'giving in' to the FND. Not really!

For some people, the act of 'forcefully controlling', 'fighting', and putting mental energy into FND may be precisely the problem that they are grappling with. Whenever people feel an FND episode or symptom coming up, they sometimes frantically try everything and grasp for any straw to stop the episode as quickly as possible. This often creates additional discomfort, anxiety, or panic (and more warning signs!), on top of the original discomfort that fuelled the episode, particularly when the strategies do not seem to work in the moment.

For these people, their psychological prescription is **to let go of controlling the warning signs** of an impending episode, for example, by saying to yourself, 'This is my Pressure Cooker chain reaction starting: I don't have to forcefully control the FND symptoms at all costs. Instead, I will let go of control by telling myself any of the following':

- 'These sensations or symptoms are not harmful to me, my mind, or my body. Let us roll with it.'
- 'Experiencing these sensations does not automatically mean that they will progress further into a full-blown episode.' (Do not assume that warning signs mean a 100% likelihood of the FND episode happening, especially if you have been practicing strategies to prolong the time between the first warning signs and the actual episode.)
- 'The tingles are back, and that is okay. I am not required to do anything right now. I don't have to engage with the symptoms or try to actively control the tingles. The only thing I have to do is to just stand back, observe them, watch, and wait.'
- 'Instead of fighting and heavily resisting the episode, I am going to ride the wave of these warning signs. I am going to accept that these sensations and perceptions are there, without attaching any meaning.'
- 'If the episode happens, so be it. I will take a break, and then I will just continue with whatever I was doing. Let it come, because I am ready to go through this. When the sensations and symptoms worsen, I will ride the wave and still not try to actively engage by controlling them. I will continue to let go of any sorts of action, effort, or control.'
- 'If I sense that my body and mind are putting a lot of effort into relinquishing control (so basically, if I notice that I am doing exactly the opposite thing to what relinquishing control means), I will stop this process with immediate effect.' (Relinquishing control means letting go – not actively holding on to control with all your might.)

This technique is probably a better technique for people who experience dissociative episodes that are of a short duration, without self-injury, and not much impact on daily functioning.

Strategy #10: tolerate and even embrace it!

What this means: tolerating, 'sitting with', actively accepting, and even positively embracing the existence of these sensations, emotions, and symptoms whilst continuing to stay with the process of feeling and experiencing them. In this way, you stop swinging the pendulum from high heat (arousal, anxiety, intense discomfort) to low heat (dissociation, cutting off emotions) but stay with the high heat and 'feel the flame' until, at some point, your body and mind will learn and notice that these feelings will slowly and gradually start to quench over time. This experience will teach you that time can be a very powerful coping tool that can help you with controlling your emotions, arousal, or discomfort.

Imagine the following scenario: you are going on an adventurous holiday to South America to hike one of the Machu Picchu trails. On day 1, you are pumped and ready to hike! However, the trail soon starts to become quite challenging: long distances to cover, rough terrain with the occasional creek to negotiate, big boulders, blisters on your feet, thin air making you tired, queasy feelings, splitting headaches, a heavy backpack to carry, and no warm shower in sight anytime soon. You are starting to feel a little disconcerted about how you are going to survive this trek!

In your mind, thoughts and feelings come up: 'My, my', you think, 'it is SO heavy. I can do this, but my muscles are aching. I can feel my back playing up a little bit. My thighs are burning. This is an awful feeling. Why am I doing this again?' A few feet further, you think, 'Aaaaah, this is too much! I can't believe I still have so much distance to cover.' You sense becoming frustrated, worried, and exhausted. You take a few breaks along the way, and with

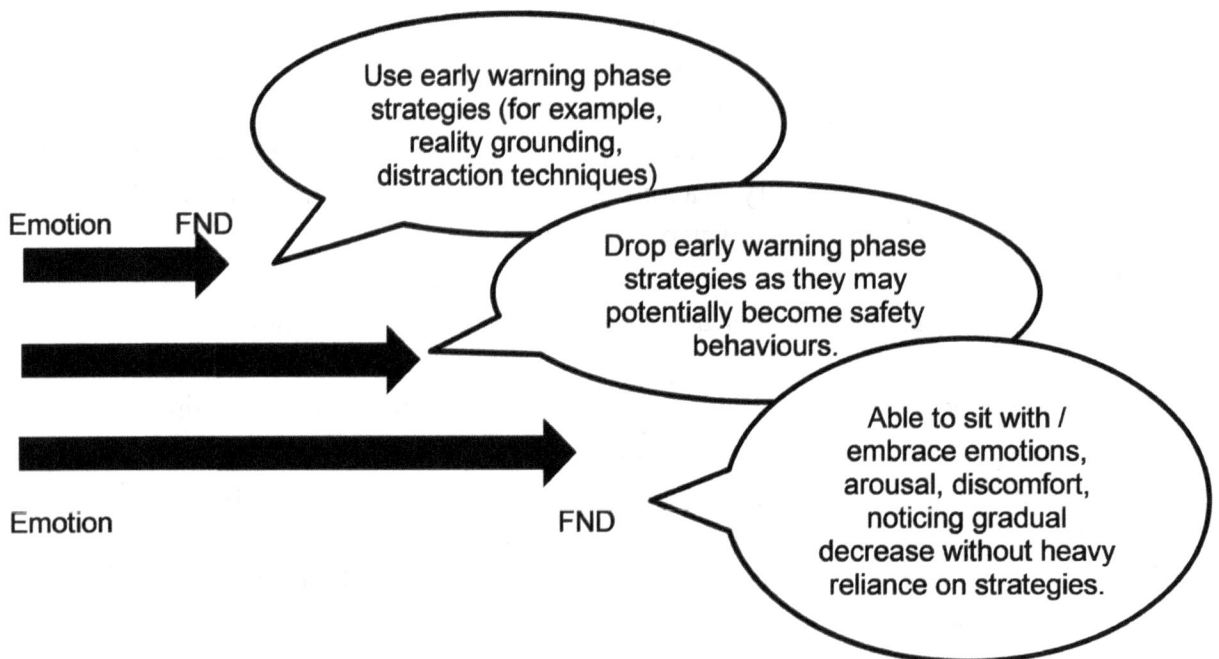

Figure 7.31 The process of sitting with discomfort in FND.

each 're-start', the negative thoughts and feelings re-emerge. Your mind is literally shouting internally, 'Wahhhh, make this stop! Can't take this any longer!'

Suddenly, you become aware of your shouty internal mind. You realise that the shoutiness is not helping you endure this already-tough journey that you are going through with your hiking mates. Is it truly making things feel better for you? Initially, you may have thought of this as a distraction technique, but you soon realise that you are feeling worse.

Instead, you decide to change tack and do something different. You say to your mind, 'I'm letting go of this fight. I am going to stop fighting right at this minute – on top of the physical and psychological stress that I am currently experiencing because of this trek. I know it will be temporary, but for now, I will need to endure the journey. The negative thoughts and feelings make things worse. They make my muscles even more tense and painful. I can feel everything amplified. Instead, I will say to myself, "I am going to accept and stay with the feelings, no matter how intense. With every step I take on the trail, I am going to notice and experience the sensations in my body and mind as they are, absorb my beautiful surroundings, accept and simply tolerate, and even embrace the sensations and feelings – without actively engaging, judging, or fighting them. I am doing well for trying! And good grief, I am on my way to Machu Picchu!"'

The following phrases may also be helpful for tolerating discomfort:

- 'I will do this by "staying with the tingles", experiencing physically, and maybe emotionally, how they feel for me at this minute.'
- 'I'm going to stick with these experiences like I'm surfing a long wave in the ocean.'
- 'I will hold on to riding that wave until I reach the shore so my body and mind can experience that the sensations and symptoms will reduce over time.'
- 'I know that the fight-flight-or-freeze response will go down eventually. That is part of our biological make-up. I just have to stick with it and ride it out, no matter how uncomfortable right now. It will take time, and that is okay. I have that time available to start feeling a reduction at some stage.'

Strategy #11: cognitive reframing of warning signs

7.24 eResource alert!

Sometimes we are so vigilant and on the lookout for the warning signs of FND that we may mistake the normal signs of the body as a warning sign for an impending dissociative episode. It is almost like our body is generating a false alarm. This 'misinterpretation' of normal body processes ('Oh, oh, feeling a slight tingle and fuzzy-headed means I am going to have another seizure.') creates turmoil and discomfort, which in turn feed into more physical symptoms, and like a self-fulfilling prophecy, it decreases the threshold for another dissociative episode. To illustrate these points better, read here first about Matt's story.

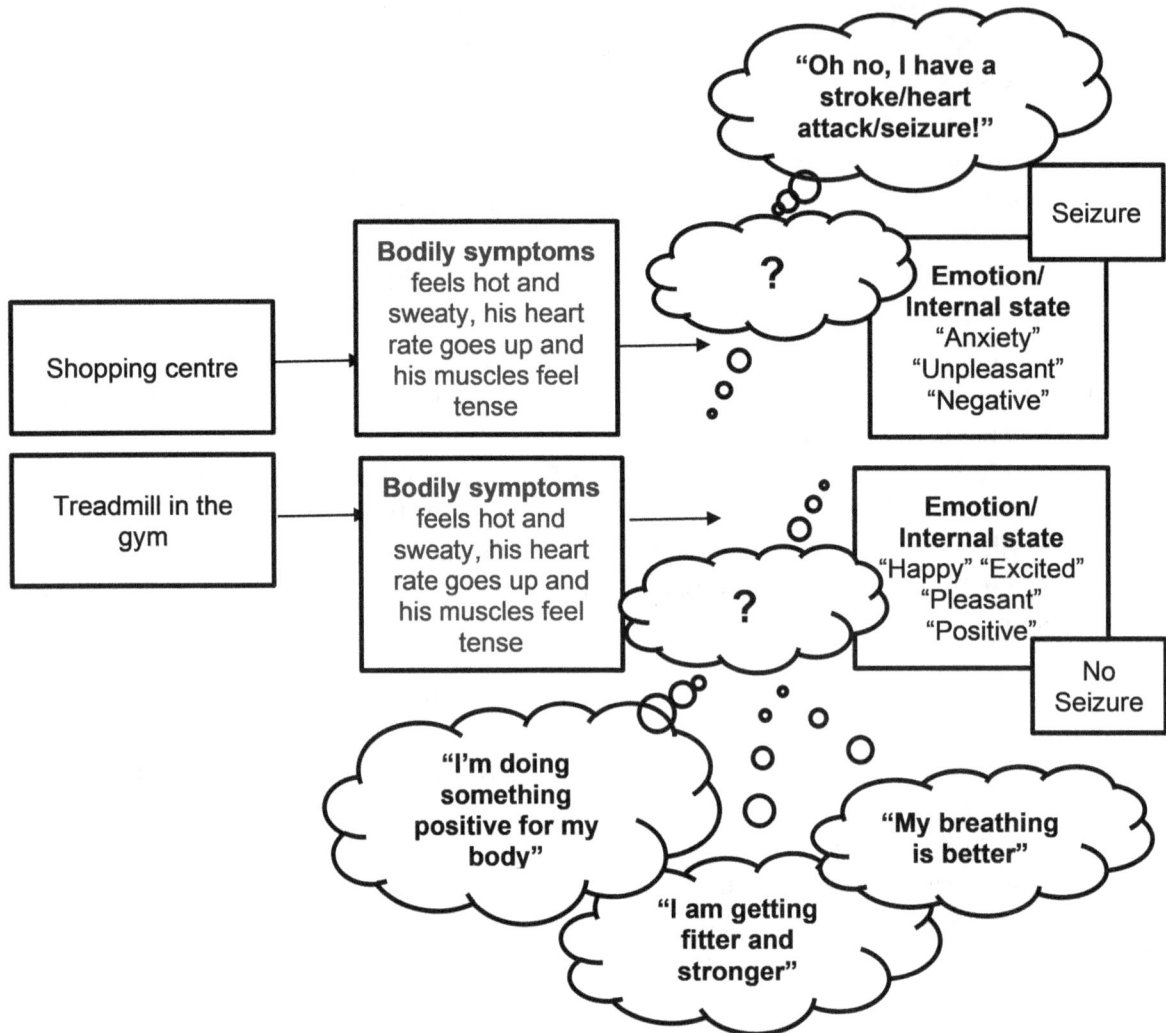

Figure 7.32 The impact of cognitive reframing on dissociative seizures.

Let us glean from a powerful technique often used in the treatment of panic attacks. Look at the two situations in Figure 7.32. Both clearly generate the same bodily symptoms, yet one situation results in **unpleasant emotions and a seizure**, while the other situation produces **positive emotions and no seizure**.

What is the difference? As you can see, it is the **thoughts** that connect the bodily symptoms with the emotions! If you interpret the bodily symptoms as non-threatening (as opposed to a misinterpretation of the symptoms as something threatening, like a stroke or a dissociative seizure), the outcomes widely differ.

Please note that it is not expected that people can just flip their thoughts at the drop of a hat. Of course not – cognitive reframing is hard work and takes effort, regular practice, and time. Figure 7.32 is there to illustrate the principle.

My FND survival kit: the pressure cooker steam diverters

A central goal in FND management is **to do something** with your state of discomfort: either 'reconnect' or 'tolerate'.

At the beginning of your recovery journey, you may find it difficult to sit with the discomfort of reconnecting or tolerating. This is where your FND survival kit comes in! Pressure cookers

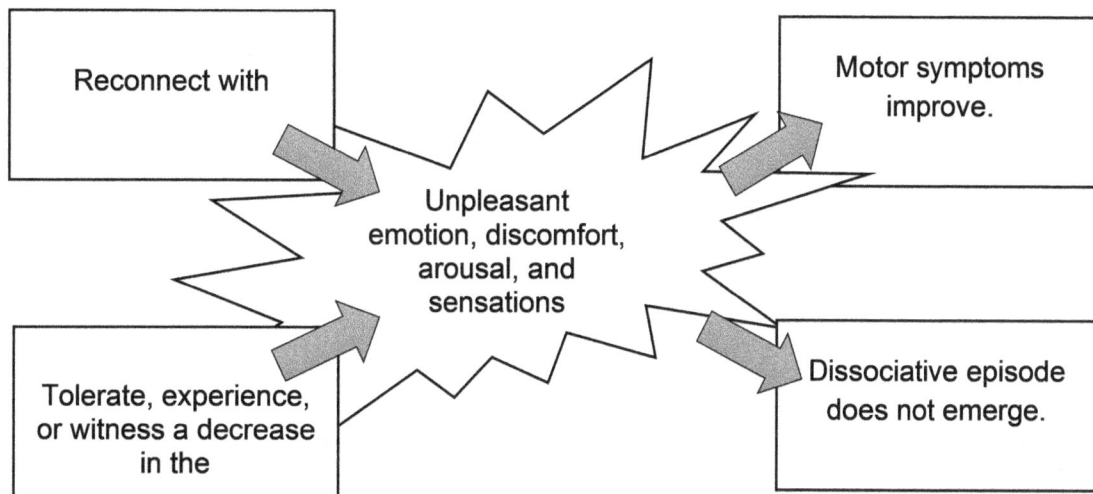

Figure 7.33 Reconnecting and tolerating in FND.

sometimes need a steam diverter, a silicone add-on that changes the direction of the steam to prevent it from going to a place where you do not want it to go or where it can cause damage, for example, a kitchen cabinet. In the same way, you can consider the FND survival kit as a steam diverter for the difficult feeling or state. Your FND survival kit can help you reconnect with or tolerate a difficult emotion or state for a period, sufficiently long enough, before a dissociative episode arrives or motor symptoms worsen. Take another look at all the strategies you have come across so far and pick your 'dream team' of steam diverters.

Carefully consider what you are doing with your attention

There is a slight caveat around some of the aforementioned strategies, particularly the strategies that require you to focus on the sensations in your body and 'ride the wave of discomfort'.

We know from the research literature and clinical practice that an increased focus of attention on symptoms and hypervigilance are maintaining factors of FND (Edwards et al., 2012). The question arises whether paying too much attention on sensations will keep the FND going. How confusing! Do I need to **distract and shift attention away** or **focus my attention**?

Keep in mind that these methods are **only intended for short-term use**: your goal is to stop the episode and symptoms from progressing further. Do not do this all day long. This attention is reserved for helping you manage the early warning signs. Constantly focusing on the FND and other bodily symptoms that you may experience is not what is meant here.

A strategy that can help you determine whether focusing your attention is helpful vs hurtful for FND is the subjective feeling it generates **in the long run**. Do you continue to feel anxious, unwell, overwhelmed, sick, or any internal state that is negative when you focus attention on your symptoms? Is the FND not subsiding or getting worse? Then it is likely not a good idea to persist. Remember, over time, strategies should make you feel better, not worse (but please note that temporarily worsening discomfort is totally expected – this is more about the long term).

If you are a partner, family member, friend, or healthcare professional of a person with FND

Each of the aforementioned strategies applies to you too! Distress, discomfort, unpleasant feelings, negative emotions, arousal, tension, and dread of seeing your loved one or client unwell **are all felt and mirrored by people in the environment.** Chapters 9 and 10 will delve more deeply into these relationships and how this maintains FND.

Strategies for the active FND phase

The active phase of FND can be defined as the **height of the symptoms**, when the symptoms are **full-blown** and **at their strongest**, and way past the early warning signs stage. For some people with FND, this can be brief (a dissociative episode lasting for a few minutes or a few hours); for other people with FND, this can take longer (losing the function of your legs lasting for days, weeks, or months). How do you manage high levels of FND symptoms and/or intense discomfort at the peak?

The Pressure Cooker chain reaction

Let us now turn our attention to a specific group of elements that make up the FND maintenance cycle. This forms the core of 'what keeps the FND and dissociation going' and is called the **'Pressure Cooker chain reaction'**, the first step of FND. Environmental and social processes determine the second step of FND and will be more closely looked at in Chapters 9 and 10.

To understand the mechanism of FND, follow the numbers in sequence (see Figure 7.34).

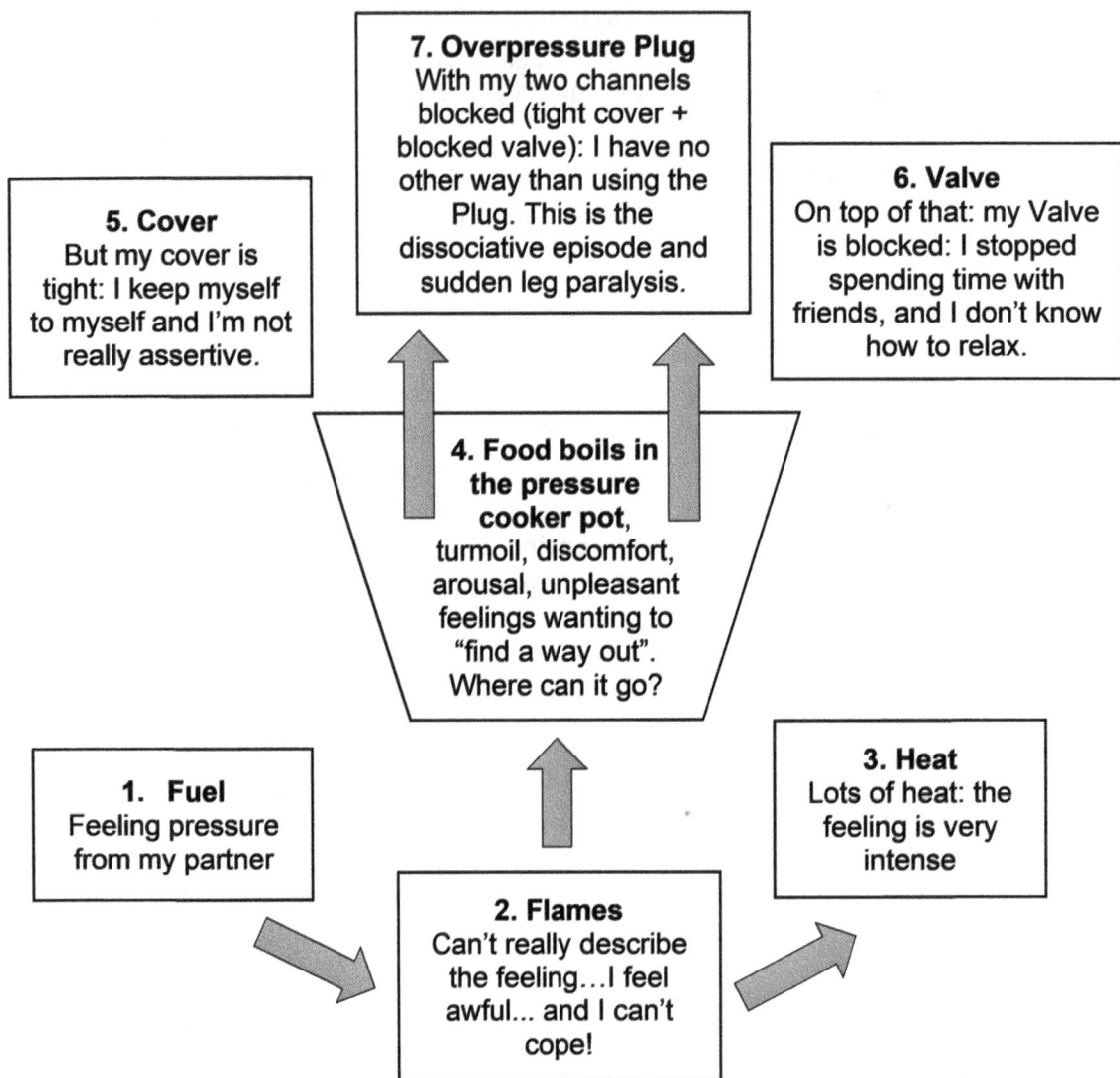

Figure 7.34 The Pressure Cooker chain reaction: assessment.

1. My fuel, the trigger for my FND, is feeling psychological pressure from my partner.
2. The fuel feeds my flames, which are my thoughts and feelings in response to the pressure. It may be difficult to describe in words what I feel, but it is unpleasant and uncomfortable.
3. The unpleasant state that I am in feels very intense, and I do not want to feel this way.
4. My pressure cooker is boiling, and the food is reaching the top of the pot. It wants to find a way out, or else, the pressure cooker might explode. In the same way, the feeling (whatever I call it: emotion, arousal, unpleasant sensations) wants to find a way out– where can it go?
5. One way of making sure the pressure cooker will not explode is to open my cover, or express and talk about my emotions with someone I feel safe with and can trust. But my cover is tight: I am someone who keeps my emotions to myself. I am not very assertive, and I do not trust anyone.
6. Another channel to let the boiling food calm down in the pot is to engage with social, enjoyable, or relaxing activities. But my valve is blocked: I stopped socialising, my social circle is small, and I do not use any relaxation strategies. Plus, my disabilities prevent me from going out much these days.

With my two regular channels blocked, how can I make sure that my pressure cooker will not explode and I can control the boiling contents in the pot?

7. I have a third channel, and that is a small plug in the cover called the overpressure plug. It is tiny and not ideal because it does not release all the steam that I have and affects my body, but it will at least release some of the pressure in the pot. The overpressure plug represents my FND symptoms, in my situation: the dissociative episode and my sudden leg paralysis. As a result of the FND, I feel very tired and have tense muscles, but that awful feeling is luckily gone.

7.25 eResource alert!

Interested in finding out how you could apply the Pressure Cooker chain reaction assessment to your own personal situation? Why not try this exercise yourself! Ask your FND ally to support you in this process.

Breaking the Pressure Cooker chain reaction

Look at Figure 7.34 again. Where in the chain could you intervene to stop or slow down the Pressure Cooker chain reaction and ensure that the overpressure plug will not be engaged? It turns out that you can use strategies **to intervene anywhere in the chain**! Figure 7.35, which follows, shows you the potential strategies that you could use to intervene in this person's Pressure Cooker chain reaction. This is not the 'perfect solution' to breaking the chain. The book describes many strategies, and you can use any strategy that you feel comfortable with.

5. Open the cover
During a calm moment, I will say to my partner how I feel about the pressure on me. I will try to set firm boundaries next time it happens again using assertiveness. I will also suggest couple's therapy to work on our long-term communication problems.

7. Overpressure plug
With my two channels re-opened (Cover + Valve): I don't need the Plug any longer. As a back-up, if I feel funny, I can use my reality grounding techniques.

6. Unblock the valve
Pick up my old hobbies again, meet up with my friends, find a community, build in more relaxation time into my busy schedule.

4. Monitor the boiling food in the pressure cooker pot
Keep observing the "bubbles" that come and go (thoughts, feelings)

1. Remove the fuel
My FND diary has demonstrated that whenever my partner puts pressure on me, I feel discomfort building up. To cope, I'll leave the room temporarily, for about 20-30 minutes to help my brain calm down. Afterwards, I'll explain the Pressure Cooker Chain Reaction to my partner to show them how 'putting pressure' on me affects and triggers the FND.

2. Extinguish the flames
Emotion detective exercise to help me label what I feel. Keep an emotion-FND voice diary tracking my emotions daily. Plan a behavioural experiment to break the link between the Flames & Plug.

3. Dialling down the temperature of the heat
Sit and tolerate the discomfort a little longer, I know it will reduce over time. Use the re-breathing technique to "take the edge of".

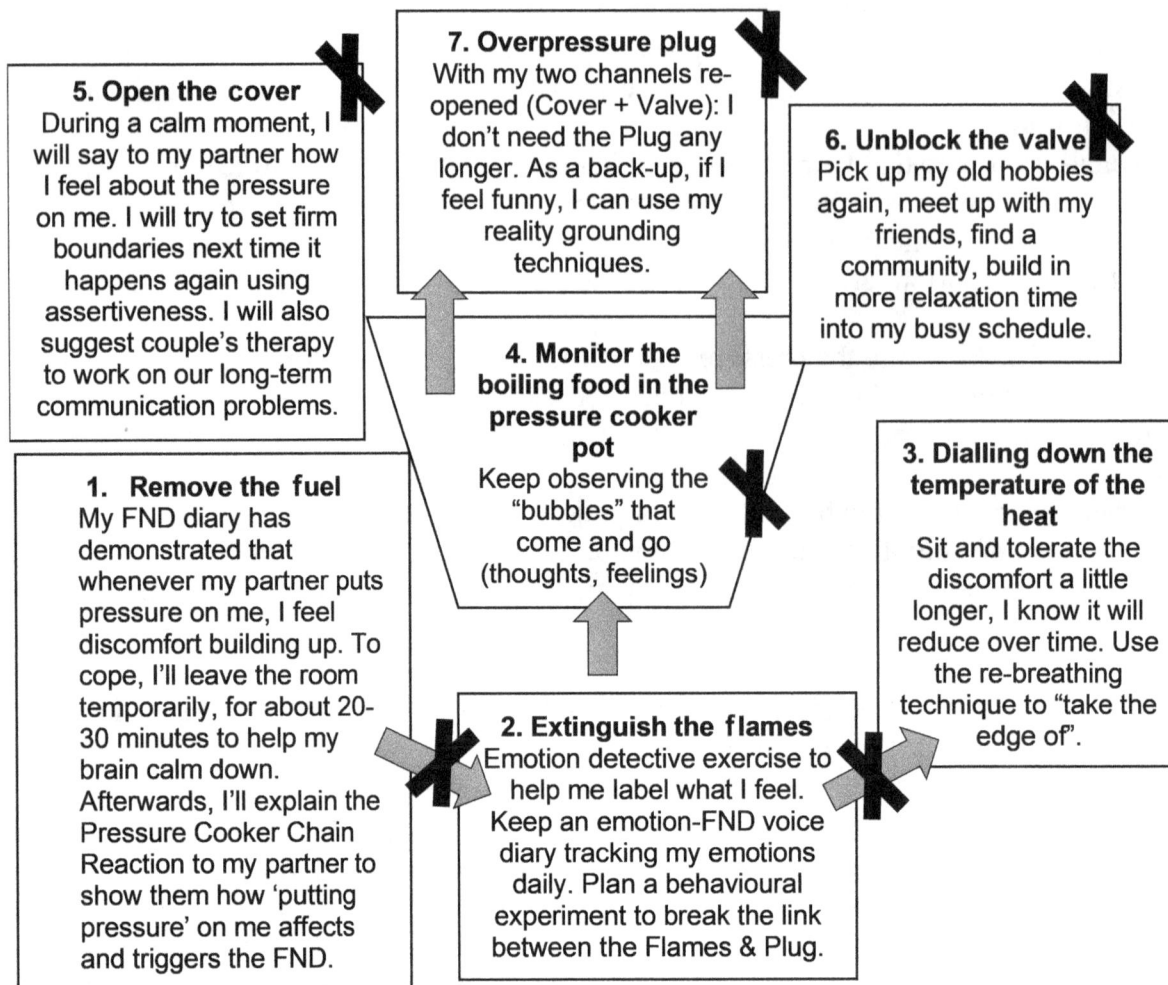

Figure 7.35 The Pressure Cooker chain reaction: intervention.

7.26 eResource alert!

If you have completed the Pressure Cooker chain reaction assessment, please have a go at thinking about the intervention next, along the lines of Figure 7.35. How can you break the links between the elements in your own situation? Please feel free to revisit earlier sections and chapters in the book to refresh your memory on helpful strategies.

The kitchen environment plays an equal role during the active FND phase

Exploring the Pressure Cooker chain reaction is not the whole story. The people in your environment play an equally important role in FND, either as a **helping hand** to support you with managing FND symptoms or as a **well-intentioned helping hand** that unfortunately keeps the FND symptoms going (more on that in Chapters 9 and 10).

Figure 7.36 outlines how your partner, family, friends, or healthcare professionals can act as a helping hand in your FND recovery by – paradoxically – gradually letting go of the support provided by your environment so that you independently learn to manage FND symptoms on your own. For more details on that process of letting go and some top tips to manage the active phase of FND, read this 7.27 **eResource**.

Phase 1:
The environment responds to the FND symptoms.
Keep the person physically safe from harm and accidental self-injury, provide practical support. Assess the Pressure Cooker Chain Reaction

Phase 2:
Collaboration between person and environment
Help establish warning signs, select and practice "early warning phase" strategies together when calm/outside dissociation. Explore alternative, more helpful coping strategies to break the links between the elements in the Pressure Cooker Chain Reaction (the top parts of the cooker are a good start: express difficult thoughts and feelings + find an enjoyable activity, reduce social isolation, and increase social connection).

Phase 3:
Apply the strategies together in the moment
Both of you: use the early warning phase skills that you both practiced together at a time **when the person starts to dissociate / experience the FND symptoms**, to help them apply the skills "in the moment" together and problem-solve any issues. Regularly offer the person a safe space to talk. You may also join the person in making links with the community for enjoyable activities and reduce social isolation.

Phase 4:
Transition from collaboration to independent practice
Gradually "disconnect" from each other: enable the person with FND to practice applying the strategies on their own when the warning signs emerge, or the episode has started to progress, **a process of "letting go"**. Support the person's confidence in pulling this off on their own and to rely on their individual skill set to manage FND– without the other person's presence and extra support.

Phase 5:
Make a move towards independent coping altogether
The person with FND is consistently practicing and applying the coping skills, either fully or mostly on their own accord with minimal support and a quick nudge from the environment, to independently manage FND symptoms as they arise ("self-regulation"). The environment should openly express confidence and belief in the person's capabilities of FND management and recovery.

Phase 6:
Consolidation of the skills
Once the person with FND has started to apply their coping skills independently, confidently, and consistently, the key is to keep practicing the skills to make them more automatic and habitual long-term. Even if the person experiences a set-back, having practiced the skills will help the person bounce back quickly.

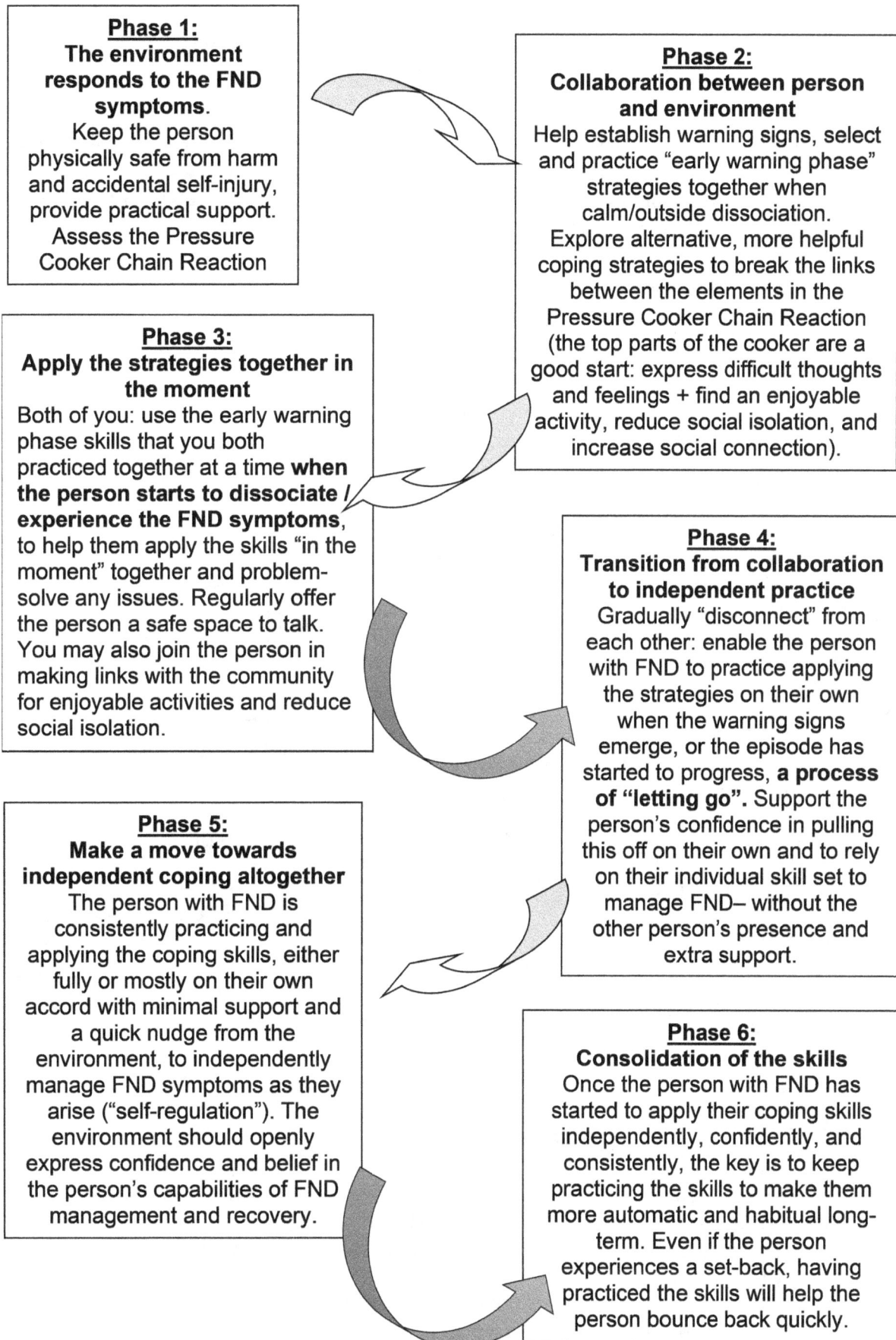

Figure 7.36 The development towards independent management of FND.

Strategies for the post-FND phase

The post-FND phase is characterised by the **end of active FND symptoms ('off peak')** and the **start of recovery**. This may look differently for different people:

- You have just experienced a dissociative seizure that lasted for a few hours. Exhausted, you end up napping afterwards for a few additional hours in the day to recharge your batteries.
- You may be emerging from a period of sleeping following a dissociative seizure, feeling a bit groggy and not entirely sure of what just happened or where you are.
- Symptoms of motor weakness may start to slowly improve. You notice less reliance on equipment and more independent activities in daily life.
- A shaking (tremor) episode, which came up earlier today, has now stopped or significantly lessened in frequency.

Hurtful vs helpful responses

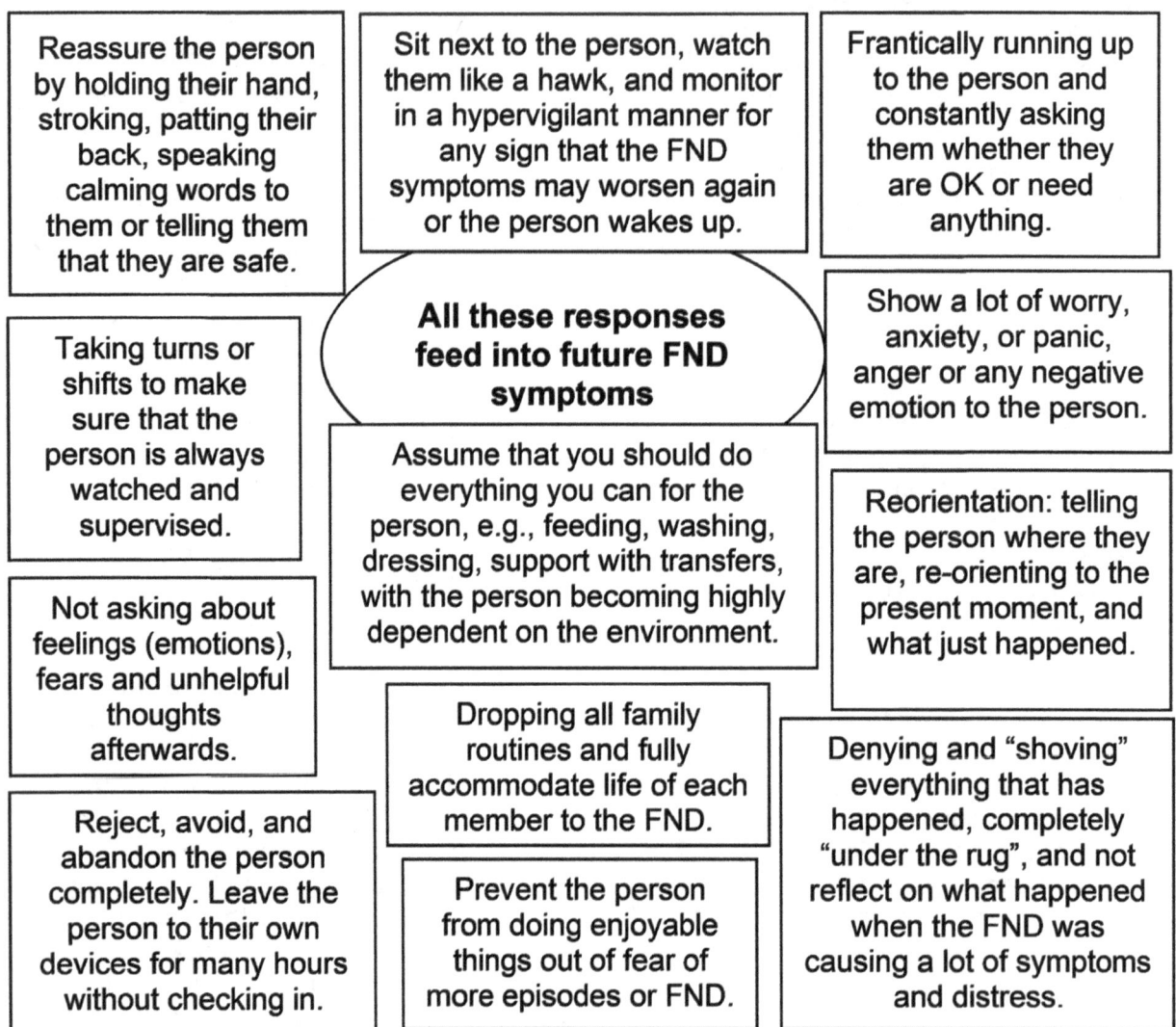

Reassure the person by holding their hand, stroking, patting their back, speaking calming words to them or telling them that they are safe.

Sit next to the person, watch them like a hawk, and monitor in a hypervigilant manner for any sign that the FND symptoms may worsen again or the person wakes up.

Frantically running up to the person and constantly asking them whether they are OK or need anything.

All these responses feed into future FND symptoms

Taking turns or shifts to make sure that the person is always watched and supervised.

Show a lot of worry, anxiety, or panic, anger or any negative emotion to the person.

Assume that you should do everything you can for the person, e.g., feeding, washing, dressing, support with transfers, with the person becoming highly dependent on the environment.

Reorientation: telling the person where they are, re-orienting to the present moment, and what just happened.

Not asking about feelings (emotions), fears and unhelpful thoughts afterwards.

Dropping all family routines and fully accommodate life of each member to the FND.

Denying and "shoving" everything that has happened, completely "under the rug", and not reflect on what happened when the FND was causing a lot of symptoms and distress.

Reject, avoid, and abandon the person completely. Leave the person to their own devices for many hours without checking in.

Prevent the person from doing enjoyable things out of fear of more episodes or FND.

Figure 7.37 Less-helpful responses in the post-FND phase.

Limit physical and verbal reassurance to stop feeding the FND. **This does not mean:** stop it forever and never reassure the person ever again!

Watch and supervise the person from eyesight distance, or with occasional checks, rather than "helicoptering" with 24-hour supervision.

Reflect on symptoms, triggers, emotions, and unhelpful thoughts afterwards using the structured FND diary.

Don't leave the person unattended for many hours assuming they'll be alright especially if there is a risk of self-injury.

"Let go" and "stand back" from symptoms, stop continuous monitoring. Sometimes, a time-out and rest is best and not just for the person experiencing the FND!

All these responses help reduce the risk of future FND symptoms

Don't be angry, frustrated, invalidating or judge the person. Be kind and compassionate, but firm.

As much as possible, try to maintain family routines and encourage each member to have some "me time" and pursue their life goals.

Encourage and help the person plan in enjoyable activities that create a sense of social belonging ("positive risk taking").

Don't be frantic, but take your time, and react calmly, instead of looking concerned, worried, anxious and full of panic that will risk causing similar emotions in the person battling the FND.

Encourage independence in daily activities as quickly as possible. Don't assume the person is unable.

Refrain from immediate re-orientation, as this may feed into FND. Better to wait until the person comes out of a dissociative episode and is able to find this information out independently.

Look at the environment's contribution to the FND and complete a double Pressure Cooker Chain Reaction: one for the person, one for the family, partner, friend, or healthcare professional.

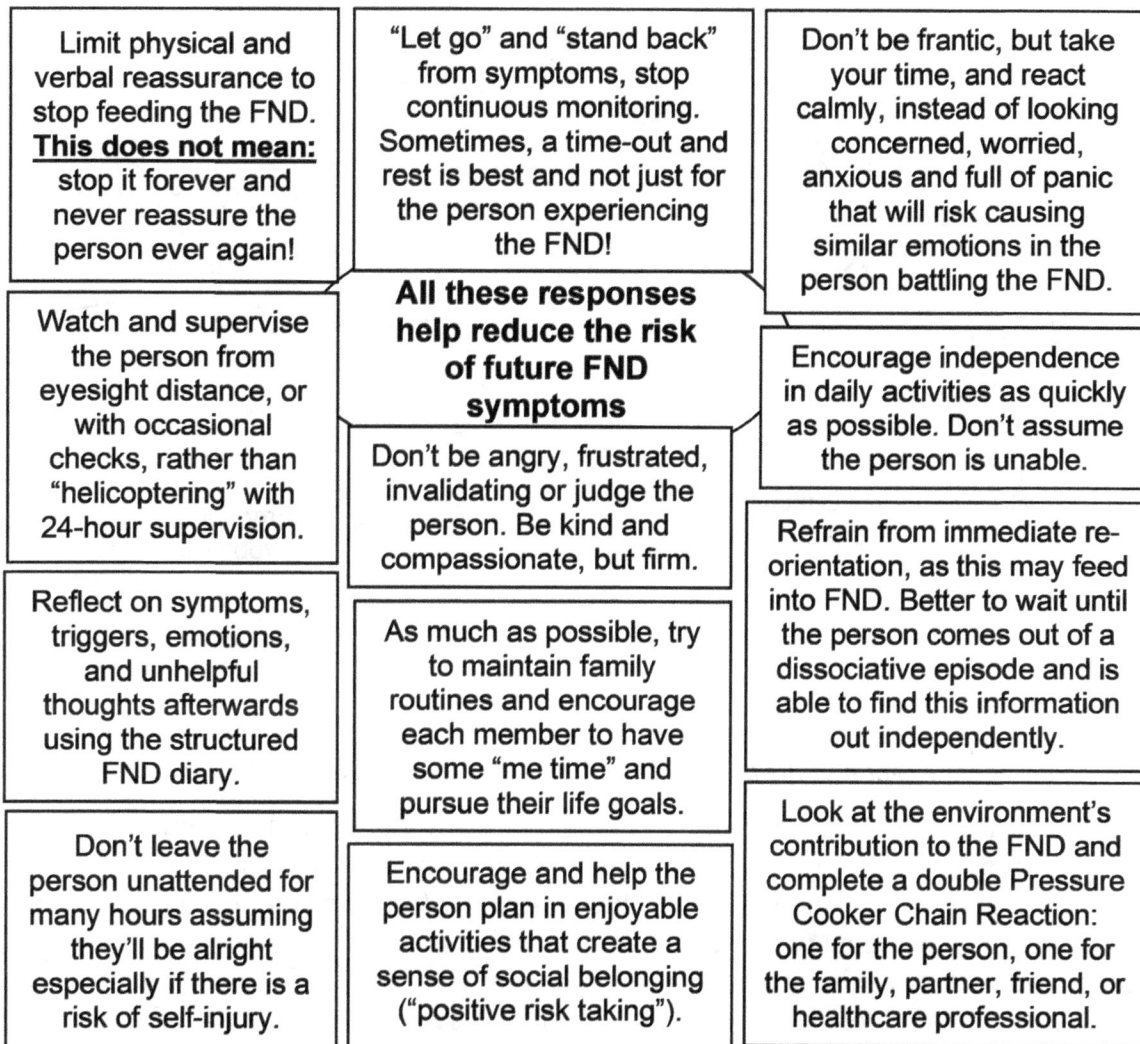

Figure 7.38 More helpful responses in the post-FND phase.

7.28 eResource alert!

Here you can find some more information on 'post-FND phase' reflection exercises and other helpful strategies for you and your partner, family, friend, or healthcare professional.

7.29 eResource alert!

Despite our individual differences, seizure guidelines applied across different people do share some commonalities. Want to find out more? Read up on useful 'rule-of-thumb' guidelines. Caution is warranted: it is strongly recommended that you and your family (healthcare professionals) complete a Pressure Cooker chain reaction each as this will give you the best chances to overcome FND; do not just assume that these guidelines 'will do'. FND recovery is hard work and requires a lot of thought, as well as constantly challenging yourself and the fine-tuning of intervention plans, with the expected emotional wobbles on the road for everybody involved in this shared process of overcoming FND.

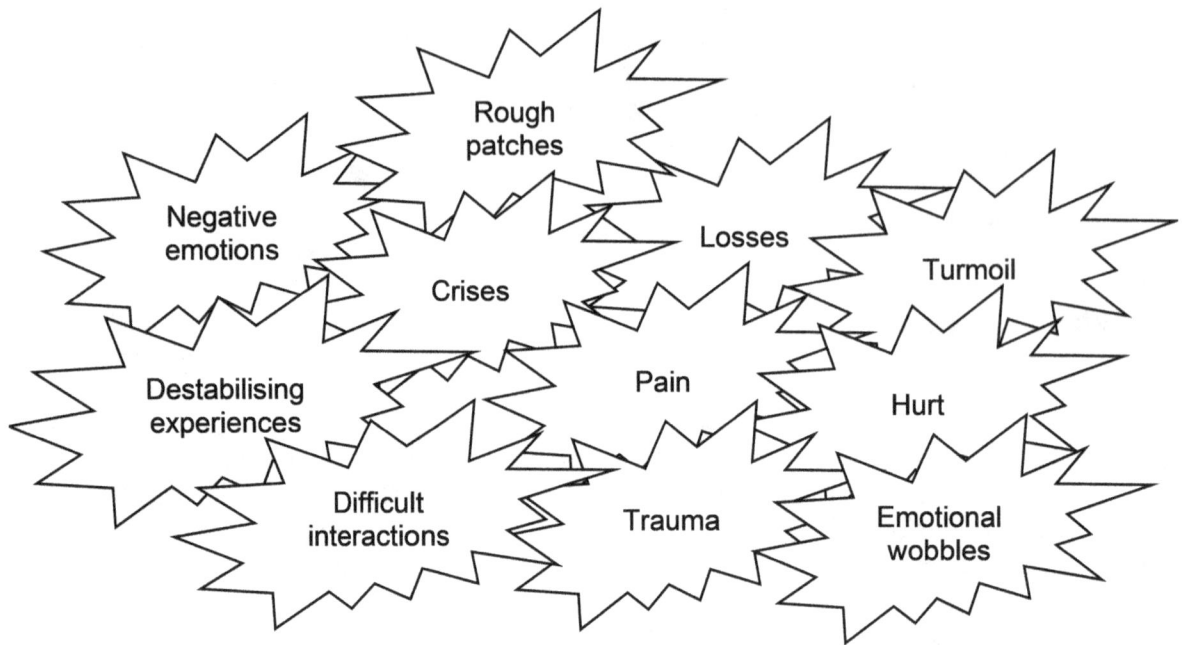

Figure 7.39 'Life'.

And a final thought: accept that the bottom parts of the Pressure Cooker Model equal life

Chapter 7 focused on the elements that make up the Pressure Cooker chain reaction: fuel, flames, heat, and the overpressure plug. The bottom parts of your Pressure Cooker Model are essentially the same thing as 'life'. We know that **life is full of stresses for everyone, FND or no FND,** with some people experiencing more of it than others (see Figure 7.39).

Stress-free lives do not exist, and no amount of therapy or avoidance will ever take stress away. It is inevitable that we must tolerate, experience, and sit with some of that distress and discomfort. We can make things easier for ourselves and take control over what life throws at us by working on starting to clean up the top parts of our Pressure Cooker Model: the cover (regularly talk to someone you feel psychologically safe with about difficult thoughts and feelings), valve (frequently release psychological pressure through enjoyable, social and stress-relieving activities), and kitchen (actively work on improving relationships and communication patterns with the people around you).

References

Adolphs, R., Tranel, D., Damasio, H., & Damasio, A. R. (1994). Impaired recognition of emotion in facial expressions following bilateral damage to the human amygdala. *Nature, 372*(6507), 669–672.

Adolphs, R., Tranel, D., Damasio, H., & Damasio, A. R. (1995). Fear and the human amygdala. *Journal of Neuroscience, 15*(9), 5879–5891.

Bakvis, P., Roelofs, K., Kuyk, J., Edelbroek, P. M., Swinkels, W. A., & Spinhoven, P. (2009a). Trauma, stress, and preconscious threat processing in patients with psychogenic nonepileptic seizures. *Epilepsia, 50*(5), 1001–1011.

Bakvis, P., Spinhoven, P., & Roelofs, K. (2009b). Basal cortisol is positively correlated to threat vigilance in patients with psychogenic nonepileptic seizures. *Epilepsy & Behavior, 16*(3), 558–560.

Bechara, A., Damasio, A. R., Damasio, H., & Anderson, S. W. (1994). Insensitivity to future consequences following damage to human prefrontal cortex. *Cognition, 50*(1–3), 7–15.

Bechara, A., Damasio, H., & Damasio, A. R. (2000). Emotion, decision making and the orbitofrontal cortex. *Cerebral Cortex, 10*(3), 295–307.

Bowman, E. S., & Markand, O. N. (1999). The contribution of life events to pseudoseizure occurrence in adults. *Bulletin of the Menninger Clinic, 63*(1), 70.

Brown, R. J., Bouska, J. F., Frow, A., Kirkby, A., Baker, G. A., Kemp, S., Burness, C., & Reuber, M. (2013). Emotional dysregulation, alexithymia, and attachment in psychogenic nonepileptic seizures. *Epilepsy & Behavior, 29*(1), 178–183.

Calder, A. J., Keane, J., Manes, F., Antoun, N., & Young, A. W. (2000). Impaired recognition and experience of disgust following brain injury. *Nature Neuroscience, 3*(11), 1077–1078.

Carlson, E. B., & Putnam, F. W. (1993). An update on the dissociative experiences scale. *Dissociation: Progress in the Dissociative Disorders, 6*(1), 16–27.

Chugani, H. T., Behen, M. E., Muzik, O., Juhász, C., Nagy, F., & Chugani, D. C. (2001). Local brain functional activity following early deprivation: A study of postinstitutionalized Romanian orphans. *Neuroimage, 14*(6), 1290–1301.

Clark, D. M., & Wells, A. (1995). A cognitive model of social phobia. In R. G. Heimberg, M. R. Liebowitz, D. A. Hope & F. R. Schneier (Eds.), *Social phobia: Diagnosis, assessment, and treatment* (pp. 69–93). New York: The Guilford Press.

Damasio, A. R., Tranel, D., & Damasio, H. C. (1991). Somatic markers and the guidance of behavior: Theory and preliminary testing. In H. S. Levin, H. M. Eisenberg & A. L. Benton (Eds.), *Frontal lobe function and dysfunction* (pp. 217–229). Oxford University Press.

Decety, J. (2015). The neural pathways, development and functions of empathy. *Current Opinion in Behavioral Sciences, 3*, 1–6.

Edwards, M. J., Adams, R. A., Brown, H., Pareés, I., & Friston, K. J. (2012). A Bayesian account of 'hysteria'. *Brain, 135*(11), 3495–3512.

Ekman, P., & Friesen, W. V. (1971). Constants across cultures in the face and emotion. *Journal of Personality and Social Psychology, 17*(2), 124–129.

Fan, Y., Duncan, N. W., De Greck, M., & Northoff, G. (2011). Is there a core neural network in empathy? An fMRI based quantitative meta-analysis. *Neuroscience & Biobehavioral Reviews, 35*(3), 903–911.

Freyd, J. J., Martorello, S. R., Alvarado, J. S., Hayes, A. E., & Christman, J. C. (1998). Cognitive environments and dissociative tendencies: Performance on the standard Stroop task for high versus low dissociators. *Applied Cognitive Psychology: The Official Journal of the Society for Applied Research in Memory and Cognition, 12*(7), S91–S103.

Gul, A., & Ahmad, H. (2014). Cognitive deficits and emotion regulation strategies in patients with psychogenic nonepileptic seizures: A task-switching study. *Epilepsy & Behavior, 32*, 108–113.

Inagaki, T. K., & Eisenberger, N. I. (2012). Neural correlates of giving support to a loved one. *Psychosomatic Medicine, 74*(1), 3–7.

Keynejad, R. C., Fenby, E., Pick, S., Moss-Morris, R., Hirsch, C., Chalder, T., Hughes, A., & Nicholson, T. R. (2020). Attentional processing and interpretative bias in functional neurological disorder. *Psychosomatic Medicine, 82*(6), 586–592.

Kross, E., Berman, M. G., Mischel, W., Smith, E. E., & Wager, T. D. (2011). Social rejection shares somatosensory representations with physical pain. *Proceedings of the National Academy of Sciences, 108*(15), 6270–6275.

Ludwig, L., Whitehead, K., Sharpe, M., Reuber, M., & Stone, J. (2015). Differences in illness perceptions between patients with non-epileptic seizures and functional limb weakness. *Journal of Psychosomatic Research, 79*(3), 246–249.

Marotta, A., Fiorio, M., Riello, M., Demartini, B., Tecilla, G., Dallocchio, C., & Tinazzi, M. (2020). Attentional avoidance of emotions in functional movement disorders. *Journal of Psychosomatic Research, 133*, 110100.

Maslow, A. H. (1943). A theory of human motivation. *Psychological Review, 50*, 370–396.

Papagno, C., Pisoni, A., Mattavelli, G., Casarotti, A., Comi, A., Fumagalli, F., Vernice, M., Fava, E., Riva, M., & Bello, L. (2016). Specific disgust processing in the left insula: New evidence from direct electrical stimulation. *Neuropsychologia, 84*, 29–35.

Pareés, I., Kassavetis, P., Saifee, T. A., Sadnicka, A., Bhatia, K. P., Fotopoulou, A., & Edwards, M. J. (2012). 'Jumping to conclusions' bias in functional movement disorders. *Journal of Neurology, Neurosurgery & Psychiatry*, *83*(4), 460–463.

Pick, S., Mellers, J. D., & Goldstein, L. H. (2018). Implicit attentional bias for facial emotion in dissociative seizures: Additional evidence. *Epilepsy & Behavior*, *80*, 296–302.

Schmahmann, J. D., & Sherman, J. C. (1998). The cerebellar cognitive affective syndrome. *Brain: A Journal of Neurology*, *121*(4), 561–579.

Selvi, Y., Kiliç, S., Aydin, A., & Özdemir, P. G. (2015). The effects of sleep deprivation on dissociation and profiles of mood, and its association with biochemical changes. *Nöro Psikiyatri Arşivi*, *52*(1), 83.

Shamay-Tsoory, S. G., Tomer, R., Berger, B. D., Goldsher, D., & Aharon-Peretz, J. (2005). Impaired "affective theory of mind" is associated with right ventromedial prefrontal damage. *Cognitive and Behavioral Neurology*, *18*(1), 55–67.

Stone, J., Warlow, C., & Sharpe, M. (2010). The symptom of functional weakness: A controlled study of 107 patients. *Brain*, *133*(5), 1537–1551.

Stone, V. E., Baron-Cohen, S., & Knight, R. T. (1998). Frontal lobe contributions to theory of mind. *Journal of Cognitive Neuroscience*, *10*(5), 640–656.

Stroop, J. R. (1935). Studies of interference in serial verbal reactions. *Journal of Experimental Psychology*, *18*(6), 643–662.

Tankersley, D., Stowe, C. J., & Huettel, S. A. (2007). Altruism is associated with an increased neural response to agency. *Nature Neuroscience*, *10*(2), 150–151.

Uliaszek, A. A., Prensky, E., & Baslet, G. (2012). Emotion regulation profiles in psychogenic non-epileptic seizures. *Epilepsy & Behavior*, *23*(3), 364–369.

Van IJzendoorn, M. H., & Schuengel, C. (1996). The measurement of dissociation in normal and clinical populations: Meta-analytic validation of the Dissociative Experiences Scale (DES). *Clinical Psychology Review*, *16*(5), 365–382.

Voon, V., Brezing, C., Gallea, C., Ameli, R., Roelofs, K., LaFrance Jr, W. C., & Hallett, M. (2010). Emotional stimuli and motor conversion disorder. *Brain*, *133*(5), 1526–1536.

Whitehead, K., Stone, J., Norman, P., Sharpe, M., & Reuber, M. (2015). Differences in relatives' and patients' illness perceptions in functional neurological symptom disorders compared with neurological diseases. *Epilepsy & Behavior*, *42*, 159–164.

Williams, I. A., Levita, L., & Reuber, M. (2018). Emotion dysregulation in patients with psychogenic nonepileptic seizures: A systematic review based on the extended process model. *Epilepsy & Behavior*, *86*, 37–48.

8 Facilitating physical factors in FND

Pot, warning light (layer 4)

The Pressure Cooker Model adopts a biopsychosocial perspective that looks at biological, psychological, and social aspects of FND. An explanation of FND without any mention of the body would not do the condition any justice. Chapter 8 focuses on two physical elements: the pot and the warning light.

Pot

Cracks and fissures in the pot do not help the FND. The pot element describes physical and medical factors that people with FND often report during therapy sessions and that may maintain the FND.

This section is not intended to minimise FND or your physical symptoms. However, these physical factors can occasionally explain some of the FND symptoms or make the FND worse. The goal of reviewing the pot element is to find out whether there are any physical factors at play that can be addressed to alleviate some of your symptoms. If, after review, you continue to experience FND symptoms, then you will be able to say that you have done a lot to address any possible physical factors that could contribute to the FND which will help you move on to focussing on more psychological and social aspects.

A helpful way to look at the important physical factors that contribute to FND is to use the following mnemonic: FND SELF-CARE. Each letter of the acronym represents a physical or medical feature that is important to FND. In the next section, each one will be described in detail.

Food fuel

Vitamins and minerals

A subset of people with FND have vitamin deficiencies. We also know that quite a large proportion experiences co-existing anxiety and depression. Did you know that psychological difficulties can indirectly but greatly influence our food intake and diets?

- If you are anxious, you may feel too nauseous to eat anything.
- Stress may cause you to reach for unhealthy foods quicker.
- If you have been feeling depressed for a long time and it has been impacting on your motivation and appetite levels, you may not take good care of yourself by eating foods with little nutritional value or nothing at all.
- Some people manage their emotions with food or alcohol overuse, which may lead to vitamin deficiencies. Eating disorders like binge eating and bulimia nervosa are relatively uncommon but can emerge and often predate the development of FND.

Furthermore, some people with FND experience such severe symptoms that it keeps them from leaving the house for a longer period of time. For example, if all your limbs are paralysed, you

DOI: 10.4324/9781003308973-8

may be bed-bound. Other people may not be able to leave the house for 'psychosocial' reasons, such as feeling anxious about having a dissociative episode in public, not feeling safe enough outside due to accidental self-injury caused by seizures or falls, social anxiety, as well as social isolation and not having anyone in your support system who could take you out to places. As a result, people may start to miss out on sufficient vitamin D, the 'sunny vitamin', because of not catching sunrays due to staying indoors.

Unfortunately, the effects of vitamin deficiencies on the body can overlap with FND symptoms. Look at the symptoms displayed in Figure 8.1, which are also commonly found as part of the FND! It is always worth checking with your medical team whether (some of) your symptoms could potentially be better explained by vitamin deficiencies, not in the least to prevent harm to your body.

A few people, with and without FND, experience dangerous levels of vitamin and mineral deficiencies, sometimes unbeknownst to them. Severe deficiencies can cause irreparable harm to your body. A good example is Korsakov's syndrome in people who consume too much alcohol and become deficient of thiamine. This can cause irreversible injuries to the memory centres in your brain, with some people requiring 24-hour care and supervision.

Another thing to think about is the fact that vitamin deficiencies can also be caused by physical illnesses that you may not know you had, or predate the FND, for example, conditions affecting the gut, such as pernicious anaemia, Crohn's disease, or ulcerative colitis.

Although these are more extreme examples, it does illustrate that it is always worth looking at your vitamin and mineral levels to check that these do not inadvertently contribute to FND; are a sign of another underlying physical condition that you may not have been aware of and needs treatment; as well as to help prevent harm to your body.

Although vitamin and mineral deficiencies can cause you to feel unwell and impact on the FND, some of these deficiencies can be reversible and treatable with vitamin supplementation and improvements made to your diet. You would not want to miss out on opportunities to feel

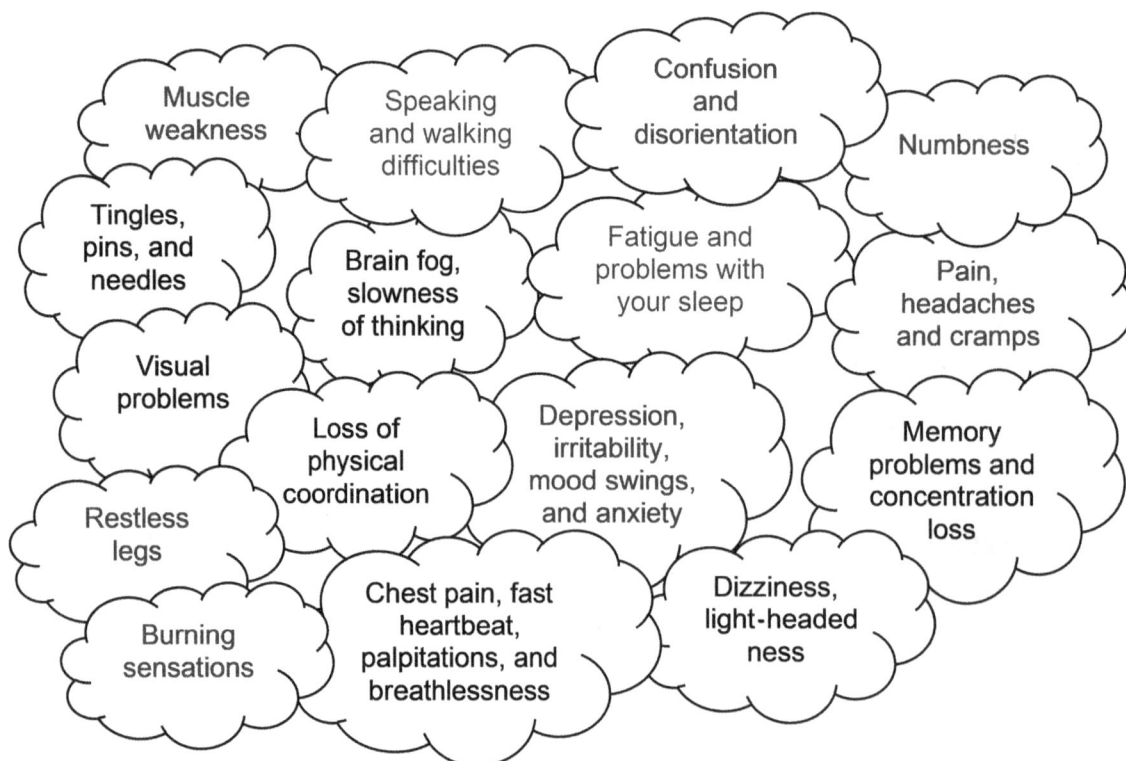

Figure 8.1 Neurological consequences of vitamin deficiencies.

better! In addition, ensuring that your body and mind are in the best state they can possibly be will help you benefit in the most optimal ways from your neurorehabilitation programme. You will have sufficient energy, motivation, and focus to tackle recovery from FND head-on.

8.1 eResource alert!

If you are interested in finding out more about vitamins, minerals, and their importance for the body, make sure to check this information out.

Our second brain: the gut–brain axis

In the previous section on vitamins and minerals, we could already see a strong link between what we eat and how that may affect our body and mind. Our gut is very long: it starts in our mouth; passes through the oesophagus, the stomach, small and large intestine; and eventually ends with the rectum. People often feel embarrassed or ashamed talking about gut-related issues, especially when they involve the lower parts of our gastrointestinal system. Although understandable, there is no need to feel this way about our bowel functioning. It is all part of nature and our biological make-up. Our bowels rightly deserve our full attention! Bowel care is an essential part of day-to-day life, and if things do not flow that well in these body areas, we need to do something about it.

Did you know that there is a strong relationship between the gut and the brain? We have about 100 to 500 million neurons in our 'enteric nervous system' (Dicks, 2022). The gut is also called our 'second brain'. It is fascinating to think that approximately 90–95% of the neurotransmitter serotonin can be found in our gastrointestinal system! (Gershon & Tack, 2007; Strandwitz, 2018). Serotonin is very important for regulating our mood and a neurotransmitter of interest in often-used antidepressants ('SSRIs', selective serotonin reuptake inhibitors).

Have a think about a time when you felt stressed, anxious, or worried. What happened to the different parts of your gut? You may have come up with the following list:

- Dry mouth.
- Possibly feeling something in your throat, like a sensation of tightness that you normally do not experience.
- Feeling butterflies in your stomach.
- Feeling nauseous, or an upset and churning stomach, perhaps having to go to the toilet to vomit.
- Having a 'knot' in your stomach.
- Not being able to eat at all.
- Or the opposite: 'stress eating', especially high-calorie and sweet foods.
- Slowing or even the cessation of digestion, involving multiple toilet visits to open your bowels.
- Your anal sphincter closing.

That is quite a big list, isn't it? A stressed-out brain clearly has a lot of influence on our gut. However, this is just one direction, from brain to gut. A less-known relationship in the opposite direction, from gut to brain, is called the **gut–brain axis**. It turns out that our gut health has a strong connection with how our brain functions and links in with the cognitive and emotional centres of the brain (what we think and how we feel). The gut communicates with the brain.

The gut–brain axis in people with FND: a new theory

Asadi-Pooya et al. (2019) hypothesised that there may be a link between unhealthy or harmful gut microbiota and emotional dysfunction in people with psychogenic non-epileptic seizures.

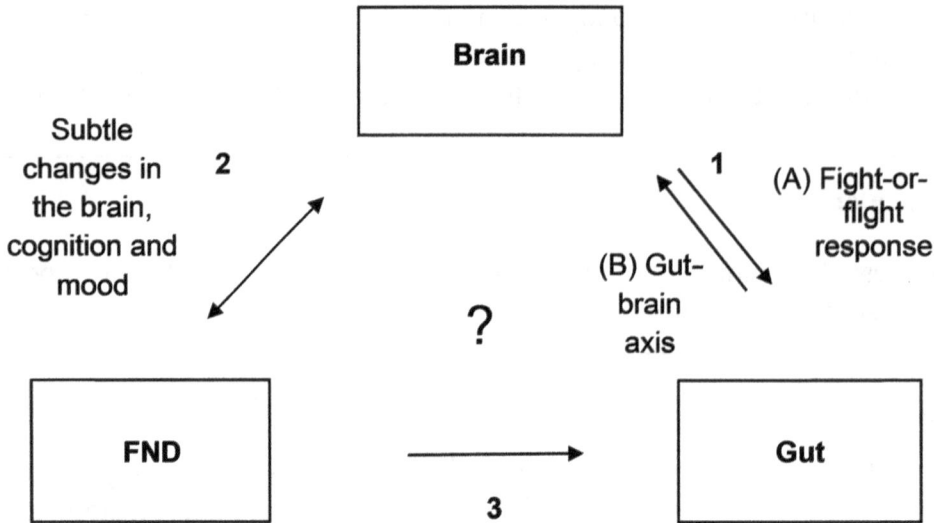

Figure 8.2 The gut–brain axis in FND.

Interestingly, these authors suggest that if this hypothesis is correct, one could think of research studies that explore the effects of probiotics in people with these seizures. Food for thought!

People with FND may report the following gastrointestinal symptoms:

- Dry mouth
- Swallowing problems ('globus sensation')
- Tight throat
- Food intolerances
- GERD (gastroesophageal reflux disease)
- Stomach butterflies
- Nausea
- Post-seizure vomiting
- Irritable bowel syndrome
- Inflammatory changes due to previous medication overdoses
- Constipation, or a problem with opening your bowels (sometimes, a person may 'hold on' to bowel contents for a prolonged period of time, which can potentially risk a 'megacolon')

Given these symptoms, could gut–brain axis dysfunction play a role in FND, and what evidence is there?

Look at the numbers in Figure 8.2. We know that there are strong relationships between the brain and the gut in opposite directions (pathways 1A and 1B). There are also clues to brain issues in people with FND, for example, subtle changes on brain scans, including in areas important for emotions, such as the amygdala; reduced thinking skills that rely on different parts of the brain; and mood problems (pathway 2). People with FND often report a range of gastrointestinal issues (pathway 3).

CAN WE THEREFORE SPEAK OF GUT–BRAIN AXIS DYSFUNCTION IN FND?

The writings seem to be on the wall: all the necessary elements of the triangle in Figure 8.2 are present (people with FND show difficulties along their gut–brain axis). Although these are exciting ideas, it is helpful to keep in mind that there are various reasons for gut problems in people with FND, including, but not limited to, medications; antibiotics that destroy the 'friendly' bacteria that help your gut; illnesses in the bowel that pre-dated the FND; lifestyle and dietary factors; lack of exercise and problems with mobility; dehydration; and psychological difficulties.

Regardless of the causes, the gut–brain axis is important for everyone, FND or not. If we pay attention to gut health, we may be able to influence our brain health, and therefore our mood and thinking skills, and eventually the FND. Although speculative, an exciting prospect could be the use of probiotics in FND. A specific type of probiotic is called 'psychobiotics' or 'psychomicrobiotics', which are probiotics that have been investigated in psychological conditions, such as anxiety and depression (see for a summary of clinical trials: Appleton, 2018). Psychobiotics improved questionnaire scores on self-reported mood and anxiety symptoms (Appleton, 2018).

8.2 eResource alert!

Quite a subset of people with FND experiences weight problems and, occasionally, co-existing eating disorders. Learn more about these important topics here.

Night rest

Why do we sleep?

- Cleans out toxic waste and debris in your brain that you have been building up during the day.
- Contributes to a healthy immune system and fighting infections.
- Repairs cells and tissues in the body.
- Supports a healthy hormone balance and blood sugar regulation.
- Supports the consolidation of memories.
- Optimises your cognitive performance during the day, productivity, efficiency, accuracy, and reaction time. A good sleep supports attentional focus on important activities in daily life, such as childcare, work and driving.
- Restores our minds and bodies: important for mood, well-being, energy levels, being 'present in body and mind' for your treatment, fully participating in rehab, and ultimately, your FND recovery.

What is the nature of sleeping difficulties in FND?

Most people with FND will report difficulties with sleeping (Bennett et al., 2021), with numbers varying between 62% (Nielsen et al., 2017), 75% (Stone et al., 2010), 80% (Goldstein et al., 2021), and 82% (Petrochilos et al., 2020). One study (Pattichis et al., 2019) found that 73% of people with dissociative seizures demonstrated significant scores on a sleep quality questionnaire indicating poor sleep – a frequency that was somewhat higher than in people with epileptic seizures (64%). People with FND report a vast array of sleeping difficulties:

- Not being able to fall asleep whatever you do, often with thoughts and worries keeping you up.
- Waking up multiple times during the night, tossing and turning in your bed for hours.
- Waking up in the middle of the night due to PTSD flashbacks and nightmares.
- Waking up very early in the morning and not being able to get back to sleep, sometimes associated with depression.
- Sleeping long hours during the night and day, more than the recommended 7–9 hours ('hypersomnia').
- Feeling very sleepy during the day ('daytime somnolence') and taking naps, which disrupts the sleep–wake cycle.

- Your breathing stopping and starting during sleeping ('sleep apnoea').
- Pain, restless legs, and physical disabilities making it hard for you to turn at night.
- Although less common, dissociative seizures can emerge at night-time.
- Not feeling refreshed after a night's sleep.

8.3 eResource alert!

We may sometimes inadvertently engage in thoughts, feelings, and behaviours that adversely impact on our sleep, without even realizing it! Complete this sleep questionnaire to help you reflect on 'pressure point' areas that may need your extra attention to improve your sleep.

Tips and tricks for a good night's sleep for people with FND

Practical solutions for a better sleep environment

- Upgrade to a **comfy bed** and mattress; use earplugs, an eye mask; put your phone away or use silent notifications; invest in a good set of curtains or blinds; change rooms to minimise distractions from the street or neighbours.
- **Associate your bed with 'sleep'** and not with 'activity'. If you have a TV in your bedroom or like to work in your bedroom, get rid of the TV or stop working in a 'place of rest' (understandably difficult if you live in a studio apartment).
- Explore whether **your 'significant other'** plays a role in your disrupted sleep. Think about relationship difficulties, or a partner with their own sleep issues.
- Request a **health review** that looks at your medications (for example, are you on sleep-inducing, or the opposite, stimulant medications that tamper with your sleep-wake cycle?), physical health, and vitamin deficiencies.

Cope with thoughts, emotions, and memories that bother you at night

- Keep a **notebook** or **voice note diary** next to your bed. If thoughts and feelings keep you up at night, 'dump' them in your notebook to free up your mind.
- Find an **emotional outlet during the day**, express your thoughts and feelings to someone you trust and feel safe with (open the cover), and/or engage in enjoyable, relaxing, and social activities (unblock the valve).
- Look out for **triggers** of poor sleep using a **sleep diary** or **phone app**, including emotions, stress, worries, and events that happened during the day.
- Check your **sleep history**: identify past triggers for poor sleep, and 'recycle' strategies that worked well for you at that time.

Watch out for understandable, but unhelpful, behaviours

- Remove anything that activates the brain right before or during sleep: listening to podcasts, music, watching TV, work, checking your phone, vigorous sports exercises.
- Stop in time and **limit your intake of caffeine**, sugary or energy drinks (including green tea and hot chocolate), as well as fluids if bladder issues wake you up at night.
- Check whether **dissociation** may account for your sleeping patterns: Do you sleep to 'forget about things'? Does sleep help cut your emotions off temporarily and take something unpleasant away? Be careful, because sleep can become a reward for your brain, increasing in frequency and length every time you feel unwell.
- **Clock-watching** when you are wide awake in bed feeds anxiety, worries, and frustration, exactly the emotions that will arouse you even more.

- FND can be exhausting, but **avoid daytime naps** that disrupt your sleep–wake cycle.
- If you happen to wake up at night, it is better to get up and **do a light activity** (read a book) until you start to feel tired again. 'Try' again to see if you fall asleep.
- Try a **pacing approach** to address exhausting boom-and-bust cycles.

Establish a sleep routine

- To help you fall asleep, create a daily **wind-down sleep ritual** before going to bed.
- Try some **relaxation exercises** right before sleep to bring physical arousal down and calm your brain.
- Stick to the same daily bedtime and wake time to ensure you clock 7–9 hours of sleep, and **build a routine** that signals to your body and mind, 'It is sleep time.'
- **Find an ally!** Agree with your partner or family to wind down and sleep within a certain 'sleep window'.

Drugs and medications

People with FND tend to be on a lot of medications. Sometimes this is called 'polypharmacy'. *Poly* means 'multiple', and *pharmacy* means 'medications'.

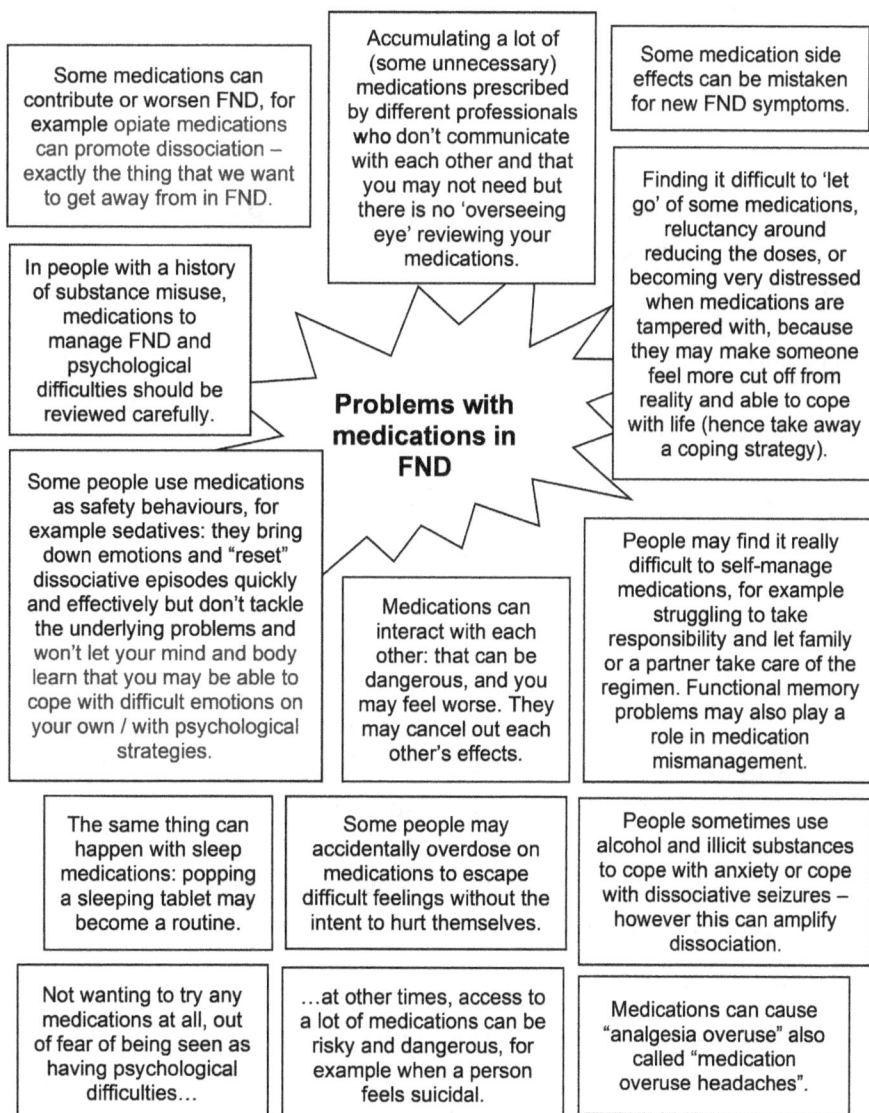

Some medications can contribute or worsen FND, for example opiate medications can promote dissociation – exactly the thing that we want to get away from in FND.

Accumulating a lot of (some unnecessary) medications prescribed by different professionals who don't communicate with each other and that you may not need but there is no 'overseeing eye' reviewing your medications.

Some medication side effects can be mistaken for new FND symptoms.

In people with a history of substance misuse, medications to manage FND and psychological difficulties should be reviewed carefully.

Finding it difficult to 'let go' of some medications, reluctancy around reducing the doses, or becoming very distressed when medications are tampered with, because they may make someone feel more cut off from reality and able to cope with life (hence take away a coping strategy).

Some people use medications as safety behaviours, for example sedatives: they bring down emotions and "reset" dissociative episodes quickly and effectively but don't tackle the underlying problems and won't let your mind and body learn that you may be able to cope with difficult emotions on your own / with psychological strategies.

Problems with medications in FND

Medications can interact with each other: that can be dangerous, and you may feel worse. They may cancel out each other's effects.

People may find it really difficult to self-manage medications, for example struggling to take responsibility and let family or a partner take care of the regimen. Functional memory problems may also play a role in medication mismanagement.

The same thing can happen with sleep medications: popping a sleeping tablet may become a routine.

Some people may accidentally overdose on medications to escape difficult feelings without the intent to hurt themselves.

People sometimes use alcohol and illicit substances to cope with anxiety or cope with dissociative seizures – however this can amplify dissociation.

Not wanting to try any medications at all, out of fear of being seen as having psychological difficulties…

…at other times, access to a lot of medications can be risky and dangerous, for example when a person feels suicidal.

Medications can cause "analgesia overuse" also called "medication overuse headaches".

Figure 8.3 Medication issues in FND.

Although medication management should always be carried out by appropriately trained healthcare professionals, the following pieces of advice have supported people with FND in the past:

- People with FND often report challenging healthcare experiences. Although it may be hard to trust healthcare providers, **it is worth trusting a professional** interested and knowledgeable in FND who can review your medications and really help you.
- In collaboration with medical professionals, think of ways that you **could limit the use of alcohol, illicit substances, and unnecessary 'polypharmacy'**, if these have become your primary, and perhaps unhelpful, coping strategies for difficult thoughts, feelings, and dissociative seizures.
- Together with professionals involved in your care, try to see how you could gradually take more responsibility for **independent medication management** – if you and your family feel low in confidence or anxious.
- A **risk assessment** is always very important to keep you safe, especially if you experience cognitive problems or suicidal thoughts that could influence medication management.

Medications . . . psychological therapy?

- Taking away a long-standing coping strategy may leave you feeling vulnerable; therefore, seek support to **develop alternative strategies**, for example, psychological techniques to help you sit with difficult feelings and manage dissociation.
- Your psychological skills, you can always carry with you, but medication prescriptions are finite: they need to be refilled and may lose their effectiveness as tolerance builds up over time for some medications.
- Medications influence neurotransmitters in our brains, but did you know that **brains** and **brain connections can change and adapt as a result of life experience due to a process called 'plasticity'**? (Even though brains have more capacity for neuroplasticity in our younger than older years, as well as a very limited ability to generate new brain cells). You can consider psychological therapy as a form of experience, and by engaging with psychological therapy, you are essentially supporting your brain functions.

Medications are still important!

In summary, this is not an 'either/or' stand-off or a dichotomous choice between either psychological therapy or medications. In clinical practice, a combination of psychological therapy and medications often achieves good results.

Sickness and physical illness

The 'S' in the FND SELF-CARE acronym represents any 'sickness' and physical conditions that are associated or co-exist with the FND. Although some people only experience FND, it is not uncommon for people to have additional physical conditions. Figures 8.4, 8.5 and 8.6 show how we can roughly divide some of these more commonly encountered physical illnesses in three different groups.

You may ask yourself why it is important to know about these three groups of co-existing physical conditions in people with FND? For many reasons!

- Some of these conditions (Ehlers–Danlos and POTS) have the potential to **increase a person's attentional focus on their physical symptoms**, for example, by having to pay a lot more attention to your joints or your heart rate, as part of treatment. Unfortunately, increased self-focused attention is one of the maintaining factors that 'feeds' the FND.

An injury and FND may cause very similar symptoms (for example, problems with mobility). However, the organic injury alone is **not capable of sufficiently explaining** the full range or severity of your physical symptoms.

For people with epileptic and non-epileptic seizures:
- A person may have had a history of childhood epilepsy that was previously well-controlled with anti-epileptic medications.
- New-onset dissociative episodes show normal tests and often associated with a difficult life event, for example a divorce.
- Non-epileptic diagnosis can be really difficult to believe and accept for the person, and a big shift to manage emotionally.

An **organic injury** in the neurological or musculoskeletal system, often predating the FND.

Group #1 "Functional overlay"

FND on top of (examples):
- Spinal issues including previous back surgery or a bulging disc.
- Epileptic seizures, as well as non-epileptic seizures in a subset of people (see D'Alessio et al., 2006; Baroni et al., 2016).
- (Mild) traumatic brain injury and post-concussional syndrome.

Treatment of people with functional overlay is often complex and **requires a careful and multidisciplinary approach** with the support of a medical team.

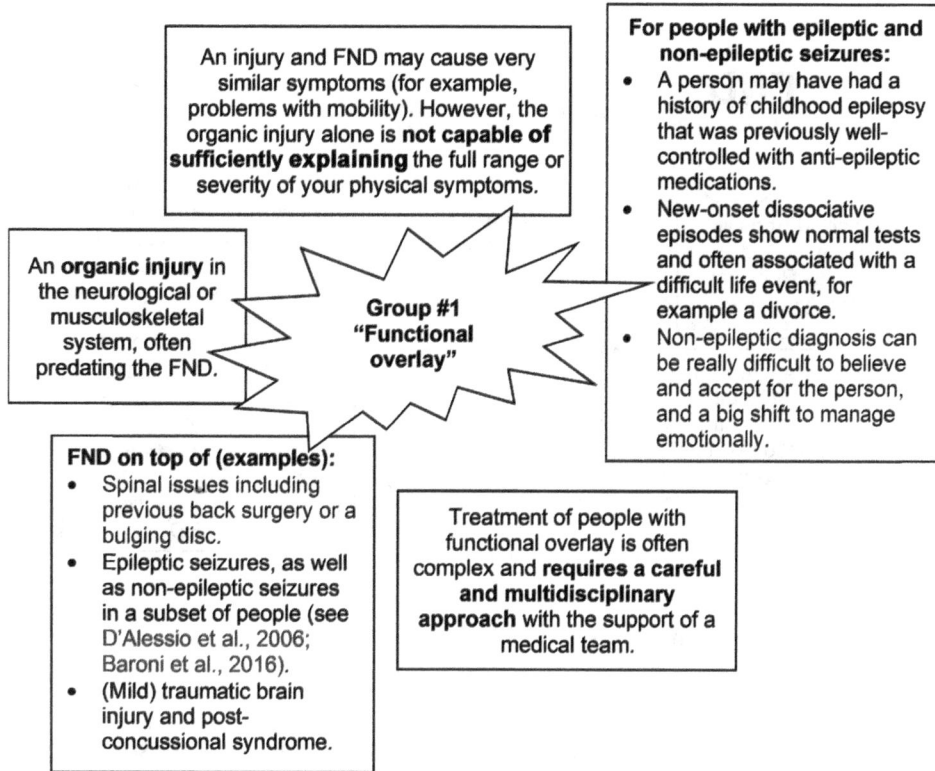

Figure 8.4 Functional overlay in people with FND.

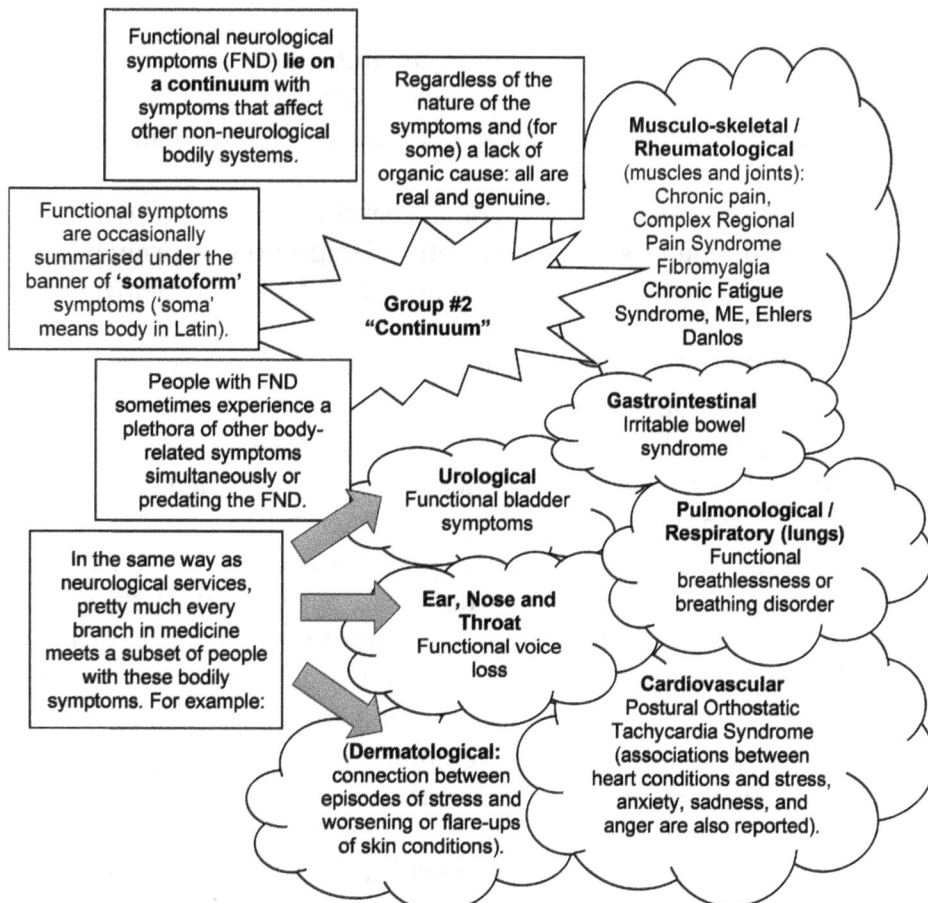

Functional neurological symptoms (FND) **lie on a continuum** with symptoms that affect other non-neurological bodily systems.

Regardless of the nature of the symptoms and (for some) a lack of organic cause: all are real and genuine.

Musculo-skeletal / Rheumatological (muscles and joints): Chronic pain, Complex Regional Pain Syndrome Fibromyalgia Chronic Fatigue Syndrome, ME, Ehlers Danlos

Functional symptoms are occasionally summarised under the banner of **'somatoform'** symptoms ('soma' means body in Latin).

Group #2 "Continuum"

Gastrointestinal Irritable bowel syndrome

People with FND sometimes experience a plethora of other body-related symptoms simultaneously or predating the FND.

Urological Functional bladder symptoms

Pulmonological / Respiratory (lungs) Functional breathlessness or breathing disorder

In the same way as neurological services, pretty much every branch in medicine meets a subset of people with these bodily symptoms. For example:

Ear, Nose and Throat Functional voice loss

Cardiovascular Postural Orthostatic Tachycardia Syndrome (associations between heart conditions and stress, anxiety, sadness, and anger are also reported).

(Dermatological: connection between episodes of stress and worsening or flare-ups of skin conditions).

Figure 8.5 A continuum of body-related symptoms in people with FND.

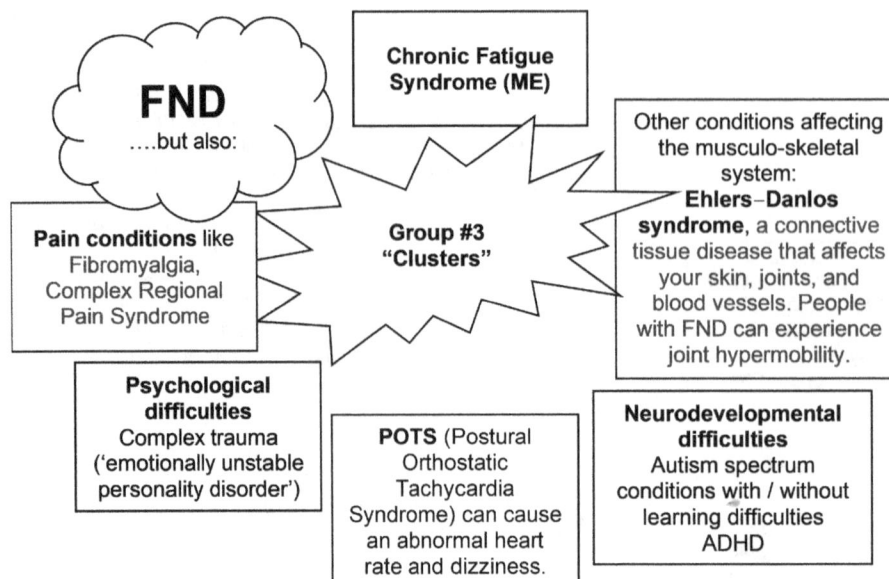

Figure 8.6 Clusters of symptoms in people with FND.

- Do you remember Chapter 2? We discussed that some people with dissociative episodes may have (had) other coping strategies that brought down unpleasant feelings quickly and effectively to achieve a state of psychological safety, including substance use, long sleeping episodes, multiple emergency room visits, 'emotional eating', and self-harm.
- In the same way, if people present with functional symptoms affecting multiple body systems, then it is sometimes more helpful to **look beyond 'contents'** (manifestation of symptoms) and **treat the 'underlying process'** (Do they achieve psychological safety? Are there possible social functions that connect these conditions?) rather than treat each condition separately.
- People with functional overlay, somatoform, or clustered symptoms present with a higher level of complexity, risks, and require **a joined-up multidisciplinary approach**, as well as **adaptations to interventions** (e.g. think about dissociative seizure management in someone with hypermobile joints or POTS).
- Physical illnesses can also contribute to the development of FND via **'modelling'**, a social learning process (Bandura et al., 1961; Bandura & Walters, 1977), that may explain why some people with epileptic seizures later go on to develop non-epileptic seizures. People who have frequently been exposed to hospital environments, surgeries, or medical procedures in childhood may have an increased risk of developing FND later in life.
- Although the mechanisms are not entirely clear and these healthcare experiences are distressing, hospitals can also be caring environments, particularly if things are difficult at home. In addition, family members may become more attentive and caring. Not knowing any different, a person's physical symptoms can inadvertently become a way of signalling to other people that the person needs help, support, and care. Rather than expressing difficult emotions verbally, the person may feel more comfortable expressing emotions in physical ways. Modelling may also explain why healthcare workers are generally at a higher risk of developing FND.
- People with FND often report an infection that set off the FND for the first time. How is this possible? We need to go back to theories of FND that emphasise the role of thinking processes in FND, including **abnormal expectations, beliefs, or misattributions** about illnesses (for example, Edwards et al., 2012).

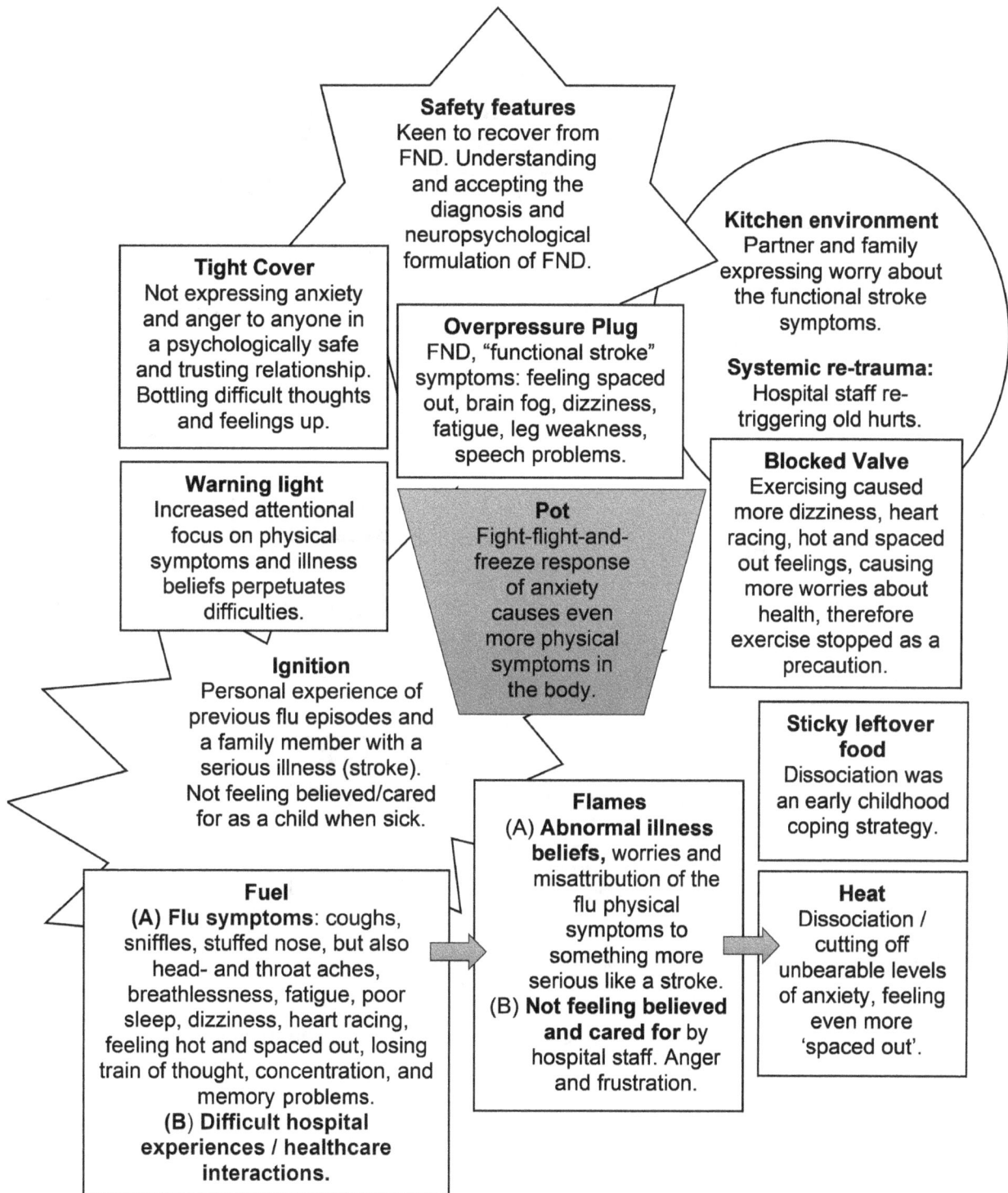

Figure 8.7 How a flu can lead to FND.

Equipment

FND comes with physical disabilities. For this reason, a lot of people with FND rely on equipment. Equipment plays an important role in the lives of people with FND, and the number of aids depends on the severity of your disabilities and care needs. Equipment can help you with various activities in daily life (ADLs), getting around in the home, going outdoors and accessing your community (see Figure 8.8).

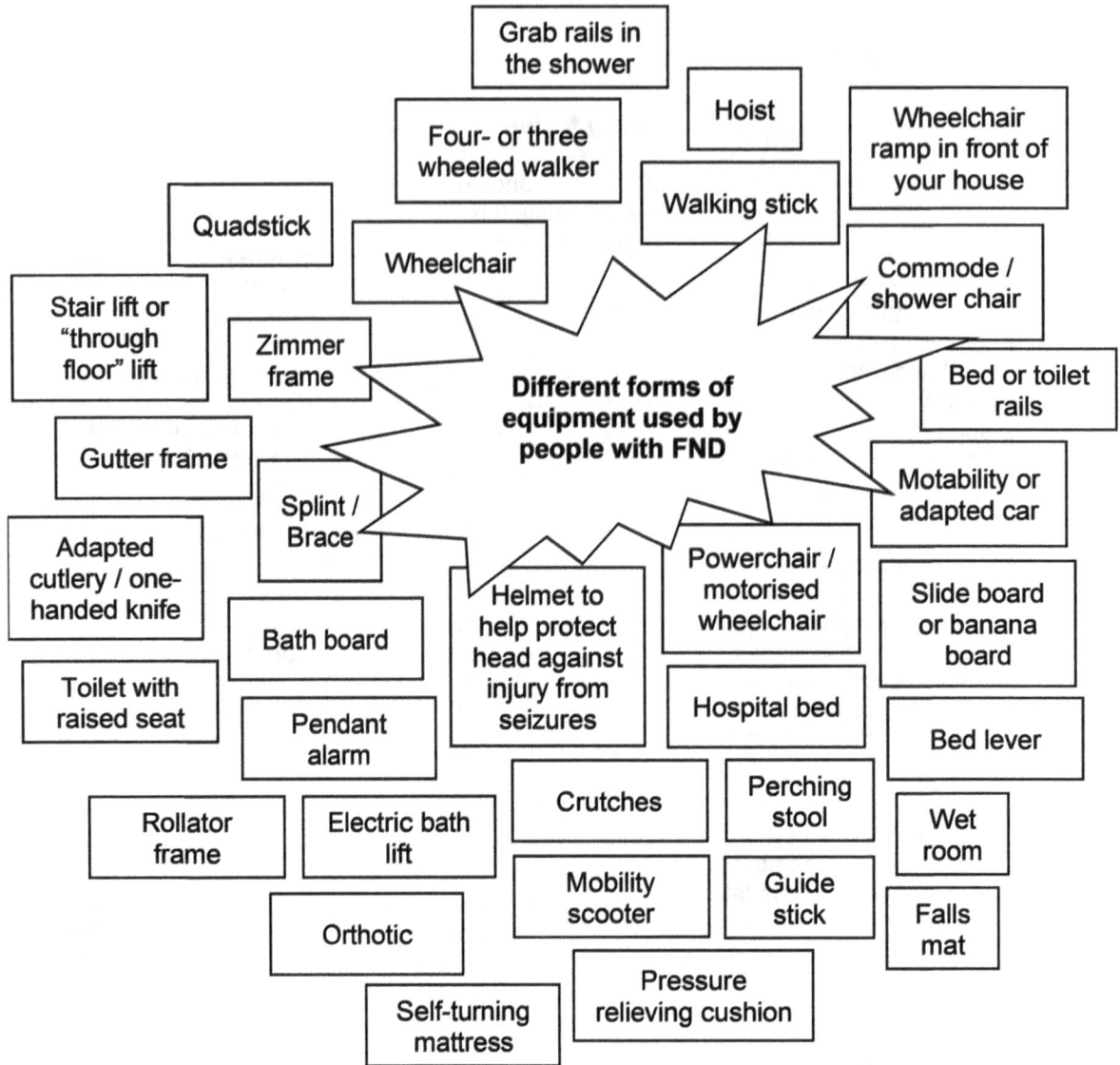

Figure 8.8 Equipment and adaptations in FND.

Equipment is not always thought to be helpful during rehabilitation of FND (occupational therapy consensus recommendations for FND; Nicholson et al., 2020):

- Stops you from improving in the future because it may negatively impact on the way you move, function in day-to-day life, or use other muscles to 'compensate' whilst 'neglecting' the muscles affected by the FND.
- Increases attention to your symptoms, a key maintaining factor of FND.
- Causes 'secondary problems' and pain in your joints. Just think about how your shoulders or your hands may feel on crutches after a while.
- Decondition your muscles and make them weak.

When we think of equipment, most people will probably think of physical aspects, for example, how it enables you to wash, dress, go outdoors, and mobilise. However, did you know that equipment is strongly associated with emotions and psychological functions?

Parting ways with equipment can be extremely difficult. In addition to losing your physical support, bearings, and possibly risking falls, stepping down equipment may also feel strange

The prospect of significant changes in your life when you are recovered from the FND and not having to rely on the equipment any longer can sometimes feel frightening and daunting.

Equipment can be a form of physical protection, anxiety coping mechanism or "psychological crutch": Some people experience worries and anxiety around hurting themselves without the equipment and making the FND worse.

Equipment (especially wheelchairs) can be a safety behaviour (like a "psychological safety blanket") and increase confidence, for example in people with social anxiety, body image issues, and fear of falling.

Psychological functions of equipment

Provides not only physical, but also psychological and social support: Kind and supportive responses that equipment often elicits from our social environment, for example people getting out of the way when seeing you in a wheelchair or tiptoeing around you and helping you to meet your physical and emotional needs better.

Some people with FND have reported that wheelchairs and other equipment make them look more inconspicuous sitting (compared to standing/walking), not having to look people in the eye due to height differences, feel less self-conscious about the body, and provide firm protection to prevent falls. Letting go of the equipment may feel like you lose this safety.

Or the opposite: receiving judgemental responses from the environment and not being believed when not needing the equipment anymore. The equipment helps to "convince" others that you have a "true, real condition".

Equipment can make people in your environment feel psychologically safe too! People worry less about falls and your dependence.

Equipment may act as a barrier towards people in your environment approaching you, particularly people you don't want approaching you. Equipment may serve as a protection mechanism for some people with FND who are in difficult home situations or relationships.

Equipment can be a way of creating social belonging, for example it can get someone, who is stuck indoors due to mobility problems, out of the house and engage with social activities.

Not feeling "whole" without it, having used the equipment for a long time, it has become part of a person's identity, with some people giving the equipment a special name.

In some people: it protects against self-harm; it restricts access to the means to hurt yourself.

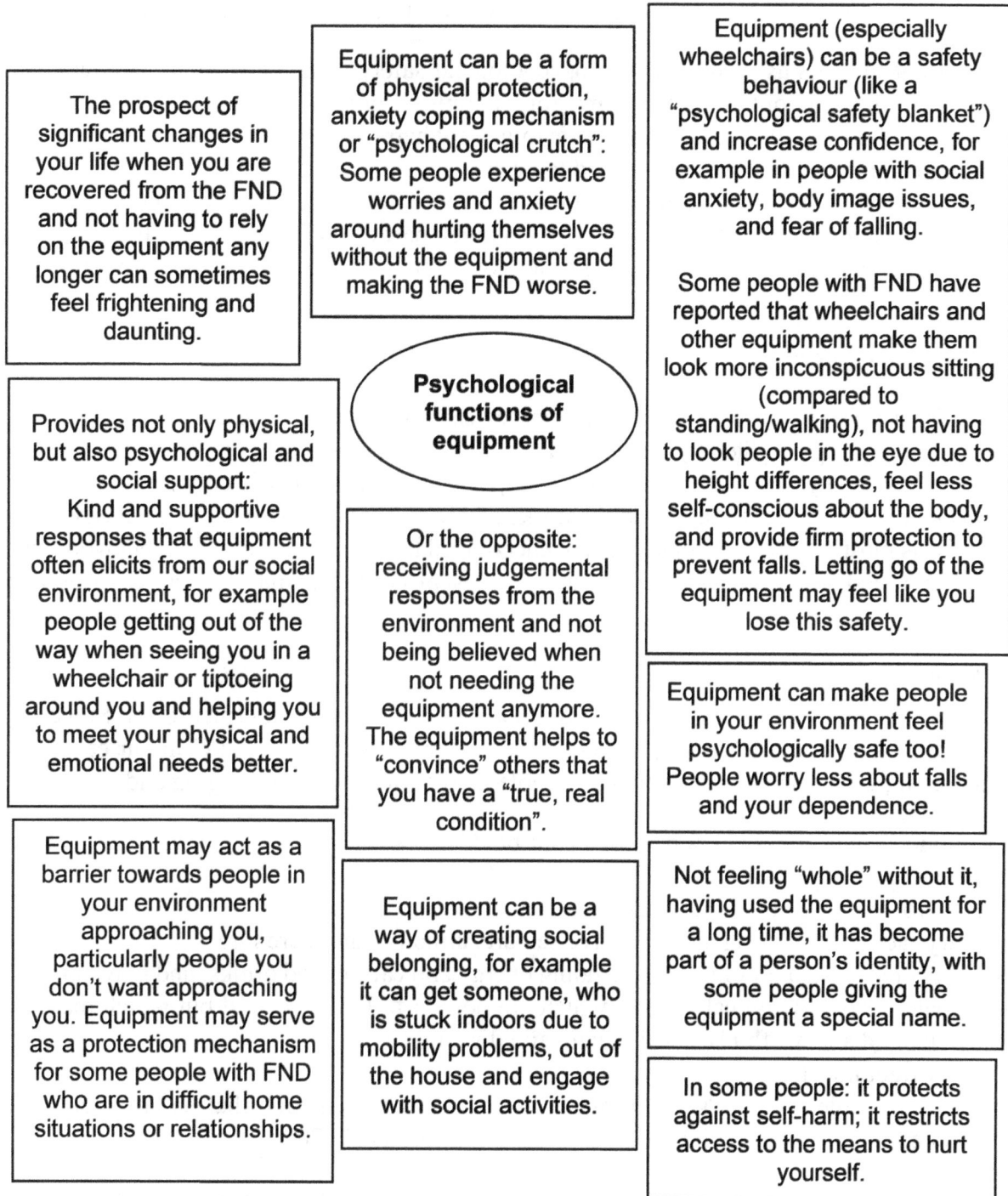

Figure 8.9 Psychological functions of equipment in people with and without FND.

in your body; you may be moving differently, using different muscles, and experience different sensations. These body changes can impact on how we feel, since the body and mind are strongly interconnected.

You may also lose your sense of psychological safety. People with FND sometimes say, 'Thanks to the equipment, I was finally able to leave my house, see people and go places, feel part of society again', 'It gave me back my independence', 'My wheelchair gave me more confidence than I had before', 'People were kind/a lot kinder to me'.

Not letting go of equipment despite the 'go ahead' from your treating team is problematic:

- Equipment may act as a physical and psychological safety behaviour. Safety behaviours can stop us from testing out our worst fears (for example, 'I will fall and injure myself'). But we will not find out that our deep-seated fears might not happen in the first place if we keep holding on to equipment that we are allowed to drop.
- Holding on to equipment for longer will make us more reliant, and the FND more entrenched. This means that the equipment has become so much part of our daily life, routines, and occasionally, identity that it becomes harder to let go and believe that you can do without.

8.4 eResource alert!

Dropping a piece of equipment can be a psychologically powerful experience, as part of positive risk-taking, to help you literally move on in life. Read here about how you can set up a behavioural experiment yourself. Please note that it is very important to closely collaborate with your physio- or occupational therapist, and that these experts have given you the 'go ahead'. This exercise is most helpful for people who are encouraged to step down equipment, but worry and feel fear around 'letting go', for example about the last piece of equipment in their rehab journey.

Liquids and bladder problems

Bladder and continence issues are quite common in people with FND (please see Stone et al., 2010; Hoeritzauer et al., 2016; Nielsen et al., 2017; Panicker et al., 2020; Gilmour et al., 2020; Bennett et al., 2021). The types of bladder problems reported are wide-ranging and include:

- Incontinence and a loss of control over your bladder.
- Not feeling an urge or sensing when your bladder is full.
- Unable to void or empty your bladder entirely.
- Urinary 'accidents' during a dissociative seizure, although these are rare.
- Some people drink a lot of fluids, including energy and caffeinated drinks, and may not be able to urinate for psychological reasons which are not yet fully understood but which make their bladders hold a lot of fluids, causing pain and discomfort.
- Urinary tract infections.
- A condition called Fowler's syndrome, a form of urinary retention that has frequently been associated with FND (Hoeritzauer et al., 2016; Gilmour et al., 2020).

Urinary issues require some people with FND to wear incontinence pads, self-catheterise, or more rarely, wear an in-dwelling or suprapubic catheter. This carries risks, requiring close monitoring for infections and skin breakdown.

Generally, bladder issues are **not always actively treated** in people with FND, unless the continence problems are severe, the main bothersome symptom of FND, result in serious and frequent infections or injuries, and require complex care and equipment.

Other reasons include:

- **Reduced awareness and knowledge** on how to treat functional bladder problems.
- **Lack of specialist continence nursing support** available for people with FND.
- The **'overshadowing'** of other FND symptoms, like dissociative seizures and limb weakness, over bladder issues. When people self-catheterise and manage relatively well without any difficulty, then clinical attention often gets geared towards treating the more urgent FND symptoms that more strongly impact on daily life.

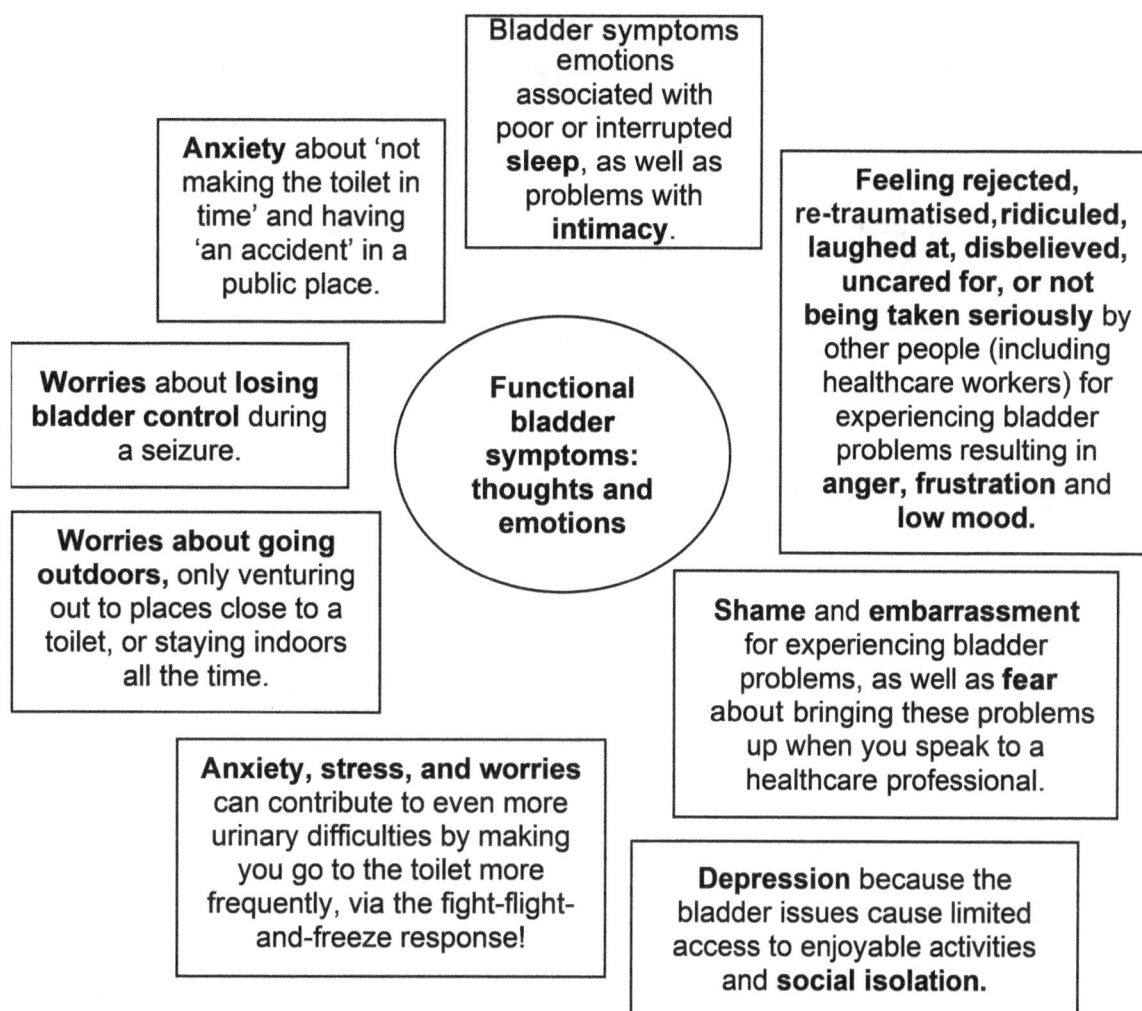

Bladder symptoms emotions associated with poor or interrupted **sleep**, as well as problems with **intimacy**.

Anxiety about 'not making the toilet in time' and having 'an accident' in a public place.

Worries about **losing bladder control** during a seizure.

Worries about going outdoors, only venturing out to places close to a toilet, or staying indoors all the time.

Functional bladder symptoms: thoughts and emotions

Feeling rejected, re-traumatised, ridiculed, laughed at, disbelieved, uncared for, or not being taken seriously by other people (including healthcare workers) for experiencing bladder problems resulting in **anger, frustration** and **low mood.**

Shame and **embarrassment** for experiencing bladder problems, as well as **fear** about bringing these problems up when you speak to a healthcare professional.

Anxiety, stress, and worries can contribute to even more urinary difficulties by making you go to the toilet more frequently, via the fight-flight-and-freeze response!

Depression because the bladder issues cause limited access to enjoyable activities and **social isolation.**

Figure 8.10 Difficult thoughts and feelings around bladder functioning in FND.

- Like the all-important topic of good bowel movements, people are often reluctant to openly discuss issues about what is happening 'down below', due to **embarrassment and shame**. There is no need to – our bladder and passing urine are all part of our biological make-up and deserve our attention!

Urinary problems are often viewed and managed from a physical perspective. But did you know that emotions play a major role in bladder issues? (see Figure 8.10).

Management of bladder difficulties in FND

- **Do not ignore!** Put any feelings of embarrassment aside, and always discuss with your healthcare provider as part of your FND care plan.
- If possible, ask for a **review with a continence nurse**, preferably specialising in FND. The continence nurse may suggest bladder scans and helpful strategies, such as:
  - Improving your bladder routine and hygiene where necessary.
  - Double voiding and sitting a bit longer on the toilet to make sure that your bladder is empty.
  - Limiting your fluid intake right before bed so you do not have to interrupt your sleep and come out of bed at night.
  - Providing 'bladder education' on poor management strategies, for example, on the harmful effects of drinking too little or too many fluids.

- Sometimes, **loved ones** can become very involved in intimate care for bladder dysfunction, even though the person may be able to do their own independent bladder management. Read more about boundaries in Chapter 10.
- Bladder problems may also take on a **social function**, for example, act like a **deterrent and protection** towards another person getting intimate or seeking proximity. In extreme and rare situations, bladder problems can serve as a **form of self-harm, control,** or **a way of communicating emotional distress** to other people, for example, by not going to the toilet after ingesting a lot of fluids.
- Sometimes, bladder problems are better viewed as **one of the many manifestations** of an underlying process of dissociation rather than focusing treatment on each symptom alone. It is not uncommon for people's bladder problems to spontaneously resolve after movement, seizures, and emotional difficulties improve. It is like tackling your main FND symptoms has a **knock-on effect** on bladder issues.

Fight-or-flight

The fight-or-flight element of the pot represents the unique physiological effects and 'biological signature' of emotions: what happens in the body when you experience an emotion (see Chapter 7). Let us take a look at one of the most commonly reported emotions in people with and without FND: anxiety.

Imagine that you are going for a hike in a remote forest

Suddenly you spot a bear. What would you do? Notice how the question was phrased: 'What would you **do**?' Most people would probably try to run away and flee the bear. A rare few people may feel brave enough to fight the bear in self-defence. But you can assume that pretty much everyone would somehow 'get into action', and quick! This is called the **fight-or-flight response**. People with FND occasionally describe a third response called **'freeze'**, where people are so anxious and overwhelmed that they are unable to move and do anything, feeling paralysed and 'frozen in fear' for a period of time.

People have recently been talking about two more anxiety- and threat-related responses called fawn and flop. **Fawn** refers to a response characterised by complying and putting other people's needs and emotions ahead of your own to protect yourself, not speaking your truth and being your authentic self, a bit like a person with a tight cover who bottles up feelings. **Flop** is quite similar to what we see in someone experiencing a dissociative seizure and falling to the floor, with floppy limbs and loss of awareness and responsiveness. Although the discussion will focus mostly on the fight-or-flight response, it is always good to keep the remaining three responses in mind because they are relevant for people with FND.

What do you think would happen if our brains had developed in such a way that we did not have a fight-or-flight response?

We would first need to try to recognise and identify what it is that we have in front of us and take some time to deliberate on the correct course of action. This would not be good for our survival in the world! By the time that we have decided that it is indeed a bear that may try to attack and eat us, it would have likely already eaten us. Our emotions, in this case anxiety, prepare our body for action (fight, flight, freeze, fawn, and flop) **without much thinking**. Emotions are therefore **protecting** us from harm.

How does the fight-or-flight response work on a more neurological level? What happens
in our brains when we feel anxiety?

An American researcher called Dr Joseph LeDoux (1996, 2003) proposed the dual pathway model of fear, which describes two routes in the brain: the **slow route** ('high road') and the **quick and dirty route** ('low road'). The best way to explain the dual pathway model is by imagining another frightening animal: a snake. One day, you are walking in a garden. All of a sudden, you see a snake in your grass patch. We have two roads in the brain: the high road and the low road. When we see a threatening object (like a snake), these two roads in our brain become simultaneously activated.

The high road is a slow road and runs through a part called the cerebral cortex. The high road helps you recognise that what you see is a snake: 'It is green and writhing on the ground. It is long and thin. Mmm, this may be a snake.' You also become consciously aware of the danger and know, 'Uh-oh, this is a snake. It is dangerous. I have got to get out now!' Just having a high road is not great for survival. Like with the bear, we would be too late with realizing that it is a snake. By that time, the snake may already have attacked and bitten us, and we may not survive.

Luckily, we also have a low road in our brain. The low road is much quicker than the high road. You see a snake and the signal is transmitted to a brain region called the amygdala.

It is almond-shaped, and we have two of them, one in each hemisphere of the brain. The amygdala is an important area for anxiety with different compartments that are crucial for the fight-or-flight response, with connections to other parts of the brain (like the periaqueductal grey) important for regulating heart rate, blood pressure, pain, as well as escape and freezing behaviours.

The amygdala activates the fight-or-flight response in the body. We do not become conscious of the snake. We do not think long and hard, 'Might this be a snake?' 'Could it be dangerous?' 'Or poisonous?' We just quickly act. This saves us time, and we have a higher chance for survival.

What happens to people without amygdalae?

There have been rare reports of people without amygdalae in the research literature who do not feel fear despite feeling other emotions (Feinstein et al., 2011) and struggle with recognising and making social judgements about whether a person is approachable and trustworthy (Adolphs et al., 1998), both skills you need for your 'survival' in day-to-day life.

Does the amygdala play a role in FND?

Yes, the amygdala appears to be quite an important structure in people with FND. The activity in the amygdala region in response to fearful faces compared to happy faces showed no difference in people with FND as compared to those without FND. People with FND also showed greater connections between the amygdala and a brain area important for the preparation of movements (Voon et al., 2010) as well as more activity in the amygdala during an experimental movement task compared to control participants (Voon et al., 2011).

Fight-or-flight in constant overdrive: panic attacks

Some people with FND may misinterpret a physical symptom that is part of the normal biological response of anxiety in the body (for example, feeling dizzy, sweaty, or shaky) as something threatening ('These dizziness, sweatiness, and shakiness symptoms mean that I am going to have a stroke/heart attack/fall down/faint/have a dissociative seizure').

What happens in the body during the fight-or-flight response?

Did you know that some of these fight-or-flight symptoms overlap with FND symptoms? Some people's FND symptoms can be fully or partially explained by this response! A hopeful message, because a lot of useful psychological strategies can help, including learning to recognise the fight-or-flight response in your own body, breathing exercises, cognitive reframing techniques, and behavioural experiments.

What do the body changes in the fight-or-flight response have to do with dissociation?

Occasionally, people with FND may experience all the physical symptoms of a certain emotion **but do not 'experience' or 'feel' the same emotion in a psychological sense.** Our body may feel it, but our mind and heart do not. **There is a disconnection between the body and the mind.**

Look back at the biological signatures of each emotion in Table 7.8 in Chapter 7. Do you notice any similarities between the physical effects of different emotions on the body? Just relying on our bodily symptoms to make sense of what emotion we are dealing with may not be the most optimal strategy. We could make errors in judging the correct emotion! Think, for example, about the difference between anxiety and anger and the impact on our body: both emotions make your heart rate go up, make you feel sweaty, warm, and hot, and make your muscles tense up. There are more similarities than differences! Therefore, it is no surprise that people sometimes mix these emotions up.

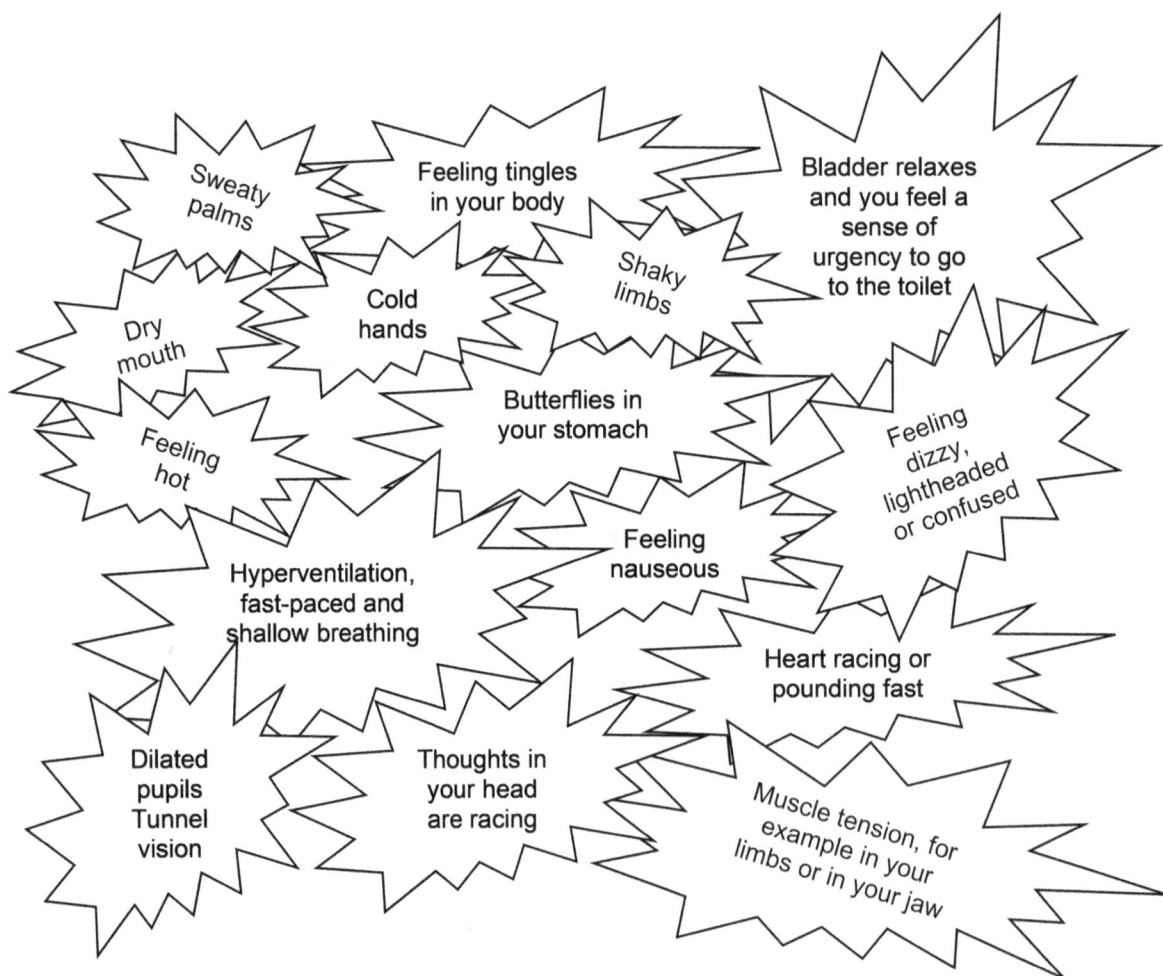

Figure 8.11 Bodily changes during the fight-or-flight response.

For the recognition of emotions, it will probably be a better strategy to not only rely on the biological signature but also somehow **try to reconnect with our emotional experience**, 'the way emotions subjectively feel'. Luckily, we can try to help 'bring emotions back' with the emotion exercises described in the 7.19 **eResource alert!** earlier.

Contacts

Another important part of the FND SELF-CARE acronym is 'contacts'. This refers to the often-increased number of contacts between people with FND, healthcare staff, and social care professionals (see, for example, Razvi et al., 2012; Nunez-Wallace et al., 2015; Merkler et al., 2016; Ladha et al., 2017; Kyle & Wu, 2020; Finkelstein et al., 2021; Stephen et al., 2021). Table 8.1 shows some of the patient- and system-related reasons that people with FND tend to be connected to so many health services.

8.5 eResource alert!

Here you can find a list of health and social care contacts that have been reported by people with FND and their families, as well as some background information on an unhelpful term often used in FND called 'healthcare utilisation'.

Emotions can increase healthcare contacts

- **(Health) anxiety** about developing a very serious illness and understandably checking out and seeking reassurance on new symptoms to ensure nothing is missed.
- Feeling **hopeless** and **powerless** about not receiving care and support for managing FND symptoms from professionals who may have discharged you, and now you are 'grasping for straws'.
- **Frustration, anger,** and **low mood** about not being believed and 'left to your own devices' in the context of previous healthcare or personal experiences. Accessing healthcare may communicate and help convince a professional about the legitimacy and justification of a person's symptoms (please note that the symptoms are still real and genuine). People with FND sometimes feel angry about healthcare professionals who attribute everything to the FND ('diagnostic overshadowing').
- **Confusion** and **mixed feelings** about the diagnosis – both from people with FND and healthcare professionals who both may seek organic/biological explanations for the symptoms. Healthcare professionals are not always up to speed with FND or may not know how to treat or what to do with a person with FND, resulting in more investigations and referrals elsewhere.
- **Compassion**, **empathy**, and **sympathy** from healthcare professionals that meet a need that is not met in other relationships in the person's life.
- **Difficult family dynamics at home** may contribute to the new or a worsening of FND symptoms, resulting in more healthcare contacts.

Increased healthcare contacts can maintain FND

Although, on the surface, you might ask yourself, 'What do healthcare contacts have to do with maintaining FND?' **Healthcare contacts are a very important part of the FND recovery journey**. Researchers have discovered unhelpful 'interaction cycles' between people with FND and healthcare professionals (Barnett et al., 2022).

- Relationships are a key area in FND – although the relationship between a person with FND and a healthcare professional is therapeutic in nature and not personal (like with a partner,

Table 8.1 Patient and system ('environmental') factors determining increased healthcare contacts for people with FND and their healthcare professionals

Patient factors	System factors
"Heterogeneity" of FND symptoms • FND affects the entire neurological system and produces a wide variety of different symptoms in people, for example tremors, weakness, seizures, brain fog. • FND is often part of a wider spectrum of functional problems that affect other bodily systems: irritable bowel syndrome, chronic pain, fibromyalgia, Ehlers-Danlos, and chronic fatigue syndrome.	**FND requires multidisciplinary treatment** • FND affects the body and mind and is often treated by a multidisciplinary team consisting of different healthcare professionals. • It is logical that with so many disciplines involved, the number of healthcare contacts also increases.
Peaks and troughs of FND • Waxing and waning, an unpredictable course and uncertainty about new FND symptoms make new investigations and healthcare visits more likely. • Imagine experiencing a set-back, like sudden leg weakness. It makes sense that you would like to check this out, in case it is something that requires urgent treatment.	**Lack of awareness, under recognition and confusion on FND in healthcare professionals.** • Although nowadays there is a lot more awareness on FND, there are still professionals who do not know or understand FND. Inappropriate referrals are made to professionals who they think may know more and can help.
New symptoms • People with FND often report new symptoms. Sometimes, FND morphs in appearance over time, for example from dissociative seizures to functional weakness. Naturally, you would like to investigate this.	**Low confidence in own skills** • Professionals may still not always feel confident about making an FND diagnosis or have faith in their own skills. They want to make sure and not miss anything, worry about misdiagnosis and order investigations just to be sure. • This lack of confidence may also result in passing a person with FND from pillar to post (avoidance). Healthcare professionals may not want or do not know how to deal with the patient, so refer them onwards to another professional.
Physical conditions predating the FND • Some people have other conditions that predate the FND, in addition to the FND, for example diabetes, high blood pressure, asthma.	**Lack of joined-up care in FND** • Multiple healthcare professionals prescribing medications, investigations or treatments without communicating to one another or being aware of each other's work on the person with FND.
A safe haven • Not knowing where else to go. Left to your own devices, A&E seems like the only option where you can get help for the symptoms.	**Lack of specialist FND services** • The system is currently not built to receive and treat the ever-increasing number of people with FND that still need treatment. People subsequently end up in other services to get help but these are often not the right services.

family member, or friend), **a healthcare relationship is still a relationship between two people** that has the potential to become a source of difficulty as well as strength.

- Good relationships are based on good communication, honesty, empathy, appropriate boundaries, as well as feeling believed, cared for, accepted, and validated. The **interactions between people with FND and healthcare professionals** are not always characterised by these features and **can break down** at times (systemic re-traumatisation; read more about this in Chapter 9).
- A **current healthcare relationship can re-trigger old hurts from past relationships**. Not feeling believed and cared for and being rejected by people may have happened to you in the past in the context of childhood, personal, and family relationships. A new relationship – including a 'healthcare relationship' – may resemble earlier traumatic or difficult relationship experiences and can **re-trigger** similar distressing thoughts and feelings, not always on a conscious level of awareness. People may feel 'irked' and psychologically unwell, uncomfortable, or distressed but unsure about underlying reasons.
- All these examples can **trigger** and **maintain FND**.

Strategies you and your family can try to improve the quality of healthcare contacts

- **Obtain an official diagnosis and a proper explanation of FND.** Factors that have been found to reduce healthcare contacts in FND include receiving a positive diagnosis of FND as well as a clear and accurate explanation of FND. Having these two conditions met is also essential for accessing the right treatment for your symptoms.
- **Allow and actively encourage your information to be shared** between all your healthcare professionals so that investigations are not unnecessarily repeated and to help improve communication by 'joining up' the dots of your healthcare.
- **Complete a structured FND diary (see the 7.5 eResource** for more information). It is not unheard of that people may experience increased or more intense FND symptoms before, during, or after a consultation with a healthcare professional. When this happens quite often, try to complete an FND diary to find out whether something about that healthcare contact and interaction may have elicited or re-triggered feelings of discomfort or distress.
- **In some situations, trying to self-manage the FND in the first instance may be more helpful**, for example, by reflecting on the strategies from the book that you have learned so far. This obviously does not mean that your symptoms are not real or should not be taken seriously.

Let us think about dissociative seizures, for which people seek medical help. Some people visit the emergency department on a weekly or monthly basis or call an ambulance every time they experience an episode – despite investigations demonstrating that the episodes are non-epileptic in nature and do not require urgent care. The person and their family may struggle to tolerate the discomfort or distress around experiencing or witnessing these symptoms.

- **Make a plan about what you will do when you develop a new symptom.** It is sensible to get yourself checked out in case the symptom is something serious that needs medical and urgent attention. You are completely right in doing that. Just because you have FND does not mean that you cannot also develop other physical symptoms. In the eyes of a healthcare professional, FND may become like a big flashing light that takes full centre stage and **overshadows** any other physical difficulties that a person may have. People worry about missing serious physical health issues, as well as not feeling believed, cared for, and validated.
- For some people, however, the number of healthcare contacts can increase quite substantially. You may find yourself visiting the accidents and emergencies department or your general practitioner on a frequent basis, with professionals telling you each time that your symptom is not life-threatening.

If this happens a lot in your life and you develop new symptoms quite regularly that have repeatedly been reassured and checked over by healthcare professionals, it may be worth thinking about whether some of these healthcare contacts have become **safety behaviours** for you and your family. After seeing a professional, people tend to feel more reassured, especially if the symptoms caused high levels of discomfort or anxiety beforehand. These visits reduce distress and discomfort in the short term but may not be a viable solution in the long term because they take away your precious time and attention from other meaningful activities and relationships in your life and do not address the real root of the problem.

Did you know that regular healthcare visits at the same locations can create a **self-fulfilling prophecy**? Every time you are sent away by a healthcare professional, or clinical service, the experience may make you feel not believed, rejected, or abandoned, and it may erode your trust in the healthcare system – exactly the things that people often fear. What is worse, **it could make it harder to overcome FND**. Some healthcare contacts will be experienced as pleasant and validating, whereas other interactions the exact opposite: unpleasant and rejecting. Not everyone in the healthcare world is kind to people with FND. This mixture of positive and negative responses can become part of what is called an **intermittent reinforcement** schedule and maintain the FND (see Chapters 9 and 10 for more information on this topic).

Ability to care for self

People with FND can struggle with any of the activities of daily living (ADLs) displayed in Figures 8.12 and 8.13 due to a variety of symptoms, including loss of function and strength in your

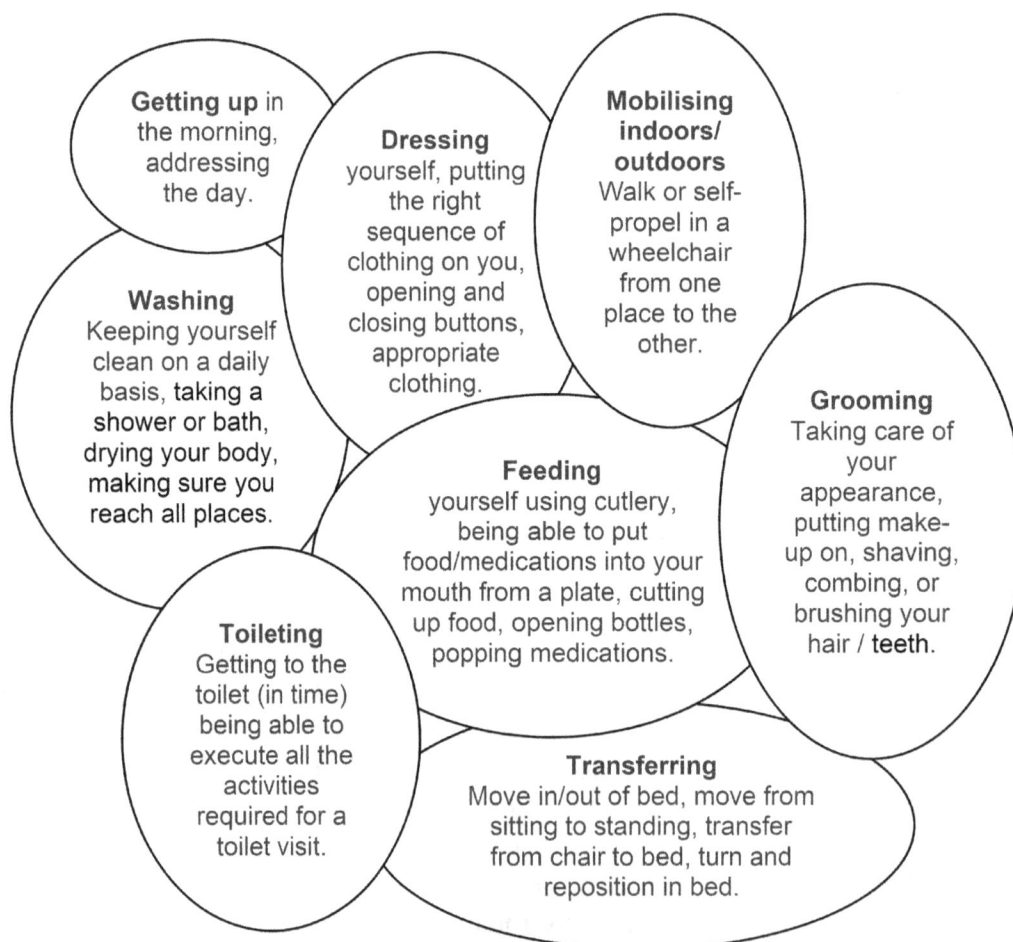

Figure 8.12 Basic/personal activities of daily living ('PADLS').

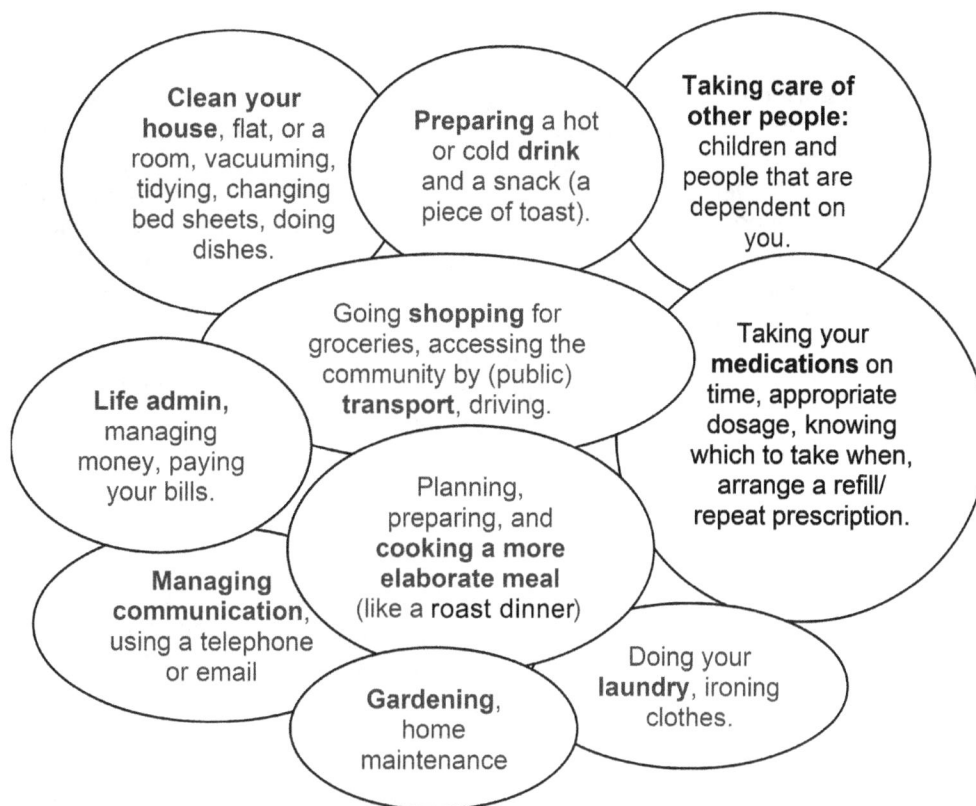

Figure 8.13 Instrumental/domestic activities of daily living ('DADLS').

limbs; restricted range of movement; shaking and jerking; dissociative seizures; problems with memory, concentration, sequencing, and brain fog; sensory sensitivities; as well as issues with balance and dizziness.

There is a wide scope of abilities ranging from fully independent, no help needed; supervision only but otherwise independent; assistance of one or two people required to complete the activity safely and effectively; and full dependency, with another person doing the activity.

Tips to improve your ADLs

- Complete a **Pressure Cooker chain reaction** for yourself and your family! Where can you break the links to reduce FND and therefore help improve ADLs? Remember, although not everyone will achieve 100% recovery, **FND is a potentially reversible condition**, and so is the quality of ADLs. For some people, it is possible to get their full "pre-FND" independence back.
- Did you know that compromised ADLs can stir up all sorts of different emotions? Vice versa, emotions can also heavily impact on disabilities in day-to-day life. Have a look at Figure 8.14 and find out about how **underlying emotions** – irrespective of whether ADLs adversely impact on how you feel or the other way around – play a role in your own ADLs. The 'direction of travel' does not really matter: any emotion, regardless of its origin, can maintain FND.
- It is not just the emotions of a person with FND that impact on ADLs. **Partners, families, and friends** can experience **very similar emotions**, including anxiety, low mood, anger, frustration, but also resentment and compassion 'fatigue'. It is equally important to watch out for a carer's own distress.

Fear and sadness around losing relationships with carers or losing a tight-knitted relationship that has grown closer and that was otherwise more distant when ADLs were less impacted.

Anxiety and fears around going out/ accessing your community: it becomes harder to 'take the plunge' leave the house and meet people.

Low mood and depression because of a lack of enjoyable/meaningful activities, mental stimulation, not being able to access the community, or connecting socially with other people in real life.

Emotions in the context of disabilities/ affected activities in daily life.

Shame / embarrassment about not being able to work and fulfil your usual family role, for example as the 'head' providing financially.

Guilt about not being able to take care of yourself, help in the household, resulting in dependency and additional stress on a "stretched" partner or family.

Very understandable feelings of **resentment**, maybe **envy**, around other people being able to do the things they can do but you are not. A desire to be able to do similar activities.

Fear of the unknown/recovery Becoming more independent with ADLs may result in a return to prior challenging life circumstances; new psychological pressure and increased demands from partners/family because you are viewed as "nearly there" or "cured". People may not see the invisible disabilities you're still grappling with.

Fear of falling Walking practice and improving independence may stall as you may not feel ready to let go of equipment or take your equipment with you at all times 'just in case' you may fall.

Lack of confidence resulting in **anxiety** and **low mood**. You may not believe in yourself that you will be able to manage activities in daily life independently without support.

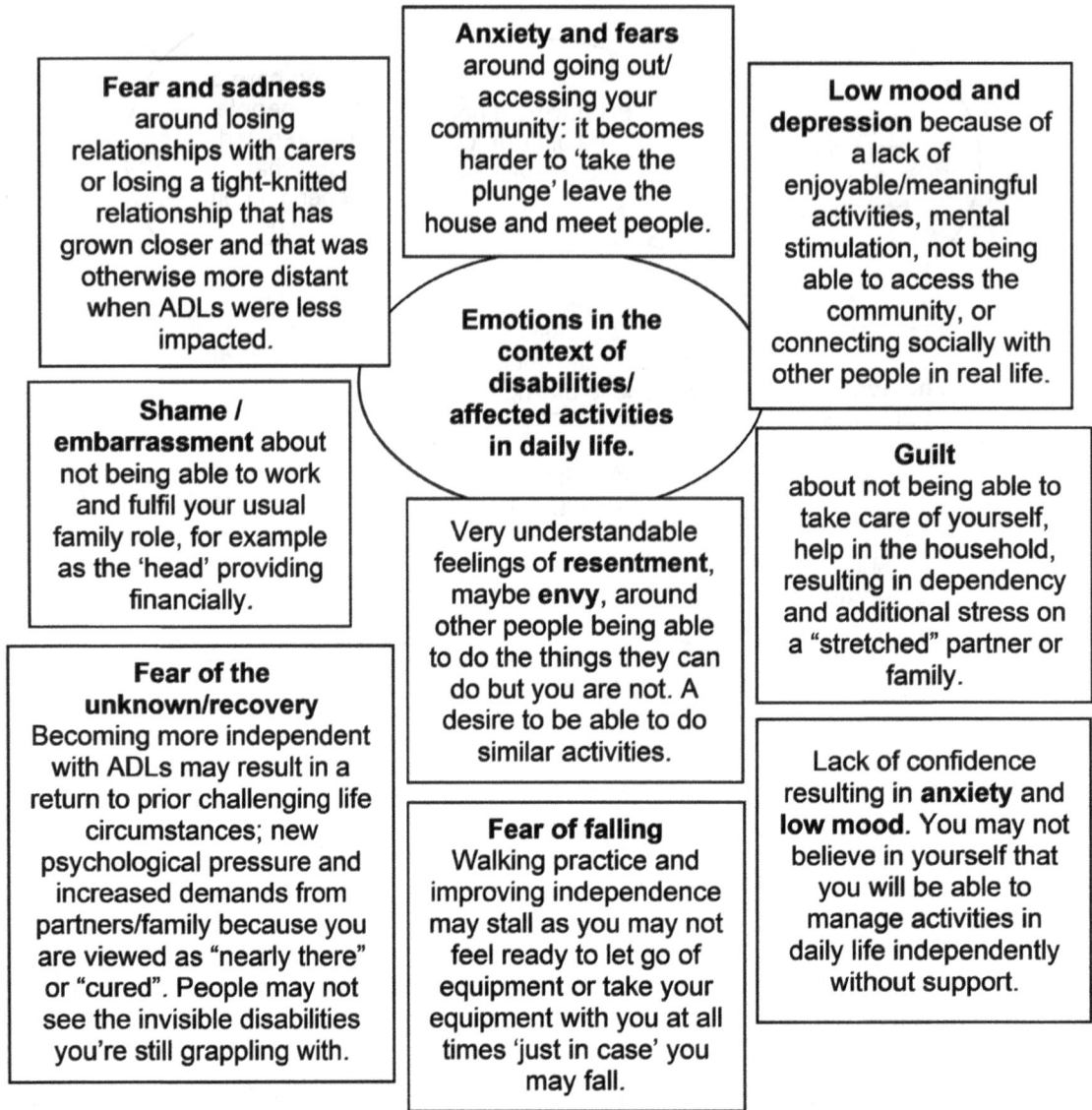

Figure 8.14 Emotions in ADLs reported by people with FND.

- Any emotion will impact on a family's own coping strategies, sometimes with unhelpful, but very understandable, responses. It is normal for family to take chores away if a person is too disabled. How else is the person going to complete their ADLs? The other side of the coin is that the people closest to you **can unintentionally maintain the FND and dependency in daily life** by exactly that: doing too much, 'always on standby', and removing opportunities that enable the person to practice skills that help towards independence and ultimately overcome the FND.

- As you can see from Figure 8.14, emotions in ADLs are often intricately linked with **relationships** between people with and without FND. Some people feel **socially isolated** because of disabilities and develop new friendships with carers or much closer ties with family. Occasionally, people struggle with increased independence and the prospect of losing those close relationships, with an increased risk of social isolation.

- You might wonder, 'There are so many ADLs – what do I start working on?'

  - Look at **quick wins**: which ADLs could quickly improve?
  - Focus on **simple ADLs** first, and master **complex ADLs** later to increase your sense of achievement and confidence in the process.

- Any **enjoyable ADLs** you have missed doing and make you feel good about yourself?
- **Urgent ADLs** that could relieve you and your family?

- **Boom-and-bust cycles** loom in the background and are often a sensitive area in FND. When you work on ADLs, always **try to pace yourself** sufficiently but to such an extent that you feel slightly out of your comfort zone and you are really **challenging yourself**.
- Over the years, some people accumulate heaps of aids and home adaptations. Totally understandable if you are dealing with disabilities on a day-to-day basis. However, equipment use in FND has its downsides too. **Equipment is intricately linked with ADLs**: the more you work on your independence, the less likely you need to rely on equipment.
- It is often very helpful to obtain advice from **specialist occupational therapists** and **physiotherapists** familiar with supporting people with FND in regaining independence in ADLs. That said, a **closely collaborating multidisciplinary team** remains the gold standard, especially if you have a care package and experience a high level of disability in your day-to-day life.

Importantly, the way that FND symptoms prevent or interrupt a person's day-to-day activities can cause risks to the person as well as people in their environment. Let us take a closer look at risks in FND in the next section.

Risks

Figure 8.16 shows some of the most common risks found for people with FND who were admitted for a period of inpatient neurorehabilitation in the context of severe and long-standing FND. Please note that this is not an unusual graph at all, as quite a few of these risks have been observed across all levels of severity and durations of FND and affect all aspects of the FND: the body, mind, as well as social and relationship functioning.

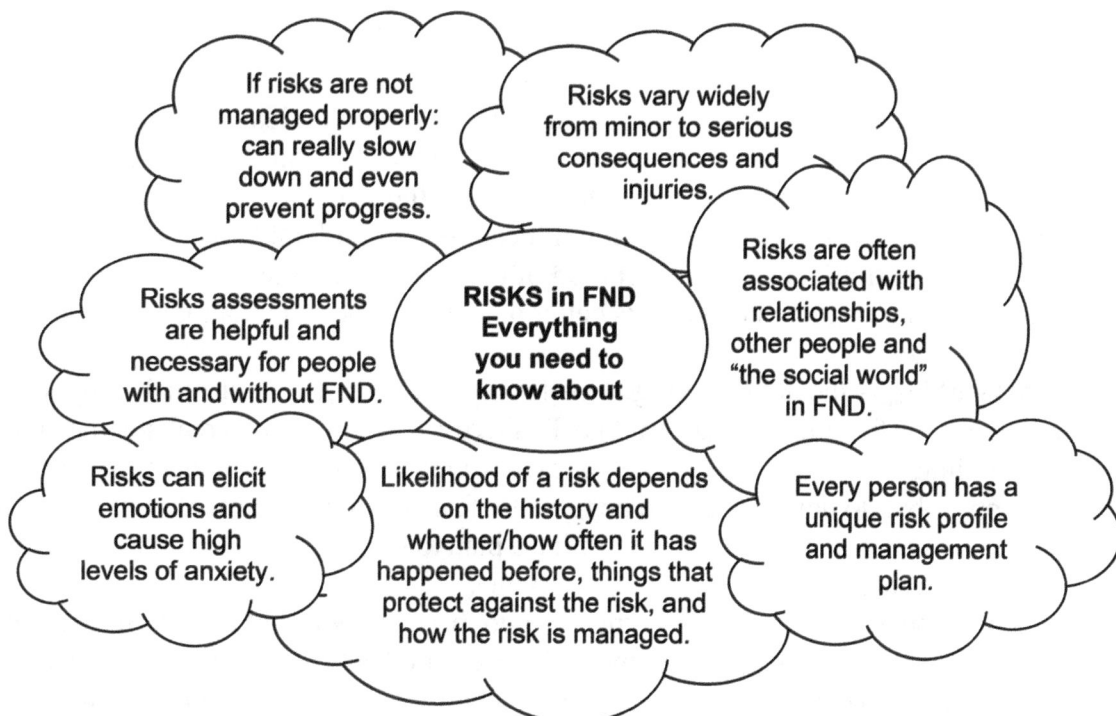

Figure 8.15 Risks in FND.

Figure 8.16 -
Top 11 most frequent risk types in FND

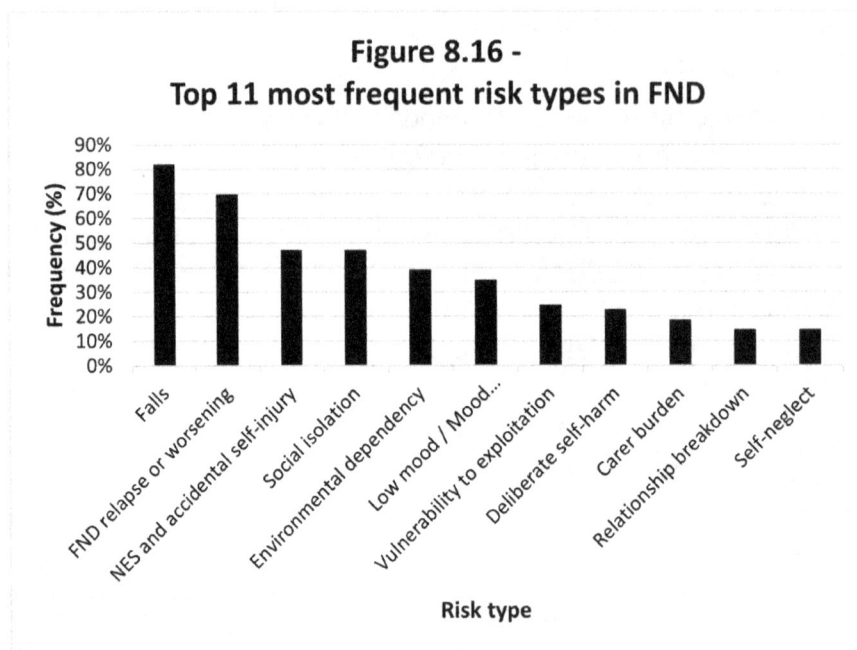

Figure 8.16 Top 11 most frequent risk types in FND.

Note: NES = non-epileptic episode; environmental dependency = reliance on family, carers, or support staff for activities in daily life.

8.6 eResource alert!

For a full list of risks described by, and observed in, people with FND, check the eResource. The list of risks is long, but that does not mean that everyone experiences all these risks. This is just to help you become aware of your personal risk profile so that you can make a clear management plan to reduce any risks to you and your family.

What can I and my environment do if we feel afraid of the risks?

- **Write down** your biggest fears about risks and their likelihood in detail, particularly for low-level risks that cause disproportionate, excessive and unnecessary anxiety. Re-read your worries multiple times and vividly experience the fears that the words may elicit in you. Learn to sit with the distress and you will see how it will become more tolerable over time.
- **Face your fears, particularly if the likelihood of the risk is managed well with a firm plan!** Dipping your toe into unknown territory is better than doing nothing about it at all and keeping the status quo.
- **Positive risk-taking** is the act of taking steps towards recovery in your rehab fully knowing that there is a chance that the risk may emerge. Positive risk-taking with a realistic management plan is a good thing as it helps you test out your fears. Get used to the idea that there is a chance that risks happen, but do not let your life be ruled by fear. **Who is in control: you or the fear?** Risk assessments are there to help you determine a plan to minimise fears around, for example, injuries. There is a safety plan out there for everyone.
- If the problem is about your family struggling to let go, **become aware of each other's emotions**. It is surprising how little we sometimes know about each other's fears and worries. Most commonly, this is because **we do not want to burden the other person**, do not know how to express our emotions, or find it a strange experience and prefer to avoid this altogether. All very reasonable, but not helping the cause. Sometimes, the act of communication is half the battle. **Communicating feared risks** ('opening the cover') can be very therapeutic and take away the edge.

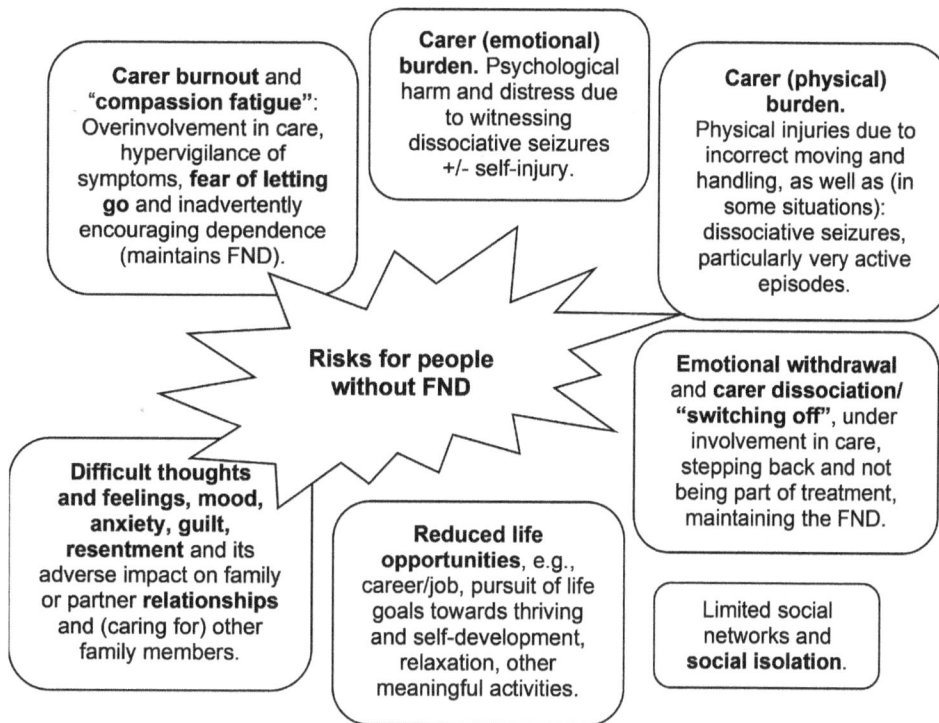

Figure 8.17 Common risks for people without FND who care for people with FND.

- **Family matters!** Risks are about people with and without FND. Did you know that risk management is a **joint undertaking** – just like everybody contributes to FND, everyone chips in and makes changes to reduce risks. For example, your physio has said you are safe to drop a piece of equipment. You need to take a 'risk', but your family equally may need to let go of their own fears and enable you to take that risk.
- **Carer self-care.** Understandably, the focus of treatment is often on the person carrying the FND symptoms. However, considering the physical, psychological, and social risks conveyed in Figure 8.17, the **well-being** of the person without FND is **equally important**. Carer strategies might involve:

  - 'Me time' for regular relaxation, social connection, or pursuit of life goals.
  - Moving and handling advice from physiotherapy and occupational therapy professionals.
  - Respite or a care package with external carers.
  - Psychological therapy for the carer themselves (though couples and family therapy is highly recommended for FND).
  - Explore the **interpersonal dynamic** between 'carer' and 'cared for'. Jump ahead to Chapter 9 and 10 explore how the concept of **reciprocal reinforcement** maintains FND and how completing two Pressure Cooker Models is always a helpful idea in the quest to overcome FND.

- **Contemplate the true risk of seizures.** Good questions to ask:

  - Is the likelihood of the risk emerging really that high and insurmountable?
  - What would be the worst thing that could happen?
  - If the worst thing would happen, what would be so bad about that?
  - If you experience brief 'switching off' seizures that no one notices, or longer episodes that people will notice but without self-injury, does it justify staying at home, or could you take a 'social risk', potentially experience the short seizure but enjoy the rest of your time out?

- Make a **family risk plan** like the one that follows (Table 8.2), and plan for the worst-case scenario if the risk occurs.

Table 8.2 Our family risk plan

Risk assessment	What is it?	Person with FND	Person without FND
Description of the risk	What exactly is the risk?	• Risk of a dissociative seizure in a shop, fall on the cold hard floor and accidentally hurting myself.	• Risk of not letting go of reassuring behaviours, prolonging the seizure.
Risk factors that increase the risk	What increases, maintains, and keeps the risk going? (Top tip: look at both of your Pressure Cooker Models!!).	• Keeping myself to myself and not speaking about my fears. • Staying at home, out of fear for a seizure and injuries. • Low self-confidence that I can manage this.	• My family hovering over me constantly, reassuring me, holding my hand. • Encouraging me to stay at home and taking chores out of my hands.
Protective factors ("Safety features")	What helps to reduce the risk?	• Good knowledge about seizure triggers, well-practiced strategies. • Treatment is effective: seizures have reduced in frequency, severity, and duration. • Fallen before but never seriously hurt myself. • No recent falls. • Learned to express difficult thoughts and feelings a little better.	• Everybody in the family is aware and fully supports the seizure management plan. • Good support network, family takes on board Pressure Cooker Model formulation. • We all have a positive mind-set.
Risk management	What strategies can I put in place to minimise the risk?	• Tell my family how I feel immediately before going into the shop. • Make a graded hierarchy: go to the corner shop with familiar and friendly staff initially rather than a big shopping centre. • Inform the shop staff in advance and share strategies ("stand back").	• Encourage the person to speak about feelings before the shop. • Don't hover like a helicopter over the person with FND but allow the person to use their own coping strategies. • Manage my own fears about the person's seizure and "stand back" to let them cope.
Emergency plan	What to do when the risk occurs?	• Make sure I am physically OK and then stand back. Something soft to protect my head. • If I hurt myself quite badly, seek medical help. • Try again and not let this hold me back!	• Briefly explain to bystanders to stand back and then continue the intervention. • Provide a seizure card, don't call an ambulance right away.

8.7 eResource alert!

Physical, psychological and social risks are common occurrences in FND. Therefore, everybody, whether you have or do not have FND, needs a proper risk assessment and management plan. Have a go at identifying your own risks, and complete a risk management plan together with your partner, family and/or friends.

Exercise, sports and movement

A tricky topic in FND

Exercise can be a difficult topic of discussion for people with FND. Some people with FND who are told to start exercising 'because [their] legs are fine' and 'there's nothing wrong with [their] nervous system' may feel not believed, invalidated in terms of their symptoms, and dismissed by healthcare professionals. Other people may have been pushed to be very active or not believed since childhood. Exercise can be a sensitive point and provoke a lot of distress for people with FND, including anger and frustration.

8.8 eResource alert!

Did you know that research studies have demonstrated increased brain activity after exercise, compared to before exercise, and that exercise just generally positively impacts on brain functioning? (see for instance the following scientific articles: Cotman & Engesser-Cesar, 2002; Crabbe & Dishman, 2004; Schneider et al., 2009). You may already know all of this, but have a read about the many physical, psychological and social benefits of exercise here.

8.9 eResource alert!

Check out some of the strategies that can help you alleviate a few of the barriers described in Figure 8.18. This is not intended to teach you about what your body can do or cannot do. It simply provides a guide to help you on the way to start thinking about or actually doing exercise.

Fear of falling

People whose FND symptoms affect their movements and walking ('motor-type FND' or FMD, functional movement disorder) can experience **falls** and report a **fear of falling**, although people with dissociative seizures are not exempt (see Figure 8.19).

8.10 eResource alert!

Read here about physical and psychological factors that make falls in people with FND more likely and, more importantly, read also about what some of the protective factors are that lower your risk against falls!

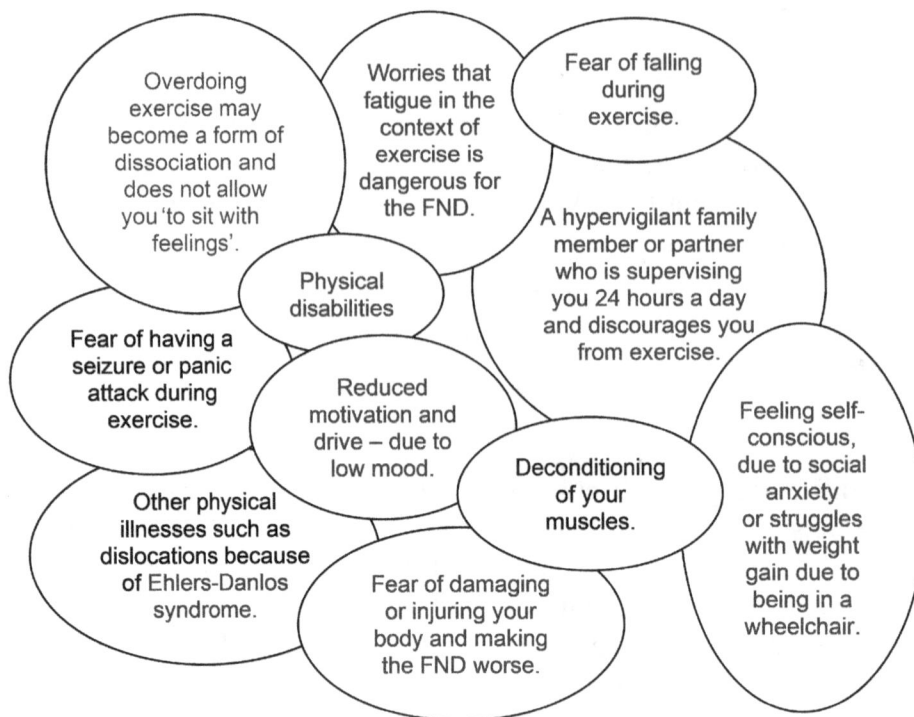

Figure 8.18 Barriers to exercise in people with FND.

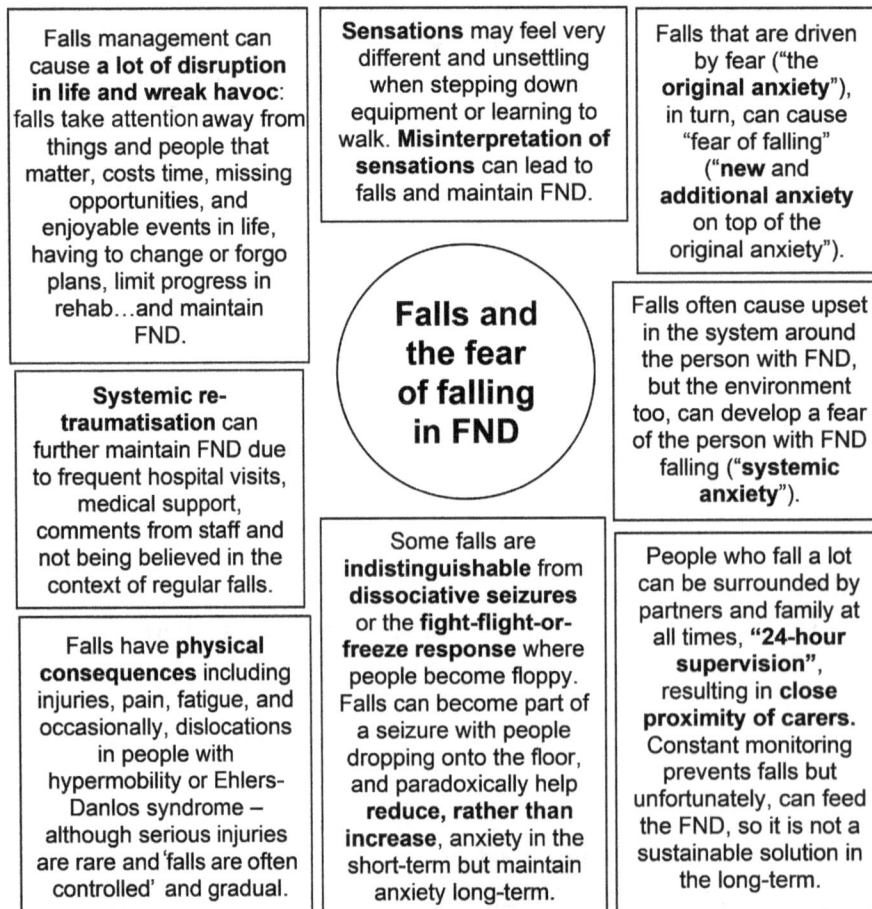

Figure 8.19 (The fear of) falling in FND.

How can the fear of falling keep the FND going?

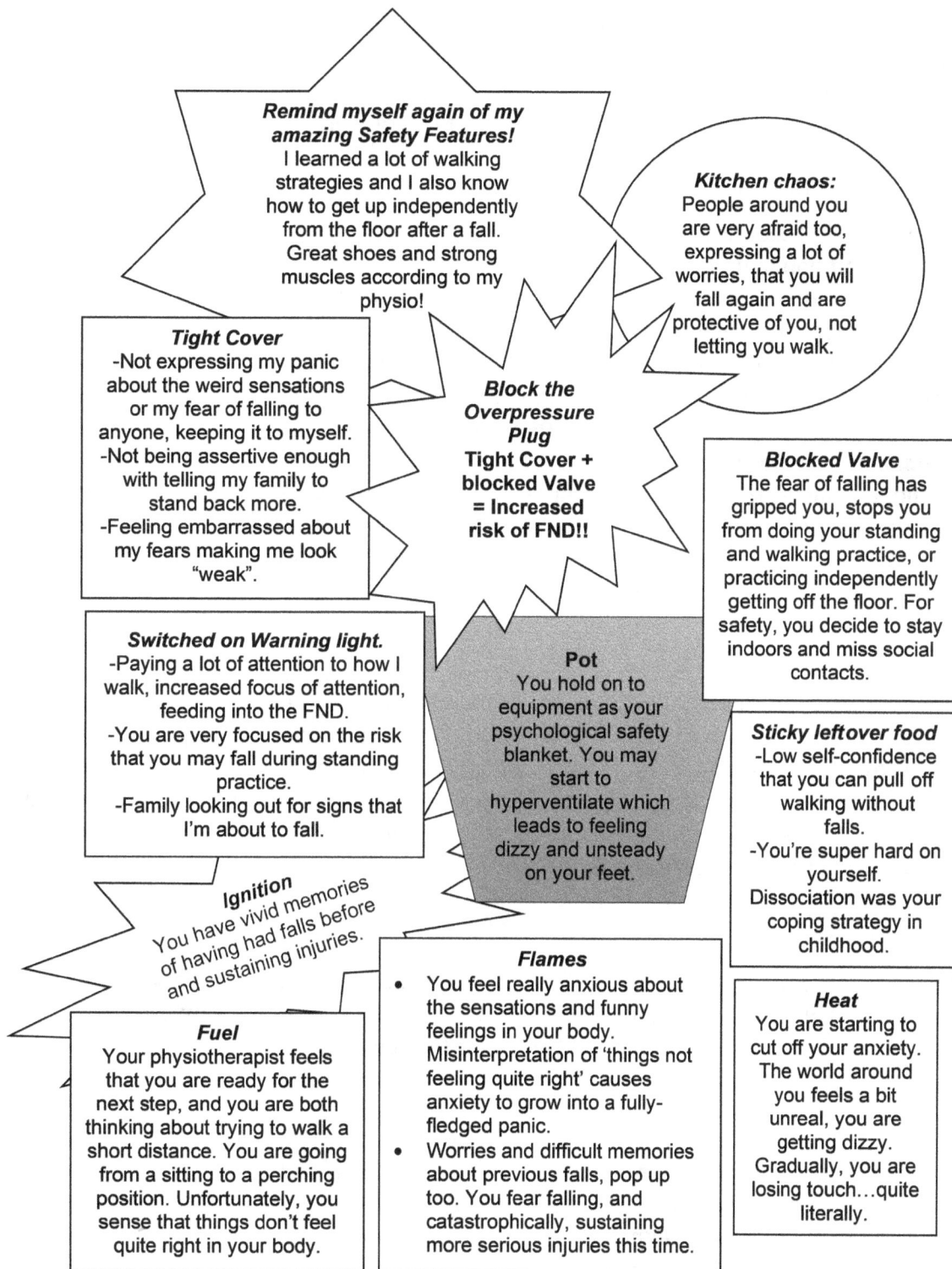

Remind myself again of my amazing Safety Features!
I learned a lot of walking strategies and I also know how to get up independently from the floor after a fall. Great shoes and strong muscles according to my physio!

Kitchen chaos:
People around you are very afraid too, expressing a lot of worries, that you will fall again and are protective of you, not letting you walk.

Tight Cover
-Not expressing my panic about the weird sensations or my fear of falling to anyone, keeping it to myself.
-Not being assertive enough with telling my family to stand back more.
-Feeling embarrassed about my fears making me look "weak".

Block the Overpressure Plug
Tight Cover + blocked Valve = Increased risk of FND!!

Blocked Valve
The fear of falling has gripped you, stops you from doing your standing and walking practice, or practicing independently getting off the floor. For safety, you decide to stay indoors and miss social contacts.

Switched on Warning light.
-Paying a lot of attention to how I walk, increased focus of attention, feeding into the FND.
-You are very focused on the risk that you may fall during standing practice.
-Family looking out for signs that I'm about to fall.

Pot
You hold on to equipment as your psychological safety blanket. You may start to hyperventilate which leads to feeling dizzy and unsteady on your feet.

Sticky leftover food
-Low self-confidence that you can pull off walking without falls.
-You're super hard on yourself. Dissociation was your coping strategy in childhood.

Ignition
You have vivid memories of having had falls before and sustaining injuries.

Fuel
Your physiotherapist feels that you are ready for the next step, and you are both thinking about trying to walk a short distance. You are going from a sitting to a perching position. Unfortunately, you sense that things don't feel quite right in your body.

Flames
• You feel really anxious about the sensations and funny feelings in your body. Misinterpretation of 'things not feeling quite right' causes anxiety to grow into a fully-fledged panic.
• Worries and difficult memories about previous falls, pop up too. You fear falling, and catastrophically, sustaining more serious injuries this time.

Heat
You are starting to cut off your anxiety. The world around you feels a bit unreal, you are getting dizzy. Gradually, you are losing touch...quite literally.

Figure 8.20 The relationship between the fear of falling and FND.

Breathing exercises

Have you noticed any problems or changes in the rate and quality of your breathing during exercises that you have been prescribed to manage the FND? Breathing difficulties are far more common in FND than people think, particularly when practicing and relearning new movements, but sometimes go unnoticed. What type of breathing problems can emerge during these exercises?

PROBLEM 1: BREATH HOLDING

This can be very uncomfortable and is often accompanied by strenuously and effortfully contracting the muscles when you are asked to do a new movement, for example, doing repeated sit-to-stand movements or lengthening the time that you are standing in a certain posture next to a plinth. People often do not realise that they have 'stopped' breathing during these exercises. This makes sense, because you may be hyper-focused on the movement that you are trying to do correctly.

WHAT CAN YOU DO TO MANAGE BREATH-HOLDING SPELLS?

The first step is to become aware that you may be inadvertently engaging in breath-holding episodes. Once you notice that you are holding your breath, the next step is to change the way you are breathing and use it in your therapy. This will not only help you feel more comfortable; it also has two other major advantages.

By becoming more aware of your breathing pattern, you can 'use' your breath to improve your movements, for example, by taking an in-breath and, on your out-breath, performing the new movement. By synching your breathing pattern with the movements you make, you can give the movement an 'extra push' to help execute it better.

The other advantage of focusing on your breathing pattern is the fact that you will not be focusing on your movement that much. Focusing more on breathing means focusing less on movement. Learn more about heightened self-focused attention, which is one of the major maintaining factors of FND, in the next section of Chapter 8.

PROBLEM 2: HYPERVENTILATION

Hyperventilation, also known as taking quick and shallow breaths, is another problem that can pop up during movement exercises. This can lead to dizziness, dissociation, and feeling unwell, which in turn can lead to you feeling more unsteady on your feet, having FND episodes, and ultimately increasing your risk of falling – all things you do not need during your recovery journey. Flick back to Chapter 7 to learn more about breathing exercises that may help you prevent becoming dizzy, including the re-breathing technique.

Body, movement . . . emotions

By now you have probably learned that there is a very strong, but certainly also highly complex, relationship between the body, movements, and emotions. Relearning movements as part of a neurorehabilitation programme can elicit difficult thoughts and feelings for people with FND. Some people report that the following events can feel surprising, distressing, and confrontational:

- Witnessing your body's movements and postures on video recordings.
- Seeing yourself in a wheelchair or other equipment in the mirror.
- Changes in your body producing changes in body image and body confidence.
- Fear of what progress in physiotherapy, improved movements, and therefore increased independence mean for the future in terms of social consequences, new responsibilities, and relationships.
- Transitions between standing, stepping, and walking that elicit new, unknown, and fear-inducing sensations.

How can psychology help when you do not feel your physical base?

Although physiotherapy and occupational therapy are crucial to help you with 'finding your feet' again, sometimes to people's surprise, psychology plays a big role in that process too.

Quite a few people with FND experience muscle weakness and sensation loss below the waist and struggle with feeling and sensing the physical base under their feet. For example, standing in between the double bars or sitting on the plinth may not feel stable, or the ground under your feet may feel very uncomfortable. Not feeling your physical base can go hand in hand with not feeling your psychological base. People with FND often report problems with 'how stable you feel in yourself', low self-esteem, and self-confidence. Since movements, postures, and emotions are associated, it is not really that surprising to expect a relationship between what is happening with your physical base and your psychological base.

Not feeling your physical base can become a problem when the next phase of your treatment is standing or stepping. Here are some useful psychological strategies to help you feel and reconnect with the sensations of your feet again:

- If you are able to **slow down the speed** of any weight-bearing exercises (for example, swinging from side to side and putting pressure on one leg and then on the other) that are recommended by your physiotherapist, this could help you become **more aware of the sensations** in your feet.
- **Try to describe** what is happening in your feet or slightly higher up in your ankles, knees, thighs if you cannot feel your feet. **Any description of a sensation** in your body is good. Be as **detailed** as possible: 'My feet feel funny' is less detailed than 'I can feel the pressure changes in the soles of my feet when I swing from side to side', 'The muscles in my ankles and calves are pulling a bit', 'I can feel slight discomfort in my back, but it is not pain', and so on.
- If you struggle with describing the sensations of touch and pressure clearly (as a subset of people with FND will do), **try describing a different object than your body** first, for example, a soft toy, a squeeze ball, or the sensation of a hairbrush on your head. Be as detailed as you can, as if an alien has landed from Mars and has never seen any of these items and wants to know how they feel: What description would you give? Once you have 'mastered' the description, try again to describe any sensations that come up in your body as you are trying to feel the base of your feet.
- **Bring into awareness any unhelpful thoughts and feelings**, especially feelings around frustration of not feeling your feet. There is no point 'forcing' to feel your feet or anxiously waiting for that moment to arrive. Keep describing the physical sensations in your body.
- **Look at the positives.** Your body may be holding you up to some degree, and there may be some movements or positions that you are able to do, no matter how small.

Warning light

What is attention?

Emotions play an important role in FND – so does attention! We need our attentional skills to function appropriately in day-to-day life:

- **Keeps us safe** and helps us **survive** in the world, for example, when we cross a busy street.
- **Stops our brains** from becoming **overwhelmed** with information. Just imagine how you would feel attending to everything that is happening around you simultaneously! Wah!
- Important for **making memories** and **learning new information** or **skills**.
- Helps you **avoid distractions**, live a productive life, and **focus on meaningful tasks**, like making a cup of tea, writing an essay, or understanding a conversation.

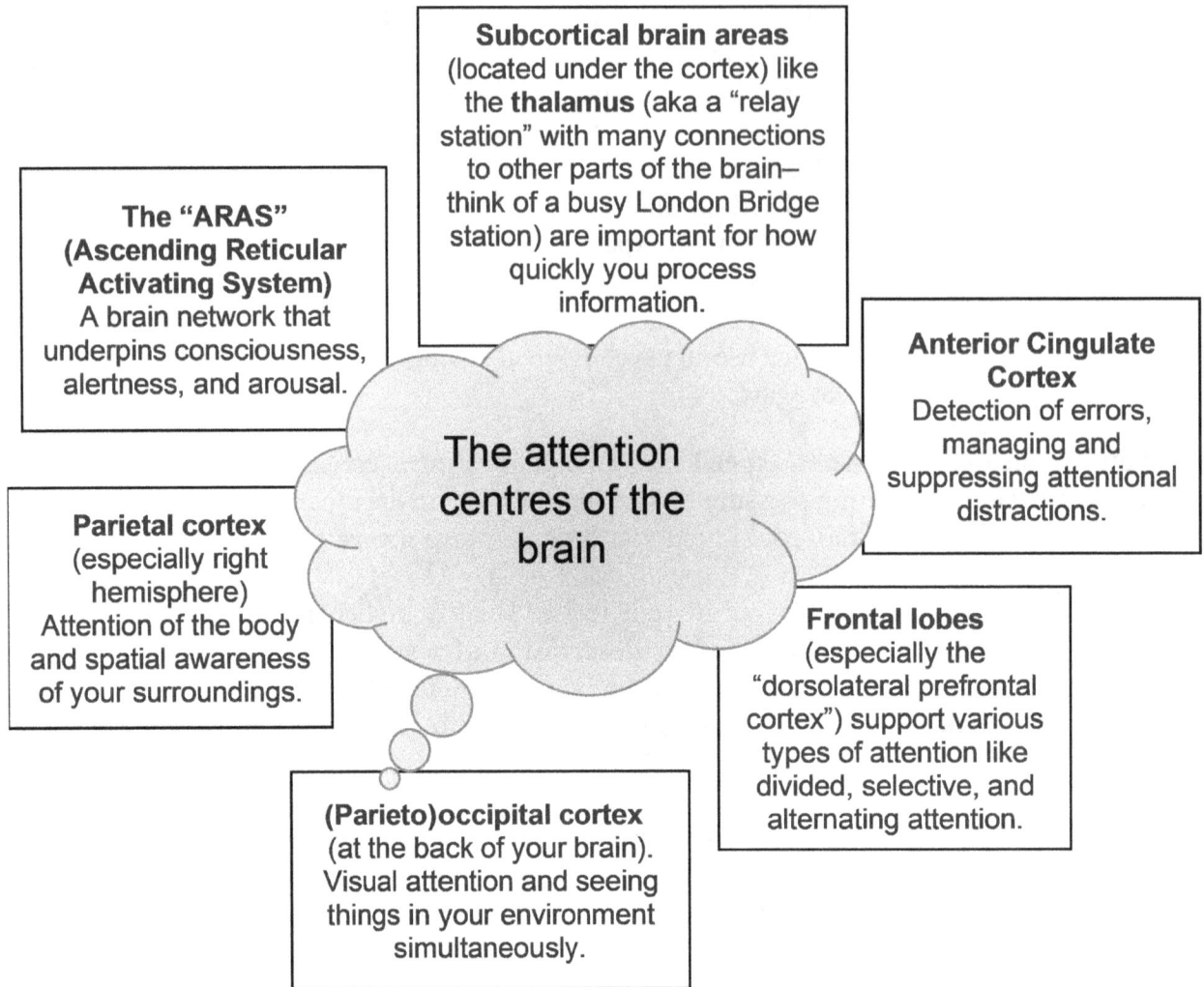

Figure 8.21 Important brain areas for attention.

- And in people with FND, attention has a special place:

  - Attention is crucial for **connecting with your emotions**. You could view dissociation as the opposite of paying attention to emotions.
  - Attention is important for **maintaining** your **physical health**.
  - In a way, FND recovery is about **redistribution of attentional resources**: a little bit more attention for emotions and a little bit less attention directed towards physical symptoms.

Increased self-focused attention in FND

Let us quite literally direct our attention now to . . . **self-focused attention on physical symptoms**, a very important concept in FND and a **maintaining factor** that can keep the FND going and 'feed the FND' (Brown, 2006; Van Poppelen et al., 2011; Edwards et al., 2012; Stins et al., 2015). Treatment programmes for FND are based on the idea of redirecting self-focused attention during movements (see for example, 'movement retraining' by Nielsen et al., 2017).

Table 8.3 Different types of attention in people with and without FND

Type of attention	What is it	Real-life examples
Focused attention	Ability to **mobilise your attentional resources and** respond to things you see, hear, or feel in your environment.	• A friend calls your name, you hear it, and turn around.
Selective attention	Ability to block out, ignore or suppress irrelevant distractions whilst applying razor-sharp focus on something else.	• Finding a friend you are meeting at a busy train station on a Friday night. • The 'cocktail party' effect: concentrating on talking to your friend at a party whilst filtering out all the hustle and bustle around you – without any difficulties.
Divided attention	Also called: dual or multi-tasking. Doing two tasks at the same time. There is often a 'performance decrement' in one of the tasks.	• Preparing a meal in the kitchen whilst watching / following the story line of your favourite television programme. • Crossing a two-lane busy roundabout in your car, paying attention to switching gears whilst checking whether and when you can switch lanes and ensuring that you are not bumping into other drivers. • Playing sports: watching a tennis ball whilst running around on the court, keeping your eye on your opponents.
Alternating attention	Ability to flexibly switch your attention between tasks or activities. Stopping one activity, then moving on to the next, maybe coming back to the original activity.	• Cooking a meal, switching back and forth between tasks: read the recipe, keep a watch on not overcooking your pasta, chopping up tomatoes. • Paying attention to multiple conversation partners and shifting between them. Operate several types of tools during a do-it-yourself assembly of a piece of furniture.
Sustained attention	Maintaining your focus on a task over a long period. Whilst trying to keep concentrated, being able to spot and look out for something meaningful that occurs on and off.	• Driving a car on a long motorway you are not too familiar with and spotting/ 'on the look-out' when your exit is. • Listening to lottery numbers being called out and spotting your lucky numbers.
Information processing speed	The speed of attention paid to information that comes in through our senses and is propagated into our brain. "How fast the cogs turn".	• Listening to a presentation, absorbing slide information, following the presenter, or a teacher explaining a difficult math problem in the classroom.
Visual attention	Being able to perceive more than one object at a time in a complex visual scene.	• Standing at Trafalgar square in London, visually scanning your environment: seeing droves of people, big red double-decker buses, cars, a fountain, Nelson's column, other statues, the pigeons.

Pressure cooker fast facts: what does self-focused attention look like in FND?

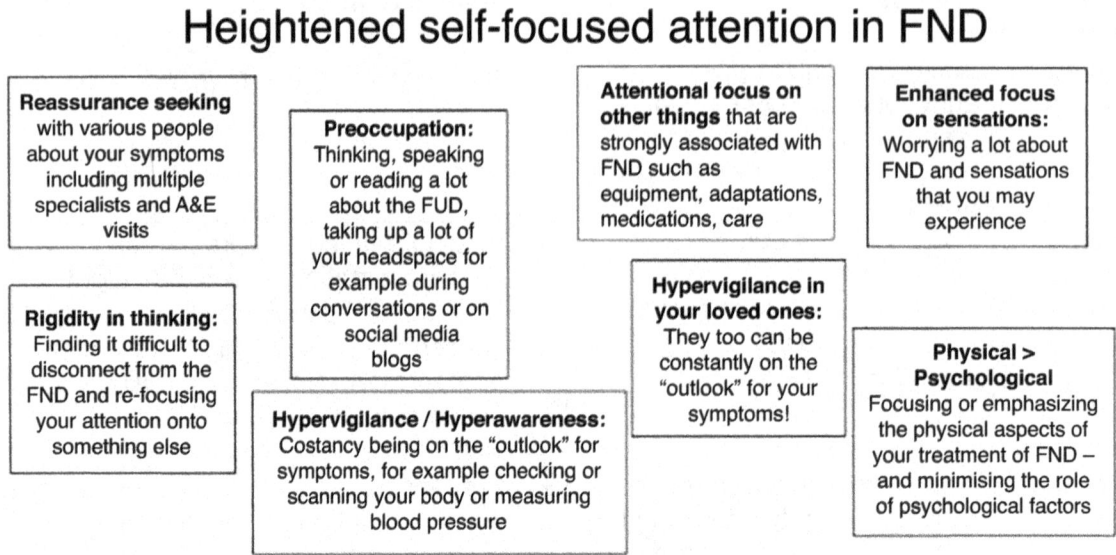

Heightened self-focused attention in FND

Reassurance seeking with various people about your symptoms including multiple specialists and A&E visits

Preoccupation: Thinking, speaking or reading a lot about the FUD, taking up a lot of your headspace for example during conversations or on social media blogs

Attentional focus on other things that are strongly associated with FND such as equipment, adaptations, medications, care

Enhanced focus on sensations: Worrying a lot about FND and sensations that you may experience

Rigidity in thinking: Finding it difficult to disconnect from the FND and re-focusing your attention onto something else

Hypervigilance in your loved ones: They too can be constantly on the "outlook" for your symptoms!

Physical > Psychological Focusing or emphasizing the physical aspects of your treatment of FND – and minimising the role of psychological factors

Hypervigilance / Hyperawareness: Costancy being on the "outlook" for symptoms, for example checking or scanning your body or measuring blood pressure

Figure 8.22 Heightened self-focused attention in FND.

Break free from increased self-focused attention and stop fuelling the FND

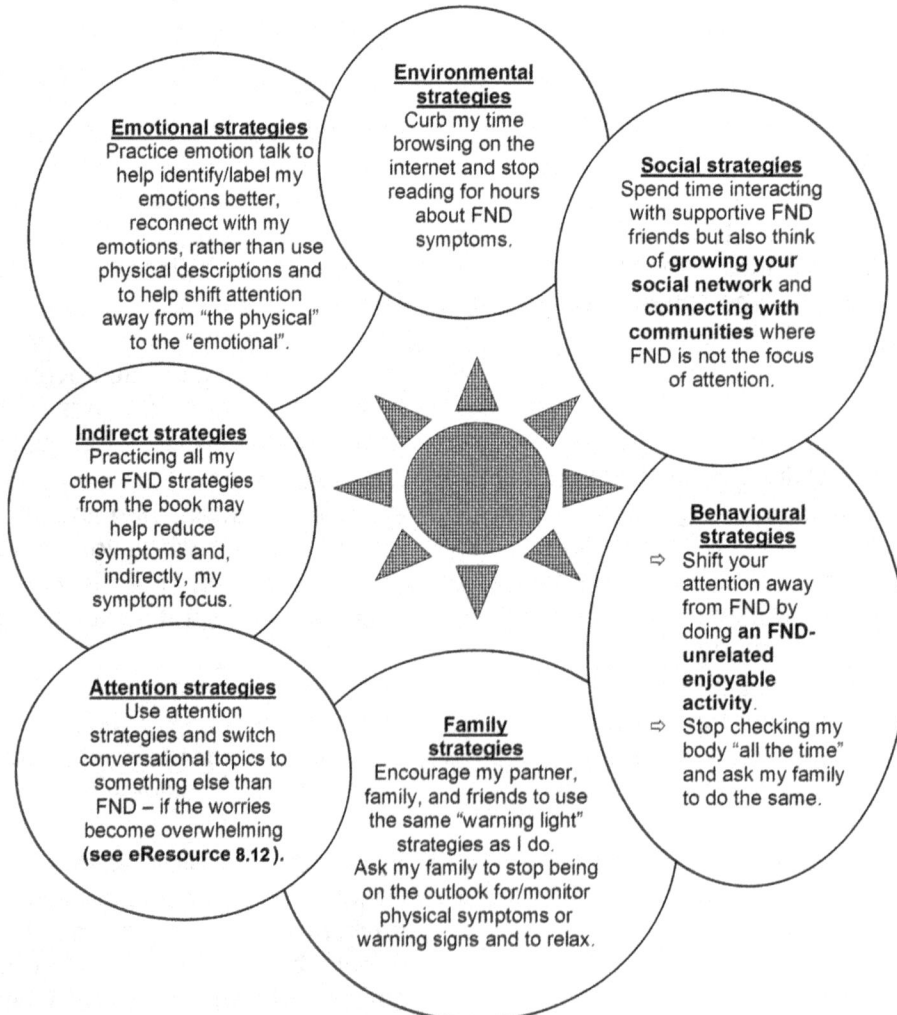

Emotional strategies Practice emotion talk to help identify/label my emotions better, reconnect with my emotions, rather than use physical descriptions and to help shift attention away from "the physical" to the "emotional".

Environmental strategies Curb my time browsing on the internet and stop reading for hours about FND symptoms.

Social strategies Spend time interacting with supportive FND friends but also think of **growing your social network** and **connecting with communities** where FND is not the focus of attention.

Indirect strategies Practicing all my other FND strategies from the book may help reduce symptoms and, indirectly, my symptom focus.

Behavioural strategies
⇨ Shift your attention away from FND by doing an **FND-unrelated enjoyable activity**.
⇨ Stop checking my body "all the time" and ask my family to do the same.

Attention strategies Use attention strategies and switch conversational topics to something else than FND – if the worries become overwhelming **(see eResource 8.12)**.

Family strategies Encourage my partner, family, and friends to use the same "warning light" strategies as I do. Ask my family to stop being on the outlook for/monitor physical symptoms or warning signs and to relax.

Figure 8.23 Strategies for switching off your warning light.

8.11 eResource alert!

Self-focused attention is consistently identified in research studies by leading scholars in the field of FND as a factor that 'keeps the FND going'. Read how you can do a self-assessment and take stock of what your situation with self-focused attention looks like at the moment.

Let us look at some strategies to help you reduce self-focused attention on physical symptoms and **switch off your warning light**. These exercises are meant for you and the people that care for you (see Figure 8.23).

8.12 eResource alert!

Do you find yourself worrying a lot about FND and spending hours thinking about your physical symptoms? Perhaps you have noticed a weird sensation in your body, and now you worry about developing a serious illness? Although being health conscious is generally a good thing, some people, rather unhelpfully, take it to the next level and worry excessively, spending hours of the day thinking about FND and health. All very understandable, and there is no judgement to anyone, but health worries, and the increased self-focused attention that comes with it, maintain FND, so let us help you exert more control over your thoughts! Read about two brilliant attention strategies: **'FND worry zones'** and **'alternating your attention with music'**. Please note that this is an **exercise for people with and without FND in your environment**.

Stirring your pot of worries: relationship with self-focused attention

In Chapter 7, you learned about typical thoughts and feelings in people with FND. One category of beliefs was left out: **worries.** Since **worries are intricately linked to self-focused attention** and worry strategies often try to shift or manipulate attention, everything you need to know about worries will be discussed here in Chapter 8.

What are worries?

- Unhelpful thinking patterns that elicit fear, stress, and anxiety.
- Pertains to future events and situations (but people also worry or 'replay' events that happened in the past).
- You feel out of control and unable to cope with the outcome.
- Some worries are realistic (plausible scary outcomes), whereas others are hypothetical (no real grounds to suspect a negative outcome).
- Can be abstract and vague without delving into specifics.

Worry fuel: what stirs the pot?

- Increased **attentional focus** and **time spent** on worry feeds worry.
- Thinking, researching, and planning for **all potential scenarios** and feared outcomes.

- Only thinking about the **worst-case scenario**.
- **Anticipatory worry:** worry a lot in advance of a feared situation because you feel that this could somehow positively influence the outcome or prepare you better if the result is not what you expected.
- **Worrying 'on purpose'** 'a lot' in advance in a bid to prevent your feared outcome.
- **Worrying** because you otherwise think if you do not worry, you may 'jinx it'.
- Feeling strange, not yourself, and as if something is wrong with you if you do not worry, particularly if worry has become an **integral part of your identity**.
- **Jumping from topic to topic** to form an unstoppable 'worry chain'.
- Sticking to high, unattainable, **perfectionist standards**.
- **Inability to sit with the discomfort** of unpredictability and uncertainty.
- **Post-morteming** and thinking for hours after an event has taken place.
- **Replaying the tapes in your head** for hours to check where you may have gone wrong.
- People in **your environment** who are always on edge, worried, and anxious.

Although these strategies feel like 'problem-solving' at first glance, unfortunately, they **create a false impression of psychological safety** and maintain, prolong, or amplify worries in the long term.

What is the worry threshold, and what happens when the worry threshold is reached?

People with and without FND can experience a lot of worries. When worries start to build up and we give them worry fuel, this could result in FND (see Figure 8.24).

Some people have strong dissociative tendencies, possibly since childhood, as a protection and survival mechanism. People with a strong propensity towards dissociation may not even realise that they experience worries. Even if you are not consciously aware of worries, one way or another, worries will find their way via different routes, especially via the body and behaviours.

Watch out for the following signs of underlying worries, especially when worries...

- Soak up a lot of attentional resources, make you distractible and lose focus on everyday tasks without knowing why.
- Strain your personal, family, and social relationships.
- Stop you from doing enjoyable, constructive, or meaningful activities.
- Make you feel unwell, distressed, and anxious.
- Provide you with a sense of powerlessness and a lack of control.
- Make you fatigued, feel painful joints and muscles, heart racing, dizzy, and sleep poorly at night. (For more information, please read the 8.13 **eResource** on 'how worries impact on our body'.)
- Make you grab for quick-acting but unhelpful means to cope, for example, binge eating, drinking alcohol, using drugs or taking extra non-prescribed medications.
- Keep making you go back to healthcare services.
- Increase your procrastination and make you put off tasks. Read the 8.14 eResource to learn more about what procrastination is. Increase your procrastination and make you put off tasks.
- Result in frequent boom-and-bust cycles or when you are simply 'boom' with your activity levels all the time. (If you struggle with your activity levels, go back to Chapter 6.)
- Are picked up by people in your environment who tell you 'you worry too much'.
- Elicit or amplify FND symptoms.

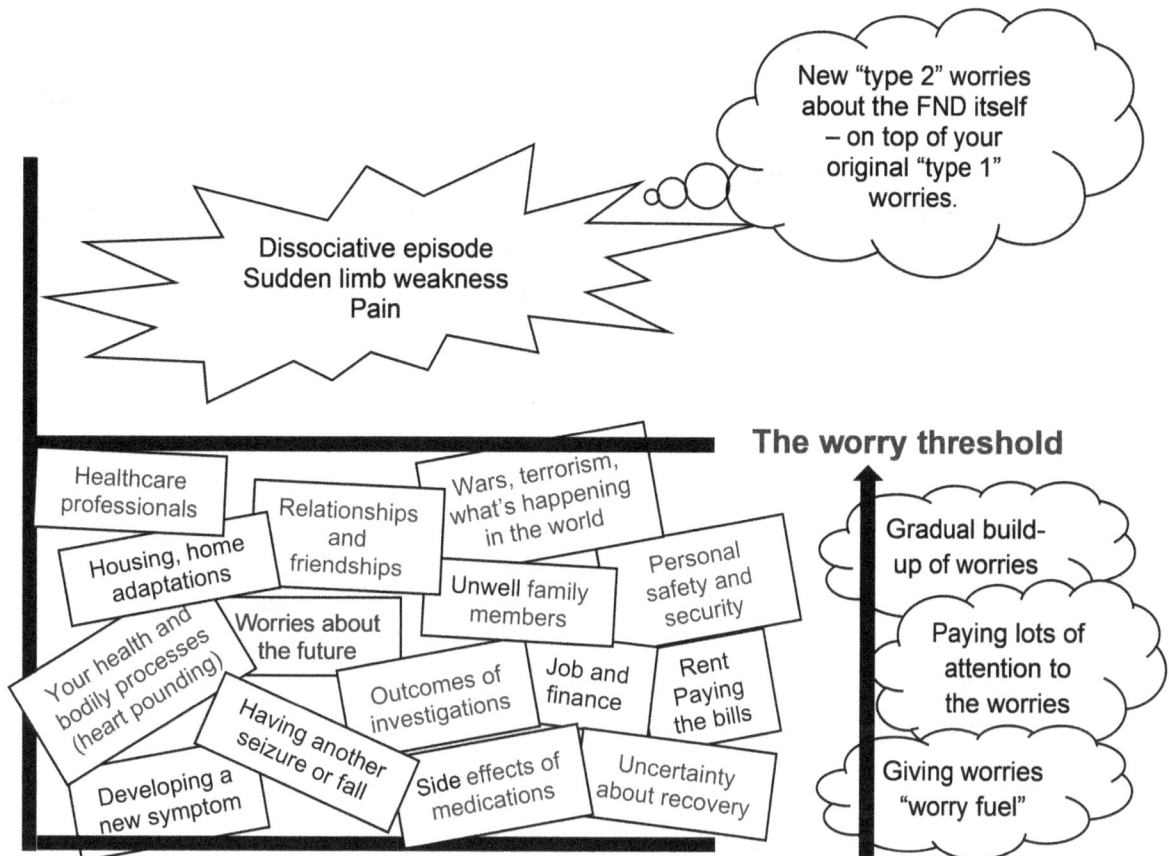

Figure 8.24 How crossing the worry threshold can lead to FND.

8.15 eResource alert!

Before exploring positive worry strategies, read this **eResource** first to learn about common but less helpful worry strategies which look beneficial at first glance but feed the worry.

Helpful worry strategies

TOP TIPS FOR MANAGING YOUR WORRIES

- Worries love it when a person is on their own. **Try not to withdraw and resolve worries in your all by yourself but talk about your worries particularly with someone in your life whom you feel 'psychologically safe' with,** and be careful about feeding worries with too much attention.
- **Cut the 'attentional supply'** to stop giving power to the worries using attention-shifting techniques.
- **Regularly link up socially with friends and people** and do an **unrelated enjoyable or social activity** to 'snap out of it'. Feeling happy is the antidote against feeling worried and anxious.
- **Watch your level of engagement with worry.** Are you *actively* pushing the worries out of your mind or *actively* attaching to worry? Both are excessive and cause your mind to still be in

overdrive. It is a good idea to challenge your worries with 'hard evidence to the contrary', but watch how long you spend on this activity and whether it makes the worries worse.

- **Sit with distress temporarily but swiftly move on.** Try to acknowledge and even embrace the presence of the worry briefly (some mind activity, but not much), and then practice with letting go by focusing on whatever activity you were doing (allocate your attentional resources to helpful, meaningful, and constructive activities – worries do not fall into that category).
- **Question the worry's worth, and shift your attention away.** We only have a limited amount of attention in our 'attention store'. What truly deserves your full attention and headspace in this moment? Worries or a constructive activity? Use the attention-shifting techniques described earlier.
- **Raise your insight.** How much time do you spend on worries? Keep a worry diary and decide: Is this worth it? People do not always notice but can spend hours thinking about a variety of worries.
- **Dump** the worries. If worries keep you up at night, consider a voice diary, a journal, or a piece of paper with a pen next to your bed. Another technique is a worry box. As soon as a worry comes up, write the worry down and 'dump' the worry so the burden is off your mind and you can try to enjoy some sleep.
- **Break the worry chain reaction** by choosing multiple deliberate 'worry slots' during the day where you purposefully worry a lot. Outside those purposeful worry moments, try to curb the worries altogether. This gives more control over your thoughts.
- **Postpone** the worries, as we have seen earlier for FND-specific thoughts. By the time you reach your postponed worry slot, you may not even need it!
- **Plan ahead.** Ask yourself: What is the worst thing that can happen, and how will I manage or control this situation, in case it will happen? Can I prepare a coping plan in advance?
- **Procrastination.** Tolerate the distress, discomfort, or uncertainty that worries may generate about the task. Try to do a little bit every day rather than postpone and do a lot in one go. Or stop thinking and dithering but just do it!
- **Think about the worry traffic jam.** Imagine that you are on your way to an important appointment. You are running late, and then, of course, of all days, you are stuck in the mother of all traffic jams. It is excruciating and only moves at snail-speed. In your mind, you want to frantically move things along. You are looking left, right, and centre at ways to escape the traffic jam. There is no escape. You are stuck and boxed in from all sides.

Will active worrying, getting frustrated, and being angry help you move the traffic faster and get you quicker to your destination? Not in any way! The best thing that you can do is to (1) 'just be' and ride it out until your traffic jam starts to gather pace again, (2) enjoy yourself (listen to music, call up a friend for a fun chat), or (3) problem-solve a potential late arrival to your appointment (calling the people who may be waiting for you). Worry does not influence the outcome.

References

Adolphs, R., Tranel, D., & Damasio, A. R. (1998). The human amygdala in social judgment. *Nature, 393*(6684), 470–474.

Appleton, J. (2018). The gut-brain axis: Influence of microbiota on mood and mental health. *Integrative Medicine: A Clinician's Journal, 17*(4), 28.

Asadi-Pooya, A. A., Asadipooya, K., & AlBaradie, R. S. (2019). Gut microbiota and psychogenic non-epileptic seizures; Are they related? *Expert Review of Neurotherapeutics, 19*(12), 1163–1163.

Bandura, A., Ross, D., & Ross, S. A. (1961). Transmission of aggression through imitation of aggressive models. *The Journal of Abnormal and Social Psychology, 63*(3), 575.

Bandura, A., & Walters, R. H. (1977). *Social learning theory* (Vol. 1). Prentice Hall: Englewood Cliffs.

Barnett, C., Davis, R., Mitchell, C., & Tyson, S. (2022). The vicious cycle of functional neurological disorders: A synthesis of healthcare professionals' views on working with patients with functional neurological disorder. *Disability and Rehabilitation*, *44*(10), 1802–1811.

Baroni, G., Piccinini, V., Martins, W. A., de Paola, L., Paglioli, E., Margis, R., & Palmini, A. (2016). Variables associated with co-existing epileptic and psychogenic nonepileptic seizures: A systematic review. *Seizure*, *37*, 35–40.

Bennett, K., Diamond, C., Hoeritzauer, I., Gardiner, P., McWhirter, L., Carson, A., & Stone, J. (2021). A practical review of Functional Neurological Disorder (FND) for the general physician. *Clinical Medicine*, *21*(1), 28.

Brown, R. J. (2006). Medically unexplained symptoms: A new model. *Psychiatry*, *5*(2), 43–47.

D'Alessio, L., Giagante, B., Oddo, S., Silva, W., Solís, P., Consalvo, D., & Kochen, S. (2006). Psychiatric disorders in patients with psychogenic non-epileptic seizures, with and without comorbid epilepsy. *Seizure*, *15*(5), 333–339.

Dicks, L. M. (2022). Gut bacteria and neurotransmitters. *Microorganisms*, *10*(9), 1838.

Edwards, M. J., Adams, R. A., Brown, H., Parees, I., & Friston, K. J. (2012). A Bayesian account of 'hysteria'. *Brain*, *135*(11), 3495–3512.

Feinstein, J. S., Adolphs, R., Damasio, A., & Tranel, D. (2011). The human amygdala and the induction and experience of fear. *Current Biology*, *21*(1), 34–38.

Finkelstein, S. A., Cortel-LeBlanc, M. A., Cortel-LeBlanc, A., & Stone, J. (2021). Functional neurological disorder in the emergency department. *Academic Emergency Medicine*, *28*(6), 685–696.

Gershon, M. D., & Tack, J. (2007). The serotonin signaling system: From basic understanding to drug development for functional GI disorders. *Gastroenterology*, *132*(1), 397–414.

Gilmour, G. S., Nielsen, G., Teodoro, T., Yogarajah, M., Coebergh, J. A., Dilley, M. D., Martino, D., & Edwards, M. J. (2020). Management of functional neurological disorder. *Journal of Neurology*, *267*(7), 2164–2172.

Goldstein, L. H., Robinson, E. J., Mellers, J. D., Stone, J., Carson, A., Chalder, T., Reuber, M., Eastwood, C., Landau, S., McCrone, P., Moore, M., Mosweu, I., Murray, J., Perdue, I., Pilecka, I., Richardson, M. P., & Medford, N.; CODES Study Group. (2021). Psychological and demographic characteristics of 368 patients with dissociative seizures: Data from the CODES cohort. *Psychological Medicine*, *51*(14), 2433–2445.

Hoeritzauer, I., Phé, V., & Panicker, J. N. (2016). Urologic symptoms and functional neurologic disorders. *Handbook of Clinical Neurology*, *139*, 469–481.

Kyle, K., & Wu, A. D. (2020). The impact of diagnosis on health care utilization in functional movement disorders. *Movement Disorders Clinical Practice*, *7*(7), 868.

Ladha, H., Gupta, S., & Pati, S. (2017). Trends in hospital inpatient costs of psychogenic nonepileptic seizures (P3. 230). *Neurology*, *88*.

LeDoux, J. (1996). Emotional networks and motor control: A fearful view. *Progress in Brain Research*, *107*, 437–446.

LeDoux, J. (2003). The emotional brain, fear, and the amygdala. *Cellular and Molecular Neurobiology*, *23*(4), 727–738.

Merkler, A. E., Parikh, N. S., Chaudhry, S., Chait, A., Allen, N. C., Navi, B. B., & Kamel, H. (2016). Hospital revisit rate after a diagnosis of conversion disorder. *Journal of Neurology, Neurosurgery & Psychiatry*, *87*(4), 363–366.

Nicholson, C., Edwards, M. J., Carson, A. J., Gardiner, P., Golder, D., Hayward, K., Humblestone, S., Jinadu, H., Lumsden, C., MacLean, J., Main, L., Macgregor, L., Nielsen, G., Oakley, L., Price, J., Ranford, J., Ranu, J., Sum, E., & Stone, J. (2020). Occupational therapy consensus recommendations for functional neurological disorder. *Journal of Neurology, Neurosurgery & Psychiatry*, *91*(10), 1037–1045.

Nielsen, G., Buszewicz, M., Stevenson, F., Hunter, R., Holt, K., Dudziec, M., Ricciardi, L., Marsden, J., Joyce, E., & Edwards, M. J. (2017). Randomised feasibility study of physiotherapy for patients with functional motor symptoms. *Journal of Neurology, Neurosurgery & Psychiatry*, *88*(6), 484–490.

Nunez-Wallace, K. R., Murphey, D. K., Proto, D., Collins, R. L., Franks, R., Chachere II, D. M., & Chen, D. K. (2015). Health resource utilization among US veterans with psychogenic nonepileptic seizures: A comparison before and after video-EEG monitoring. *Epilepsy Research*, *114*, 114–121.

Panicker, J. N., Selai, C., Herve, F., Rademakers, K., Dmochowski, R., Tarcan, T., von Gontard, A., & Vrijens, D. (2020). Psychological comorbidities and functional neurological disorders in women with idiopathic urinary retention: International Consultation on Incontinence Research Society (ICI-RS) 2019. *Neurourology and Urodynamics*, *39*, S60–S69.

Pattichis, A., Sivathamboo, S., White, E., Rychkova, M., Perucca, P., Kwan, P., Goldin, J., & O'Brien, T. (2019, October). Subjective sleep quality is not reflected in objective sleep measures in an epilepsy population. *Journal of Sleep Research*, *28*, 111 (RIVER ST, HOBOKEN 07030–5774, NJ USA: Wiley).

Petrochilos, P., Elmalem, M. S., Patel, D., Louissaint, H., Hayward, K., Ranu, J., & Selai, C. (2020). Outcomes of a 5-week individualised MDT outpatient (day-patient) treatment programme for functional neurological symptom disorder (FNSD). *Journal of Neurology*, *267*(9), 2655–2666.

Razvi, S., Mulhern, S., & Duncan, R. (2012). Newly diagnosed psychogenic nonepileptic seizures: Health care demand prior to and following diagnosis at a first seizure clinic. *Epilepsy & Behavior*, *23*(1), 7–9.

Stephen, C. D., Fung, V., Lungu, C. I., & Espay, A. J. (2021). Assessment of emergency department and inpatient use and costs in adult and pediatric functional neurological disorders. *JAMA Neurology*, *78*(1), 88–101.

Stins, J. F., Kempe, C. L. A., Hagenaars, M. A., Beek, P. J., & Roelofs, K. (2015). Attention and postural control in patients with conversion paresis. *Journal of Psychosomatic Research*, *78*(3), 249–254.

Stone, J., Warlow, C., & Sharpe, M. (2010). The symptom of functional weakness: A controlled study of 107 patients. *Brain*, *133*(5), 1537–1551.

Strandwitz, P. (2018). Neurotransmitter modulation by the gut microbiota. *Brain Research*, *1693*, 128–133.

Van Poppelen, D., Saifee, T. A., Schwingenschuh, P., Katschnig, P., Bhatia, K. P., Tijssen, M. A., & Edwards, M. J. (2011). Attention to self in psychogenic tremor. *Movement Disorders*, *26*(14), 2575–2576.

Voon, V., Brezing, C., Gallea, C., Ameli, R., Roelofs, K., LaFrance Jr, W. C., & Hallett, M. (2010). Emotional stimuli and motor conversion disorder. *Brain*, *133*(5), 1526–1536.

Voon, V., Brezing, C., Gallea, C., & Hallett, M. (2011). Aberrant supplementary motor complex and limbic activity during motor preparation in motor conversion disorder. *Movement Disorders*, *26*(13), 2396–2403.

9 Environmental and interpersonal factors in FND

The kitchen (layer 5)

You made it to the kitchen environment, the final part of the Pressure Cooker Model! Every pressure cooker pot lives in a kitchen environment. But what exactly is the kitchen in the Pressure Cooker Model? Look at Figure 9.1. We do not exist in a social vacuum; we are surrounded by people with their own pressure cookers. The kitchen represents all the people, social interactions, relationships, and systems around the person with FND.

FND is a two-step process

To understand the kitchen environment better, let us jump back to Chapter 7. Do you remember the Pressure Cooker chain reaction? ('what keeps the FND and dissociation going')? You learned that this was **the first step of FND**.

Imagine the following situation:

A person experiences a dissociative seizure in response to a heated family argument, psychological pressure, and lots of demands placed on the person (i.e. interpersonal triggers). The person **felt psychologically very unsafe**, but the seizure helped the person cut off their feelings temporarily and switch off from intolerable distress and arousal (via the Pressure Cooker chain reaction). The dissociative episode **supported the person to achieve a state of psychological safety**, provided a sense of relief from inner turmoil, and restored stability. Therefore, the seizure **met an internal emotional need**. This process is called the **internal regulation function of FND**. The FND symptoms support the person to cope with something unpleasant happening **inside the individual (or internally)** to regulate back to a state of psychological safety again. The person is also **doing this on their own without help or reliance on other people**, hence the name 'internal regulation'.

However, there is also a second step in FND that is determined by **environmental and social processes**. In our example earlier, the dissociative seizure had social functions:

- The heated argument, psychological pressure, and demands stopped immediately.
- People started reassuring and caring for the person rather than screaming and putting pressure ('uncaring').
- The person finally felt noticed and respected, and was able to make themselves heard by communicating through the dissociative seizure ('Stop putting pressure on me!').
- The seizure helped keep more arguments at bay, at least for the foreseeable future. The environment was extra careful and walked on eggshells to not provoke another seizure.

As you can see, the FND came with **social consequences**. The environment somehow interacted with the FND symptoms, and this interpersonal dynamic helped the individual cope with their internal state. This is called the **external regulation function** of FND.

DOI: 10.4324/9781003308973-9

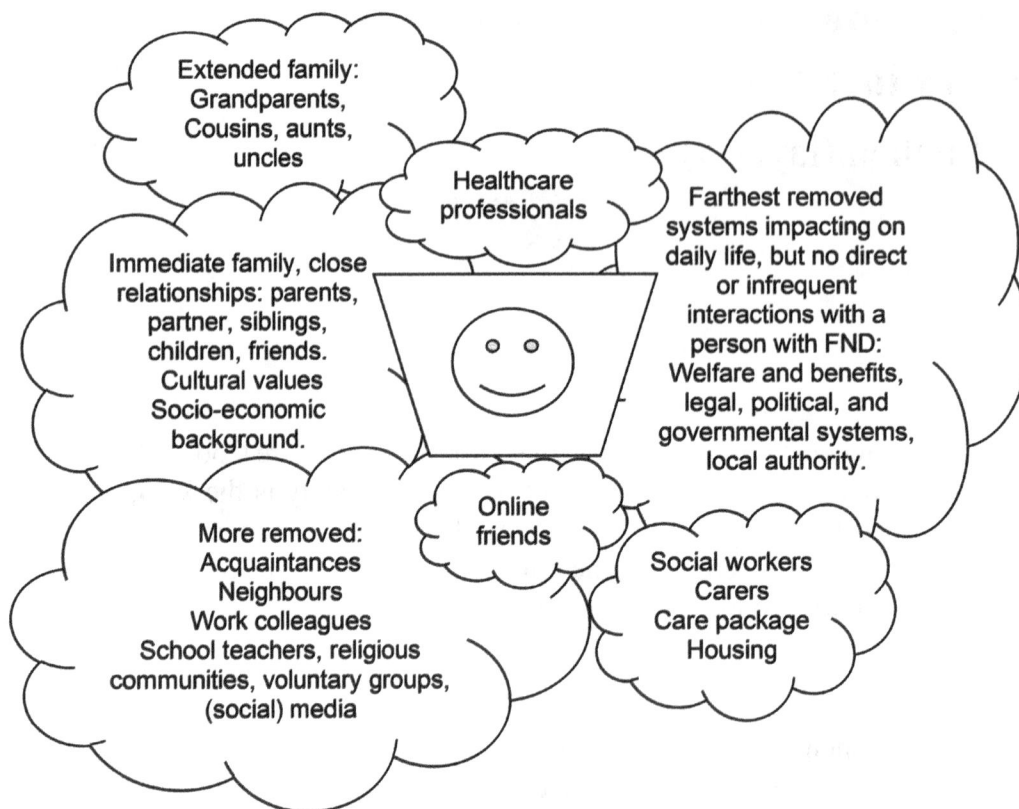

Figure 9.1 The kitchen: multi-layered social systems in FND.

Our example shows that FND is not just about the person with FND. It turns out that **everybody has a Pressure Cooker chain reaction**, whether you experience FND or not! Stay tuned, because later in Chapter 9, you will learn how the person with FND and their environment both achieve a state of **interpersonal psychological safety through their pattern of responding and relating.**

From secondary gains to social functions of FND

In the literature, the second step in FND is often called **'secondary gains'**. Why does the term *secondary gains* pose a problem for FND?

- Old-fashioned and pejorative.
- Implies that symptoms are generated on purpose and put on by a person with FND to gain something from their environment, often something socially or morally 'unacceptable' in society (people with FND receiving welfare benefits and attention with some people in the environment sadly not viewing this as 'justified' due to the nature of FND symptoms).
- Makes the person not believed, uncared for, and feel disrespected.
- Creates a false impression of a one-way street; however, **an interaction between people is always a two-way street**.

The Pressure Cooker Model has rebranded this second step as something radically different. Rather than 'secondary gains', **FND is viewed as having social functions** and **meeting basic human needs in two directions**. Not only is the person with FND gaining something from the environment, but also vice versa, people surrounding the person with FND, such as family, friends, and healthcare professionals, are equally gaining something from the person, **and all that keeps the FND going.**

Social functions of FND: straight out of the clinic

Please keep in mind that the **social consequences of FND** are often unintentional, inadvertent, and operate on an unconscious level.

Most people will be kind, caring, compassionate, and supportive to a person feeling unwell, in pain, and not in their best physical and emotional state. These are normal and natural automatic responses from our environment.

The social functions of FND need our compassion and understanding because they meet unmet needs in the moment. The term 'social functions' does not imply that people with FND are putting their symptoms on, should not be believed, or are doing this for attention. **None of these statements are true, and they have no place in FND.**

Examples of the social functions of FND for the person with FND

- **'Build a wall.'** FND can be a **deterrent** or **a protective barrier** against something unpleasant in the environment, for example, arguments, strife, unwanted intimacy, proximity, or emotional connection/reaction from a person.
- **'Letting off the hook.'** To **stop people from putting psychological pressure** or **making unreasonable demands** on you – often in the context of long periods of having to cope with high pressure, demand, and responsibilities in your life.
- **'Off-duty port of call.'** FND can help a person, normally the family's 'first point of contact' during crises, to temporarily 'bow out' and protect them from the constant emotional overwhelm and burden that other family members pose on this individual.
- Provides **a sense of control in a complicated and unpredictable life situation**, for example, when arguments and conflicts in the home immediately stop following a seizure.
- FND can **distract** from unhelpful or unhealthy family and partner dynamics – and keep the peace – because all the focus is shifted to the person's health issues.
- **'Family glue.'** In a person with an unreleased, unspeakable dilemma, the FND can protect an entire family structure from falling apart.
- **'Safety blanket.'** FND may **bring or keep someone emotionally and physically close and show their care and compassion**, either a loved one or a person who has otherwise been quite distant, avoidant, estranged, or unavailable. This social function of FND happens in some people with a complex trauma background whose physical and emotional needs were not, or were inconsistently, met in childhood.
- It should be noted that connecting and wanting to feel close to other people is a basic human need that everybody in the world experiences: FND or not. When those needs are not sufficiently met, perceived as unmet, and people struggle with identifying emotions and putting those needs into words, a person may try to find a sense of closeness in other understandable but probably less helpful ways, which contributes to communicating needs in a more physical manner.
- **'Make noise.'** FND may help make a person feel cared for, heard, noticed, taken seriously, respected, validated, believed, treated with kindness and compassion, with people becoming more careful and sometimes walking on eggshells; it stops people in their tracks to become more responsive and sensitive to someone's needs, particularly if life before FND was quite challenging.
- FND can **convince** other people **of the person feeling unwell** who would otherwise not believe or take the person seriously and keep placing demands.
- FND can **communicate a symbolic message, emotion, or difficult situation** that is hard to put in words to others. Think (for example) about someone with functional speech problems which may symbolically reflect 'I don't feel that I have a voice in the family, and my ideas often get dismissed by others'. FND can paradoxically **improve communication** with important people in your life, who will **finally take time to listen to you.**

- FND may provide a sense of **identity, meaning**, or **purpose** and increase **self-esteem** in some people.
- **FND can support the expression of distress** in ways that are **more socially acceptable** and less stigmatised: experiencing physical symptoms is less 'frowned upon' by society than experiencing distress or mental health problems.

Examples of the social functions of FND for the person without FND

An important and recurrent theme in FND is care. No, wait a second – care and relationships are a **universal theme for everybody**!

- Wanting to feel cared for is a basic human need.
- Vice versa, caring for another person meets that need for the person who wants to feel cared for.
- This may also serve to meet another **unmet need in the carer** who, like the person with FND, experiences a lack of psychological safety.

What needs, beliefs, and emotions may someone who cares for a person with FND experience? Here are some clinical examples of the social functions of FND **for the person without FND**:

- **Reassurance and caring can reduce the carer's anxiety and discomfort** in response to witnessing FND symptoms and distress ('This is too hard to watch').
- **Feeling sympathy, sadness, and sorry for the person** and wanting to express that through caring activities.
- **Guilt.** Some people with FND may have missed out on care, support, and validation by their parental caregivers or other family members **in the past**. The family may now make this up by engaging in excessive caring.
- Caring activities around FND have **become a part of a carer's identity and purpose** in life by creating dependency in the person with FND.
- A carer **can show affection** to the person with FND **through caring**, in more practical rather than emotional ways, by meeting a person's care needs with washing, dressing, preparing meals, accessing the community, and many other practical day-to-day activities.
- If a carer feels **embarrassed** or **ashamed** of the person's FND symptoms (for example, a dissociative episode in a public place), reassurance and care will quickly reduce these symptoms and, with that, the carer's emotions.
- A carer's **worries and anxiety** around the lack of knowledge and confidence about whether they are doing the right thing in FND and are able to cope as a carer ('What if I make the FND worse?'): intuitively believing that excessive caring is what is helpful.
- **Fear of abandonment by keeping the person close** and not wanting other people to seek proximity to the person with FND. This can be for protective purposes, for example, worries about the person not receiving the correct care from healthcare and social care professionals and wanting to do a better job. This can also be for control purposes and, in rare instances, may have a coercive nature.
- Sometimes, in present times, people may **unconsciously replay past difficult experiences** where they felt not cared for by a parent or a family member. Often outside of their awareness, people apply sometimes excessive caring behaviours to other people in need of care that they would have wished for had they been in that same situation. Perceiving a lack of care in others may retrigger these memories of what you missed during childhood. By caring for another person, it is like your compassionate adult self is able to emotionally make up and compensate for the lack of care that you may have experienced in the past and that you are now providing to another person who symbolises your younger self.

What is reciprocal reinforcement?

Family and healthcare professionals are often inclined to focus assessment and treatment on the person with FND, who is viewed as 'the problem', especially when the symptoms are obvious and severe, for example, dissociative episodes with accidental self-injury that stop the individual from functioning in day-to-day life. That seems understandable and makes initial sense because it is the person who 'carries' and is impacted by the FND. However, given what we have just learned about the 'two-way street' of social functions in FND, the question is whether this is the correct approach.

Reciprocal reinforcement (RR)

- A psychological process in FND that unfolds between the person with FND and individuals in their environment.
- Reciprocal means 'in both directions'.
- Reinforcement suggests that there is something rewarding or relieving that keeps this psychological process going.
- According to this definition, this means that **everybody has a Pressure Cooker chain reaction, not just the person with FND**.
- RR can be viewed as a safety behaviour that helps **everyone involved in FND** feel psychologically safe and secure in each other in understandable yet unhelpful ways.

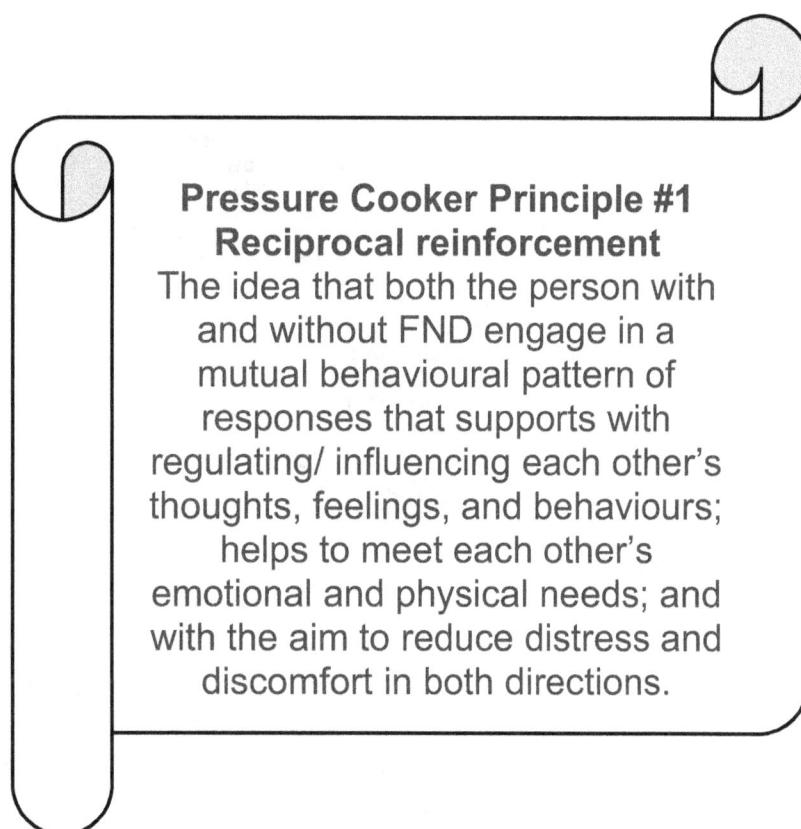

Pressure Cooker Principle #1
Reciprocal reinforcement
The idea that both the person with and without FND engage in a mutual behavioural pattern of responses that supports with regulating/ influencing each other's thoughts, feelings, and behaviours; helps to meet each other's emotional and physical needs; and with the aim to reduce distress and discomfort in both directions.

Figure 9.2 Reciprocal reinforcement.

Reciprocal reinforcement: an example

The example displayed in Figure 9.3 is probably the most commonly encountered RR pattern between a person with FND and a person in their environment.

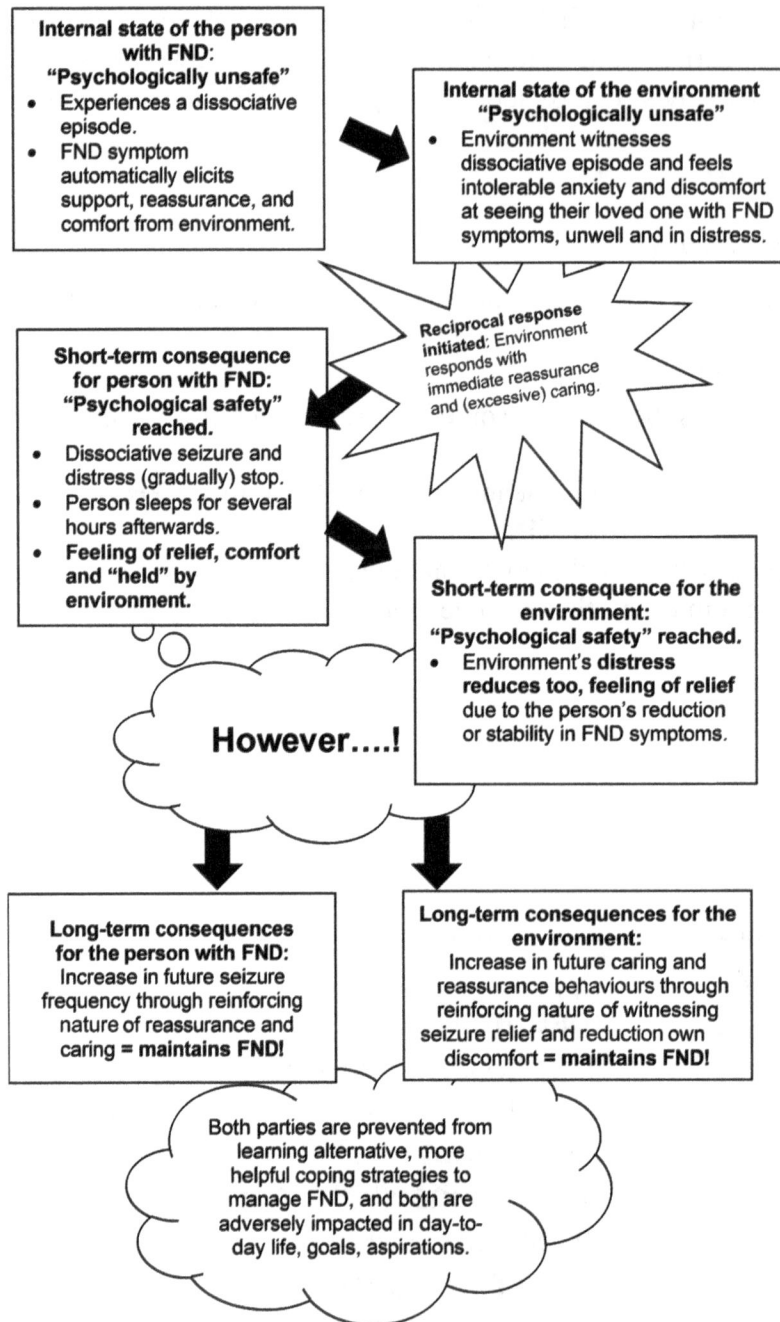

Internal state of the person with FND:
"Psychologically unsafe"
- Experiences a dissociative episode.
- FND symptom automatically elicits support, reassurance, and comfort from environment.

Internal state of the environment
"Psychologically unsafe"
- Environment witnesses dissociative episode and feels intolerable anxiety and discomfort at seeing their loved one with FND symptoms, unwell and in distress.

Reciprocal response initiated: Environment responds with immediate reassurance and (excessive) caring.

Short-term consequence for person with FND:
"Psychological safety" reached.
- Dissociative seizure and distress (gradually) stop.
- Person sleeps for several hours afterwards.
- **Feeling of relief, comfort and "held" by environment.**

Short-term consequence for the environment:
"Psychological safety" reached.
- Environment's **distress reduces too, feeling of relief** due to the person's reduction or stability in FND symptoms.

However....!

Long-term consequences for the person with FND:
Increase in future seizure frequency through reinforcing nature of reassurance and caring = **maintains FND!**

Long-term consequences for the environment:
Increase in future caring and reassurance behaviours through reinforcing nature of witnessing seizure relief and reduction own discomfort = **maintains FND!**

Both parties are prevented from learning alternative, more helpful coping strategies to manage FND, and both are adversely impacted in day-to-day life, goals, aspirations.

Figure 9.3 An example of reciprocal reinforcement.

Problems with reciprocal reinforcement (RR)

RR is an understandable, intuitive, and natural response to someone unwell, in distress, and suffering. It makes complete sense to respond with care. RR is driven by the best intentions, human needs, and emotions. However, RR is not a helpful strategy in the longer term because:

- Although RR provides **relief** and **psychological safety** in the short term, RR directly **maintains** and **prolongs FND** in the long term via a reinforcement loop.

- RR stops you from addressing and independently managing underlying **emotions** that contribute to FND. For example:
  - A healthcare professional quickly discharging a person with FND out of fear and avoidance rather than clinical rationale is not dealing with their own anxiety.
  - A frustrated family member engaging in excessive reassurance during a dissociative episode is not sitting with their own discomfort.
- RR makes it easy for existing **unhelpful coping strategies**, such as reduced verbal emotional expression (tight cover) and enjoyable activities (blocked valve), to persist.
- RR prevents everyone involved from learning, testing out, and practicing new opportunities for **more helpful** and **less-disruptive coping strategies**.
- RR promotes **dependency**, **limits progress** towards **recovery**, and **restricts** a person's **social world**.
- RR can impact on your **self-esteem** and **confidence in managing FND**.
- RR greatly **affects relationships**, blurs the line between family and caring roles, and impacts on privacy and dignity.
- The longer the process of RR continues, the more **rehearsed**, well-practiced, and ultimately **entrenched** these unhelpful strategies become as **fixed habits**.
- RR **takes precious time away** from meaningful and constructive day-to-day activities and stops us thriving in life and stands in the way of living life to the full.
- **Prolonged RR has a dark side and** causes even deeper issues (see Figure 9.4). This is called a partial or intermittent reinforcement schedule (Wagner, 1961; Kendall, 1974).

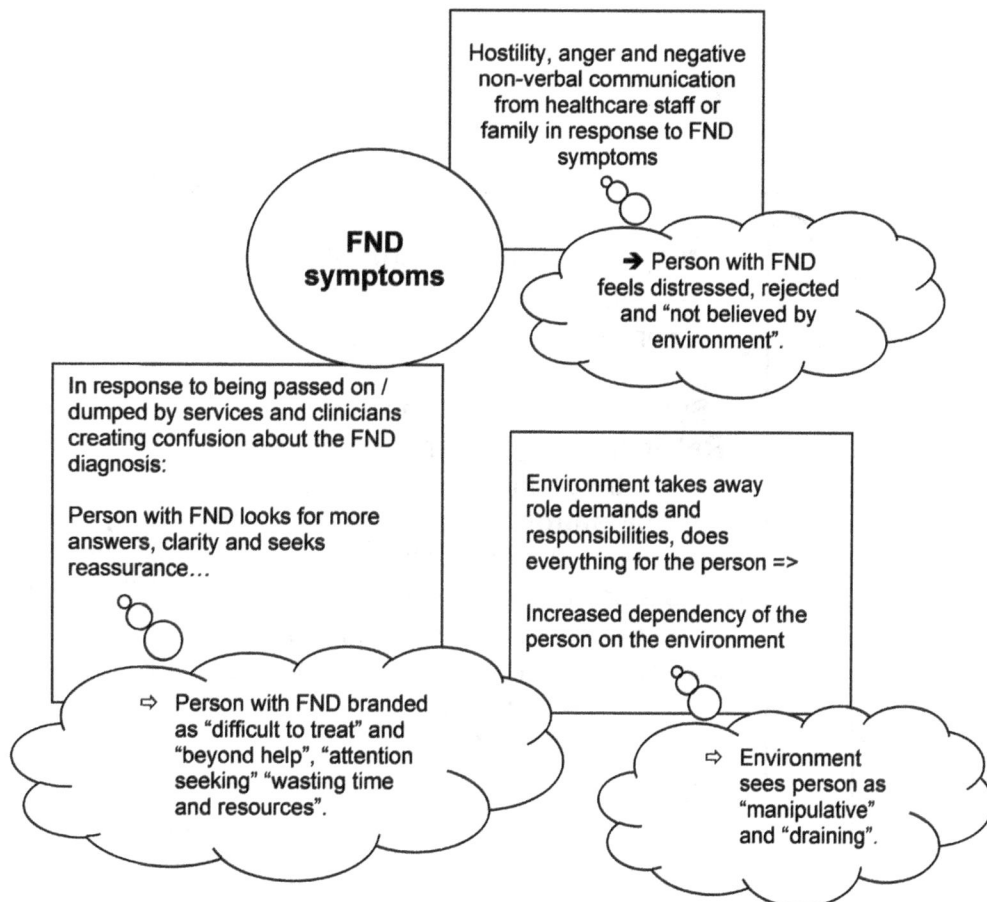

Figure 9.4 RR and intermittent reinforcement in FND.

Imagine a gambling machine. Every so often, the machine rewards a pull with a small amount of money, but not all the time. When you do receive a reward, it is kinda exciting, and you are keen for another one. This increases the chances you are staying and playing on. Unfortunately, this type of reinforcement schedule is one of the most difficult to break (but not impossible).

As you can tell, FND is not always met with kind and caring responses. In fact, nearly everybody reports difficult family and healthcare interactions. This **mixed messaging** of both acceptance and rejection fuels intermittent reinforcement, a more difficult type of learning process to overcome (but not impossible), and ultimately maintains FND.

Another issue with RR and intermittent reinforcement is that those people who experience strong fears around rejection and abandonment can start to experience their worst-case scenario – **a self-fulfilling prophecy of actual rejection further prolonging FND**. Look at the bottom parts of Figure 9.4 for an example of a family starting to distance themselves from the person with FND after initially showing care, support, and compassion.

Systemic re-traumatisation

Another dark side of RR is the increased risk of the person with FND being viewed by their environment as manipulative, needy, attention-seeking, or putting the symptoms on for attention – particularly in the context of patient–healthcare provider relationships. This is called **systemic re-traumatisation (SR)**. SR has detrimental effects on relationships in the healthcare system and, more importantly, is another maintaining factor of FND.

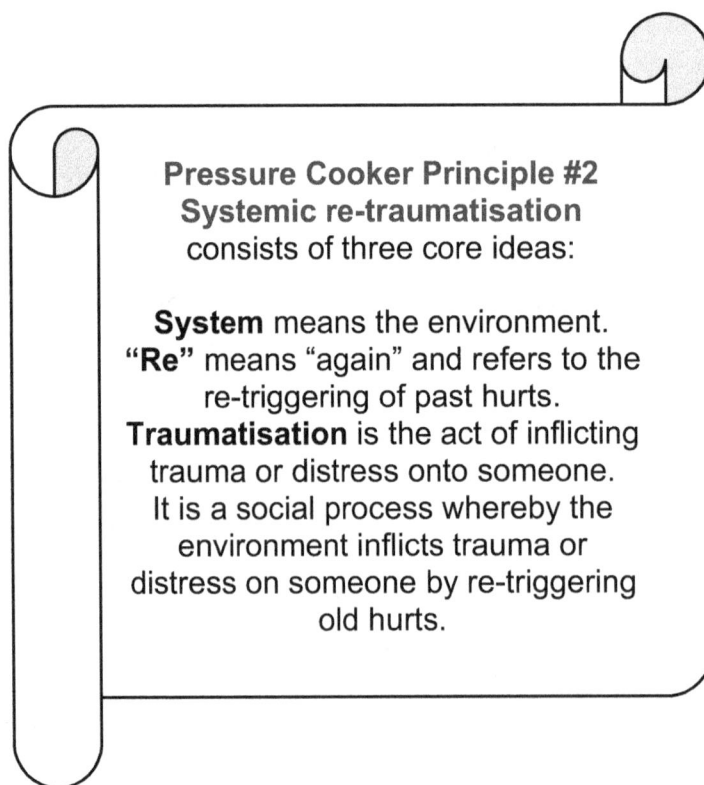

Pressure Cooker Principle #2
Systemic re-traumatisation
consists of three core ideas:

System means the environment.
"Re" means "again" and refers to the re-triggering of past hurts.
Traumatisation is the act of inflicting trauma or distress onto someone. It is a social process whereby the environment inflicts trauma or distress on someone by re-triggering old hurts.

Figure 9.5 Systemic re-traumatisation.

Systemic re-traumatisation in the clinic: reciprocal reinforcement unravelled

Do you remember our discussion on reciprocal reinforcement (RR) earlier? You learned that both people with and without FND experience thoughts, feelings, responses, and needs that maintain FND. RR consists of a series of steps that both the person and their environment equally contribute to – not just the person with FND.

However, there was **one last step missing** from those sequences. In a way, you could view the process of systemic re-traumatisation as **'reciprocal reinforcement unravelled'**. We are now getting at the heart of systemic re-traumatisation. Figure 9.6 shows you the last missing piece of the puzzle.

Figure 9.6 reveals that the responses and actions from the environment cause a normal and logical response from the person with FND, yet it is often the person who ends up being labelled, judged, and blamed by the environment for their behaviours and symptoms, even though both the person and the environment clearly contribute to FND.

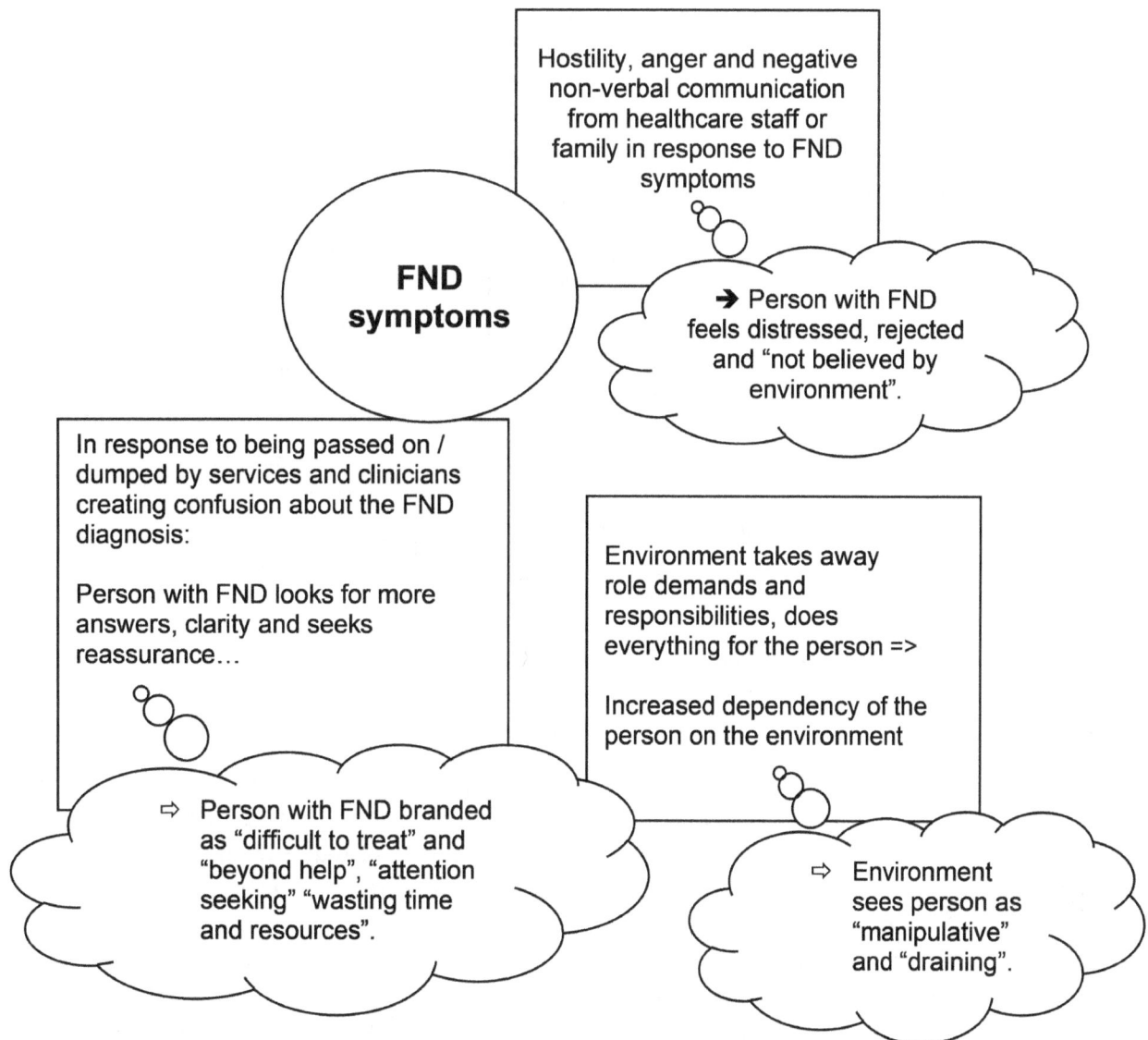

Figure 9.6 Systemic re-traumatisation in clinical and family environments.

Negative consequences of systemic re-traumatisation and reciprocal reinforcement

Research studies and clinical experiences have unveiled the many detrimental effects of the negative beliefs, emotions, and actions that result from RR and SR interactions between people with FND and their environment (see Figure 9.7).

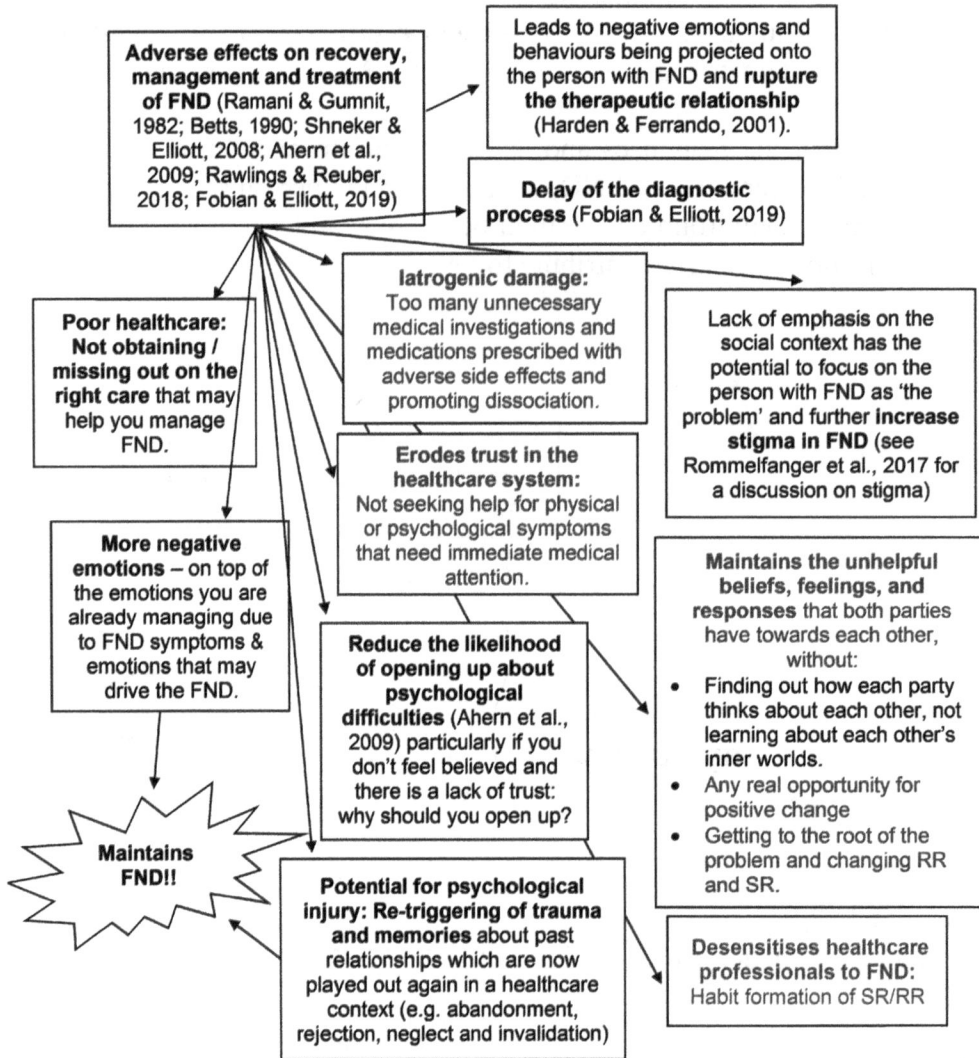

Figure 9.7 Consequences of RR and SR in the world of healthcare.

The FND mirrors: more evidence for similarities between people with and without FND!

A mirror is an item that reflects an image due to the special glass it uses. When we look in the mirror, we see our own reflection. Imagine that the mirror is not an item made of glass but, instead, is another person or a prior relationship. When we look at the other person, we may see our own qualities and characteristics in that person. A large amount of research has described the healthcare experiences of people with FND and healthcare staff who work with people with FND . . . for the groups separately.

No one thought about considering the results of all these studies together. When we link these two sets of study results, we find that there is a relationship between the experiences reported by people with FND and their healthcare workers. It turns out that the features (or themes) of these experiences mirror each other! To illustrate this point further, look at Table 9.1.

Table 9.1 Beliefs, emotions, and actions of people with FND vs staff treating people with FND in relation to each other

People with FND	Mirror	Staff treating people with FND
"Staff don't believe me"	**#1 Believing FND symptoms**	"Symptoms are not real"
Worries about negative judgements from staff, e.g. crazy, faking, seeking attention.	**#2 Negative judgements**	"They are faking, seeking attention, waste time, difficult to treat, beyond help…"
Perceived lack of support from staff.	**#3 Lack of support**	Not providing support: rushed approach to patient, rudeness, negative interactions.
Worries about relationship with staff.	**#4 Patient-staff relationship**	Worries that patient does not believe staff member, patient losing trust, saying the wrong thing.
Confusion about diagnosis.	**#5 Confusion**	Confused about FND: Limited confidence in diagnosis, management and treatment of FND, low self-perceived knowledge on FND
Feeing dumped, rejected, abandoned.	**#6 Rejection and abandonment**	Staff abandoning/dumping: Referrals to other healthcare professionals, passing patient on.
Anger, distress, hostility to staff.	**#7 Negative emotions**	Anger, frustration, irritation, distress before consultation, hostility to patients.

Note: Please see eResource 9.2 for references of peer-reviewed publications supporting this table.

9.1 eResource alert!

To show that all of us fall into similar 'thinking traps' from time to time, please read more about common thinking traps in people with FND and their healthcare professionals in the context of shared healthcare experiences. Reflection point: Do you notice any similarities between the two groups?

Now that you have learned about relationships in FND, let us focus on how to improve interactions and build better interpersonal dynamics between people with and without FND, in our final chapter of this book. Nearly there!

References

Ahern, L., Stone, J., & Sharpe, M. C. (2009). Attitudes of neuroscience nurses toward patients with conversion symptoms. *Psychosomatics, 50*(4), 336–339.

Betts, T. (1990). Pseudoseizures: seizures that are not epilepsy. *Lancet (British edition), 336*(8708), 163–164.

Fobian, A. D., & Elliott, L. (2019). A review of functional neurological symptom disorder etiology and the integrated etiological summary model. *Journal of Psychiatry and Neuroscience, 44*(1), 8–18.

Harden, C. L., & Ferrando, S. J. (2001). Delivering the diagnosis of psychogenic pseudoseizures: Should the neurologist or the psychiatrist be responsible? *Epilepsy & Behavior, 6*(2), 519–523.

Kendall, S. B. (1974). Preference for intermittent reinforcement. *Journal of the Experimental Analysis of Behavior, 21*(3), 463–473.

Ramani, V., & Gumnit, R. J. (1982). Management of hysterical seizures in epileptic patients. *Archives of Neurology, 39*(2), 78–81.

Rawlings, G. H., & Reuber, M. (2018). Health care practitioners' perceptions of psychogenic nonepileptic seizures: A systematic review of qualitative and quantitative studies. *Epilepsia, 59*(6), 1109–1123.

Rommelfanger, K. S., Factor, S. A., LaRoche, S., Rosen, P., Young, R., & Rapaport, M. H. (2017). Disentangling stigma from functional neurological disorders: Conference report and roadmap for the future. *Frontiers in Neurology, 8*, 106.

Shneker, B. F., & Elliott, J. O. (2008). Primary care and emergency physician attitudes and beliefs related to patients with psychogenic nonepileptic spells. *Epilepsy & Behavior, 13*(1), 243–247.

Wagner, A. R. (1961). Effects of amount and percentage of reinforcement and number of acquisition trials on conditioning and extinction. *Journal of Experimental Psychology, 62*(3), 234.

10 Improving pressure cooker dynamics

Building better relationships

The urge to bond, care, socially connect, and feel secure with another individual is hardwired and primal. Relationships are the core in the existence and survival of many species.

Look at the following example: Imagine a bunch of buffalos on a savanna plain. A buffalo on its own is quite vulnerable to predators. A group of cheetahs circling around a single buffalo would likely be the end. Have you noticed that buffalos always move in herds? A big herd ensures that the species survive: together the buffalos are strong, and no predator would dare to come close – they look pretty intimidating as a group! Being part of a herd, a flock, or a social group is protective for survival. In the same way, as humans we herd together, and we have an intrinsic need towards socially connecting, belonging, and playing a meaningful part in a group, including a family and in society.

If these bidirectional bonds and relationships between people are less than optimal, dysfunctional, or broken in some way or we become socially isolated and lack any sense of belonging to a group, the environment, or society that the 'ill' individual with FND is part of, they should be considered just as ill, with exactly the same levels of illness as the person that is targeted as 'the problem'. By ignoring the concept of systemic illness in FND, the road to recovery will less likely be fully or satisfactorily achieved. To start FND recovery is to start repairing relationships and to consider FND as a manifestation of systemic illness.

An environmental approach to FND: building better relationships

Hopefully by now you have learned that the Pressure Cooker Model views FND as a multi-layered condition that involves social connections with many people: everybody contributes to FND, and everybody is responsible for recovery. Although a person just so happens to experience the actual symptoms, FND manifests, at least partly, because of underlying relationship dynamics that is the combined product of the person and the environment. That is why focusing on the environment and relationships is so important and brings longer-lasting changes in FND: all aboard the same train, please! Figure 10.1 displays the ways in which you, your partner, your family, your friends, and your healthcare professionals can repair relationships to manage FND.

10.1 eResource alert!

Reflection point: Take a good look at your social environment and the people who surround you. Whom do you interact with on a regular basis, and importantly, do any of these social systems potentially contribute to the FND? Find out more by doing this exercise, which will help you map out and redo your 'kitchen' environment, if needed. It can be helpful to do this exercise with someone trustworthy and who knows you well.

Chapter 10 outline: the big kitchen clean-up

If we presume that FND is, at least partially, driven and maintained by relationship factors, then it makes sense to explore areas that can break reciprocal reinforcement patterns between the person and

DOI: 10.4324/9781003308973-10

the system. If the only thing that you remember from Chapter 10 is, 'FND care is a family, couples, and environmental intervention', you have won more than half the battle! Let us explore the following areas:

- Establish for yourself: What exactly makes a **good relationship** and creates **psychological safety**?
- Increase your **awareness into what is going on in FND relationships.**
- How can you guard and adjust blurred **relationship boundaries**?
- Complete a **Pressure Cooker Model** and **stop reciprocal reinforcement.**

Pressure cooker fast facts: what makes a good relationship and creates psychological safety?

If we want to build better relationships to manage FND, we probably need to start with a discussion around what normal relationships look like in the first place. But what is 'normal', anyways? To some degree, every relationship is a mix of positive qualities and aspects that are probably less helpful. There is no such thing as 'the perfect relationship'. Bear in mind also that not everyone has had the opportunity to learn the 'relationship basics' of a healthy and secure relationship for reasons outlined in Chapter 5. Although the list of positive relationship qualities displayed in Figure 10.1 is not exhaustive, it is a useful guide because some people with FND and their environment experience difficulties in several of these areas.

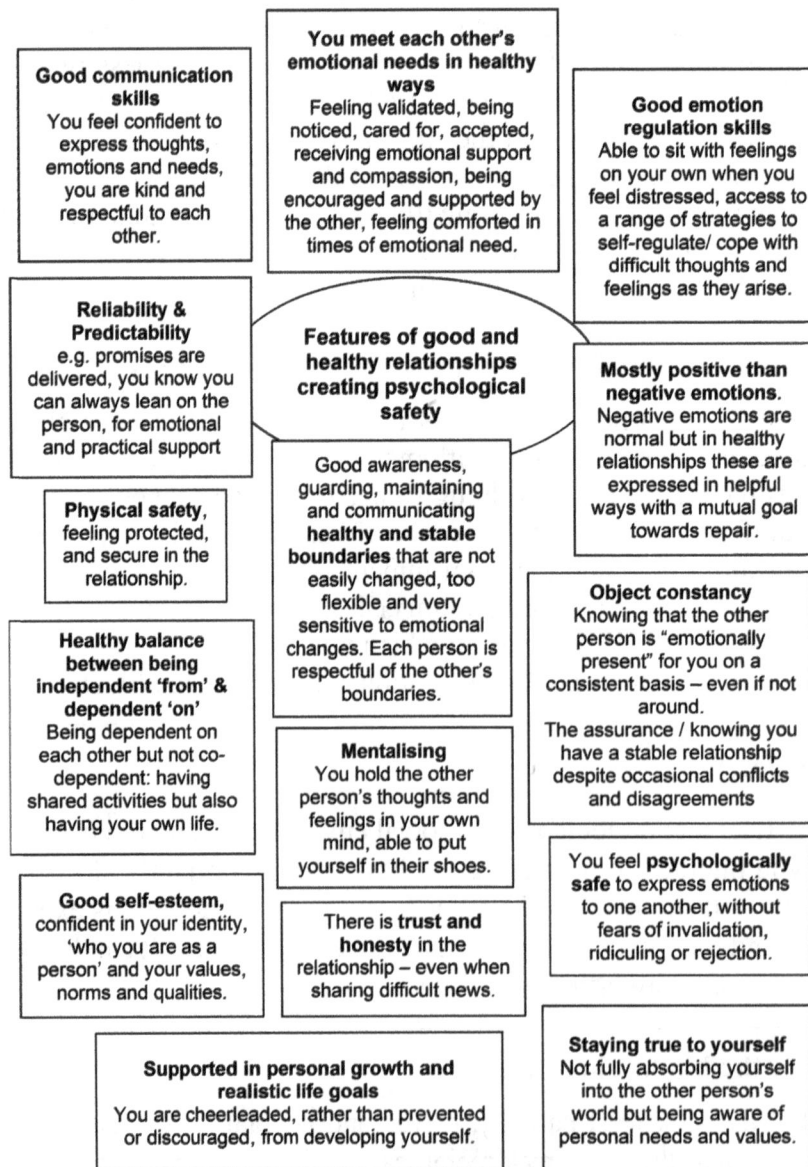

Figure 10.1 A few important building blocks of a high-quality relationship.

Increase your awareness into what is going on in FND relationships

Reciprocal reinforcement (RR) greatly impacts on the quality of relationships and redefines the roles between a person with FND and their partners, family members, friends, and healthcare professionals, in both directions. Let us review some common ways in which RR changes the nature of personal and family relationships.

FND may become part of the **family's identity**: the family's time, resources, attention, and energy become entirely focused on the person with FND (see Figure 10.2).

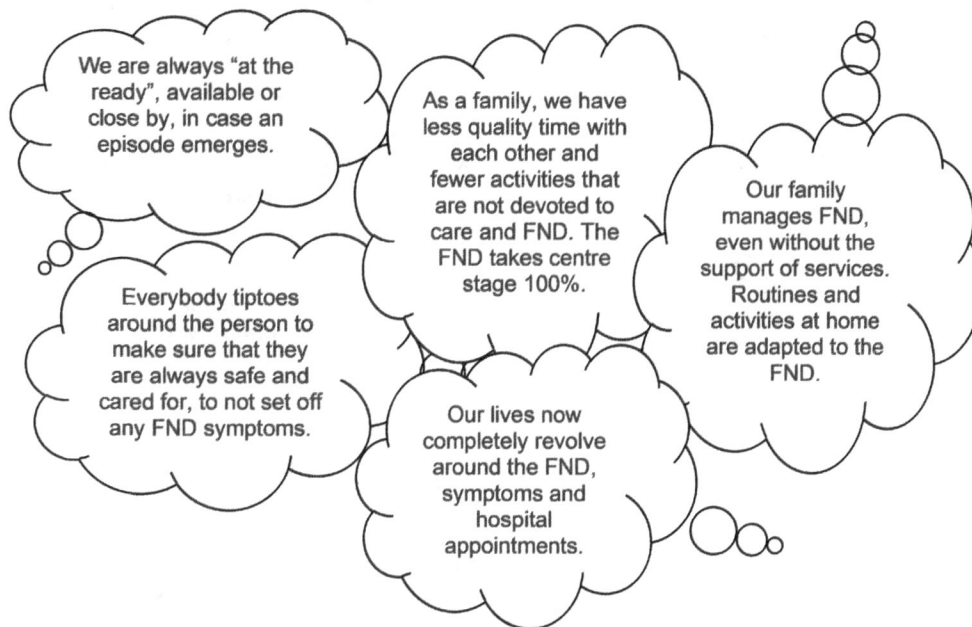

Figure 10.2 The impact of FND on family identity and functioning.

Emotions in the family that contribute to FND and/or emotions that arise because of the FND affect the quality of caring activities and family relationships (see Figure 10.3), often resulting in role changes in the family (see Figure 10.4).

Although not often a topic that is explored in sessions or spontaneously mentioned during consultations, it is nevertheless really important. What can we say about sexual relations in FND?

Top 10 most common relationship difficulties that maintain FND

1. Problems with **assertiveness** and **expressing needs** in personal relationships.
2. Difficulties with **recognising** and regularly **expressing emotions**.
3. Mismatch in **emotion communication** between partners or family members.
4. Unhelpful boundaries: **co-dependency**, enmeshed, hypervigilant, and overprotective.
5. Unhelpful boundaries: **overly distant** relationship characterised by unmet or insufficiently met emotional needs.
6. **Social isolation**, with only the immediate family or social media as the main emotional support network.
7. Relationship dynamics in the context of loss, absence, or abandonment through **separation, divorce, or death**.
8. Relationship dynamics due to threats towards social losses, potential rejection, or abandonment, for example, through an **unreleased unspeakable dilemma** or **psychological pressure**.
9. Constant **strife and arguments** in the relationship.
10. **Domestic violence** and **coercive control** in the relationship – less common but far-reaching consequences for a person's life if present.

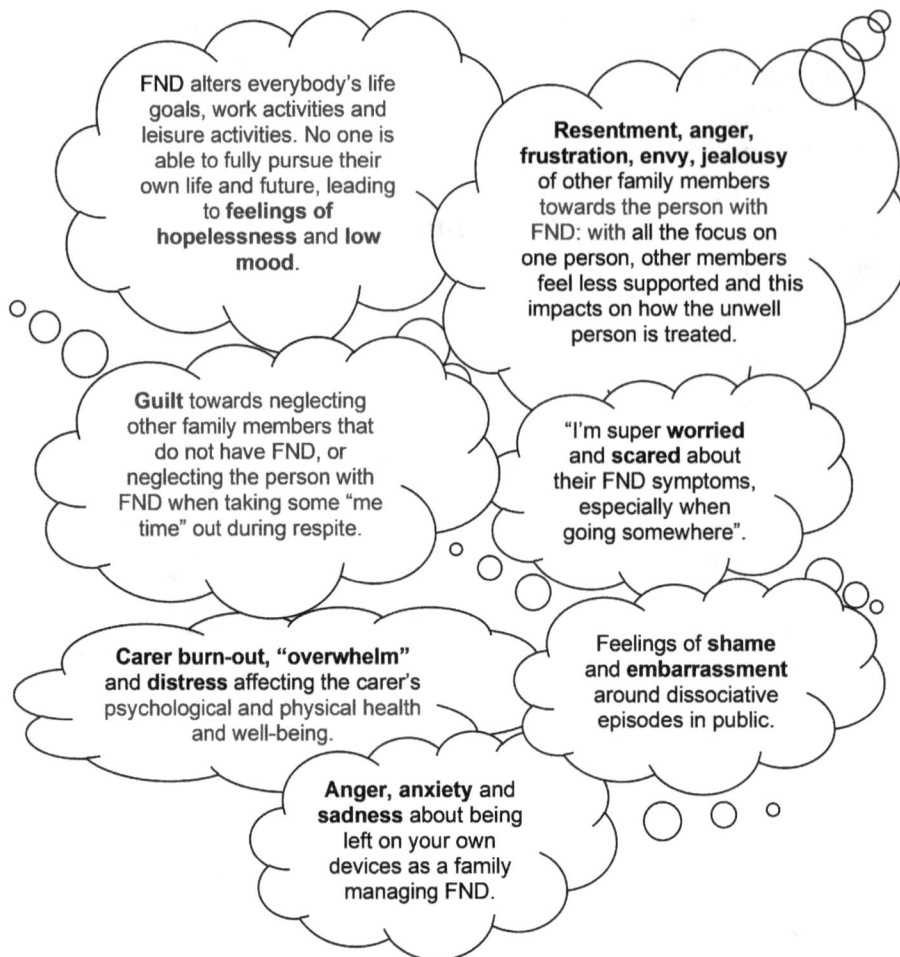

Figure 10.3 The variety of difficult emotions experienced in families with FND.

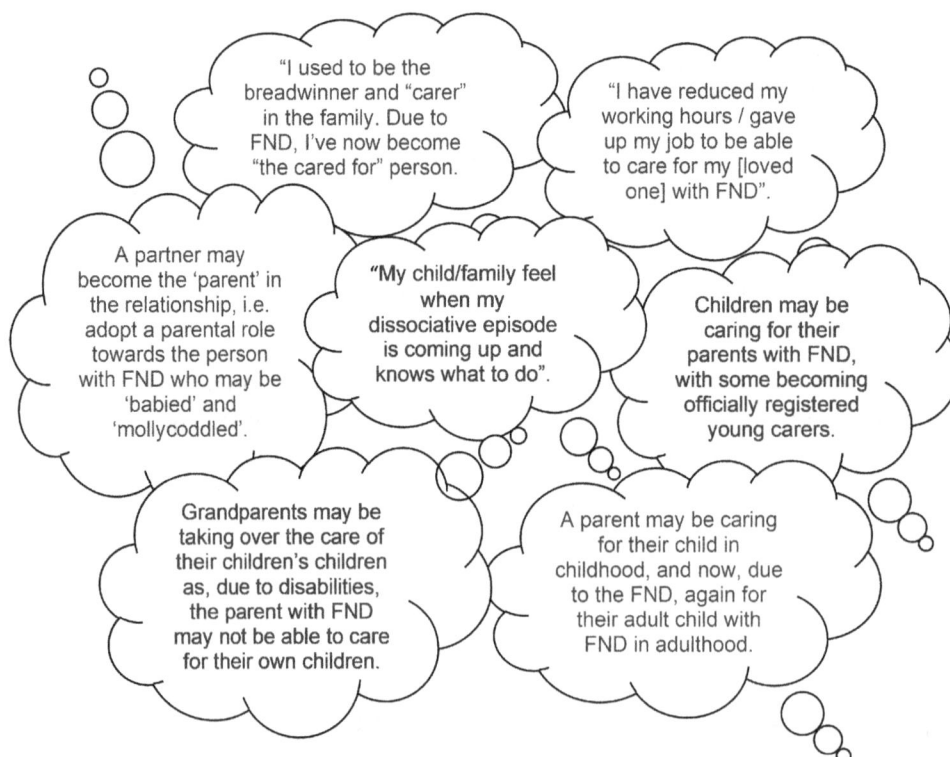

Figure 10.4 Role changes and role reversals in families with FND.

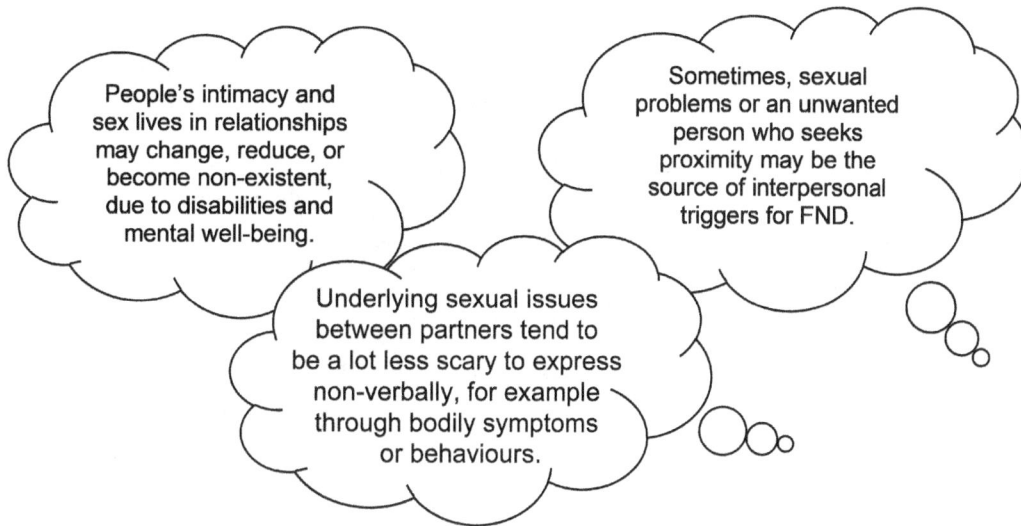

Figure 10.5 FND and sexual intimacy, a sensitive but important topic.

10.2 eResource alert!

For more details and background reading on these relationship difficulties in FND, check out this eResource to bring you up to speed.

How do we discern and guard relationship boundaries in FND?

That is a good question. When is too little 'too little', too much 'too much', or perhaps out of the ordinary? Who decides that you have reached the point where caring patterns adversely affect the FND in your own family and personal relationships? Better questions to ask are: **Am I hurting or helping? Is this more about me or the other person?**

Compare caring to eating, another basic human need. We eat and drink every day to sustain ourselves. In the same way, as humans we need care and validation to sustain ourselves psychologically and function in life. We cannot just withdraw all care for the rest of our life to stop FND! This is not about encouraging people to stop caring altogether. Caring is about quantity, quality, timing, and placing appropriate boundaries by all parties involved.

Care patterns at either extreme are not helpful and are associated with the maintenance of FND symptoms. Treatment often consists of finding a middle way between these two extremes: a combination of **self-regulating** our emotions on our own vs **co-regulating** with other people in our environment, as well as discovering and learning new ways of caring and relating to one another.

The following **relationship checklist** may help you and your loved ones determine whether it is useful to think about changing the way you care and relate to one another in the context of managing FND. If you tick quite a lot of boxes, then you might want to look further into the environment's contribution to FND:

- Can you detect a **reciprocal reinforcement pattern**, in particular, are the FND and caring patterns somehow regulating everyone's emotional needs and achieving a state of psychological safety between people?

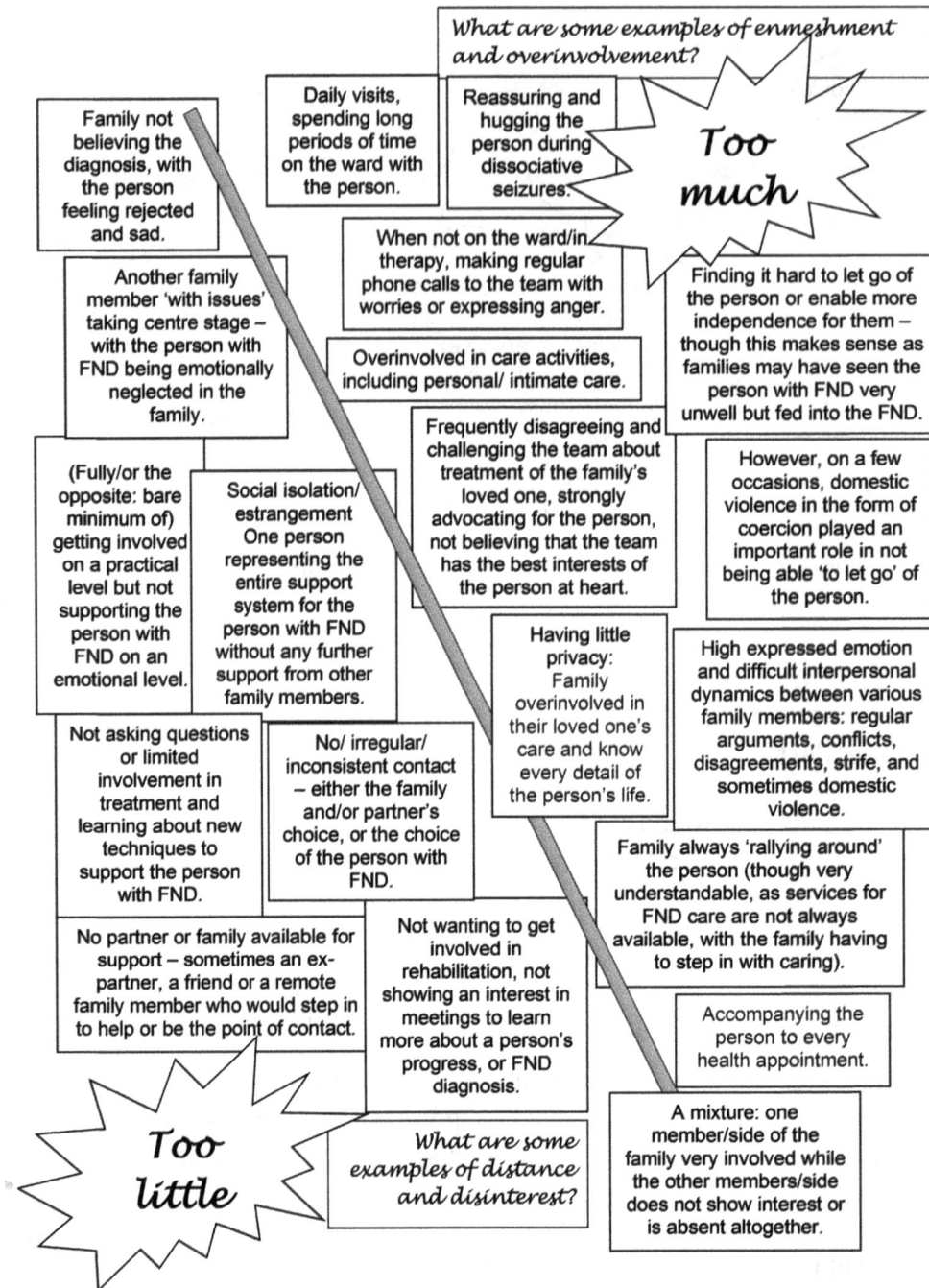

Figure 10.6 What do boundaries sometimes look like in FND?

- Is the relationship otherwise characterised by **frequent distress**, discomfort, negative emotions, and unhelpful thoughts for one person or everyone involved?
- Has the relationship between *the person being cared for* and *the person who is caring for* become **entrenched, long-standing, and intertwined** with **people's identities**? Does everybody's life revolve around the FND and caring activities?
- Do these care patterns **absorb time, effort, and resources**; adversely impact on day-to-day activities; and push away other valuable life roles? Think of fulfilling family roles (being a partner, mother, father, grandparent, sister, brother, daughter, son, and so forth) or other meaningful life roles (work, friendships, 'me time', pursuing life goals, hobbies, and interests).
- Are **care needs and disabilities increasing** rather than decreasing over time?
- Is there a risk of **carer fatigue** or burnout? Does it feel physically and emotionally heavy and overwhelming?

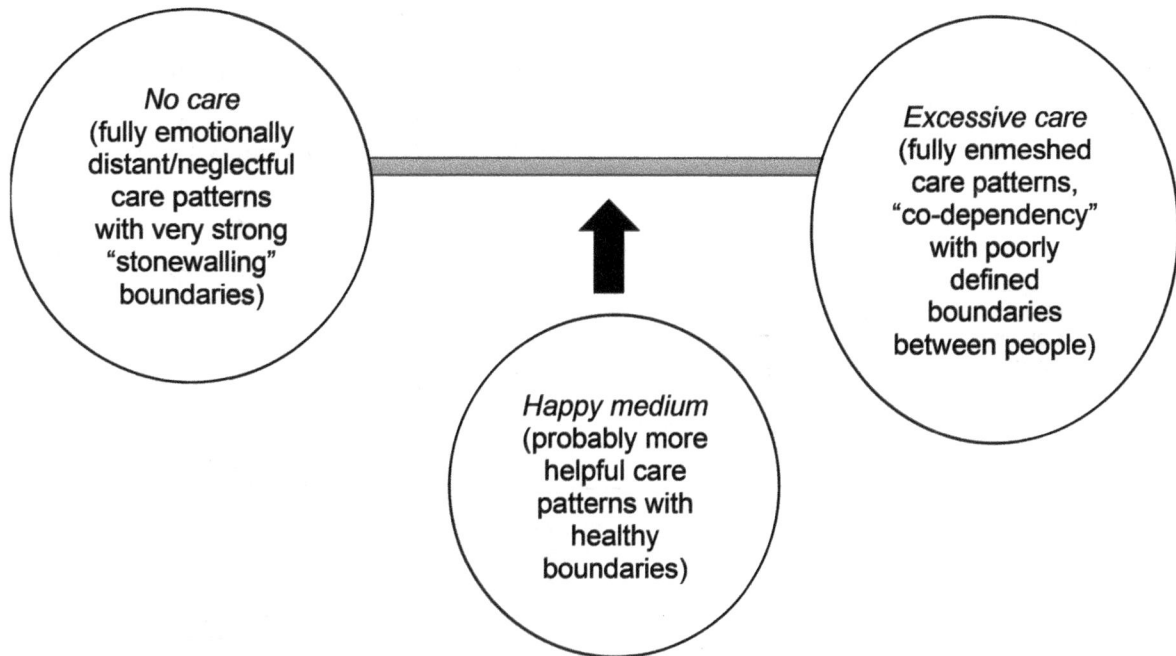

Figure 10.7 Thinking of 'caring for another person' as being on a continuum.

10.3 eResource alert!

This exercise will help you gauge the level of emotional closeness and distance in your relationships and support you with gaining some insight into whether your relationships could be helpful or hurtful to FND.

Since we arrived at the point of carer fatigue and burnout . . .

Imagine sitting on a plane on a long-haul intercontinental flight towards a tropical destination somewhere far away. There is quite some turbulence, the warning lights switch on, and suddenly the breathing masks drop. Panic ensues. Your partner sitting next to you is starting to feel very uncomfortable and is struggling to put their mask on. What do the flight attendants normally recommend during the safety briefing at the beginning of your flight? Something along the lines of:

'Put on your own mask first before helping others to put on theirs.'

Imagine running out of oxygen and passing out because you are trying to help someone else put their mask on. Now there are two people passing out.

Depending on the level of disability, caring for someone with FND can be an intense, challenging and sometimes tiring experience – of no fault at all to anyone involved.

For some people, the reality of caring is full on: daily personal care, repositioning, medication management, meal preparation, toileting, driving to hospital appointments, seizure care, and so forth.

FND SELF-CARE is not just about the person with FND but for everyone involved in the person's life. Just like with the plane masks, in order to care in the best way for another human being, you first need to ensure that you are caring for yourself. You could become a 'super carer' for the other person by meeting your own physical and emotional needs with the necessary self-care first.

Social media system: helpful or hurtful?

A system that is often reported by people with FND as positive, supportive, and informative is the **social media system**. In recent years, a large number of FND communities, fora, blog posts, web pages, social media outlets, and networking accounts have arisen for people with FND.

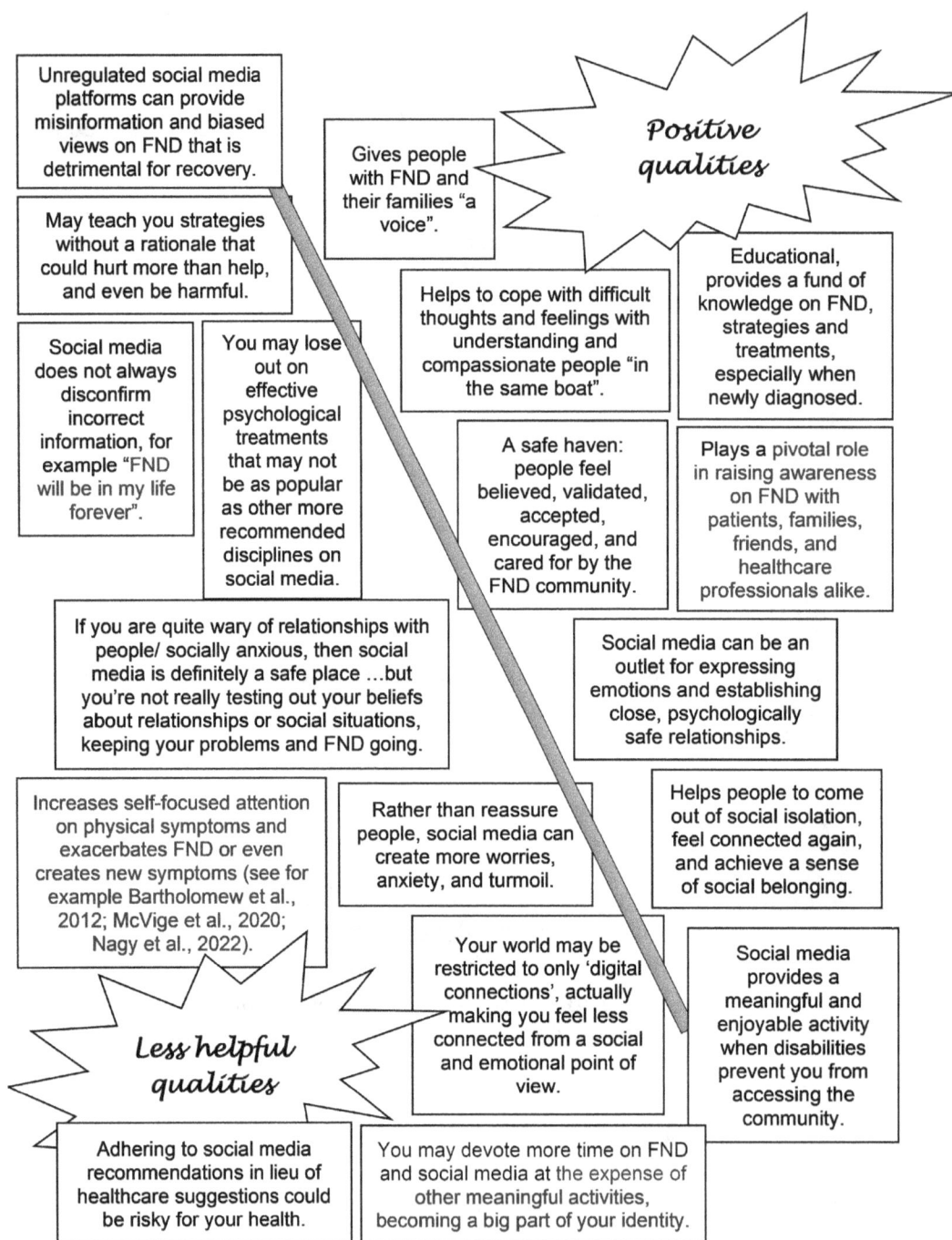

Figure 10.8 Social media in FND.

10.4 eResource alert!

Read about the FND SELF-CARE 'family version' and the 'environmental valve' on the Pressure Cooker Model to learn about common issues for carers who care for a person with FND.

10.5 eResource alert!

Figure 10.8 has hopefully given you a balanced view on social media use and FND. To help you decide on whether social media is helpful or hurtful, read here about its positive qualities as well as the red flags.

We have arrived at Pressure Cooker rehab!

Let us get down to business and help you overcome the FND! But before we start, this is the plan:

- Everybody, both people with and without FND, will complete a Pressure Cooker Model.
- Everybody will be asked to check out their own Pressure Cooker Model. Do not worry if the structure of the Pressure Cooker Model looks daunting. It will look a bit much initially!
- Here is what you can do instead. Look at Figure 10.9 and decide for yourself what challenge level you find yourself at currently and follow the accompanying instructions.
- Whatever you decide, start somewhere. It does not matter where that somewhere is. As long as you start.
- Once you have decided on your level of challenge, re-read the chapters that explore these elements and have a freestyle brainstorm to select your strategies.

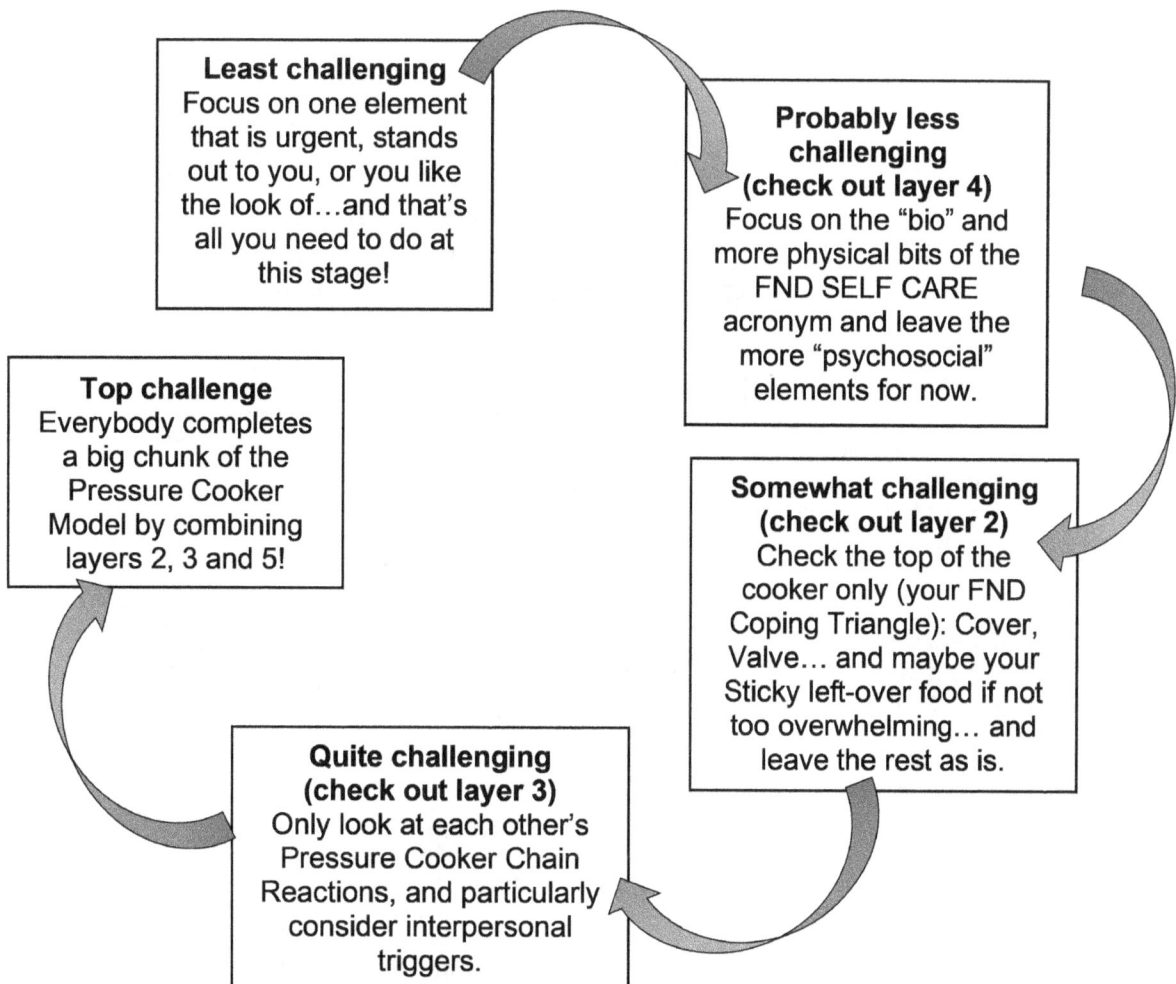

Least challenging
Focus on one element that is urgent, stands out to you, or you like the look of…and that's all you need to do at this stage!

Probably less challenging (check out layer 4)
Focus on the "bio" and more physical bits of the FND SELF CARE acronym and leave the more "psychosocial" elements for now.

Top challenge
Everybody completes a big chunk of the Pressure Cooker Model by combining layers 2, 3 and 5!

Somewhat challenging (check out layer 2)
Check the top of the cooker only (your FND Coping Triangle): Cover, Valve… and maybe your Sticky left-over food if not too overwhelming… and leave the rest as is.

Quite challenging (check out layer 3)
Only look at each other's Pressure Cooker Chain Reactions, and particularly consider interpersonal triggers.

Figure 10.9 Different Pressure Cooker Model challenges for different needs.

My pressure cooker fact-finding and story ('assessment' and 'formulation')

Do you remember the story of Daniel and Kayleigh from Chapter 2? The couple is now officially in 'Pressure Cooker rehab'. With the facts from Chapter 2 on hand, Daniel and Kayleigh are ready to create their joint FND story of how these facts hang together and contribute to FND. In terms of difficulty level (Figure 10.9), this is probably classified as a 'top challenge': the whole Pressure Cooker Model will be completed by Daniel and Kayleigh together. However, rest assured, you are not expected to follow suit. As was highlighted before, pick your difficulty level and just roll with it! Starting is half the battle.

10.6 eResource alert!

Check out these handy questions to guide you through the process of completing the elements.

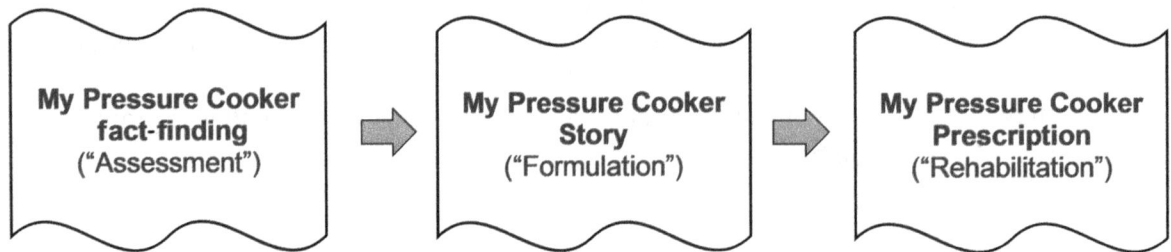

My Pressure Cooker fact-finding ("Assessment") → **My Pressure Cooker Story** ("Formulation") → **My Pressure Cooker Prescription** ("Rehabilitation")

Figure 10.10 My Pressure Cooker rehab.

The five-layer system of the Pressure Cooker Model

Remember discussing 'psychological formulation' in Chapter 1? A good way of looking at how the biological, psychological, and social elements tie together into one Pressure Cooker Model to create your own personal story of FND is to organise the elements into layers.

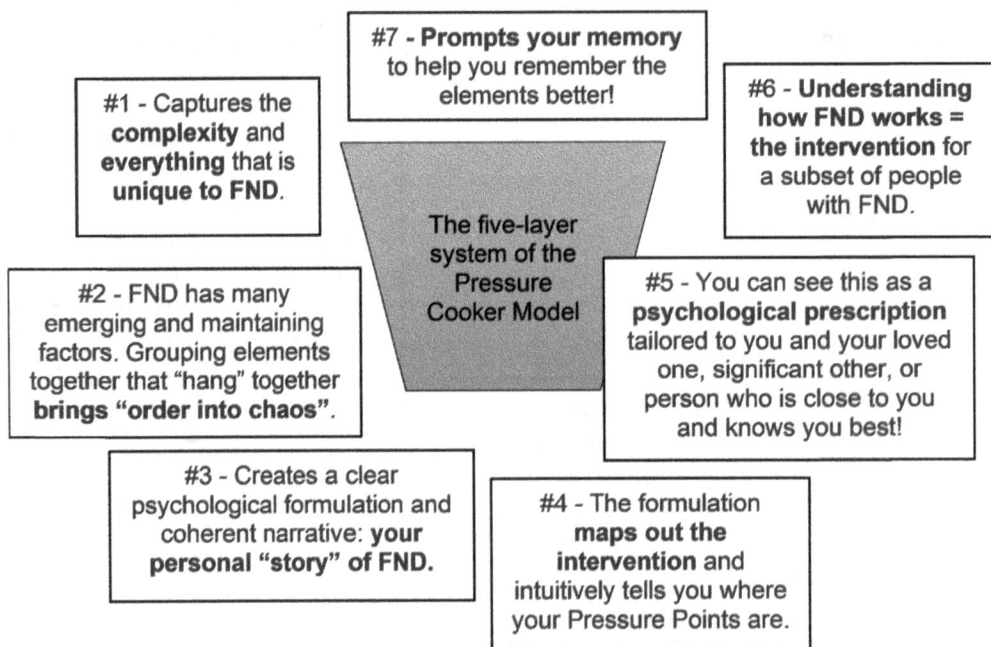

#7 - **Prompts your memory** to help you remember the elements better!

#1 - Captures the **complexity** and **everything** that is **unique to FND**.

#6 - **Understanding how FND works = the intervention** for a subset of people with FND.

The five-layer system of the Pressure Cooker Model

#2 - FND has many emerging and maintaining factors. Grouping elements together that "hang" together **brings "order into chaos"**.

#5 - You can see this as a **psychological prescription** tailored to you and your loved one, significant other, or person who is close to you and knows you best!

#3 - Creates a clear psychological formulation and coherent narrative: **your personal "story" of FND**.

#4 - The formulation **maps out the intervention** and intuitively tells you where your Pressure Points are.

Figure 10.11 Reasons for using a five-layer system in the Pressure Cooker Model.

What made Daniel vulnerable to develop FND?

- Some difficult childhood experiences had happened that involved rejection, like bullying at school.
- Furthermore, his parents argued a lot, were quite strict and invalidated his emotions.
- To protect himself from all this psychological hurt and survive in childhood, Daniel had learned to keep quiet about emotions, suppress emotions, and push on with activities. It was the best thing he could do at the time.

How did Daniel cope with difficult thoughts and feelings throughout his life before the FND?

- For many years, Daniel managed to carry these secrets without much impact on his life.
- His coping mechanism of working very hard and always being on the go helped him to cut difficult thoughts and feelings off.
- Over the years, these coping mechanisms started to become less effective in managing his feelings. They became a bit rusty.

Ignition

But why did the FND develop now? What sparked the FND off in Daniel's life? ("Critical incident")

- When Daniel experienced increased stress at work and in his family ("one stressor too many"), his rusty coping mechanisms (on the go, cutting off emotions, bottling up) that worked so well over the years, started to lose their effectiveness.

Unfortunately, Daniel's old coping mechanisms were insufficient to deal with the upsurge of stress in his life. Daniel started to dissociate and cut off his emotions more strongly, which ultimately led to the development of an almost a more pronounced form of dissociation: dissociative seizures.

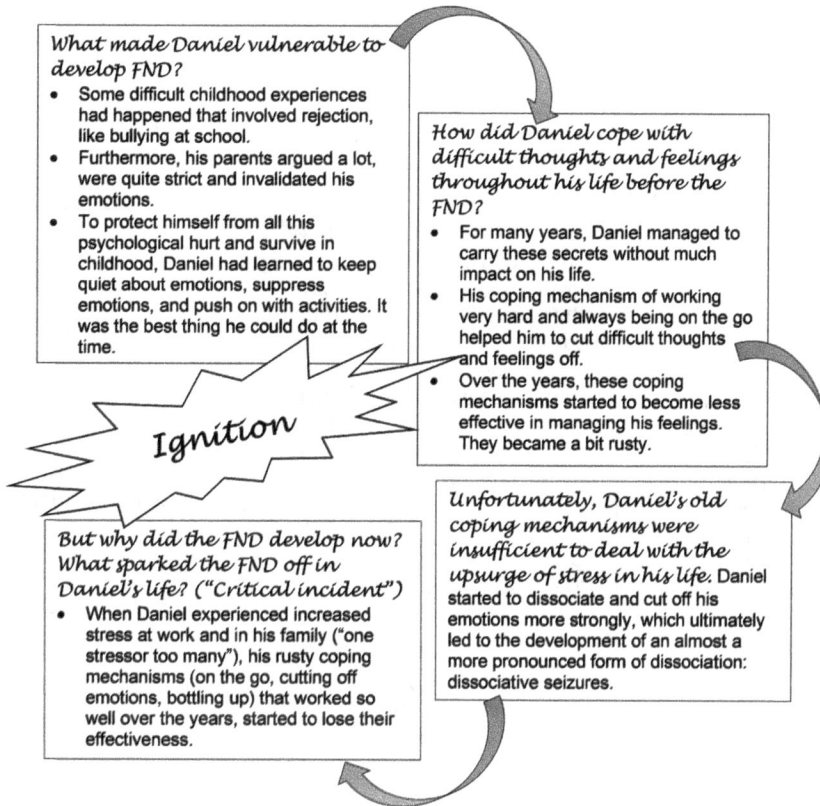

Figure 10.12 Daniel and Kayleigh's story: layer 1 (ignition).

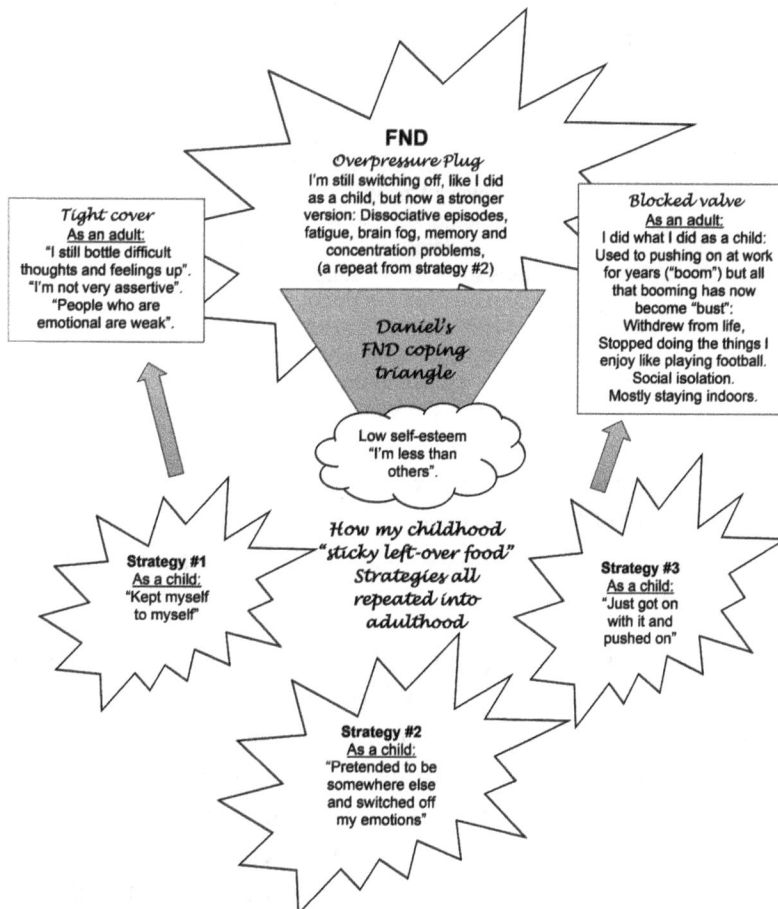

FND
Overpressure Plug
I'm still switching off, like I did as a child, but now a stronger version: Dissociative episodes, fatigue, brain fog, memory and concentration problems, (a repeat from strategy #2)

Daniel's FND coping triangle

Tight cover
<u>As an adult:</u>
"I still bottle difficult thoughts and feelings up". "I'm not very assertive". "People who are emotional are weak".

Blocked valve
<u>As an adult:</u>
I did what I did as a child: Used to pushing on at work for years ("boom") but all that booming has now become "bust": Withdrew from life, Stopped doing the things I enjoy like playing football. Social isolation. Mostly staying indoors.

Low self-esteem "I'm less than others".

How my childhood "sticky left-over food" Strategies all repeated into adulthood

Strategy #1
<u>As a child:</u>
"Kept myself to myself"

Strategy #3
<u>As a child:</u>
"Just got on with it and pushed on"

Strategy #2
<u>As a child:</u>
"Pretended to be somewhere else and switched off my emotions"

Figure 10.13 Daniel's FND coping triangle: layer 2 (cover, valve, and sticky leftover food).

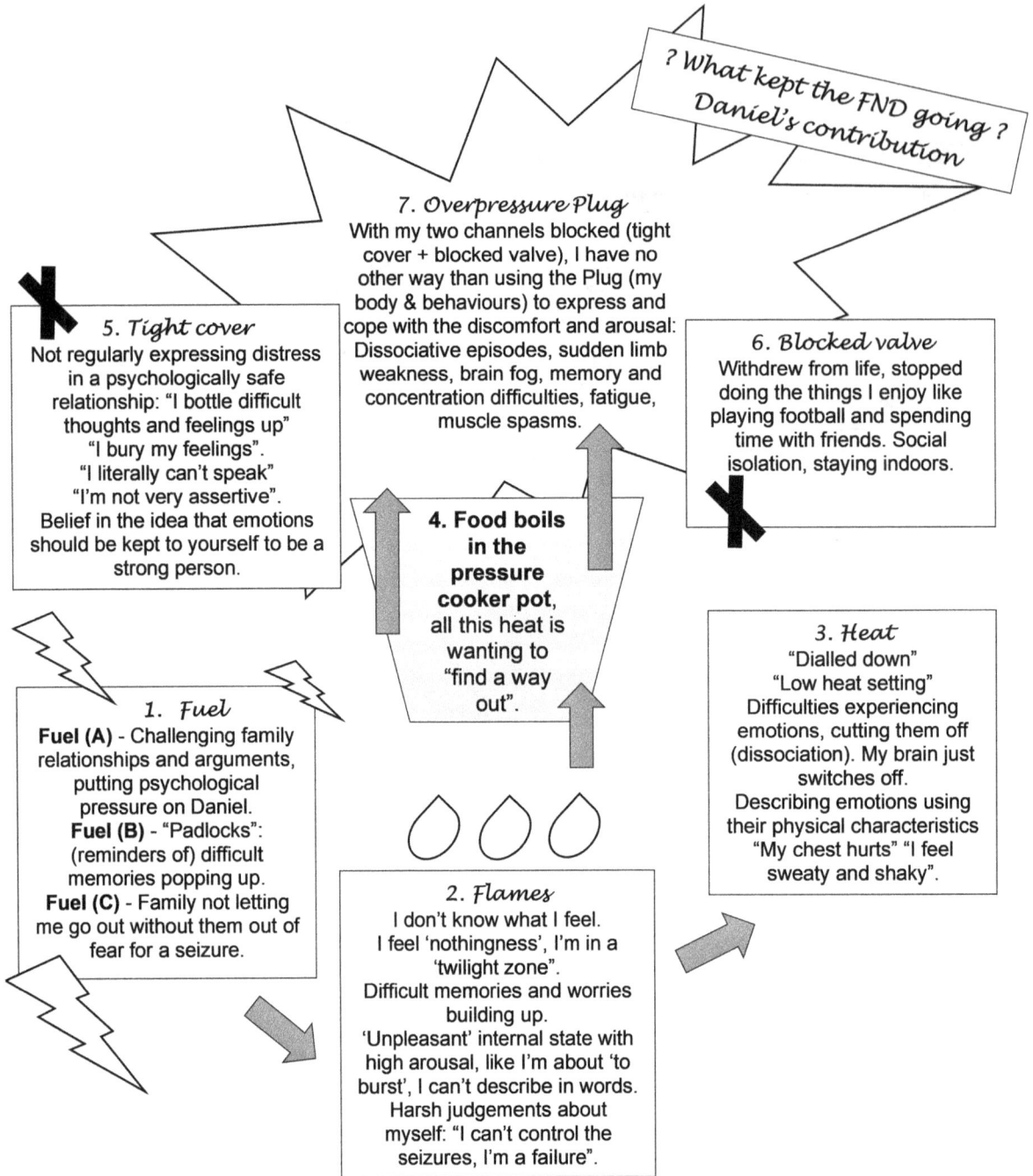

Figure 10.14 Daniel's FND maintenance cycle, a.k.a. 'the Pressure Cooker chain reaction' (layer 3: fuel, flames, heat, and overpressure plug).

Note: Start with #1 (fuel) and follow the numbers, one by one, to go through the entire FND mechanics, ending with #7 (overpressure plug).

Figure 10.15 shows you how witnessing Daniel's seizures and suffering causes a sense of fright, panic, and embarrassment in Kayleigh ('fuel A'). Note how Kayleigh has exactly the same coping strategies as Daniel: dissociation (low heat), keeping self to self (tight cover), and no enjoyable activities to release difficult thoughts and feelings (blocked valve).

Like Daniel, Kayleigh's two channels of emotional expression are blocked. Kayleigh has no other option than to cope the way she does and has worked in the past: rallying around Daniel, keeping a close eye on him, and providing lots of reassurance. Although in the short term this stops Daniel's seizures eventually, providing him with relief, in the long term, the system has become Daniel's main coping strategy for seizures, leading to full dependency and missing out

7. Overpressure Plug
With my two channels blocked (tight cover + blocked valve), I have no other way than using the Plug (my body & behaviours) to express and cope with Daniel's seizures and my own discomfort and arousal: **Enmeshed and "too much" caring: 24-hour supervision, "baby-ing", guarding for hours, verbal/physical reassurance, sense of urgency, system jumping to the rescue, taking all chores out of Daniel's hands.**

? What kept the FND going? Kayleigh's contribution

5. Tight cover
Same as Daniel: Not regularly expressing distress in a psychologically safe relationship: "I don't want to burden Daniel so I keep myself to myself" "Keeping up appearances and say everything is fine to make sure people don't see we are crumbling".

6. Blocked valve
Same as Daniel: withdrew from life, stopped doing the things I enjoy like shopping and spending time with friends. Social isolation, staying indoors, caring for Daniel.

4. Food boils in the pressure cooker pot, all this heat is wanting to "find a way out".

3. Heat
Same as Daniel: "Dialled down" "Low heat setting" Difficulties experiencing emotions, cutting them off (dissociation). My brain just switches off. Describing emotions using their physical characteristics "My chest hurts".

1. Fuel
Fuel (A) – Witnessing Daniel's seizures, breathing difficulties, pain, hurt and losing his dependency, and other people seeing it too.
Fuel (B) – Challenging interactions with Daniel, as well as family relationships and arguments.
Fuel (C) – Stress of sole childcare responsibilities, finances, big life decisions, and running the household.
Fuel (D) – "Missing out" on life and pursuing goals/hobbies.

2. Flames
Fuel (A) thoughts/feelings:
Fright, panic, shock, and embarrassment "oh no, not another seizure!" "This needs to stop asap" "what will other people think?"
Other thoughts and feelings (Fuel B, C and D):
Low mood and compassion for Daniel's suffering/ missed life opportunities but feeling hopeless and trapped in my own situation. Frustration, anger and resentment about losing my old life "can't do this anymore!". Worries about future, ability to cope, and impact of seizures on children. Mixed feelings about Daniel's condition. Guilt for daring to think all these things.

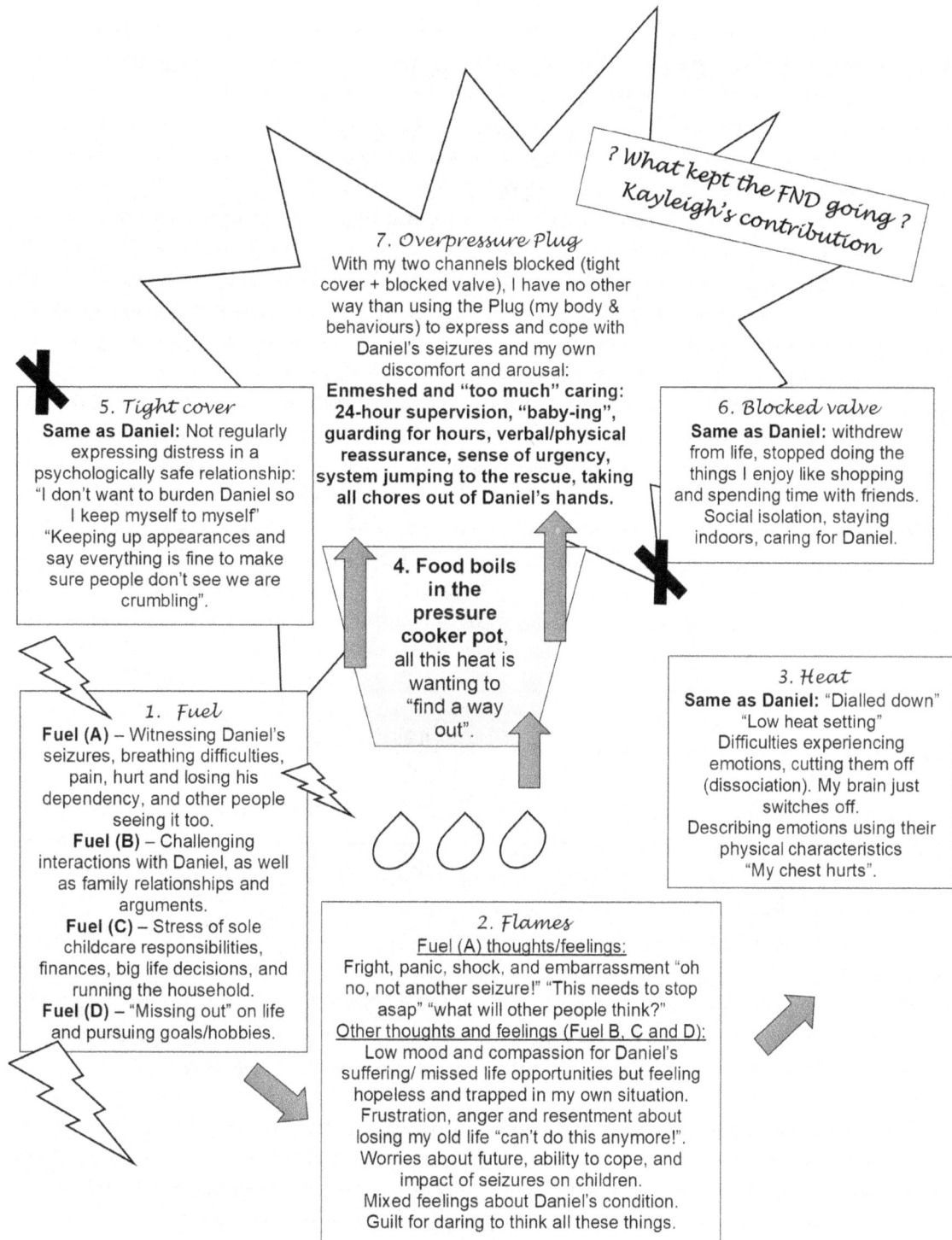

Figure 10.15 Kayleigh's FND maintenance cycle, a.k.a. 'the Pressure Cooker chain reaction' (layer 3: fuel, flames, heat, and overpressure plug).

Note: Start with #1 (fuel) and follow the numbers, one by one, to go through the entire FND mechanics, ending with #7 (overpressure plug).

opportunities to regulate emotions on his own. This is also called 'reciprocal reinforcement', and later you will learn strategies to break this interpersonal reinforcement loop.

Hopefully, you have learned that people with and without FND are really not that different from one another!

Table 10.1 Facilitating physical factors in FND: the pot (layer 4a)

Letter	FND SELF CARE element	How does it maintain the FND in Daniel's situation?
F	Food Fuel	Daniel had several vitamin deficiencies that could contribute to his brain fog, memory, concentration, speech, and sleep problems, as well as his pain, spasms, muscle weakness, breathlessness, weird physical sensations ("electrical currents"), tiredness.
N	Night rest	Daniel's long sleeping episodes, daytime napping, post-seizure naps and "feeling wiped out" helped recovery but were also a form of dissociation and avoidance of emotions.
D	Drugs and medications	Daniel's medications made the dissociation/FND worse. Quickly taking medications to reset a seizure, prolongs FND in the future: Daniel was not learning to tolerate difficult feelings without seizures by relying on medications. The avoidance was also not getting at the root of his problems.
S	Sickness and physical illness	Because of fibromyalgia and POTS, Daniel was paying a lot more attention to his body, joints, and heart rate. This increased self-focused attention, one of the maintaining factors that "feeds" the FND.
E	Equipment	Wheelchair and home adaptations, as a "safety blanket", but maintaining the FND.
L	Liquids	Not drinking enough fluids due to excessive sleep. Dehydration caused brain fog and clouding of Daniel's mind.
F	Fight-Flight-or-Freeze	Daniel's FND symptoms overlapped with the **F=Fight-Flight-or-Freeze** response. Daniel described the physical side of emotions but did not connect psychologically with the emotional experience.
C	Contacts	Multiple ambulance calls and visits to A&E for the seizures, with mixed reactions from hospital staff, making Daniel feel not believed, re-traumatising him, worsening FND.
A	Ability to care for self	Daniel received full support for all daily activities, all chores were taken out of his hands, leading to more dependency and less confidence in his own ability.
R	Risks	• **FND risk #1:** Low mood and reduced psychological well-being. • **FND risk #2:** Accidental self-injury and compromised physical safety (bruises and cuts). • **FND risk #3:** Social isolation. • **FND risk #4:** Slowed-down recovery due to missing out on rehab. • **FND risk #5:** Deteriorated family and healthcare relationships, increased systemic re-traumatisation = more FND.
E	Exercise and movement	Daniel spent days or weeks in bed in "recovery mode" causing deconditioning of his muscles and more difficulties mobilising.

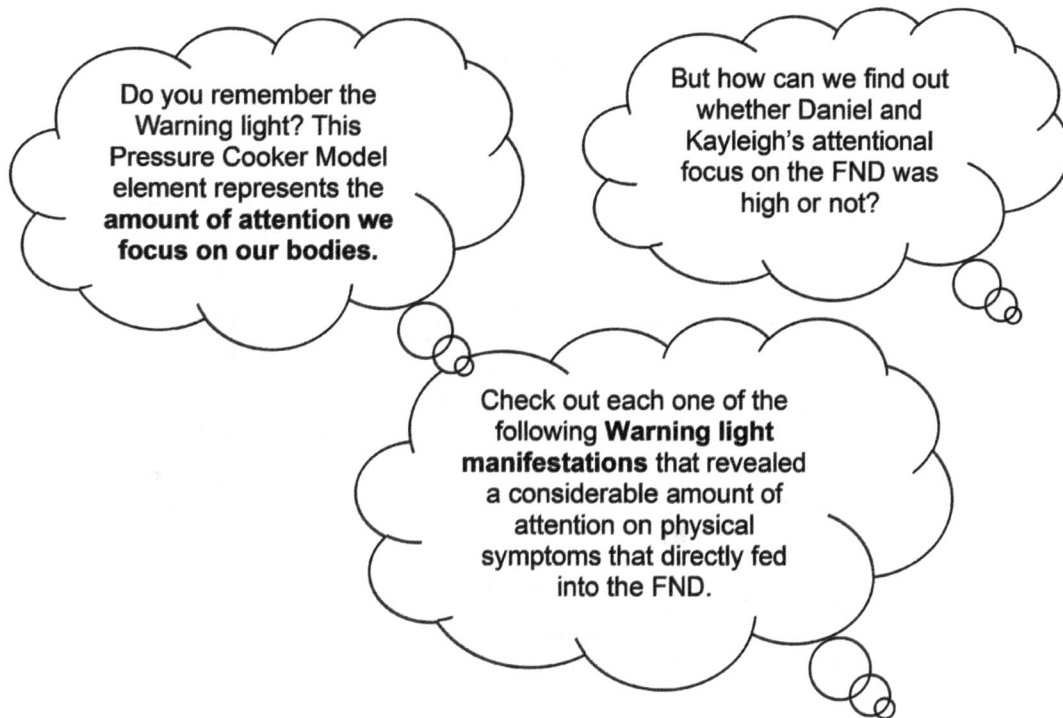

Figure 10.16 Facilitating physical factors in FND: the warning light (layer 4b).

- **'Do we spend time *thinking* about physical symptoms?'** Everybody spent a lot of time on the internet and social media blogs to read and frequently look up Daniel's physical symptoms. Understandably, Daniel and his family worried and struggled to disconnect from FND.
- **'Do we *speak* about physical symptoms in conversations?'** Although Daniel and Kayleigh never minimised psychology, Daniel's emotional lingo mostly revolved around providing physical descriptions of his underlying distress. This was the only 'emotional currency' he knew but kept the FND going.
- **'Do physical symptoms define our *identity*?'** FND gradually became an integral part of Daniel and Kayleigh's identity. Every thought, activity, and conversation in the couple's life revolved around FND, and both were active participants of FND communities online and in real life.
- **'What role do physical symptoms play in our *healthcare relationships*?'** Healthcare contacts were constant reminders of FND. Daniel and Kayleigh attended frequent hospital appointments, called an ambulance, and regularly visited A&E for the seizures for reassurance that it was not something more urgent, like a stroke.
- **'Do *people in our environment* focus on physical symptoms?'** Although Daniel was very focused on checking his body for physical symptoms, bodily sensations, and the FND, Kayleigh, his family, his friends, and yes, even his healthcare professionals were just as focused, if not more! Everybody was always on the lookout for warning signs and on tenterhooks, waiting for seizures to happen.
- **'Does our *physical environment* put the attentional spotlight on FND?'** There was quite a bit of equipment present around Daniel; his home was fully adapted, all constant reminders of the FND symptoms and physical disabilities.

As you can see from Figure 10.17, Daniel and Kayleigh have a lot of (mostly healthcare) contacts. But every contact has its own Pressure Cooker Model too! Daniel is no different from anyone else. Figure 10.18 shows you how all these interpersonal relationships and interactions directly contribute to FND via two key processes: **systemic re-traumatisation** and **intermittent reinforcement**.

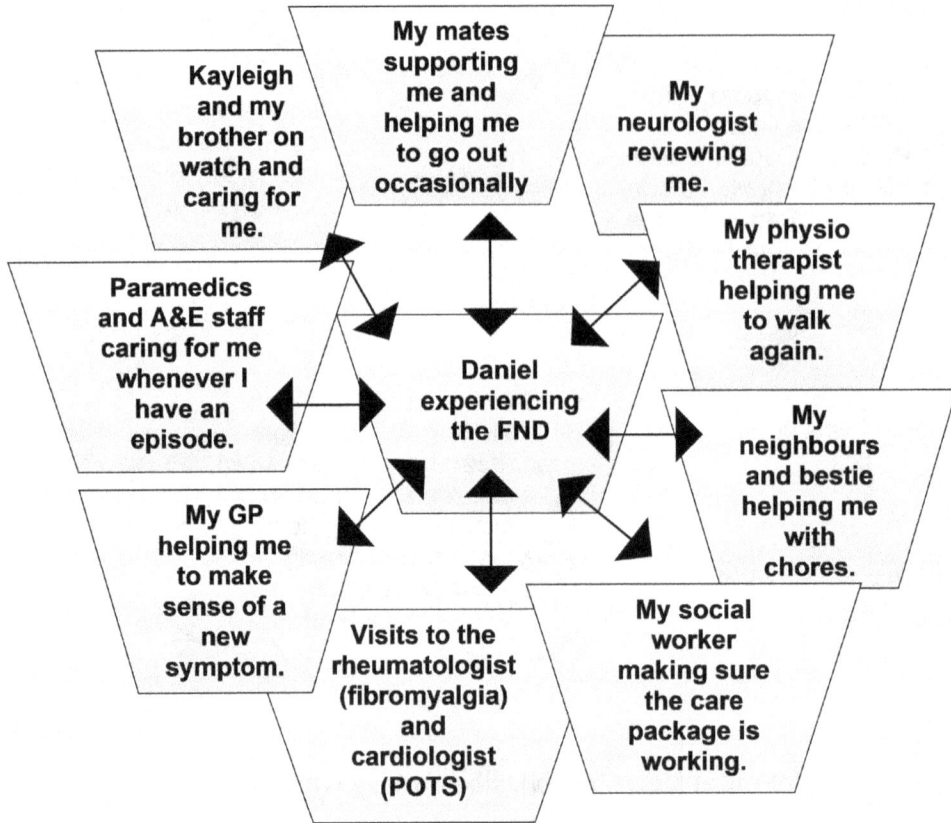

Figure 10.17 Daniel and Kayleigh's kitchen environment: relationships, social, and healthcare contacts in FND (layer 5).

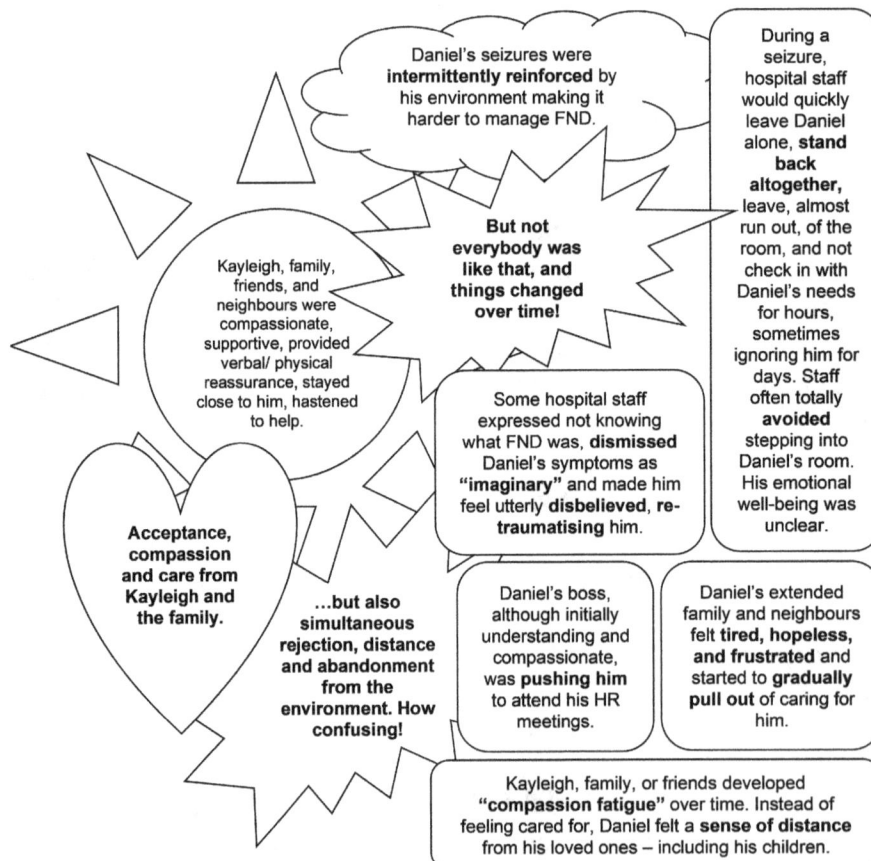

Figure 10.18 Systemic re-traumatisation and intermittent reinforcement by Daniel's environment.

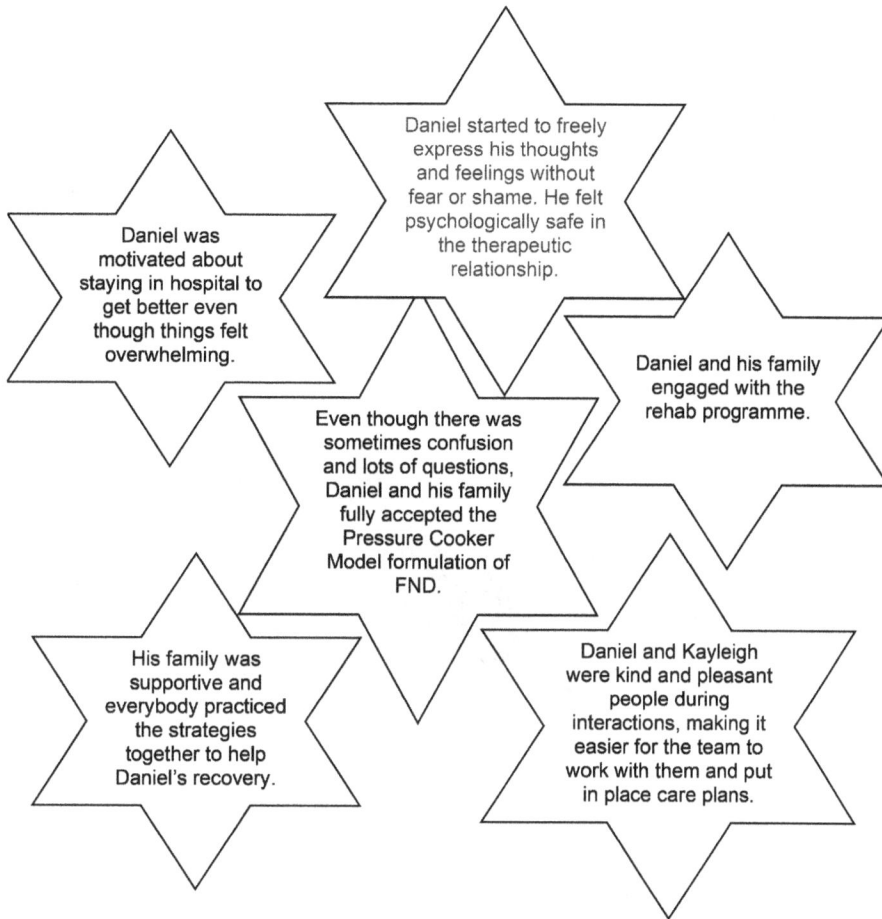

Figure 10.19 Daniel's and Kayleigh's 'safety features': positive qualities supporting neurorehabilitation.

10.7 eResource alert!

Every element of the Pressure Cooker Model of FND can be completed with details from your own situation. How about giving it a go yourself? This exercise is for the person with and without FND! Do not worry if it feels too daunting; you can complete whatever you feel comfortable with or do not do it at all at this stage.

Servicing and repairing a pressure cooker at home

The beauty of the Pressure Cooker Model is that **knowledge gives you the power** to start thinking about **where to intervene and overcome FND!** Remember the 'regular' home pressure cooker? Figure 10.20 shows you how you could intervene in every part of that home pressure cooker to prevent an explosion from taking place.

In the same way as with the home pressure cooker, you can intervene in your own pressure cooker to reduce or stop the FND. Remember Daniel's and Kayleigh's Pressure Cooker Models? Look carefully at the information again for a few minutes. Imagine that Daniel and Kayleigh are your friends or family members whom you deeply care about. For each element, think what strategies you could advise the couple for the element to improve?

For example, to open the cover, you could advise Daniel to express his thoughts and feelings directly to Kayleigh, perhaps keep a daily thought diary, and recommend a good assertiveness course. Have a look at the **eResource** 10.8 for Daniel and Kayleigh's full 'Pressure Cooker Model prescription' based on their FND story.

Safety features
Pressure regulators that make sure that the pressure in the pot doesn't become too high. Leaky lid detectors.

Kitchen environment
Go for a deep clean. Remove the entire pressure cooker from the kitchen environment. Make sure the kitchen is organised and not chaotic, to prevent further damage to the pressure cooker and the environment in case the pressure cooker would explode.

Overpressure Plug
Plug the overpressure plug with a cork. Attach the steam diverters which will not remove the steam but will divert it away so it won't affect your kitchen. cabinets or walls.

Cover
Make sure the sealing ring is sufficiently sealing but the cover is not too tight or even locked.

Valve
Unblock and clean out the valve. Regulate the valve better so that the steam is released more evenly. Reduce the use of the valve, if it is in overuse.

Warning light
Check whether the batteries are working and recharge or replace the batteries if running on empty.

Pot
Repair the cracks and fissures in the pot.

Ignition
Put the lighter away and remove it from the kitchen area so that no one can use it to spark off a flame.

Sticky left-over food
Buy a heavy-duty surface cleaner that can remove tough dirt.

Fuel
Turn off the gas main. Call the utility company to shut off the gas supply. In this way, the gas won't flow to the gas hob.

Flames
Throw baking soda or salt on the flames. Smother the flames with a wet towel. Use a fire extinguisher.

Heat
Turn the dial down of the temperature regulator.

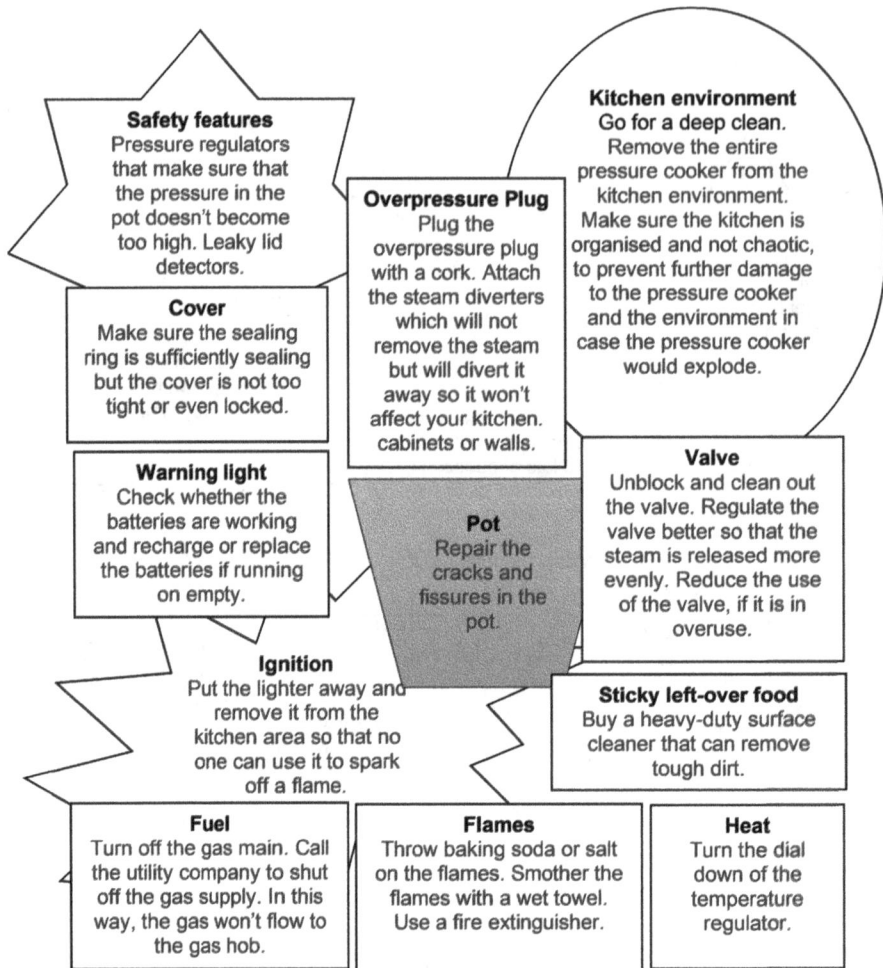

Figure 10.20 Intervention strategies to stop a pressure cooker at home from exploding.

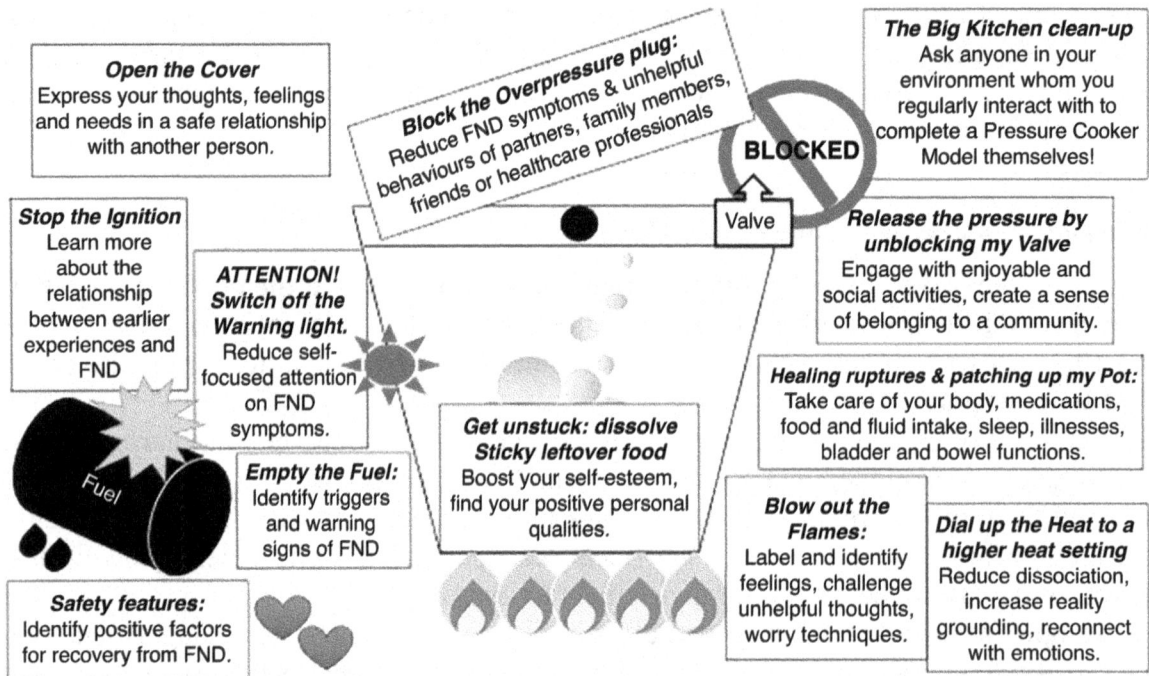

Open the Cover
Express your thoughts, feelings and needs in a safe relationship with another person.

Block the Overpressure plug:
Reduce FND symptoms & unhelpful behaviours of partners, family members, friends or healthcare professionals

The Big Kitchen clean-up
Ask anyone in your environment whom you regularly interact with to complete a Pressure Cooker Model themselves!

BLOCKED

Valve

Stop the Ignition
Learn more about the relationship between earlier experiences and FND

ATTENTION! Switch off the Warning light.
Reduce self-focused attention on FND symptoms.

Release the pressure by unblocking my Valve
Engage with enjoyable and social activities, create a sense of belonging to a community.

Empty the Fuel:
Identify triggers and warning signs of FND

Get unstuck: dissolve Sticky leftover food
Boost your self-esteem, find your positive personal qualities.

Healing ruptures & patching up my Pot:
Take care of your body, medications, food and fluid intake, sleep, illnesses, bladder and bowel functions.

Fuel

Safety features:
Identify positive factors for recovery from FND.

Blow out the Flames:
Label and identify feelings, challenge unhelpful thoughts, worry techniques.

Dial up the Heat to a higher heat setting
Reduce dissociation, increase reality grounding, reconnect with emotions.

Figure 10.21 What Pressure Cooker rehab most often entails.

My pressure cooker prescription ('rehabilitation')

Do you remember Figure 10.9 and the different 'Pressure Cooker Model challenges' that you can take on? The challenges ranged from 'least challenging' to 'top challenge'. Let us start with the 'least challenging' approach to Pressure Cooker rehab and inspect what Daniel and Kayleigh could do about addressing the problems found on layer 4 ('physical factors contributing to FND'; check out the FND SELF-CARE acronym – simply ignore the rest).

The Pressure Cooker Model challenge: probably less challenging

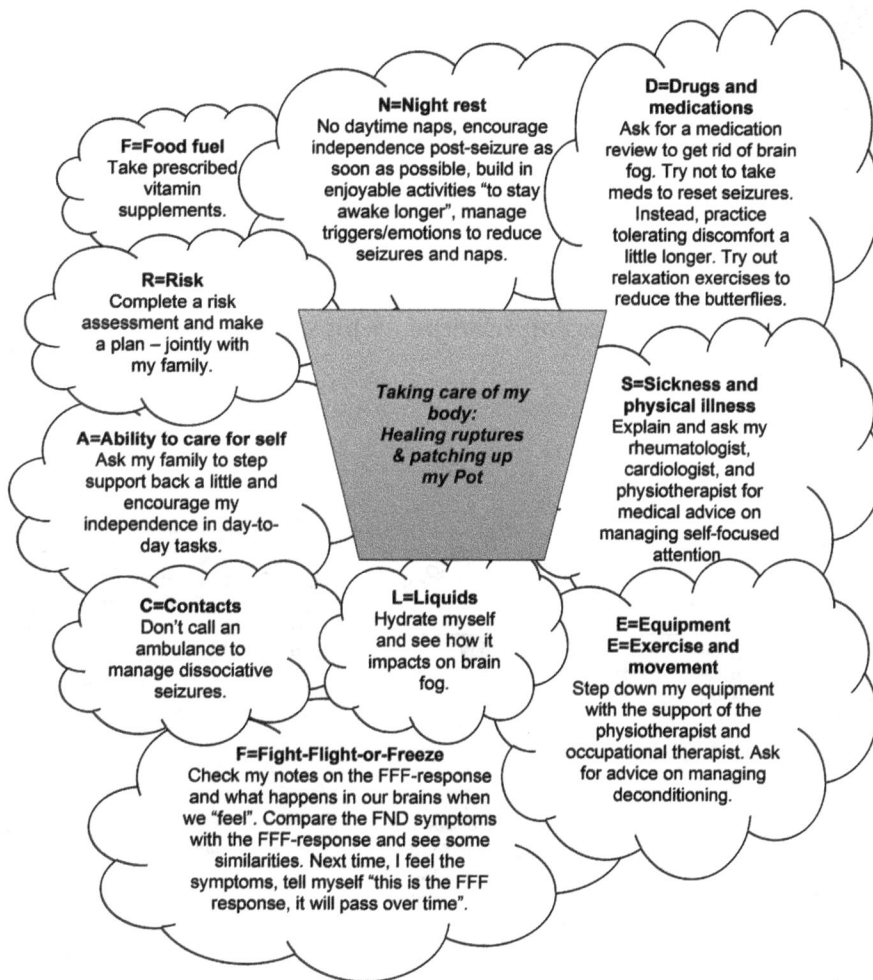

F=Food fuel
Take prescribed vitamin supplements.

N=Night rest
No daytime naps, encourage independence post-seizure as soon as possible, build in enjoyable activities "to stay awake longer", manage triggers/emotions to reduce seizures and naps.

D=Drugs and medications
Ask for a medication review to get rid of brain fog. Try not to take meds to reset seizures. Instead, practice tolerating discomfort a little longer. Try out relaxation exercises to reduce the butterflies.

R=Risk
Complete a risk assessment and make a plan – jointly with my family.

Taking care of my body: Healing ruptures & patching up my Pot

S=Sickness and physical illness
Explain and ask my rheumatologist, cardiologist, and physiotherapist for medical advice on managing self-focused attention.

A=Ability to care for self
Ask my family to step support back a little and encourage my independence in day-to-day tasks.

C=Contacts
Don't call an ambulance to manage dissociative seizures.

L=Liquids
Hydrate myself and see how it impacts on brain fog.

E=Equipment
E=Exercise and movement
Step down my equipment with the support of the physiotherapist and occupational therapist. Ask for advice on managing deconditioning.

F=Fight-Flight-or-Freeze
Check my notes on the FFF-response and what happens in our brains when we "feel". Compare the FND symptoms with the FFF-response and see some similarities. Next time, I feel the symptoms, tell myself "this is the FFF response, it will pass over time".

Figure 10.22 Daniel's and Kayleigh's strategies to tackle layer 4 (physical factors in FND).

In addition to the FND SELF-CARE acronym, layer 4 also consists of the warning light. To reduce the attentional focus on FND, Daniel, Kayleigh, and the wider family used the strategies outlined in Chapter 8 to switch off everybody's warning light.

The Pressure Cooker Model challenge: somewhat challenging

Explore Daniel's remedies in Figure 10.23 to extinguish his FND coping triangle:

What can Daniel do to open the top of his cooker? (Check out layer 2 only, 'the FND coping triangle' – ignore everything else).

Cover/sealing ring:

BLOCKED

Valve:

Valve

Fuel

Sticky left over food:

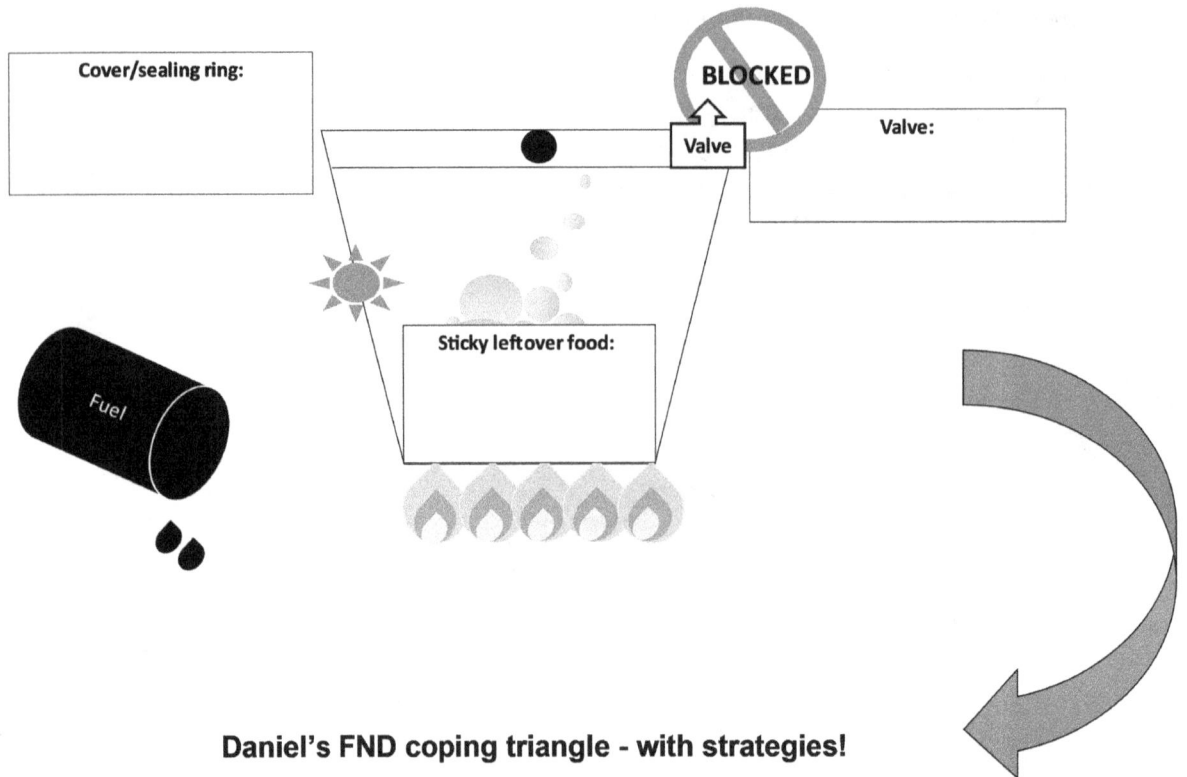

Daniel's FND coping triangle - with strategies!

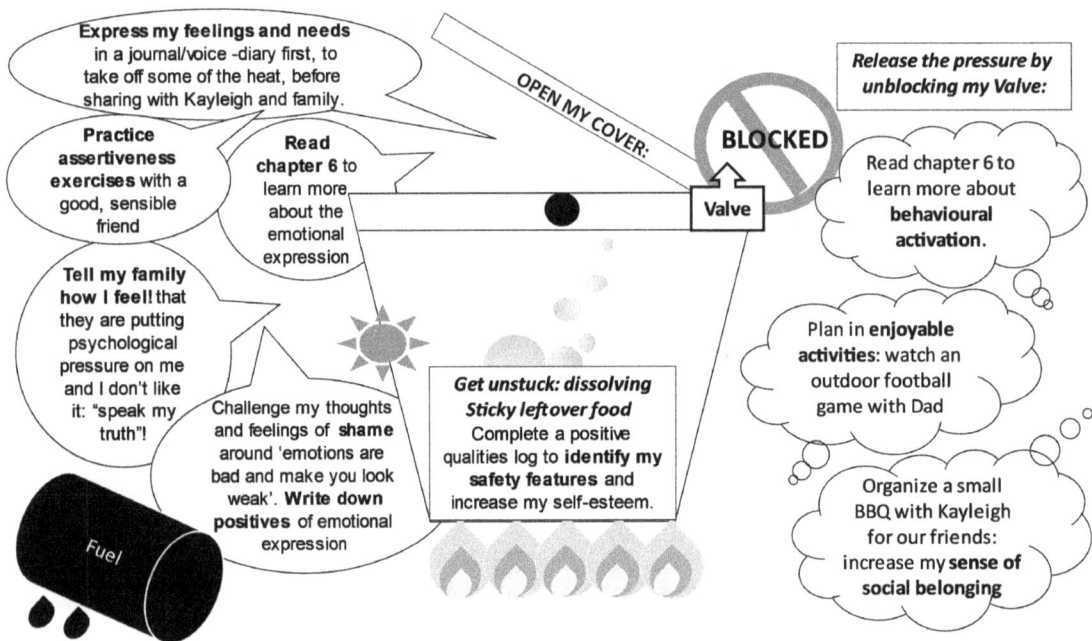

Express my feelings and needs in a journal/voice-diary first, to take off some of the heat, before sharing with Kayleigh and family.

Practice assertiveness exercises with a good, sensible friend

Read chapter 6 to learn more about the emotional expression

OPEN MY COVER:

BLOCKED

Valve

Release the pressure by unblocking my Valve:

Read chapter 6 to learn more about **behavioural activation**.

Tell my family how I feel! that they are putting psychological pressure on me and I don't like it: "speak my truth"!

Challenge my thoughts and feelings of **shame** around 'emotions are bad and make you look weak'. **Write down positives** of emotional expression

Get unstuck: dissolving Sticky left over food Complete a positive qualities log to **identify my safety features** and increase my self-esteem.

Plan in **enjoyable activities**: watch an outdoor football game with Dad

Organize a small BBQ with Kayleigh for our friends: increase my **sense of social belonging**

Fuel

Figure 10.23 Daniel's FND coping triangle.

However, Daniel is not the only one with an FND coping triangle! Check out Kayleigh's remedies in Figure 10.24 to extinguish her FND coping triangle: What can Kayleigh do to open the top of her pressure cooker?

Figures 10.23 and 10.24 show how Daniel and Kayleigh can both open the top of their pressure cookers and practice new, more helpful ways of expressing emotions.

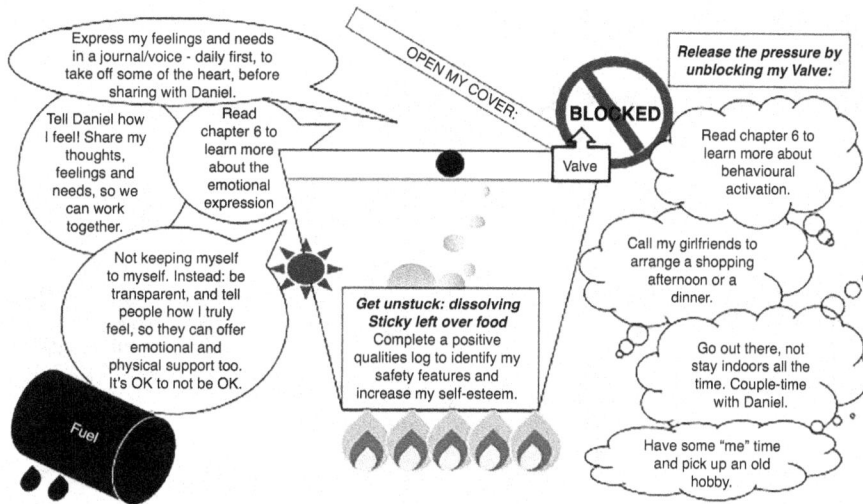

Figure 10.24 Kayleigh's FND coping triangle – with strategies!

Daniel and Kayleigh's no-FND equation

keep opening up about how we both feel (open the cover) + plan in sufficient enjoyable activities, keep a normal routine, and do not overdo it (unblock/regulate the valve) = reduces the risk of FND (with those two channels working, there is no need to use the overpressure plug any longer)

The Pressure Cooker Model challenge: quite challenging

Daniel and Kayleigh are now only going to look at each other's Pressure Cooker chain reactions and particularly consider their interpersonal triggers (check out layer 3 – leave the rest as is). How can Daniel and Kayleigh break their Pressure Cooker chain reactions? Look at just the four elements of the chain reaction in Figure 10.25. Daniel can intervene at different points in the chain to stop 'combustion'. At any point in the chain reaction, Daniel has options, no matter how 'far into the chain' he finds himself.

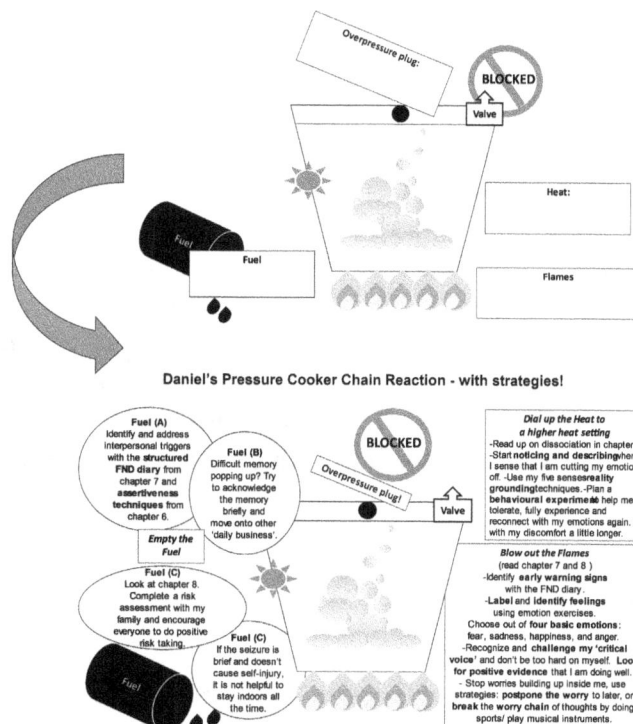

Figure 10.25 Daniel's Pressure Cooker chain reaction.

However, in order for Daniel to enable to break the links in his own chain, Kayleigh needs to come on board simultaneously! It is not just down to Daniel to sort out his chain reaction – Kayleigh, too, contributes to Daniel's recovery.

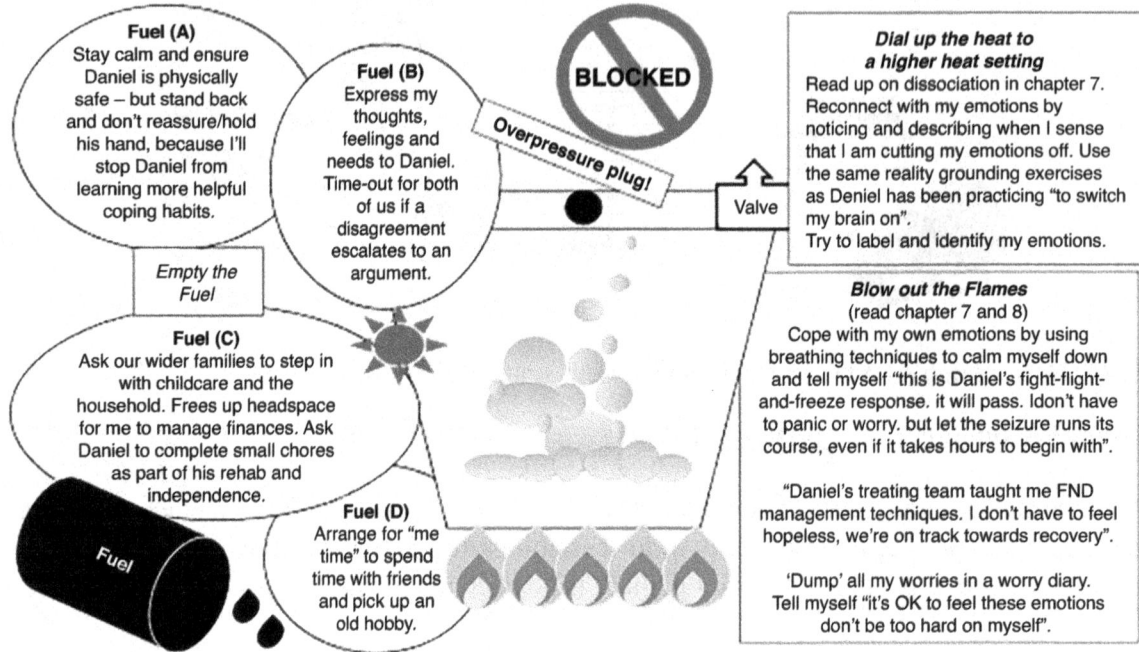

Figure 10.26 Kayleigh's Pressure Cooker chain reaction – with strategies!

The Pressure Cooker Model challenge: top challenge

Figure 10.27 shows two interlinked Pressure Cooker Models comprising of the FND coping triangle, the Pressure Cooker chain reaction, and the kitchen (combine layers 2, 3, and 5 – leave layers 1 and 4 for what they are).

For the big kitchen clean-up

Daniel and Kayleigh read up on Chapter 9 again. Together, the couple agreed that everybody in their environment should adopt the **same approach to the seizures**: keep Daniel physically safe but stand back and leave Daniel to it so that he can ride out the episode. The couple shared this approach with wider family and healthcare professionals to **stop intermittent reinforcement**, which would otherwise make it harder for Daniel to overcome the FND, as well as to educate healthcare professionals who felt less confident managing FND and who often inadvertently contributed to Daniel's symptoms through **systemic re-traumatisation**. Both Daniel and Kayleigh **completed two interlinked Pressure Cooker Models** for themselves, too, to look at their own thoughts, feelings, and responses and finally **break the reciprocal reinforcement loop** once and for all.

10.8 eResource alert!

For Daniel and Kayleigh's full Pressure Cooker Model prescription, with all elements completed, please check the eResource to learn what strategies the couple used to overcome the FND.

Social functions

- Excessive caring reduced Daniel's FND and distress, and therefore: Reduced Kayleigh's own anxiety about seeing Daniel with FND symptoms and distress too!

Reciprocal reinforcement: Seizure, psychological pressure, and disagreement stops as well as everybody's anxiety, discomfort, arousal, and panic reduce temporarily...until a new one is triggered.

Social functions

- Reducing Daniel's own discomfort as soon as possible. Not being able to tolerate this feeling as it feels so horrible.
- Feeling supported and cared for by Kayleigh, throughout his ordeal.

Valve
Bust-after-Boom

9/Kayleigh's Overpressure Plug
Quickly runs to Daniel to provide physical and verbal reassurance. (Helps Daniel with washing, dressing, all ADLs, taking every chore out of Daniel's hands.

Tight Cover
Keep self to self, not speaking about anxiety to Daniel to not burden him and make him worried

Kayleigh

Sticky leftover food
Low confidence in managing Daniel's FND symptoms. Keeps self to self.

8/Heat
Kayleigh experiences high heat, "I feel terrified" Anxiety level is a 10 out of 10

7/Flames
Kayleigh feels panic, fright: "I need to help to quash the seizure as quickly as possible".

6/Fuel
...Kayleigh witnessing Daniel's FND episode and distress.

5/...but Daniel's seizure has impact on Kayleigh

3/Heat
High heat, intense negative feeling that I want to get rid of.

Valve
Bust-after-Boom

4/Daniel's Overpressure Plug
Full-blown dissociative seizure....

Tight Cover
Keep self to self, not assertive and speaking my truth about how I feel about my family.

Daniel

Sticky left-over food
Low self-esteem Kept myself to myself as a child.

2/Flames
Pressure building up inside me, I can't really explain how I feel but it's unpleasant.

1/Fuel
Perceived psychological pressure / disagreement with Kayleigh and family.

Start here with #1 (Daniel's triggers for seizures). Then follow the numbers.

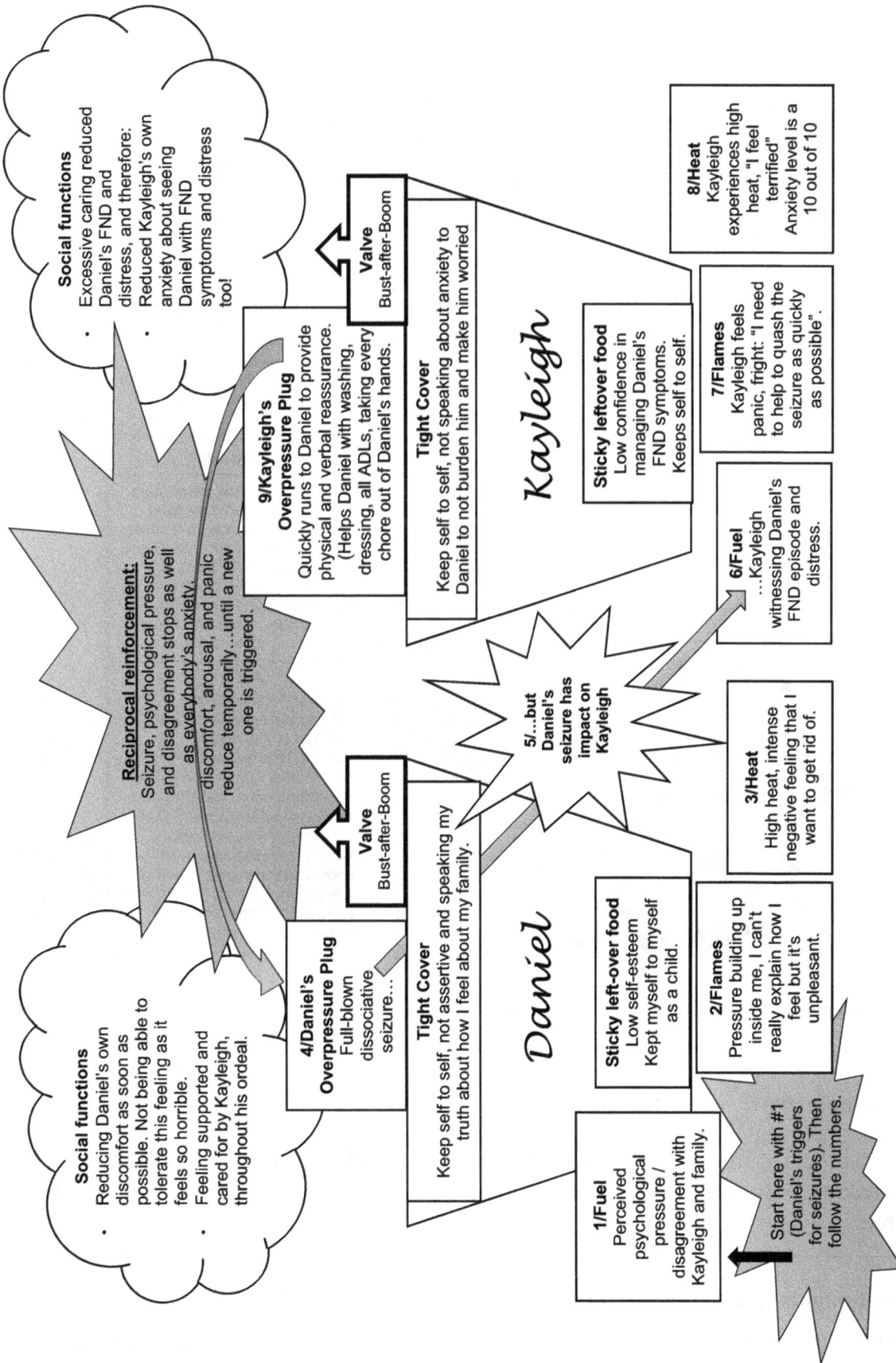

Figure 10.27 Daniel and Kayleigh's Pressure Cooker Model prescription.

Remind myself again of our amazing Safety Features!
Daniel and Kayleigh greatly valued neuropsychology, willing to give it a try. Motivated. Supportive family

The Big Kitchen clean-up:
Daniel and Kayleigh's relationship was much improved, with sufficient "couple time" and better communication with the wider family.

Opened the Cover
Daniel learned to 'relate' and connect with other people and verbalise emotions in safe, trusted relationships with staff members. Daniel was able to express his needs more assertively to his family and talk about the padlocks without experiencing FND symptoms.

Block the Overpressure Plug
Most FND symptoms improved. Brain fog disappeared, Daniel was sharp. Successfully applied new strategies (open the cover, unblock the valve) in the face of a new set-back and overcome FND.

Release the pressure by unblocking our Valves
The couple built a routine with social activities. Daniel checked out football and reconnected with old sports friends, Kayleigh reconnected with her own friends, both created a good sense of social belonging separately and together.

ATTENTION! Switched off the Warning light.
Much less focused on physical symptoms, and more able to use emotion words over physical descriptions. Less symptom checking on the internet.

Daniel and Kayleigh's Pressure Cooker Rehab Outcomes

Get unstuck: dissolving Sticky leftover food
Although his low self-esteem had slightly improved, Daniel struggled with being kind to himself and completing a log tracking his positive qualities. Work was ongoing in this area.

Stop the Ignition
Increased insight into the association between early experiences, FND, emotions and relationships.

Empty the Fuel
Both identified and managed triggers for Daniel's FND symptoms and Kayleigh's unhelpful behaviours.

Blow out the Flames
Restored mood Able to identify emotions better – though more work needed.

Dial up the Heat to a higher heat setting
More in touch with emotions, less dissociative moments.

Fuel

Pot
- Fewer ambulance calls.
- Medications and vitamin levels reviewed by the doctor.
- Sleeping returned to normal.
- Independent with personal care, meal preparation, and shopping.
- Improved walking pattern, Daniel got rid of most equipment.
- Risks all reduced: improved mood, relationships and social connection, full engagement with rehab programme, no further injuries.

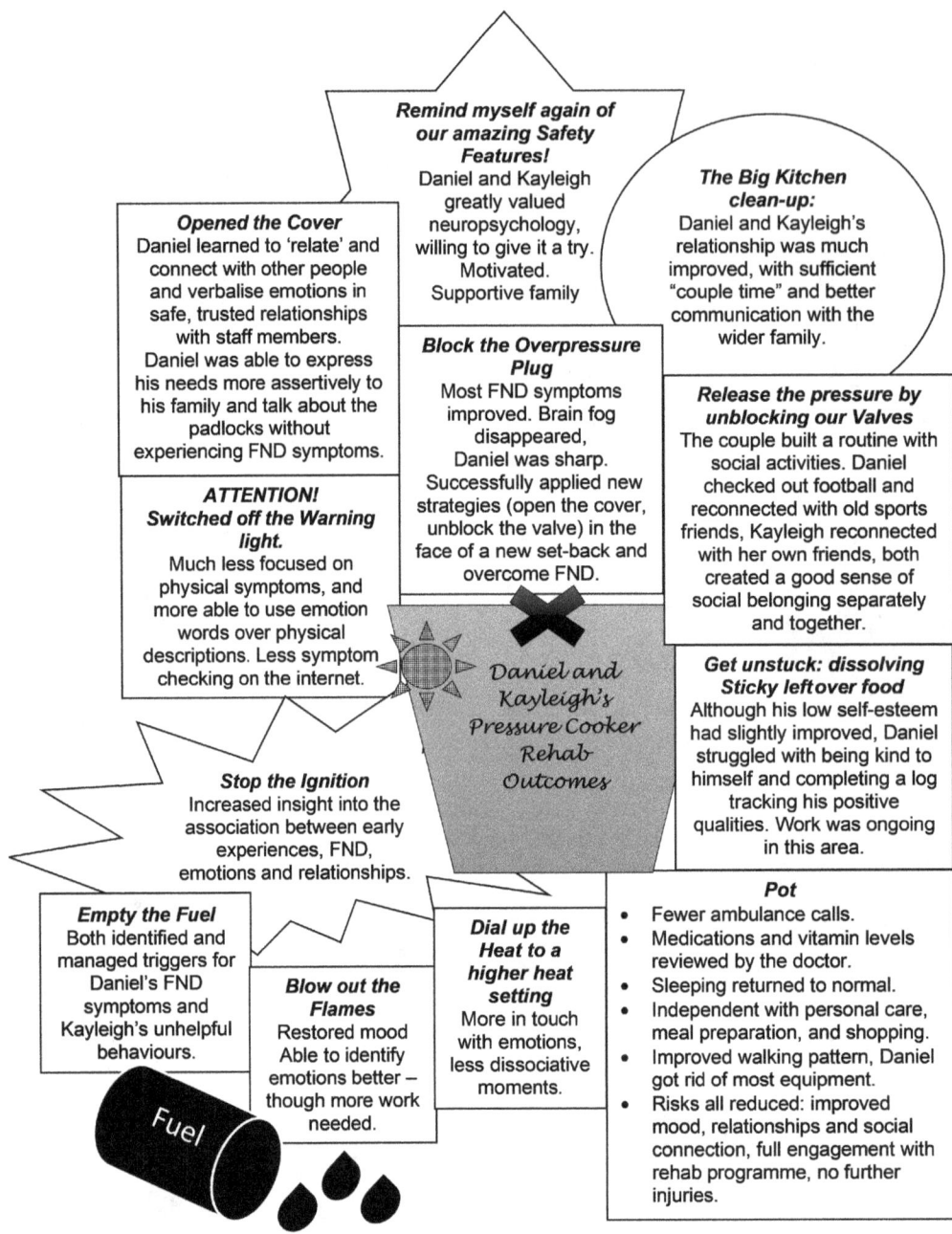

Figure 10.28 Daniel and Kayleigh's Pressure Cooker rehab outcomes.

10.9 eResource alert!

Your partner, family, friend, or healthcare professional, or all of you together, can now have a go at creating your own joined-up FND management plan with plenty of ideas from this eResource.

Some final thoughts: the Pressure Cooker values

Wonderful! You have made it to the end of *A Patient's Workbook for Functional Neurological Disorder*! The goal of the book was to help you and every person around you – partners, family members, friends, healthcare professionals, and anyone else you are close to and interact with on a regular basis – **to understand and manage FND together**. Hopefully by now everyone will have learned that FND is a shared endeavour, and every person involved in FND, symptoms or no symptoms, needs help too. Let us leave you with some final thoughts to reflect and spread the word!

Pressure Cooker value #1: There is no division between the mind vs body. The Pressure Cooker Model views FND as truly biopsychosocial in nature and does not attempt to separate the mind from the body.

Pressure Cooker value #2: There is no distinction between people. In the Pressure Cooker Model, 'everybody has FND': there are hardly any differences between people with and without FND.

Pressure Cooker value #3: FND deserves compassion and understanding. The Pressure Cooker Model provides a more balanced and compassionate view on FND: friendly language ('no stigma'), focus on social functions ('two-way street'), highlighting the role of the environment ('the system'), and generating descriptions of people's positive qualities and protective factors ('what is going well').

Pressure Cooker value #4: A coherent, neuropsychology-led formulation is a powerful tool in FND. Multidisciplinary treatment for FND should always be based on a coherent narrative that ties together the multiple strands involved in FND care using the same language.

Pressure Cooker value #5: Your personal FND narratives will inform your treatments. Developing your and your family's personal Pressure Cooker Model stories simultaneously will guide and map out the right treatment necessary for FND recovery.

Pressure Cooker value #6: And the individual is just as important! Although relationships between people play a central role in FND, the Pressure Cooker Model views key individual factors, like a person's tendency for dissociation, capacity for emotional expression, heightened self-focused attention on physical symptoms, and boom-and-bust cycles, as equally important agents and targets for treatment in FND.

Pressure Cooker value #7: FND recovery starts by an in-depth review of the social environment. Although FND links in with emotions and other psychological processes, ultimately, it is the social environment and relationships that greatly impact on how the FND starts and why it keeps going.

Pressure Cooker value #8: Everyone contributes to FND. Even though the person with FND experiences, carries and manifests the symptoms, the Pressure Cooker Model believes that both the person and the environment equally contribute to FND. Recognizing everyone's contribution to FND will help you prepare for the biggest chances of recovery.

Pressure Cooker value #9: Relationships are central in FND. The golden treatment formula for FND focuses on improving relationships and fostering collaboration, joining up your care, and above all, reducing confusion. Learning 'life-long' strategies to repair relationships and relate better to one another may give hope for a different future in FND.

Pressure Cooker value #10: Always pay attention to the impact of healthcare experiences on FND. The Pressure Cooker Model is the only framework that looks at and treats the detrimental impact of a special type of relationship on FND recovery: difficult healthcare experiences. Although this may surprise you, people with and without FND – including healthcare professionals – mirror each other's thoughts, feelings and actions.

Pressure Cooker value #11: Everyone is responsible for FND recovery. Moving the focus from 'the individual' to 'the individual-in-the-environment' releases the psychosocial pressure on the person with FND to take full responsibility 'to fix FND' and holds the 'key' to radically transform FND recovery.

Pressure Cooker value #12: FND recovery is always a joint effort. FND recovery was never about walking the path alone but a collective journey, requiring everyone to be on board. Treatment is neither 'my responsibility' nor 'their responsibility' but always a 'shared responsibility'.

Pressure Cooker value #13: The ultimate key to FND is to fully embrace the influence of the social world. If the only thing that you remember after reading this book is the importance of relationships and impact of the social world on FND, you have won more than half the battle!

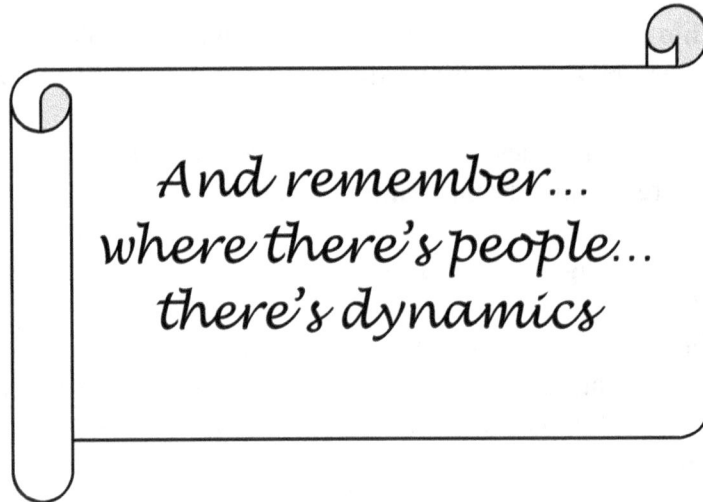

And remember…
where there's people…
there's dynamics

Index

Note: Numbers in **bold** indicate a table. Numbers in *italics* indicate a figure.

For Product Safety Concerns and Information please contact our EU
representative GPSR@taylorandfrancis.com
Taylor & Francis Verlag GmbH, Kaufingerstraße 24, 80331 München, Germany

www.ingramcontent.com/pod-product-compliance
Lightning Source LLC
Chambersburg PA
CBHW081508290326
41932CB00051B/3087